Improve International

MANUAL OF SMALL ANIMAL CARDIOLOGY

Improve
Veterinary Education

First published 2023

Published by
Improve International Ltd.
Alexandra House, Whittingham Drive
Wroughton, Swindon,
Wiltshire SN4 0QJ
United Kingdom

Tel: +44 (0) 1 793 759 159
https://improveinternational.com/uk/

Important note
Medicine is an ever-changing science, so the contents of this publication, especially recommendations concerning diagnostic and therapeutic procedures, can only give an account of the knowledge at the time of publication. While utmost care has been taken to ensure that all specifications regarding drug selection and dosage and treatment options are accurate, readers are urged to review the product information sheet and any relevant material supplied by the manufacturer, and, in case of doubt, to consult a specialist. From both an editorial and public interest perspective, the publisher welcomes notification of possible inconsistencies. The ultimate responsibility for any diagnostic or therapeutic application lies with the reader.

A Catalogue record for this book is available from the British Library

ISBN: 978-1-913352-15-8

Copywriter: Dr. Pippa Elliot
Illustrator: Elaine Leggett
Photos by the authors unless otherwise indicated.

Prologue

Small animal cardiology has established itself as one of the most prestigious specialties within veterinary medicine due to the work and research, both clinical and experimental, that specialists have been conducting for more than 25 years. In fact, the evolution of imaging techniques and, especially, echocardiography has meant significant advances in the diagnosis and treatment of heart disease, allowing multicentre studies of great relevance on diverse therapeutic strategies.

This book was initially written to contribute to the training of veterinarians interested in small animal clinical cardiology, as well as those who are undertaking a postgraduate training program such as the Improve International course, which leads to obtention of the General Practitioner Certificate in Cardiology granted by the ISVPS (International School of Veterinary Postgraduate Studies). However, given the result, the publication could be useful to veterinary students and veterinarians in general practice.

The authors who contributed to this book have been specialising in small animal cardiology for many years, in various centres (private and university hospitals) and in different countries. This has contributed to the compilation of up-to-date information on the main heart diseases in this publication, which has been compiled from a clinical point of view, with great scientific rigor and always according to evidence-based medicine. The book is organized into three sections: the initial chapters cover embryology, anatomy, and physiology of the cardiovascular system. The following chapters include the main methods and complementary examinations for cardiac evaluation. The last section consists of detailed information on major syndromes and specific cardiovascular diseases, their aetiology, pathophysiology, clinical evaluation, and the treatments which can be used. In addition, a wide range of diagrams are included in each chapter that provide a better understanding of diseases and are of use in daily practice. The bibliographical references for each chapter, although not exhaustive, are the most relevant and representative, so that the reader can use them to complement the specific and detailed information already provided.

In addition, this publication includes, both self-assessment questions at the end of each chapter and clinical cases covering the most common heart diseases, oriented to the individual training of the reader and as an aid in daily clinical practice.

The information included in this book is up to date at the time of writing, but medicine is an area that is constantly changing and therefore readers should periodically update their knowledge and ensure that the medications and doses to be used in each patient are those indicated by the company that manufactures the product.

The authors would like to thank the veterinary centres where they have worked and/or work, their colleagues, clients, and animals and everything else that has been a part of their lives, study, and work and that has contributed, both directly and indirectly, to the writing and content of this book.

Likewise, the authors would like to thank the Publisher, as without their collaboration it would not have been possible to bring this work to fruition.

Finally, we hope that the reader enjoys this text and that it contributes to further training in cardiology and in daily practice.

Mª Josefa Fernández-del Palacio,
PhD, Dipl. ECVIM-CA (Cardiology)

Authors

Mª Josefa Fernández-del Palacio (coordinator)

PhD, Dipl. ECVIM-CA
Dr Mª Josefa Fernández-del Palacio is a Professor of the Department of Animal Medicine and Surgery and responsible for the Cardiorespiratory Service of the Veterinary Hospital of the University of Murcia. She is also a diplomate of the ECVIM-CA (Cardiology) specialising in cardiology. She has published numerous book chapters and articles on cardiology in both national and international journals. Her fields of interest are cardiology and nephrology.

Domingo Casamián Sorrosal

DVM, Cert SAM, DVC, Dipl. ECVIM-CA, MRCVS
Domingo has a double diploma in veterinary cardiology and internal medicine of small animals and currently works as head of the cardiology and cardiopulmonary service at Southfields Veterinary Specialists (United Kingdom) referral centre. He is also a lecturer and clinician in cardiology and respiratory medicine at the Referral Hospital and the Faculty of Veterinary Medicine of the Universidad Católica de Valencia.

He graduated from Zaragoza and completed an internship at the Animal Medical Centre in Manchester in 2000. From 2001 to 2005 he worked in two hospitals in the UK, combined with long stays at the Cardiorespiratory Centre in Kenilworth. During this time, he obtained the British certificates in Cardiology and Internal Medicine. In 2006 he joined the University of Bristol as a resident and completed his training as a specialist in Internal Medicine (3 years) and then in Veterinary Cardiology (4 years) subsequently staying on as a clinician and then head of the service until 2016.

Domingo holds a diploma and is a specialist of the British College of Veterinary Cardiology and the European College of Small Animal Internal Medicine. He has published numerous articles in scientific journals and is a regular reviewer in journals such as JVIM, JFMS or JSAP. He has been a speaker at numerous national and international congresses. His main areas of interest include arrhythmias, pacemaker therapy and interventional cardiology.

Oriol Domenech

DVM, MS, Dipl. ECVIM-CA
Oriol obtained his degree in veterinary medicine in 1996 from the Universidad Autónoma de Barcelona. From 1996 to 1997 he worked as a veterinarian at the veterinary clinic Mediterrani Veterinaris in Reus (Tarragona). From 1997 to 1999 he completed the three Veterinary Cardiology courses from the ESAVS (European School for Advanced Veterinary Studies). Between 1998 and 2000 he worked at the Urgencias Veterinarias y Referenwcia Centre (Survet) in Barcelona as head of Cardiology. He completed the ECVIM-CA internship and residency program specialising in Cardiology between 2000 and 2004 and obtained the ECVIM-CA diploma for the specialty of Cardiology in 2006.

From 2006 to February 2011, he worked as a specialist in Internal Medicine and Cardiology at the Gran Sasso Veterinary Clinic in Milan (Italy) and at the Survet Diagonal clinic (Servei d'Urgencies Veterinaries and Referrals) in Barcelona. He earned his Master of Science degree in 2008 and won the Luera prize in 2009. In 2011 he became the head of the Department of Cardiology and Interventional Cardiology, as well as coordinator of the cardiac surgery and extracorporeal circulation group, at the Istituto Veterinario di Novara (Italy). He has been a member of the examination committee and is currently a member of the credentials committee for the ECVIM-CA (Cardiology). Since 2014 he has been director of the residency program in Cardiology for the ECVIM-CA at the Istituto Veterinario di Novara. He is the author of articles, chapters of various books and numerous studies.

Gemma Fraga Veloso

LdaVet, MSc, Dipl. ECVIM-CA (Cardiology)
Gemma graduated in veterinary medicine from the UCH in Valencia in 2003. She completed a two year internship at the veterinary hospital of the Faculty of Veterinary Medicine of Lugo at the University of Santiago de Compostela. At the same University she then completed a Master's degree in companion and exotic animals in addition to a Diploma of Advanced Studies. Gemma then completed a three year residency in cardiopulmonary medicine at the Small Animal Hospital at the University of Edinburgh. In 2012 she became a diplomate of the European College of Internal Medicine – Companion Animals (ECVIM-CA) specialising in cardiology. Gemma has worked as a clinical lecturer of cardiology at the University of Liverpool and then continued her career in various veterinary referral hospitals in the south of England. In 2017 she joined the Animal Bluecare referral hospital in Málaga.

Andrew Francis

BVSc, Cert VC, Dipl. ECVIM-CA (Cardiology), MRCVS
Andrew Francis graduated from the University of Bristol in 2002 and worked at a veterinary hospital in Devon over the next four years. During the following five years he completed a rotating internship, which continued with a research grant and cardiopulmonary medicine residency, at the University of Edinburgh. He received the certificate of specialization in Cardiology from the RCVS in 2007 and became a diplomate of the ECVIM-CA in Cardiology in 2012.

After working for three years in veterinary industry, he joined Anderson Moores Veterinary Specialists, near Winchester as one of the cardiology specialists.

Stefano Nicoli

MedVet, MSc, MRCVS
Stefano graduated from the University of Bologna in 1994. From 1994 to 2004 he worked as a general practitioner at the San Geminiano Veterinary Hospital in Modena. From 2004 onwards he developed his professional career in areas related to soft tissue surgery with special interest in urinary tract surgery, endocrine surgery, vascular surgery, microsurgery and interventional radiology.

From 2008 to 2012 he worked at the veterinary clinical hospital of the University of Turin and from 2014 he has worked at the University of Parma. He has also carried out vascular surgery work at the veterinary hospital of Reggio Emilia. He has combined his work with training periods in Europe and the United States. In 2015 he became a member of the RCVS and in 2016 he obtained a Master II livello in Nefrologia e Urologia del Cane e del Gatto of the University of Pisa qualification.

He currently divides his professional activities between Italy (Istituto Veterinario Novara and Clinica Veterinaria Roma Sud), Spain (Cardiosonic, Madrid, and Clínica Veterinaria Valencia Sur, Valencia), United Kingdom (The Veterinary Referral Centre, Godstone) and Denmark (AniCura Aarhus Dyrehospital, Aahrus). He directs the Unità Operativa per l'Incontinenza Urinaria del Istituto Veterinario Novara and the Unità Operativa per le patologie Surrenaliche e Ipofisarie at the Centro Clinica Veterinaria Roma Sud. He is author and coauthor of a wide range of publications in international journals (Journal of the American Veterinary Medical Association, Journal of Feline Medicine and Surgery, The Veterinary Journal, Veterinary Surgery, Journal of Small Animal Practice, Veterinaria) and was president of the Società di Chirurgia de SCIVAC from 2014 to 2017.

Pedro Oliveira

DVM, MRCVS, Dipl. ECVIM-CA (Cardiology), RCVS and EBVSR European Veterinary Specialist in Small Animal Cardiology and Head of Cardiology
Pedro obtained his degree in Veterinary Medicine from the Universidad do Porto (Portugal) in 2005. From 2004 to 2006 he completed an internship and worked in the Department of Cardiology of the Gran Sasso Veterinary Clinic in Milan (Italy). From 2006 to 2009 he worked in general practice and cardiology referral services in Portugal. In 2009 he returned to Milan to do the three year residency for the ECVIM-CA, specialising in cardiology, under the supervision of Claudio Bussadori (Dipl. ECVIM-CA, Cardiology) and Oriol Domenech (Dipl. ECVIM-CA, Cardiology), as well as at the École Nationale Veterinaire de Lyon (France) under the supervision of Professor Jean-Luc Cadoré (Dipl. ECVIM-CA, Internal Medicine). From 2011 he has worked in interventional cardiology services in Porto and Barcelona and joined the Davies Veterinary Specialists Cardiology Service in October 2012.

Dolores María Porteiro Vázquez

DVM, Dipl. ECVIM-CA (Cardiology)
Dolores graduated in 2005 from the Faculty of Veterinary Medicine Lugo, University of Santiago de Compostela. From 2005 to 2011 she worked at different practices in Madrid, mainly in internal medicine and diagnostic imaging. From February 2012 to July 2013 she completed an internship, specialising in Cardiology with Dr. Claudio Bussadori and Roberto Santilli in Milan (Italy). In August 2013 she started the European residency programme in Cardiology under the supervision of Dr. Santilli (ECVIM-CA Cardiology) and has recently become a diplomate. She is head of the Cardiology Service of the Puchol Veterinary Hospital (Madrid) and collaborates with the ecgontheweb Telemedicine Service (Milan). She is the author of numerous publications in national and international journals, has presented at national and international congresses, has collaborated in the writing of several chapters on veterinary cardiology books and is editor of the book "Clinical Cardiology in Dogs and Cats". Her main areas of interest are the diagnosis and treatment of arrhythmias.

Giorgia Santarelli

DVM, MSc, Dipl. ECVIM-CA (Cardiology),
MRCVS, European Specialist in Veterinary Cardiology
Giorgia Santarelli graduated cum laude in Veterinary Medicine from the University of Bologna in 2008, she then obtained Master's degree in Reproduction Technology and Diagnosis in Veterinary Medicine from the University of Murcia in 2011. After completing a two-year internship in the Cardiorespiratory Service of the Clinical Veterinary Hospital at the University of Murcia, she completed a residency in the same department and in the Internal Medicine services of the Universities of Utrecht, Barcelona and Bologna. During all this time, she completed her doctoral studies at the University of Murcia. She obtained the diploma of the European College of Veterinary Internal Medicine (subspecialty Cardiology) in 2018. Giorgia is currently working as a clinician in the Cardiorespiratory Service of the Veterinary Hospital at the University of Edinburgh (United Kingdom).

Ashley B. Saunders

DVM, Diplomate ACVIM (Cardiology)
Dr Ashley Saunders is a professor of cardiology and assistant department head at Texas A&M University. She is certified as a cardiology specialist by the American College of Veterinary Internal Medicine. Dr Saunders holds a PG Cert Vet Ed from the Royal Veterinary College in London and is a member of the Academy of Higher Education and the Michael E. DeBakey Institute for Comparative Cardiovascular Science and Biomedical Devices. Dr Saunders received the Teaching Award from the Texas A&M Alumni and Universities Association. Her research and publication interests are cardiovascular imaging, intervention techniques for congenital heart disease, management of heart failure and new teaching methods.

Contents

Pathophysiology, Diagnosis, and Management of Heart Failure

Andrew Francis

Acquired Valvular Disease

Andrew Francis

Syncope

Mª Josefa Fernández-del Palacio

Pulmonary Hypertension and *Cor Pulmonale*

Mª Josefa Fernández-del Palacio

Cardiac Biomarkers

Ashley B. Saunders

Congenital Cardiac Pathologies

Oriol Domenech

Canine Myocardial Disease

Pedro Oliveira

Feline Cardiomyopathies

Mª Josefa Fernández-del Palacio, Giorgia Santarelli

Pericardial Diseases and Cardiac Neoplasms

Domingo Casamián Sorrosal

Arrhythmias: Cardiac Rhythm Anomalies and Treatment

Gemma Fraga Veloso and Dolores Porteiro Vázquez

Cardiac Surgery

Oriol Domenech and Stefano Nicoli

Cardiovascular Anatomy and Embryology

Pedro Oliveira

An accurate assessment of the cardiovascular system and its associated diseases depends on a **sound knowledge of cardiovascular anatomy and physiology**.

This chapter reviews the anatomy of the cardiovascular system, as appropriate for a clinical cardiologist, and where appropriate highlights the idiosyncracies of feline anatomy. Also, the basic concepts of cardiac embryology are discussed as an aid to understanding the aetiology of congenital heart defects.

Cardiovascular Anatomy

The cardiovascular system is comprised of the heart and a network of blood vessels through which bloods circulates around the body to transport oxygen, nutrients, cells, waste products, hormones, and other substances. The circulation is divided into **two separate circuits**: namely the pulmonary and systemic circulation.

- The **right-sided heart chambers** act as a pump for the pulmonary circulation, pushing blood through the lungs where it is oxygenated and returns to the left side of the heart.
- The **left-sided heart chambers** pump blood through the rest of the body (systemic circulation) and back to the right side of the heart for another cycle.

Oxygenated blood exits the left heart through arteries which divide and become progressively smaller (arterioles) to eventually form capillary vessels, with the latter allowing gas and nutrient exchange between the circulation and the body's cells. Blood then proceeds through progressively larger vessels (venules and veins) and returns to the heart.

The Heart

The heart is a muscular organ located inside the thorax. It is located in the middle of the thorax, approximately level with the **third to sixth ribs**, and is surrounded by the lungs. The base of the heart is oriented dorsocranially and the apex directed ventrocaudally and slightly to the left of the transverse plane (Figure 1).

The heart consists of **four separate chambers**, with the two chambers on the left, separated from the two chambers on the right by a septum. On each side the upper chambers are called atria, and are separated from the lower chambers (ventricles) by the atrioventricular valves. The atria are separated from each other by a wall (atrial septum).

- **Right atrium** receives blood from the **systemic circulation**.
- **Left atrium** receives blood from the **pulmonary circulation**.

The two lower chambers are called **ventricles** and possess muscular walls responsible for pumping blood away from the heart into the pulmonary (right) and systemic (left) circulations. They are separated from each other by the **ventricular septum**. The right and left atria are separated from the right and left ventricles respectively by atrioventricular valves: the **tricuspid** (right side) and **mitral** (left side) **valves**.

Surface Anatomy and Orientation

Fundamental to interpreting thoracic radiographs and cardiac ultrasound images is an understanding of the heart's position and orientation in relation to other intra-thoracic structures (Figures 1, 2 and 3).

The heart is located:

- mid thorax: between third and sixth ribs
- **base**: directed dorsocranially (upwards and towards the patient's head)
- **apex**: directed ventrocaudally (downwards and towards the tail) and to the left of midline
- the **long axis** of the heart is inclined at an angle of approximately 45° from the vertical plane in most cases.

The **feline heart is consistantly positioned** as above, in contrast to dogs with their wide diversity of thoracic conformations. For example, radiographs of deep-chested dogs, e.g. Dobermann, show the heart as being positioned more vertically, whilst wide-chested breeds, e.g. English Bulldog, show the heart lying along the sternum.

Age, body condition and pathological processes may also influence the position and orientation of the heart in the chest. This is a particularly important consideration when interpreting thoracic radiographs e.g. in some older cats the heart appears in a more horizontal position.

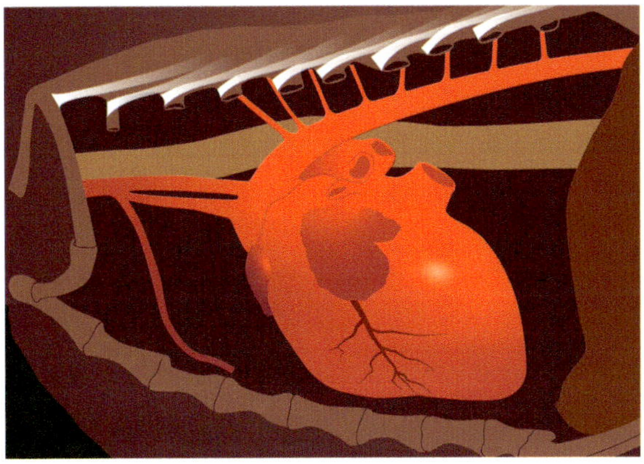

Figure 1. Orientation of the heart in the thorax.

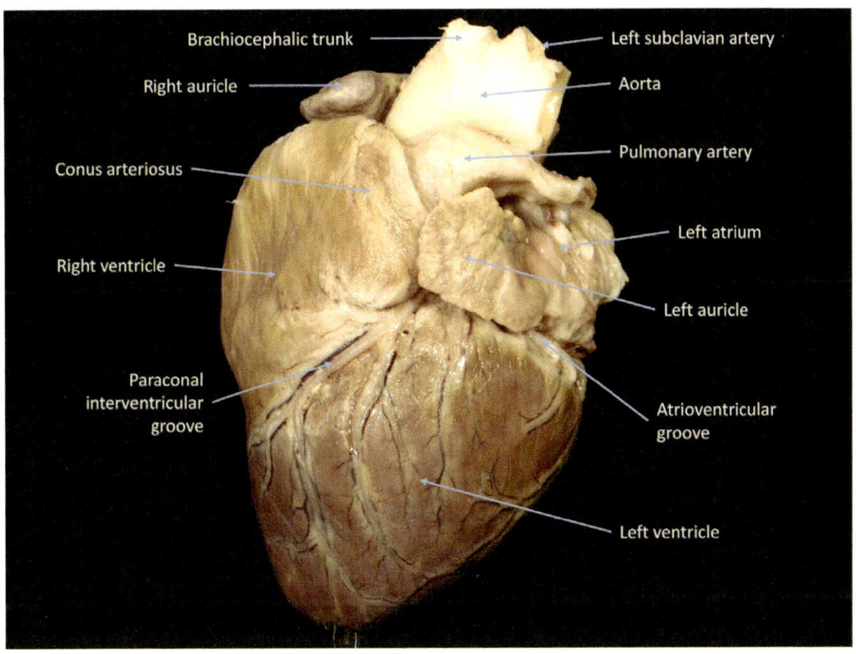

Figure 2. The surface of the heart (left side). Courtesy of Dr. Claudio Bussadori, Clinica Veterinaria Gran Sasso, Milan (Italy).

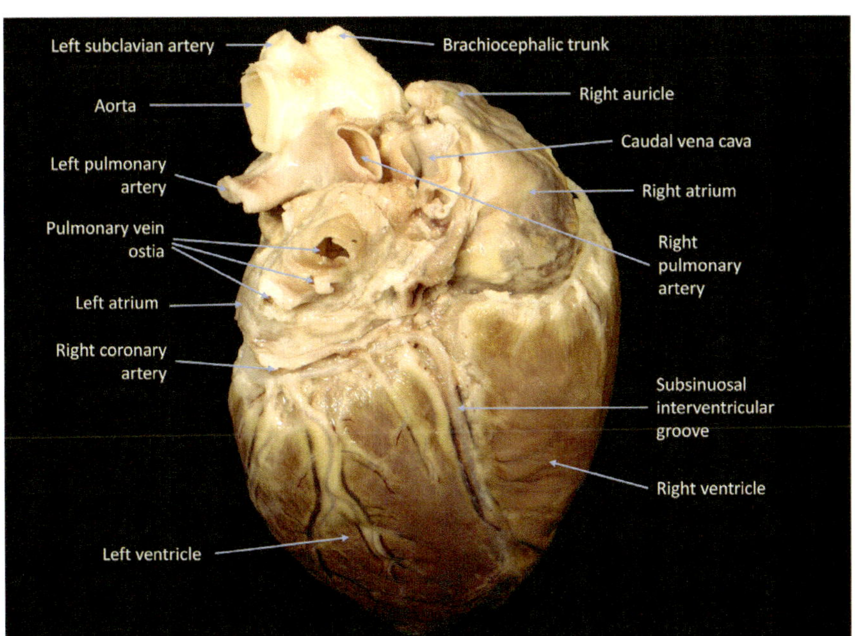

Figure 3. The surface of the heart (right side) Courtesy of Dr. Claudio Bussadori, Clinica Veterinaria Gran Sasso, Milan (Italy).

To appreciate the orientation of the heart in the chest, **the position of the auricles is a useful reference point**. The auricles are cul-de-sac appendages of the atria and project cranially from the heart base. A good learning exercise is to hold a heart model (or a real heart) in the palm of the hand and study the different structures of the heart and their positioning.

- The **auricles** face forward with the right ventricular outflow tract in-between them, positioned slightly towards the left side.
- The **base of the heart** points dorsally and cranially with the axis of the heart at approximately a 45° angle.
- The **aorta** is seen in the middle of the heart with the right auricle "hugging it" from the right side and the pulmonary trunk by its side on the left.
- The **left auricle** is seen immediately to the left of the pulmonary trunk and slightly more caudally and is easily seen from the left side of the heart, in contrast to the tip of the right auricle that appears more cranially, in front of the heart.
- The **coronary grooves**, where the arteries and veins run, mark the limits between the atria and ventricles, with the atria above and the ventricles below. They encircle the heart (except cranioventrally) and contain fat around the coronary vessels. This is often referred to as the atrioventricular groove.
- **Additional grooves** are seen originating from the coronary groove on both sides. These are **interventricular grooves** and demarcate the limits of the right and left ventricles, signalling the position of the interventricular septum. The coronary vessels are visible along these grooves, in contrast to the coronary groove, as less fat is present.
  - **On the right side** the subsinuosal interventricular groove appears as a short straight furrow on the dorsocaudal surface of the heart (Figure 3).
  - **On the left**, the paraconal interventricular groove starts on the caudodorsal side of the conus arteriosus (the infundibulum from which the pulmonary trunk arises) underneath the left auricle and runs ventrally until just before the apex (Figure 2).
  - The largest vein in the heart – the **great cardiac vein** – is located in the paraconal groove and drains into the coronary sinus.
- The cardiac apex is formed by the left ventricle, which is the most prominent chamber, and is located caudal and to the left of the right ventricle. The right ventricle can be viewed as a "pocket" wrapped cranially around the left ventricle with the inlet area sitting cranially on the right side and the outflow tract appearing on the left side. The right ventricular free wall extends approximately two thirds to three quarters of the distance from the coronary groove to the apex of the heart.

The **great vessels in the heart base are also useful in terms of orientation**.

- The cranial and caudal vena cava enter the cranial and caudal margin of the right atrium on the right side allowing identification of the right atrial limits.
- The pulmonary veins enter the left atrium on its dorsal aspect.

Atria

Right Atrium

The **right atrium receives blood returned from the body** via the vena cava and from the heart via the coronary sinus. The right atrium empties into the right ventricle via the atrioventricular orifice and through the tricuspid valve. Its anatomy is relevant from a clinical perspective as several important structures are located in the right atrium, such as the sinus node, the atrioventricular node, the terminal crest and the coronary sinus opening.

The right atrium lies cranially and dorsally to the right ventricle. It is composed of a main part (sinus venarum cavarum) and an appendage which projects cranially, ventrally and slightly to the left (right atrial appendage or auricle).

Three or four openings exist in the right atrium.

1. The **caudal vena cava** enters the right atrium caudally and returns blood from the abdominal viscera, the abdominal wall, and pelvic limbs.
2. The **cranial vena cava** enters the right atrium cranially and dorsally, and returns blood from the head, neck, thoracic limbs, ventral thoracic wall and adjacent part of the abdominal wall.
3. The **coronary sinus** is the smallest opening, entering the atrium caudally and from the left, just ventral to the opening of the caudal vena cava.
4. The **azygous vein** enters the cranial vena cava dorsally, although occasionally may enter the atrium directly. It drains blood from the lumbar region and caudal three-quarters of the thoracic wall. The interatrial septum extends from the opening of the coronary sinus to the opening into the right auricle. Between the two caval openings there is a small transverse ridge of tissue called the intervenous tubercle where blood flow converges into the right ventricle. Just caudal to this ridge, a slitlike depression exists in the atrial septum called the fossa ovalis with a crescent-shaped ridge of muscle that projects from the intervenous tubercle called the limbus *fossae ovalis*. The *fossa ovalis* may vary in size from one to several millimetres in depth in dogs and the septal wall is thin and translucent when illuminated.

During foetal life, a communication exists in the area between the right and left atria, called the ***foramen ovale***. Its purpose is to allow blood to bypass the non-functioning foetal lungs by flowing directly from the right to the left atrium.

The *foramen ovale* closes shortly after birth although it may remain patent in some dogs.

The right auricular appendage or right auricle is ear-shaped and extends cranioventrally to the left with its tip sitting just cranial and to the right of the pulmonary trunk. The inner surface is laced with multiple muscle strands called the pectinate muscles that extend from a semilunar ridge of muscle called the terminal crest or **crista terminalis**. The terminal crest marks the separation of the atrium and the auricle. The inner surface of the right atrium is smooth in contrast to the auricle. Additional features of right atrial anatomy are discussed later in this chapter when the conduction system is described.

Left Atrium

The **left atrium receives blood from the lungs** via the pulmonary veins and empties into the left ventricle through the mitral valve (Figure 5). It is located on the left dorsocaudal portion of the heart base. The pulmonary veins enter the atrium dorsally with **the number varying in dogs from five to six**. Two or three veins originate from the right lung and course dorsal to the right atrium, entering the craniodorsal part of the left atrium. Three veins originate from the left lung and enter the left atrium caudodorsally.

The **left auricle** is similar in shape, size and structure to the right auricle. It extends cranially and to the left, with its tip lying over the proximal end of the paraconal interventricular groove. The tips of the left and right auricles are separated from each other by the conus arteriosus and pulmonary trunk.

Pectinate muscles are also present in the left auricle with a smooth inner left atrial surface similar to the right atrium.

A thin concave flap of tissue may be seen in the cranial part of the interatrial septum where the valve of the *foramen ovale* was located.

Ventricles

Right Ventricle

Blood from the systemic circulation enters the right atrium and then passes into the right ventricle, from where it is pumped into the lungs through the pulmonary arteries. The right ventricle lies cranioventral to the left atrium and forms a triangular shaped "pocket" wrapped around the left ventricle. In cross-section, it has a crescent shape and the inflow (inlet) and an outflow (outlet) portions can be distinguished

The **inflow area** is dominated by the atrioventricular *ostium* or orifice between the cusps of the tricuspid valve. The **outflow area or tract** is funnel-shaped, and located at the craniodorsal aspect of the right ventricle on the left between the right auricle cranially and the left auricle caudally. This area is called the conus arteriosus and is separated from the inflow area by a ridge of muscle called the supraventricular crest or crista supraventricularis (Figures 2 and 4). The pulmonary trunk arises from the conus arteriosus and the two are separated by the **pulmonic valve**.

The inner surface of the ventricle possesses several muscular ridges, called trabecula carnae, which project into the lumen mainly from the outer wall. Additionally, muscular projections called **papillary muscles** exist in both ventricles to which chords that support the valve leaflets named ***chordae tendineae*** are attached. In dogs, there are usually three

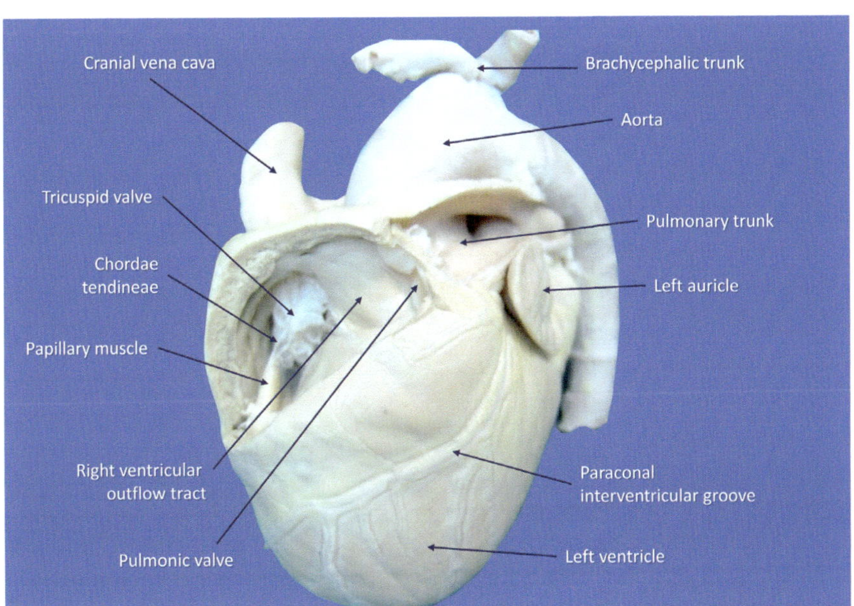

Figure 4. The right ventricle, tricuspid and pulmonic valves. Courtesy of Dr. Claudio Bussadori, Clinica Veterinaria Gran Sasso, Milan (Italy).

main papillary muscles in the right ventricle which arise from the septal wall, although there is a large amount of variation among individuals.

A single or branched muscular strand crosses the lumen of the right ventricle running to the outer wall; this originates from the septal wall near or from the base of the largest papillary muscle. It branches repeatedly as it merges with the outer wall. This structure is called the trabecula septomarginalis dextra and carries cardiac conduction fibres from the right bundle branch that supply the free wall of the right ventricle. It was previously known as the moderator band.

Left Ventricle

Blood from the pulmonary circulation enters the left atrium and passes into the left ventricle, from where it is pumped via the aorta into the systemic circulation. The left ventricle is conical in shape and is the largest chamber in the heart with thick muscular walls (Figure 5). Two openings exist with one between the left atrium and ventricle – the atrioventricular *ostium* or opening, and another between the ventricle and the aorta – the aortic *ostium*. The mitral and aortic valves control blood flow through the atrioventricular and aortic ostia respectively.

The left ventricle has two large **papillary muscles** originating in the outer wall where the *chordae tendineae* supporting the mitral valve are attached. One of the papillary muscles is positioned more cranially at the level of the auricular appendage and near the subsinuousal interventricular groove – the subauricular papillary muscle. The other papillary muscle is more caudal and closer to the paraconal interventricular groove – the subatrial papillary muscle. A fine network of muscular strands can be seen originating from the septal wall close to the base of the subatrial papillary muscle – the left **septomarginalis trabeculae** – and are thought to contain cardiac conduction fibres from the left bundle branch.

The interventricular septum is divided into two separate portions.

1. **The muscular septum** formed of adjacent muscle from both the right and left ventricles extends approximately two thirds of the way from the apex to the base of the ventricle.
2. **The membranous septum** forms the upper third of the interventricular septum, is the last part of the septum to be formed, and is thin and less muscular.

Fibrous Base

The fibrous base or cardiac skeleton separates the atria from the ventricles. It is made of fibrous tissue and collagen, and is where the atrial and ventricular muscle attach whilst keeping them separate. This is important as it ensures the **atria and ventricles are isolated from an electrical point of view**, with the atrioventricular node as their only electrical connection. The fibrous base includes **four openings** or rings where the two atrioventricular valves, the aortic and the pulmonic valves are attached. The aortic and pulmonic openings are round and well-defined whilst the atrioventricular ones are more oval-shaped.

Atrioventricular Valves

Mitral Valve

The **mitral valve divides the left atrium and ventricle** to ensure that during ventricular systole blood does not flow backwards into the atrium. It is composed of **two leaflets or cusps** (Figure 5). The cusp that is attached to the septal part of the fibrous ring is called the septal cusp whereas the cusp that attaches to the free wall side is the parietal cusp. The septal cusp is larger and wider than the parietal cusp. Since the septal cusp in humans is positioned anteriorly (in front or closer to the sternum) and the parietal cusp is positioned more posteriorly (behind the septal cusp) the terms **anterior and posterior leaflets** are often used and have filtered into veterinary medicine. These terms are not anatomically correct in quadruped patients and the terms septal and parietal are preferred.

The valve leaflets are composed of three distinct layers, arranged from top to bottom as follows.

1. The **atrialis** faces the atrium and possesses an abundance of loose collagen and the protein elastin, which allows the valve to undergo considerable stretching and then recoil back to its original shape.
2. The **spongiosa** is rich in glycosaminoglycans and proteoglycans providing the valve with compressive strength.
3. The **fibrosa** is the thickest layer and is composed of dense collagen aligned circumferentially, providing the valve with tensile strength.

Several chords extend out from the edges of the cusps to the papillary muscles. These are called ***chordae tendineae*** **and their function is to hold the valve in place** during ventricular systole and prevent the cusps being pulled back into the atrium. They are arranged in larger strands attached to the papillary muscles which form multiple ramifications, becoming progressively smaller until they attach on the ventricular side of the valve. This arrangement may be compared to a tree trunk and its branches and ensures a balanced distribution of the mechanical forces among the chordae. Histologically, *chordae tendineae* appear as thin tendons made of dense connective tissue.

Tricuspid Valve

The **tricuspid valve divides the right atrium from the right ventricle** (Figure 4). The name suggests the presence of three separate cusps or leaflets, but this is derived from human medicine and does not hold true for dogs and cats. In these species, the tricuspid valve is usually composed of two main cusps, and occasionally two or three additional smaller cusps.

- The septal cusp attaches to the septal part of the fibrous ring.
- The parietal cusp attached to the free wall side.
- Angular cusps refer to the additional smaller cusps which may be found at the angles of the main cusps.

Chordae tendineae emerge from the ventricular side of the valve leaflets and attach to the papillary muscles in the same arrangement described above for the mitral valve.

Semilunar Valves

Aortic Valve

The **aortic valve controls the exit of blood from the left ventricle** via the aorta into the systemic circulation. It is formed of **three semilunar (crescent-shaped) cusps** which can be distinguished as a **right, a left and a septal cusp** (Figure 5). At the level of this valve the aorta bulges outwards to form three sinuses called the **Valsalva sinuses**, situated laterally to each cusp. They are termed right and left sinuses and this is where the right and left coronary arteries originate from. The third sinus is termed the non-coronary sinus.

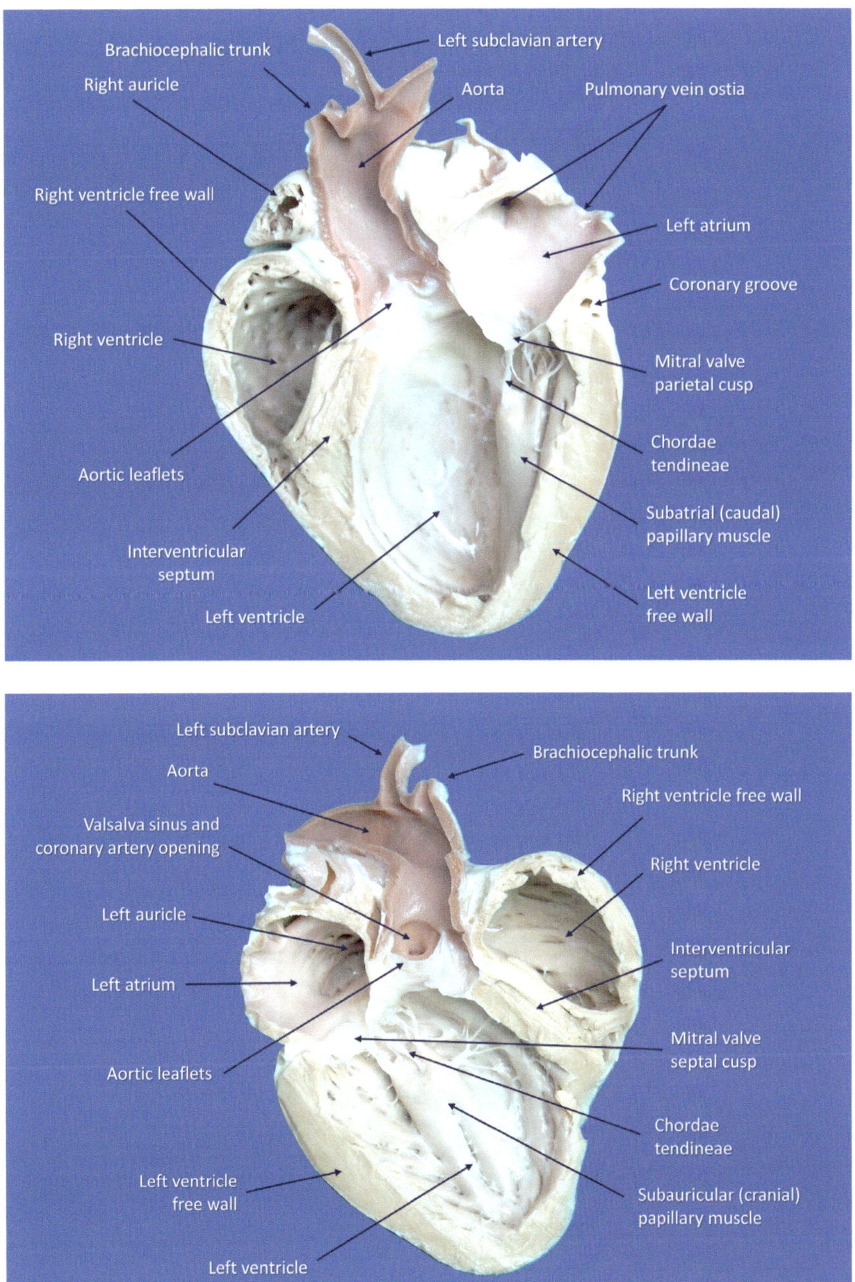

Figure 5. The left heart chambers and valves. Courtesy of Dr. Claudio Bussadori, Clinica Veterinaria Gran Sasso, Milan (Italy).

The area where the aorta becomes tubular is called the **sinotubular junction**. The cusps are attached in a semilunar shape to the aortic root extending from the fibrous ring at the level of the *annulus* and up to the level of the sinotubular junction on both sides. The semilunar hinge lines of adjacent cusps meet at the sinotubular junction forming the commissures.

Histologically the aortic valve is composed of a fibrous stroma with a layer of endocardium on both sides.

Pulmonic Valve

The **pulmonic valve controls the exit of blood from the right ventricle** via the main pulmonary artery into the pulmonary circulation. Its anatomy and histological characteristics are similar to the aortic valve (Figure 4). The cusps are divided into a right, a left and an intermediate cusp.

Cardiac Vasculature

Coronary Arteries

The **coronary arteries supply oxygenated blood to the heart**. There are both left and right coronary arteries, which originate from the aortic root (from the left and right aortic sinuses respectively) (Figure 6).

Left Coronary Artery

The **left coronary artery** is short and wide and ramifies into the circumflex and paraconal branches, as well as a septal branch in many dogs. It runs underneath the left auricle.

Circumflex Branch

The **circumflex branch** lies in the coronary groove to the left and runs dorsocaudally over to the right across the caudodorsal surface of the heart. When it reaches the subsinuosal interventricular groove it runs ventrally toward the apex of the heart as the **subsinousal interventricular branch**.

Several branches originate from the circumflex branch and run ventrally towards the apex. The longest of these branches is the left marginal branch that runs parallel to the subsinuosal interventricular branch. Branches of the circumflex artery also extend to the atria to supply the atrial muscle.

Paraconal Interventricular Branch

The **paraconal interventricular branch** is the same width as the circumflex branch and runs obliquely and distally from left to right in the paraconal interventricular groove. It extends around the apex of the heart and gives off several left ventricular, right ventricular and septal branches.

Right Coronary Artery

The right coronary artery measures approximately 1.5 mm in diameter and 5 cm in length. It is located between the pulmonary trunk and the conus arteriosus cranially on the left and underneath the right auricle. It runs towards the right side of the heart and lies in the fat in the coronary groove. It supplies blood to a large proportion of the right ventricular wall, the right atrium, and parts of the aorta and pulmonary trunk. In approximately 20% of dogs an accessory right coronary artery may arise close to the right coronary sinus and extend approximately 2 cm distally on the conus arteriosus. Several branches of the right coronary artery extend into the right ventricle and atrium.

Cardiac Veins

The **cardiac veins run alongside the coronary arteries** but are given different names to their counterparts. **They drain into the coronary sinus** which is located in the dorsal part of the coronary groove on the right side and opens into the right atrium ventral to the caudal vena cava. There is a great deal of variation between dogs in the number and size of cardiac veins but two are consistently present.

1. The **great cardiac vein** arises near the apex of the heart and ascends towards the base of the heart in the paraconal interventricular groove and then circles the caudal surface of the heart from the left in the coronary groove to join the coronary sinus.
2. The **middle cardiac vein** that ascends in the subsinuosal interventricular groove.

These veins collect blood from numerous tributaries along their course.

Conduction System

The conduction system of the heart is responsible for generating and transmitting electrical stimuli to the whole heart in a specific and ordered fashion.

The **sinus node acts as pacemaker** to the heart as it possesses specialised "pacemaker" cells generating electrical impulses,which are capable of spontaneous depolarisation. These impulses are then transmitted quickly to the other parts of the heart via pathways formed of cells organised in bundles which allow quick conduction of the electrical stimuli. These structures are present in the walls of the heart interwoven with the myocardial tissue itself. They include the internodal pathways, the interatrial pathways, the atrioventricular node, the bundle branches, and the Purkinje network (Figure 7).

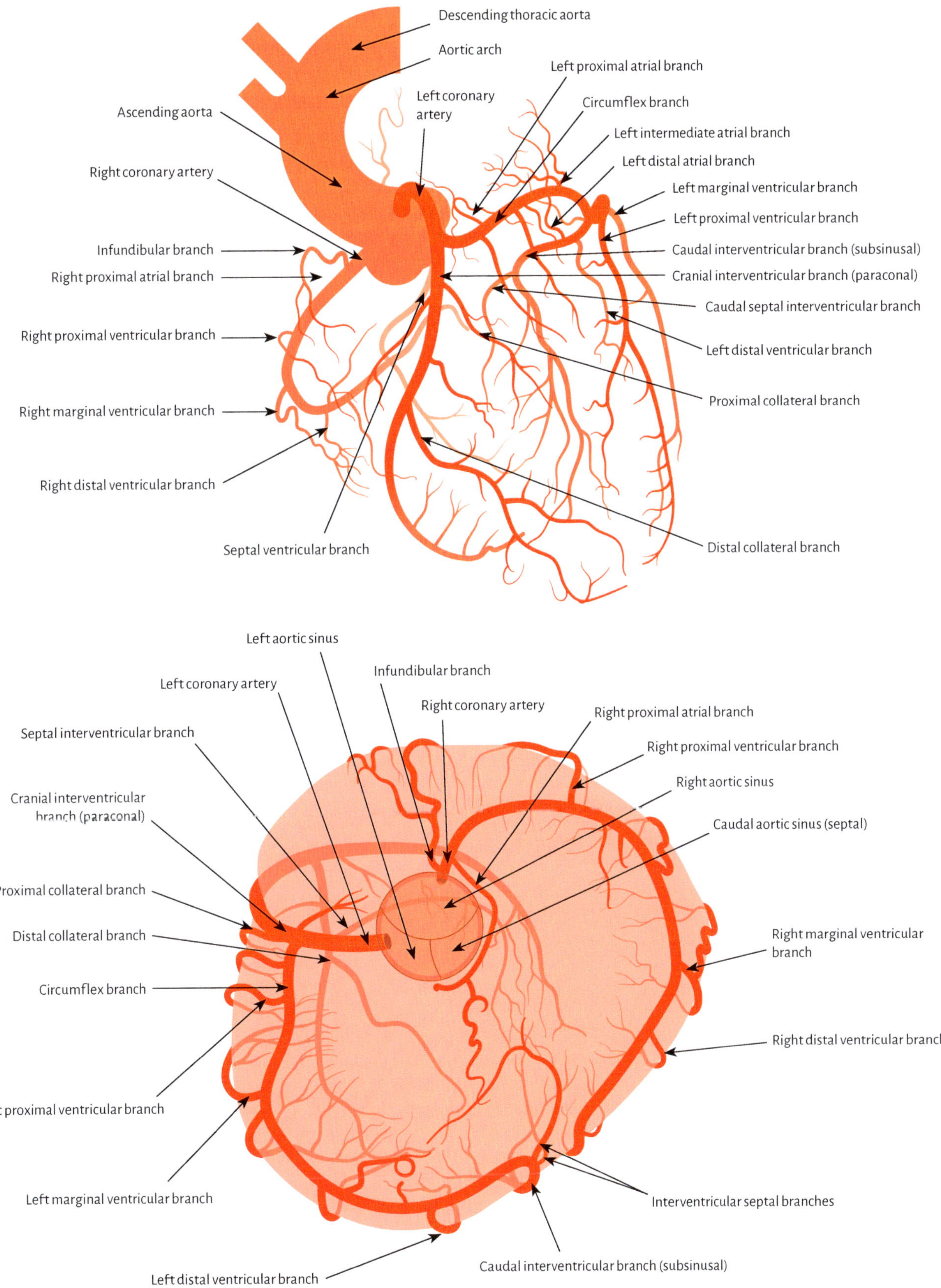

Figure 6. The coronary system.

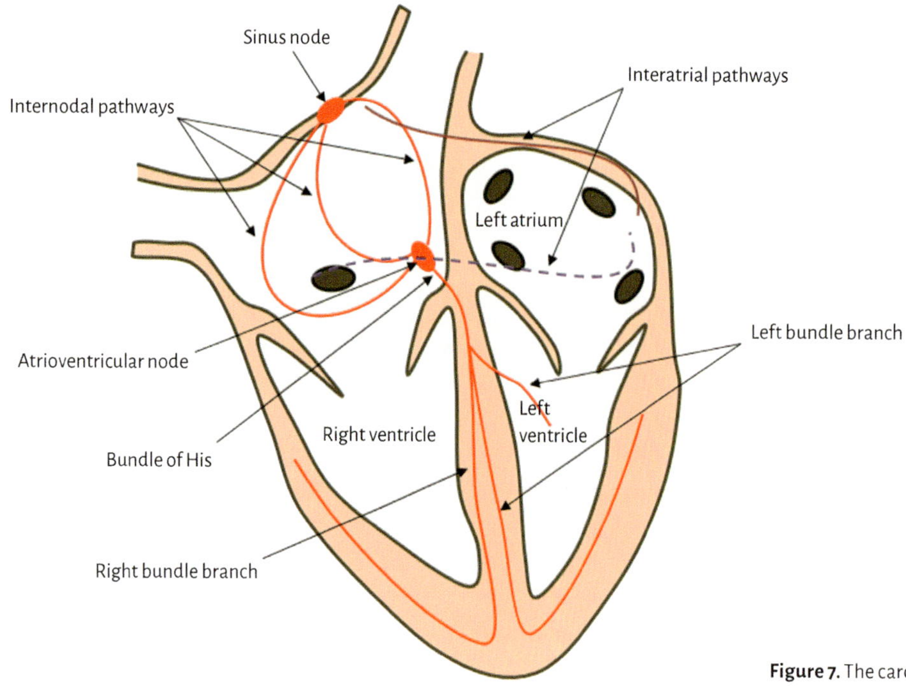

Figure 7. The cardiac conduction system.

Sinus Node

The **sinus node, also known as the sinoatrial node, is found in the wall of the right atrium** where it joins the cranial vena cava in the upper portion of the terminal groove (sulcus terminalis).

In dogs, it lies less than 1 mm beneath the epicardium and occupies almost the entire thickness of the atria. Up to 3–4 cm between both venae cavae has been reported, although there appears to be great individual variation. In cats, a triangular or ellipsoid shape of approximately 6.6–8.1 mm by 2.1–2.3 mm, with a thickness of 0.4 mm has been described. Histologically, the sinus node is composed of specialised muscle fibres arranged in a network.

Three different types of cells are present:

1. normal working **myocardial cells**
2. **transitional cells**
3. **P (pacemaker) cells**.

The P cells are capable of spontaneously generating electrical stimuli and represent approximately 50% of the cells in the sinus node. They are organised in small units of approximately five cells surrounded by connective tissue.

Atrioventricular Node

As mentioned above the atrial and ventricular myocardium are separated by a fibrous skeleton that ensures that they are electrically isolated from each other. The **only point of electrical connection is provided by the atrioventricular node** which is a specialised conduction structure that traverses the central portion of the fibrous skeleton – the central fibrous body.

The atrioventricular node (AVN) may be divided into three different portions based on histological differences between each area:

1. the atrionodal region
2. the compact node
3. the distal atrioventricular bundle.

For this reason, the term atrioventricular junction is often used instead of node as the latter is misleading and often confused with the compact node.

These structures are located on the floor of the right atrium in an area known as the **triangle of Koch**. The base of the triangle is limited by the opening of the coronary sinus and the apex is formed by the junction between the fibrous tendon (tendon of Todaro) and the septal leaflet of the tricuspid valve. In dogs, the AVN has an elongated shape with a concave surface facing the central fibrous body measuring approximately 2–4 mm in length, 2 mm in width and 0.5–1 mm thick. In cats, an elongated oval shape has also been reported measuring approximately 1.2–1.8 mm in length, 0.2–0.5 mm in width, and 0.4–0.6 mm thick.

The **atrionodal region** is formed from bundles thought to be the continuation of the internodal bundles which converge into a single proximal atrioventricular bundle which is in turn continuous with the compact node. The compact node is located on the atrial aspect of the central fibrous body and is approximately 1–1.5 mm in length in the dog. It is composed of closely interwoven fibres within a sparse collagen framework. The cells of the compact node possess characteristics similar to the pacemaker cells in the sinus node and the relevance of this becomes obvious in the next chapter. They perform the important function of **slowing down conduction just enough to allow atrial depolarisation** (and therefore contraction) to occur a few milliseconds before ventricular depolarisation.

This is in contrast with the rest of the conduction system that is designed to conduct electrical impulses quickly and highlights the importance of this being the only point of electrical connection between the atria and the ventricles. The **distal atrioventricular bundle** extends from the compact node a few millimetres until it branches at the cranial edge of the tricuspid septal leaflet at the apex of the triangle of Koch. It penetrates the *septum fibrosum* effectively bridging the atria and ventricles. It is commonly referred to as the bundle of His after its discovery by Wilhem His Jr.

Internodal Pathways

The existence of internodal pathways is still the subject of debate although there is anatomical and electrophysiological evidence to support their presence in dogs. They connect the sinus node to the atrioventricular node allowing rapid conduction of the electrical impulse between these two structures. Three distinct pathways have been described in dogs.

1. The **anterior internodal pathway** courses through the cranial aspect of the vena cava where it bifurcates into the Bachmann's bundle and then courses ventrally though the cranial part of the atrial septum.
2. The **middle internodal pathway** originates in the sinus node and courses ventrally and cranially to the *fossa ovalis* until it reaches the atrioventricular node.
3. The **posterior internodal pathway** courses downwards along the crista terminalis through the caudal portion of the atrial septum and past the opening of the coronary sinus until it joins the caudal aspect of the atrioventricular node.

Interatrial Pathways

As the name suggests **interatrial pathways provide rapid conduction of electrical impulses from the right atrium to the left atrium**. They possess cells similar to those found in Purkinje fibres in the ventricles.

At least four connections have been described but two are particularly important.

1. **Bachmann's bundle** or interatrial band splits from the anterior internodal pathway close to the sinus node and traverses the upper portion of the atrial septum towards the left auricle.
2. A connection exists along the coronary sinus wall with a proposed ending within the ligament or **vein of Marshall** in the left atrium (a remnant of the left cranial *vena cava*) – the term inferior interatrial pathway has been proposed by some authors for this connection.

Bundle Branches

Shortly after reaching the ventricular domain, the distal atrioventricular bundle divides into several branches which carry electrical impulses to both ventricles. These branches are formed of specialised conduction cells called **Purkinje cells** which are capable of very rapid electrical conduction. They are called the **bundle branches** and commonly divided into a **right and a left bundle branch**, although much individual variation exists. This division occurs in the upper portion of the interventricular septum just below the non-coronary and right aortic leaflets.

- The **right bundle branch** runs on the right side of the interventricular septum, underneath the subendocardium. Initially it is chord-like until it reaches the cranial papillary muscle of the right ventricle where it branches into three ramifications that travel towards the conus arteriosus, the septum, and the right ventricular free wall. The branches supplying the free wall form bridges from the septum to the free wall.
- The **left bundle branch** runs on the left side of the interventricular septum in the subendocardium. The initial part is brush-like and ramifies into two main groups of peripheral branches.
  - The cranial group (commonly referred to as the **anterior fascicle**) which supplies the cranial left ventricular area.
  - The caudal group (commonly referred to as the **posterior fascicle**) which supplies the caudal areas of the ventricle.

The Purkinje Network

Cells called **Purkinje cells** form bundle branches which ramify into numerous small branches and spread all over the subendocardium of both ventricles to form a network connecting the conduction system to the working myocardium.

Cardiac Innervation

The heart is innervated by the **autonomic nervous system.** Plexuses of neuron ganglions are present in several locations in the atria and the ventricles. The **sinus node** and **atrioventricular node** are richly innervated and are the most susceptible to autonomic tone. The sinus node is particularly responsive to parasympathetic tone whereas the atrioventricular node is more influenced by sympathetic tone.

- **Sympathetic innervation** to the sinus and atrioventricular nodes is provided by efferents from the ansae subclaviae via branches of the cervicothoracic ganglia and the middle cervical ganglia.
- **Parasympathetic innervation** to the sinus node is provided by the right vagus nerve, whereas the atrioventricular node receives input from both the left and right vagus nerves.

The Pericardium

The pericardium is a **fibroserous sac** which encloses the heart. Its most obvious function is to protect the heart from rubbing against the lungs and other thoracic structures, and to prevent possible infections in these neighbouring structures from spreading to the heart. The pericardium serves other purposes which are discussed in other sections of this text.

The pericardium is formed of **two layers**:

- a tough outer fibroserous membrane called the **parietal pericardium**;
- an inner serous membrane called the **visceral pericardium** (Figure 8).

The parietal pericardium attaches to the adventitia of the large vessels at the heart base and extends to the diaphragm to form the **phrenopericardial ligament** at the apex. The visceral pericardium lines the internal surface of the parietal pericardium and the external cardiac surface where it is called the **epicardium** and is tightly adhered to the myocardium. It is composed of mesothelial cells overlying a fibroelastic stroma. Numerous microvilli and long cilia exist to increase the surface area, enhance fluid transport, and facilitate movement of the serosal surfaces during cardiac movement. The space between the two pericardial layers is called the **pericardial cavity** which is filled with a small amount of phospholipid rich fluid (≈0.25 ml/kg). This fluid lubricates the exterior surfaces of the heart.

Embryology of the Heart and Great Vessels

A basic knowledge of embryology is necessary to understand the origin of congenital cardiac defects. In this section, a brief description of the formation of the heart chambers, heart valves, and great vessels is provided.

Formation of the Heart

The origin of the heart starts as **a pair of structures in the splanchnic mesoderm** which eventually become the **myocardium**.

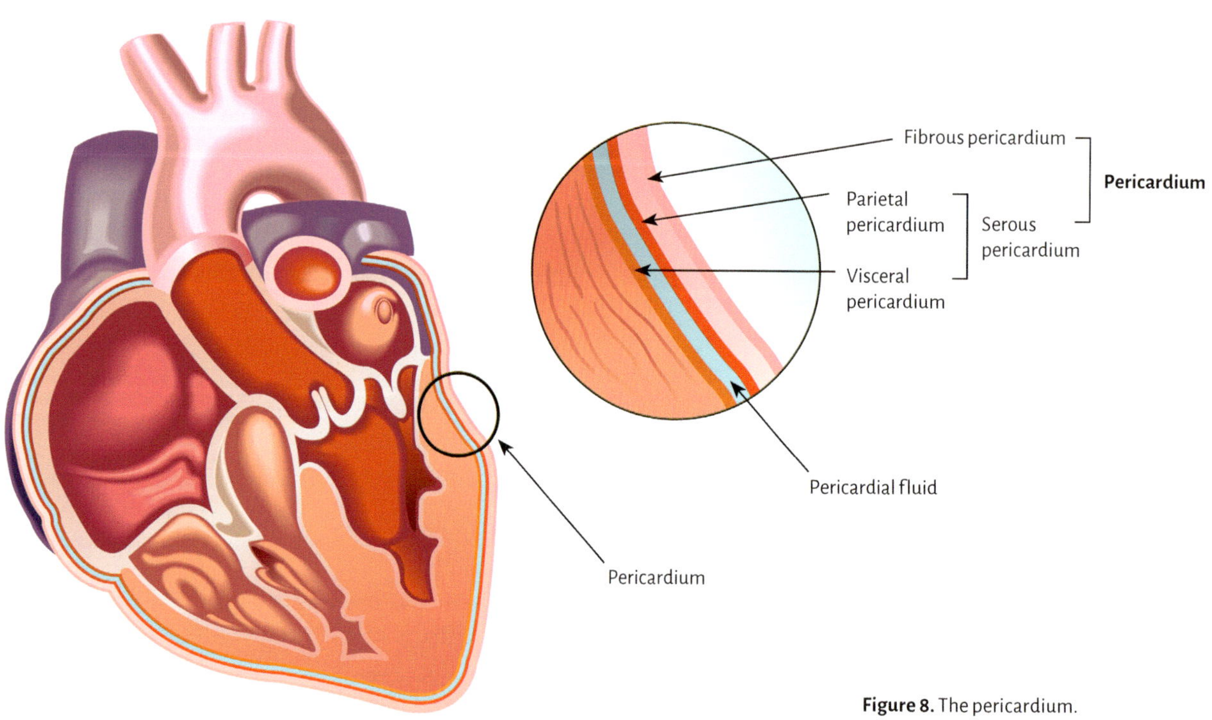

Figure 8. The pericardium.

This tissue is subsequently joined by endocardial tissue which also originates from the mesoderm to **form a pair of endocardial tubes**. The endocardial tubes then **migrate to the centre of the body** and fuse to form a single cardiac tube formed of myocardium, endocardium and extracellular material.

The cardiac tube is straight initially and has a **ventral aorta** at the anterior end (facing the front of the body) and the **omphalomesenteric veins** at the posterior end (facing the back of the body). Over time this tube bends progressively and folds over itself to form the cardiac loop.

Distinct structures can be distinguished within the cardiac loop:

1. the sinus venosus
2. the atrium
3. the ventricle
4. the *bulbus cordis*
5. the *truncus arteriosus* (Figure 9).

The **sinus venosus collects blood from the whole embryo** which then flows to the atrium, ventricle and out of the heart via the *bulbus cordis* and *truncus arteriosus*. The sinus venosus is separated from the single atrium by the sinoatrial sulcus which is the site of the future sinoatrial node. The atrium sits dorsally and cranially to the ventricle and both structures are separated by a distinct atrioventricular canal. The ventricle is separated from the *bulbus cordis* by the bulboventricular sulcus.

Cardiac Septation

After the loop stage is complete, **a series of partitions are formed separating the heart into right and left-sided chambers** (Figure 10). The sinus venosus becomes separated from the left atrium by deepening of the atrioventricular sulcus and opens only into the right atrium. The venae cavae open separately into the right atrium and part of the sinus venosus becomes the coronary sinus. At the same time the pulmonary veins open into the left atrium.

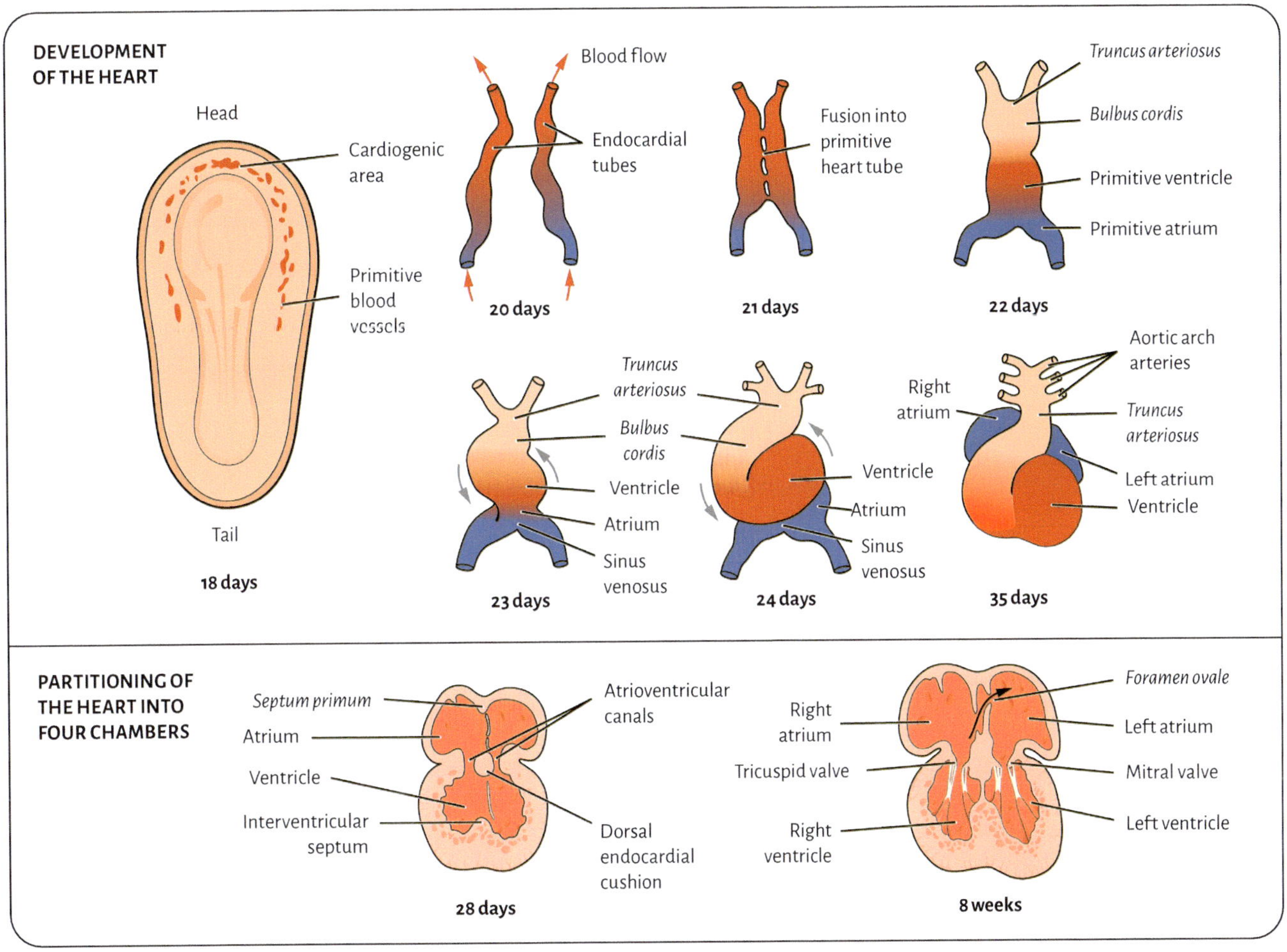

Figure 9. Development of the heart. Top: cardiac loop formation. Bottom: cardiac septation. Download for free at http://cnx.org/content/col11496/latest/.

By the end of the loop stage the atrium develops two lateral lobes that will become the left and right atria and auricles. The smooth portion of the left and right atria are derived from the sinus venosus and the rest from the primordial atrium. The caudal end of the *bulbus cordis* gives rise to the left and right ventricular outflow tracts. The cranial end of the *bulbus cordis* and *truncus arteriosus* give rise to the aorta and pulmonary trunk.

Atrial Septum

Separation between both atria occurs when the septum extends from the dorsal wall of the atrium toward the atrioventricular canal where it fuses with the endocardial cushions. This is the ***septum primum* or first septum**. The opening that exists in the ventral area of the septum before it fuses with the endocardial cushions is called the *ostium primum*. If the *septum primum* fails to merge with the endocardial cushions an *ostium primum* type **atrial septal defect is present**. Another opening exists in the upper part of the *septum primum* called the *ostium secundum*. It is formed via a series of perforations of the *septum primum* which coalesce to form this *ostium*. Its purpose is to **allow direct passage of blood from the right to the left atrium during foetal life** to avoid the non-functioning lungs.

A **second septum** called the *septum secundum* forms from the dorsal wall of the atrium to the right of the *septum primum* and merges with the endocardial cushions of the atrioventricular canal. Both septa merge and become a single atrial septum. An opening also exists in the *septum secundum* called the *foramen ovale*. It is slightly offset from the *ostium*

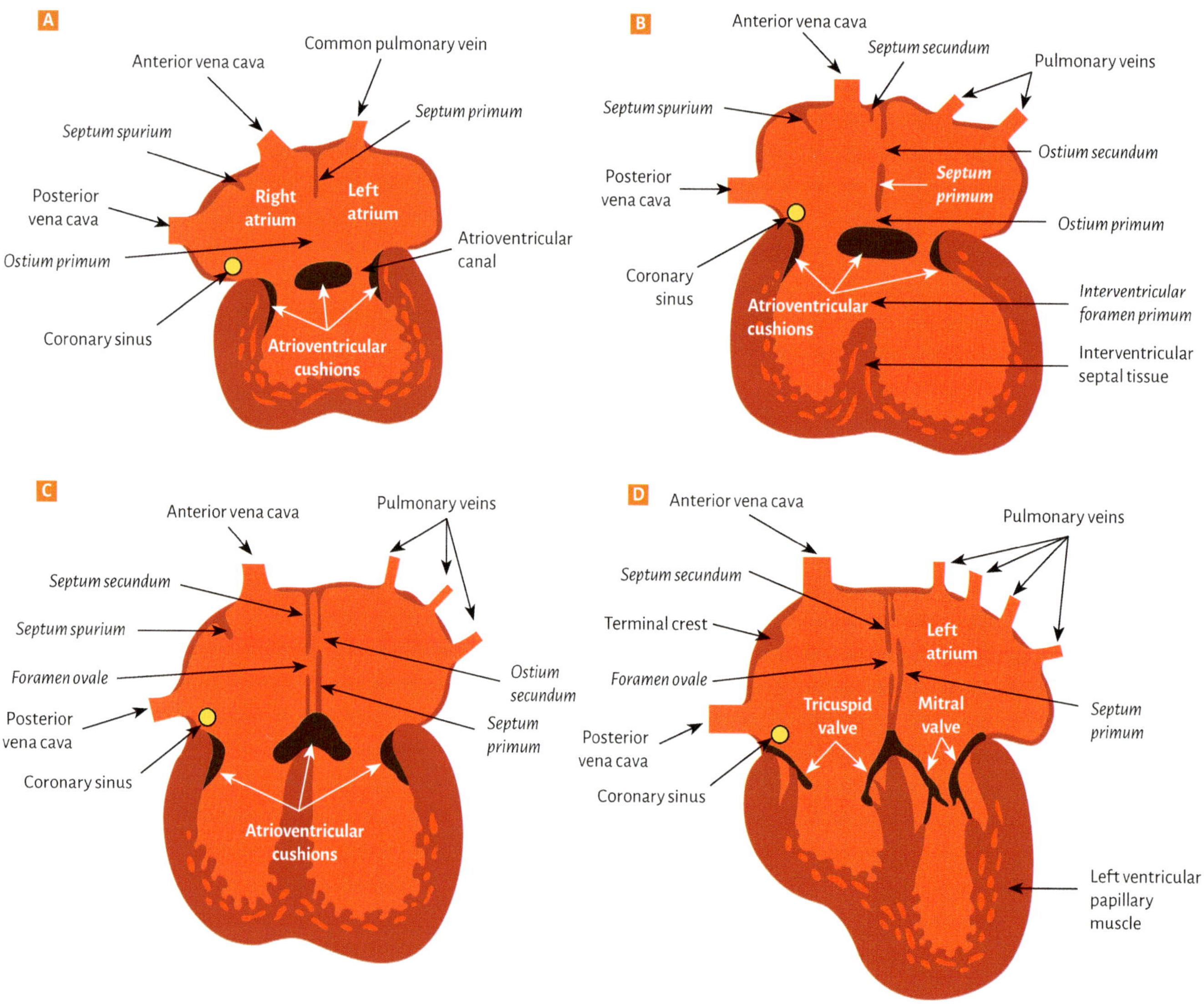

Figure 10. Cardiac septation development.

secundum so that it is covered by the *septum primum* forming a valve that only opens towards the left atrial side. This is important as it allows **passage of blood from the right to the left atrium during foetal life** but closes as soon as left atrial pressure becomes higher than in the right atrium at birth. This mechanical closure at birth is followed by fusion of the *septum primum* and *septum secundum* in this area leaving a depression called the *fossa ovalis* where the *foramen ovale* was located. In some individuals, fusion of the septa does not occur and the *foramen ovale* remains patent – **patent *foramen ovale***. If the *septum primum* is not large enough to cover this area an *ostium secundum* type **atrial septal defect** exists.

Ventricular Septum

The ventricular septum grows from the apex towards the base by extension of the tissue growth that forms the ventricular myocardium. It does not reach the atrioventricular canal and forms the **interventricular foramen**. This section of interventricular septum is known as the **muscular septum**. Connective tissue originating from the atrioventricular endocardial cushions eventually merges with the septal tissue closing the interventricular foramen, completing the separation of both ventricles. This area of the septum is referred to as the **membranous septum**. Ventricular septal defects (VSD) located in the muscular septum are called muscular VSDs and those in the membranous septum are called **perimembranous VSDs**.

Formation of the Aorta and Pulmonary Trunk

The aorta and pulmonary trunk originate from the *truncus arteriosus* and part of the *bulbus cordis*. Two distal ridge-like thickenings project into the lumen of the *truncus arteriosus* called the bulbar and the truncal ridges. They extend in a spiral course towards the proximal end of the *truncus arteriosus* and eventually fuse to form the aorticopulmonary septum, effectively forming the aorta and the pulmonary trunk. A simplistic way to describe this process is to imagine a tube that is twisted into a spiral and divided from the inside to form two separate tubes placed almost perpendicular to each other.

Abnormalities at this stage of development may result in **tetralogy of Fallot**, transposition of the great arteries, and persistent *truncus arteriosus* (common arterial trunk or simply *truncus arteriosus*). The latter consists of complete failure of this stage where the aorta and pulmonary artery do not form. One single common arterial trunk is present that provides mixed blood to the pulmonary arteries, coronary vessels and systemic circulation.

Formation of the Heart Valves

The heart valves are formed after the cardiac septation stage is completed. The atrioventricular valve cusps are formed from tissue folds derived from the atrioventricular endocardial cushions and the ventricular wall. Perforations of the cusps coalesce to form the *chordae tendineae* and the papillary muscles. Developmental abnormalities at this stage result in valve abnormalities that may affect any part of the valve apparatus and in severe forms are also accompanied by failure of closure of the *ostium primum* and the membranous portion of the interventricular septum. They are generally called **endocardial cushion defects or atrioventricular defects**.

The semilunar valves form from three swellings or cushions that develop inside the pulmonary trunk and the aorta. The cusps form via a process of excavation of these cushions, which are formed of cardiac jelly and mesenchymal cells covered with endothelium. Valvular stenosis is attributed to abnormal development of the *bulbus cordis* from which these swellings originate. Subvalvular stenosis may occur with abnormal partitioning of the *bulbus cordis* and supravalvular stenosis may be due to abnormal formation of the distal *truncus arteriosus*.

Formation of the Main Vessels

The circulatory system in the foetus initially consists of a pair of dorsal and ventral aortae joined by six pairs of aortic arches (Figure 11). These vessels give rise to the arteries of the neck and head, aorta and pulmonary arteries.

- The first, second and fifth pairs of arches **regress early** in the developmental stage.
- The third pair and the cranial part of the dorsal aortae become the **internal and external carotid arteries**.
- The right fourth arch forms part of the **right subclavian artery** whilst the caudal part of the right dorsal aorta disappears.
- The left fourth arch forms part of the **aortic arch** and continues distally with the left dorsal aorta to form the remaining part of the adult aorta.
- The sixth aortic arches form the **pulmonary arteries** with part of the left sixth arch retaining its connection to the dorsal aorta to form the *ductus arteriosus*. This connection disappears shortly after birth.

Abnormalities at this stage of development may result in **vascular ring anomalies** of which the persistence of the right fourth aortic arch is the most common in dogs.

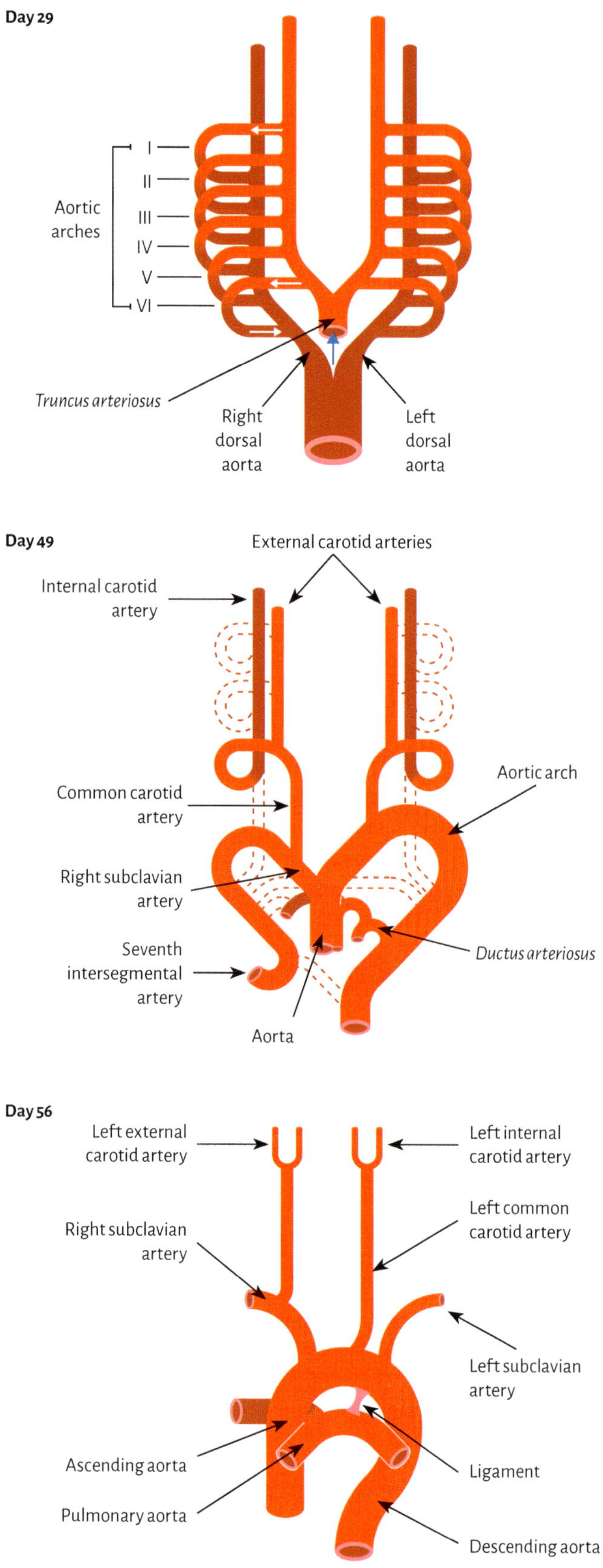

Figure 11. Formation of the great vessels. The aortic arches.

Bibliography

- Bezuidenhout, A. (2013) The Heart and Arteries. In: Evans HE & LaHunta A de (eds) *Miller Anatomy of the Dog*. St Louis: Elsevier, pp. 408–441.
- Bishop, S.P. (1999) Embryologic Development: The Heart and Great Vessels. In: Fox PR, Sisson D & Moise SN (eds) *Textbook of Canine and Feline Cardiology: Principles and Clinical Practice*. Philadelphia: Saunders, pp. 3–12.
- Fox, P.R. et al. (1999) Cardiovascular Anatomy. In: Fox PR, Sisson D, & Moise SN (eds) *Textbook of Canine and Feline Cardiology: Principles and Clinical Practice*. Philadelphia: WB Saunders Company, pp. 13–24.
- Kienle, R.D. & Kittleson, M.D. (1998) Cardiac Embryology and Anatomy. In: Kittleson MD & Kienle RD (eds) *Small Animal Cardiovascular Medicine*. St. Louis: Mosby, Inc, pp. 1–10.

Test

Answers on Page 18

1. The boundary on the inner surface of heart between the atrium and the right atrial appendage is marked by:

a. The intervenous tubercle.
b. The crista terminalis.
c. The coronary sinus groove.
d. The *fossa ovalis*.

2. Taking into account the anatomy of the outer surface of the heart, the tips of the left and right atria extend cranially and are separated from each other by:

a. The aortic trunk.
b. The cranial vena cava.
c. The conus arteriosus and the pulmonary trunk.
d. None of the above.

3. The left ventricle has large papillary muscles that originate from the outer wall where the *chordae tendineae* that support the mitral valve join it. Which of the following statements correctly describes its anatomy?

a. There are usually three main papillary muscles that arise from the septal wall.
b. The subatrial papillary muscle is located at the level of the left atrial appendage.
c. The subauricular papillary muscle is located cranially, close to the subsinusal interventricular groove.
d. The subauricular papillary muscle is located caudally and is closer to the paraconal interventricular groove.

4. Specialised conduction pathways provide rapid conduction of the electrical impulse between the right and left atrium. Of the options listed below, which pathway(s) are responsible for interatrial conduction?

a. The anterior, middle and posterior internodal pathways.
b. Bachmann's bundle.
c. The inferior interatrial pathway.
d. Options a, b, and c are correct.

5. The pericardium is a fibrous sac that contains the heart. Which of the following statements is correct regarding its anatomy?

a. The visceral pericardium adheres to the adventitia of the great vessels at the base of the heart and extends to the diaphragm to form the phrenic pericardial ligament at the apex.
b. The pericardium is made up of three layers: the parietal pericardium, the visceral pericardium, and the epicardium.
c. The visceral pericardium lines the inner surface of the parietal pericardium and the outer cardiac surface, where it is called the epicardium.
d. The parietal pericardium is composed of mesothelial cells that cover a fibroelastic stroma with numerous microvilli and long cilia.

6. Which of the following statements is correct regarding the process of formation of the atrial septum during cardiac development?

a. The *septum secundum* develops from the atrioventricular canal towards the dorsal wall of the atrium.
b. If the *septum primum* does not fuse with the endocardial cushions, there is an *ostium primum* type atrial septal defect.
c. The *foramen ovale* is an opening located in the perimembranous septum, covered by the muscular septum.
d. If the *septum secundum* is not large enough to cover the *foramen ovale*, there is an *ostium secundum*-type atrial septal defect.

Correct Answers:

1. b
2. c
3. c
4. d
5. c
6. b

Notes

Cardiovascular Physiology

Pedro Oliveira

This chapter discusses the basic concepts of cardiovascular physiology required to understand the function of cardiac cells, the heart, and circulatory system. For clinicians this is the first step to understanding the pathophysiology of various cardiovascular diseases and how the available treatment options influence its function.

Overview of the Cardiovascular System

The cardiovascular system consists of **a pump (the heart) and a circulatory system** composed of vessels through which blood flows around the body, to transport and transfer gases (oxygen and carbon dioxide), nutrients, waste products, hormones, and other substances (Figure 1).

The circulatory system is divided into two major circuits arranged in series (blood flows through one and then the other).

1. The **pulmonary circulation** includes the pulmonary arteries, capillaries, and veins.
2. The **systemic circulation** includes all other arteries, capillary beds and veins.

Blood is pumped into the **pulmonary circulation by the right ventricle via the pulmonary artery**. In the lung capillaries, gas exchange occurs replenishing the oxygen in red blood cells whilst carbon dioxide is excreted. **Oxygenated blood is returned to the heart via the pulmonary veins which drain into the left atrium**. The left ventricle then pumps this blood around the rest of the body, via the aorta, into the systemic circulation. Each organ or tissue is supplied by a number of arteries which ramify into progressively smaller vessels called arterioles, which are in turn connected to numerous **tiny vessels called capillaries**.

Gas and nutrient exchange occurs via the capillaries with various types of cells. The blood is then collected by small veins called **venules** into progressively larger veins until it is finally returned to the heart.

The various **circuits that supply the body's organs are arranged in parallel** and not in series (blood is distributed to the different organs without going through each organ one after the other). The **arteries possess thick walls with significant**

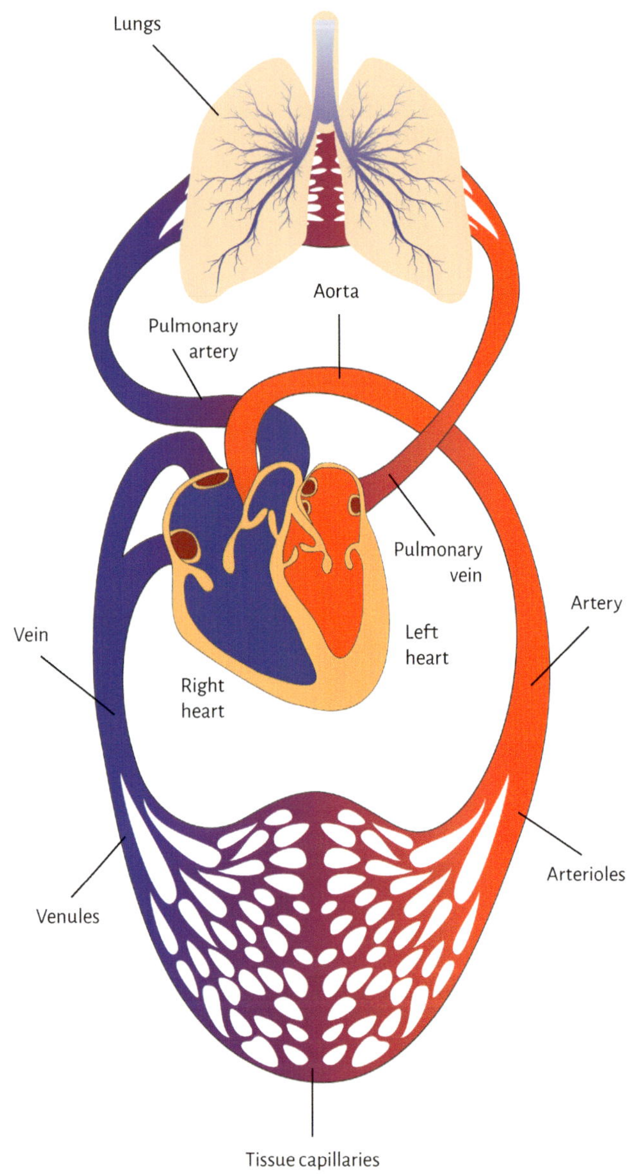

Figure 1. The cardiovascular system. The heart pumps blood through the circulatory system to provide the cells with nutrients, oxygen, hormones, and remove waste products such as carbon dioxide. There are two different circulatory systems arranged in series: 1) the pulmonary circulation and 2) the systemic circulation. Blood is pumped into the pulmonary circulation by the right ventricle via the pulmonary artery. In the lung capillaries, gas exchange occurs replenishing red blood cells with oxygen whilst carbon dioxide is excreted. Oxygenated blood is returned to the heart via the pulmonary veins which drain into the left atrium. The left ventricle then pumps this blood to the rest of the body via the aorta into the systemic circulation. Every organ in the body is supplied with oxygenated blood via arteries and this blood is subsequently collected by veins and returned to the heart for another cycle.

amounts of muscle and elastic fibres so as to withstand the high pressure generated by the heart. The elastic fibres contribute to elastic recoil in large arteries, which continues to propel the blood forward after the heart has stopped contracting.

In contrast, the **veins have thin walls with less muscle and elastic fibre** as the pressure within these vessels is low. Large veins also have valves within them, which help keep blood flowing towards the heart. Veins act as low pressure conduits and also as an important reservoir of blood in the body. Approximately **65% of the whole blood volume is present in the systemic veins** at any given time. Venodilation or constriction can shift large amounts of blood to and from different parts of the circulation.

Of the total blood volume in the body, approximately:

- 10% is found in the systemic arteries and arterioles
- 5% in the systemic capillaries
- 65% in the systemic veins
- 5% is found in the heart
- 15% in the pulmonary circulation.

The **systemic circulation is a high-pressure system** in comparison to the pulmonary circulation. The mean blood pressure is approximately 100 mmHg in the systemic circulation and only 15 mmHg in the lungs. The muscular content and anatomy of the ventricles reflects this difference; the **left ventricle is larger and more muscular than the right**. The higher blood pressure in the systemic circulation is important as some organs are dependent on it for adequate perfusion (e.g. brain, heart and kidneys). **Systemic arterioles are responsible for most of the resistance to blood flow** as they are much smaller (30 μm) than small arteries (4 mm). Additionally, the size of the arterioles can change in response to contraction or relaxation of smooth muscle in their walls with a profound impact on systemic blood pressure. Drugs used in the treatment of cardiovascular disease that influence the diameter of arterioles are often used to target this response (e.g. vasodilators).

The cardiovascular system is designed to maintain systemic blood pressure at a level that ensures all organs and tissues have an adequate blood supply. In addition, hydrostatic pressure on both arterial and venous sides should not exceed a certain level to avoid harmful systemic hypertension or venous congestion.

The three basic functions of the cardiovascular system are:

1. to maintain **blood pressure**
2. to maintain normal **blood flow** to tissues
3. to maintain normal **hydrostatic pressure** in capillaries and veins.

If the cardiovascular system is not able to perform these functions (such as occurs due to heart failure) **elements are sacrificed based on their order of importance for the survival of the individual**. For example, in the case of heart failure, venous pressures are allowed to increase causing venous congestion, ensuring blood pressure is maintained above the minimum required to perfuse vital organs such as the brain, heart and kidneys.

The Cardiac Cycle

Every time the heart beats, the **heart muscle contracts and ejects blood from the heart (systole)**, and then **relaxes so that the heart can fill with blood again (diastole)** in anticipation of the next beat. This sequence of events is called the **cardiac cycle**. Separate systolic and diastolic events occur for the atria and ventricles. The sequence of events during the cardiac cycle is listed below and illustrated in Figure 2.

Atrial Contraction

Electrical Events

Atrial contraction follows depolarization of the atrial cells, which is **represented by the P wave on the electrocardiogram**.

Mechanical Events

Atrial contraction forces extra blood into the ventricles before ventricular contraction. This amounts to up to 15% of the blood present in the ventricle just before systole and becomes particularly important during tachycardia when there is less time for the ventricles to fill with blood. The pressure inside the atria increases slightly during contraction to approximately 8 mmHg in the left atrium and 4 mmHg in the right atrium and then drops again. This increase in pressure is represented by the A-wave on the atrial pressure curve and is reflected back in larger veins as may be seen on the venous pulse trace.

Clinical Facts

Right ventricular filling pressure may be indirectly estimated from the size of the jugular veins. Increased right atrial pressures lead to jugular distension and in some cases even pulsation (pronounced A-wave). An additional heart sound – fourth heart sound (S4) – may be audible during atrial contraction against a distended ventricle causing a gallop sound.

Ventricular Contraction (systole)

Electrical Events

Ventricular contraction follows depolarization of the ventricular cells, represented by the QRS complex on the electrocardiogram. Ventricular systole occurs from the start of the QRS complex until the end of the T wave.

Mechanical Events

Ventricular contraction forces blood out of the heart into the pulmonary and systemic circulations. The description below focuses on the left ventricle and the systemic circulation.

At the end of diastole the pressure inside the left ventricle is normally approximately 8 mmHg. When contraction begins, this quickly increases to a maximum of around 120 mmHg at its peak before falling again to almost zero. The pressure inside the aorta during ventricular diastole and just before systole is approximately 80 mmHg. This means that the aortic valve only opens for blood to flow when the pressure inside the ventricle builds up to more than 80 mmHg. This period is called the **isovolumetric contraction period**.

Once the aortic valve opens, the pressure in the aorta is the same as in the ventricle, peaks and then drops until the ventricular pressure is no longer high enough to keep the aortic valve open, at which point it closes. A notch is seen in the aortic pressure curve at this point after which the aortic pressure slowly falls again to around 80 mmHg. The time between the opening and closure of the aortic valve is called the **ejection period**.

The initial part of the ejection phase is rapid until the pressure reaches its peak and then becomes slower. These changes

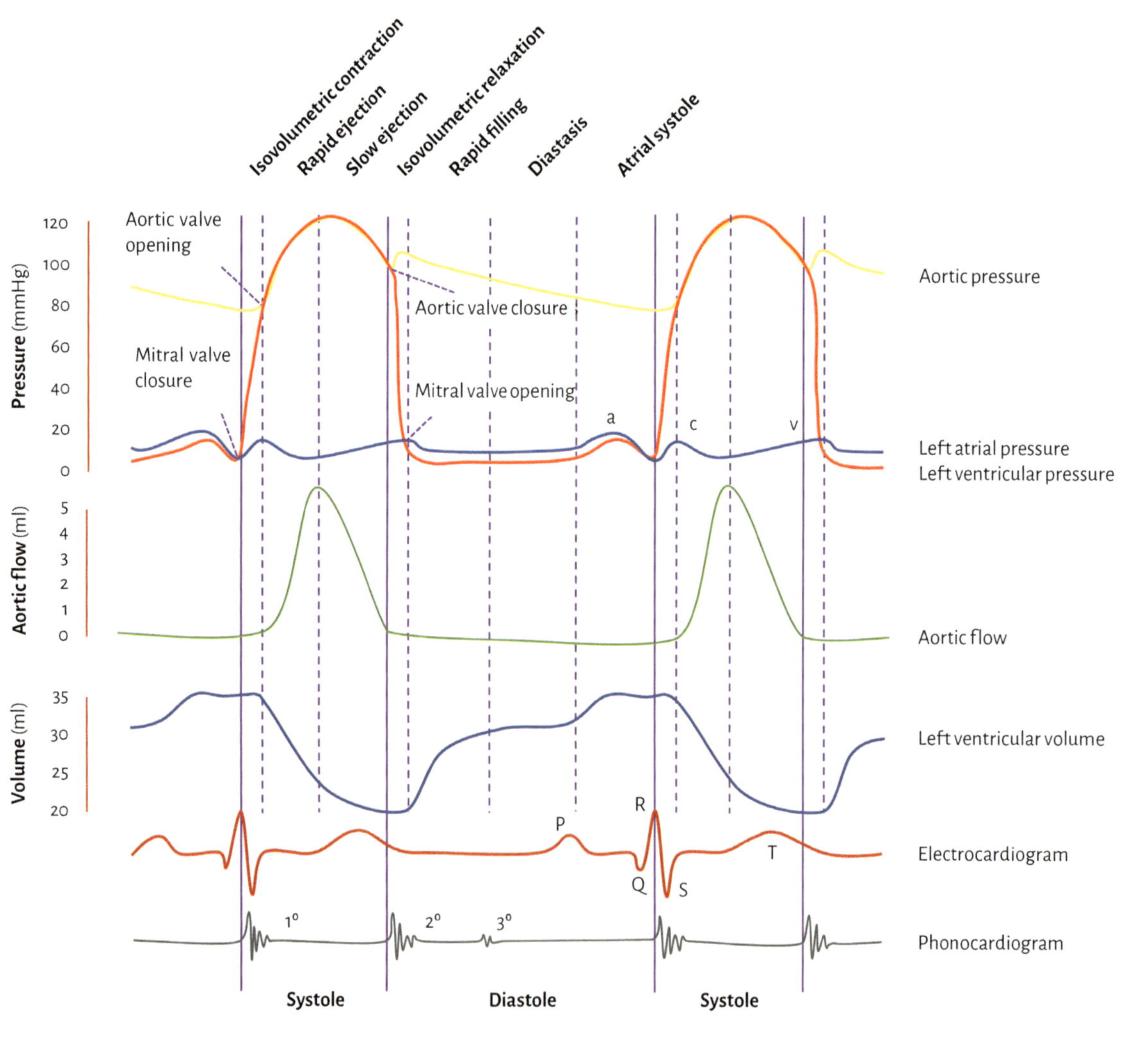

Figure 2. The cardiac cycle (see text for explanation).

can be seen in the aortic flow graph as an initial rapid increase, up to 5 l/min that then slowly reduces until it becomes zero again. The same is seen with the reduction of ventricular volume. The closure of the aortic valve marks the end of ventricular systole and the start of diastole.

Atrial pressure increases slightly as ventricular contraction starts, with blood forcing the atrioventricular valves to shut and falls quickly when the semilunar valves open. It then increases slowly again as the atria receive blood from the venae cavae and the pulmonary veins. On the atrial pressure curve this is represented as a C and a V-wave where c stands for ventricular contraction and v marks the end of ventricular systole.

Clinical Facts

- Closure of the atrioventricular and the semilunar valves is accompanied by audible heart sounds on auscultation.
  - The **first heart sound (S1)** is heard when the atrioventricular valves close.
  - The **second heart sound (S2)** is heard when the semilunar valves close.
  - These sounds are not actually produced by closure of the valves but are rather the result of blood and tissue vibrations during these events.
- The study of systolic function is an important part of clinical cardiology. Echocardiography is used to assess several systolic parameters. The volume of blood just before systole – end diastolic volume (EDV), and at the end of systole – end systolic volume (ESV) can be estimated to determine the proportion of blood ejected – ejection fraction (EF). Echocardiography is also used to estimate the volume that leaves the heart with each beat-stroke volume (SV), the isovolumetric contraction time and the ejection time.

Ventricular Diastole

Electrical Events

Ventricular diastole is the interval between the end of one systolic event and the start of another. On the electrocardiogram, this corresponds to the interval from the end of the T wave to the start of the next QRS complex.

Mechanical Events

As mentioned above **the closure of the semilunar valves marks the end of systole and the start of diastole** although the end of muscular contraction occurs slightly before this. The pressure inside the ventricles quickly drops until it is lower than the pressure in the atria and the atrioventricular valves open. The period from the closure of the semilunar valves to the opening of the atrioventricular valves is called the **isovolumetric relaxation time.** As the name suggests, **the volume of blood inside the ventricles does not change during this period**.

Once the atrioventricular valves open, blood flows into the ventricles from the atria. Atrial pressure drops slowly and equalizes with the ventricular pressure. When examining the ventricular volume curve an initial rapid filling phase is seen followed by slower ventricular filling, also known as diastasis, until atrial contraction occurs.

Clinical Facts

Echocardiography is used to assess several diastolic parameters.

- **Isovolumetric relaxation time** is determined from the study of aortic and mitral valve flows or tissue Doppler imaging of the ventricles.
- The flow of blood into the ventricles during rapid diastolic filling and diastasis (E wave) and atrial contraction (A wave) is assessed by analysing the **mitral inflow pattern**.

Cardiac Ultrastructure and Function

The heart is composed of different cell types with specific functions. The building blocks of cardiac muscle are called cardiomyocytes and are the most abundant cell in the heart. They contain numerous myofibrils within the sarcoplasm which contain **contractile elements called sarcomeres**. These cells are responsible for muscle contraction and for this reason the term working myocardium is used to distinguish them from conduction fibres, and the specialised cells in the sinus and atrioventricular nodes.

Myofibrils constitute approximately 50% of the cardiomyocyte and are incompletely separated by clefts of cytoplasm containing mitochondria and membranous T tubules. Each cell has one or two nuclei, a complex sarcoplasmic reticulum, and numerous mitochondria.

Cardiomyocytes are **tightly connected via special disks called intercalated disks**. These are composed of specialised structures – desmosomes and fascia adherens that create a strong mechanical link between each cell and other structures – the nexus or gap junction that provides a functional connection between cells.

The intercalated disks serve as strong physical connectors, ensuring cells do not become separated during contraction and allow passage of ions between cells guaranteeing that when one cell becomes depolarised the depolarization wave sweeps through all the neighbouring cells until the whole myocardium has depolarised and contracts as one. Cardiomyocytes are said to be arranged as a syncytium (from Greek meaning all cells together).

The Sarcomere

The sarcomere is the contractile unit of the cardiomyocyte. Multiple sarcomeres are arranged in series to form the myofibrils of the cardiomyocyte. Each sarcomere is composed of two main components:

1. thin filaments containing two strands of actin and regulatory proteins
2. thick filaments made of myosin.

Figure 3 illustrates the ultrastructure of the sarcomere as seen under the electron microscope. Thick lines are visible where two sarcomeres are connected to each other – these are called **Z lines**. The thin actin filaments extend from the Z lines and project towards the centre of the sarcomere. The thick myosin filaments project from the centre of the sarcomere outwards and are arranged longitudinally, intercalated with the actin filaments. The actin and myosin overlap and the interactions between them allow the sarcomere to shorten during contraction.

The myosin filaments are composed of myosin molecules arranged in parallel. Each myosin molecule has a tail that confers stability and a head that interacts with the actin filaments in response to ATP hydrolysis. Each head has a site for actin interaction and a site for ATP hydrolysis. In the absence of ATP, myosin and actin bind avidly to each other. Myosin filaments are anchored to Z discs by titin, which is responsible for the passive elasticity of the muscle, acting as a molecular spring, holding the myosin in place during contraction.

The thin filaments contain two strands of actin and two regulatory proteins called tropomyosin and troponin. Tropomyosin is an actin-binding protein that is positioned laterally along the actin filaments. It modulates actin-myosin interaction by changing its conformation. In other words, it controls when actin and myosin can interact. **Troponin is a globular protein which contains three distinct peptides**:

1. troponin T (cTnT) which attaches troponin to tropomyosin
2. troponin C (cTnC) which binds calcium causing a conformational change in tropomyosin, allowing actin-myosin interaction
3. troponin I (cTnI) which inhibits ATPase function in the myosin head.

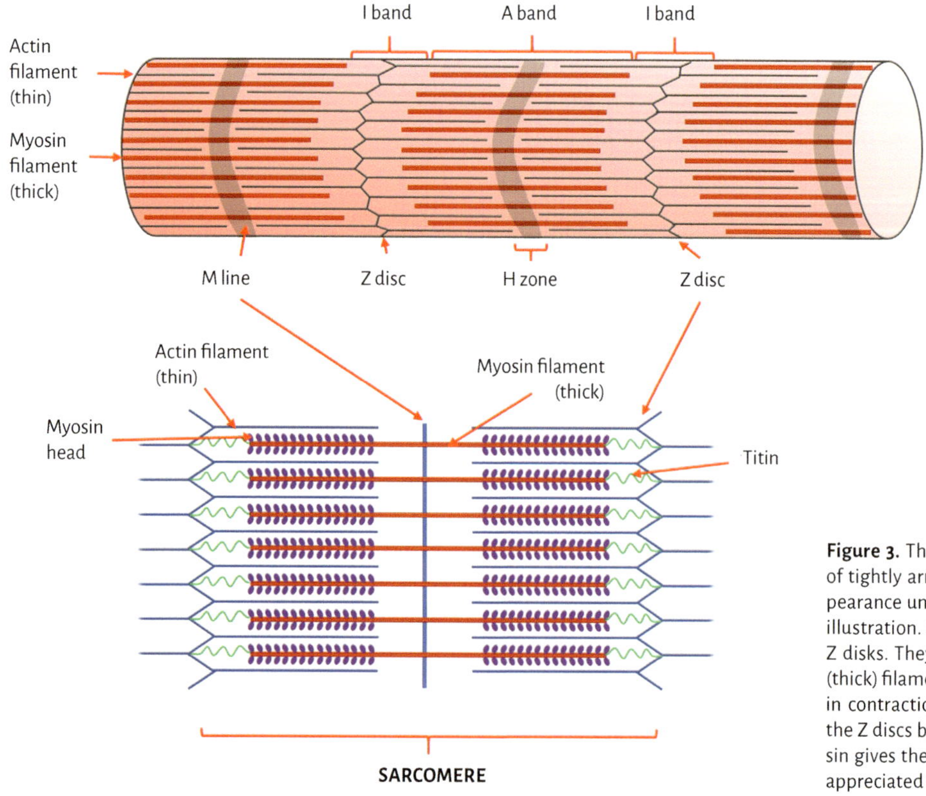

Figure 3. The sarcomere. Cardiac muscle is composed of tightly arranged subunits called sarcomeres. Its appearance under the electron microscope is seen in this illustration. Sarcomeres are tightly joined together by Z disks. They are composed of actin (thin) and myosin (thick) filaments that interact with each other, resulting in contraction. The myosin filaments are anchored to the Z discs by titin. The arrangement of actin and myosin gives the muscle a striated appearance that can be appreciated in the top picture (see text for more details).

Troponin is located at regular intervals along the actin filaments. In a clinical setting Troponin I levels in blood plasma are used in to assess the presence and degree of myocardial damage.

Sarcomere Contraction

Once familiar with the structure of the sarcomere the way it contracts can be explained. In the resting state tropomyosin blocks the myosin binding sites on the actin filaments. The release of calcium from the sarcoplasmic reticulum triggered by cell depolarization leads to binding of calcium to the troponin C peptide, which in turn displaces troponin I. This causes a conformation change in the tropomyosin which allows access to the myosin binding sites on the actin filaments, as well as allowing hydrolysis of ATP in the myosin head. The myosin head binds to the actin sites and when ATP hydrolysis occurs it loses affinity and the myosin moves on to find another actin binding site further along the actin filament. This cycle is repeated numerous times effectively resulting in shortening of the sarcomere. Once calcium levels in the cell drop as calcium returns to the sarcoplasmic reticulum, calcium is displaced from the troponin C peptide causing tropomyosin to block the myosin binding sites on the actin filaments, allowing the sarcomere to relax and return to its resting length.

Two aspects of this process are worthy of note.

1. Actin and myosin interaction is dependent on the concentration of calcium in the cell sarcoplasm.
2. ATP hydrolysis is necessary for release of the myosin and actin. If calcium levels are low (e.g. severe hipocalcemia, as a result of medications) contraction will be weak or will not occur. If ATP hydrolysis does not occur (e.g. severe hypoxia, ischaemia or death) actin and myosin bind avidly to each other (e.g. rigor mortis). Additionally, the degree of sarcomere contraction depends on the number of interactions possible between the myosin heads and actin (more details in a later section on contractility).

The Cardiac Action Potential and Cell Depolarisation

Cells generate and propagate electrical impulses by the movement of electrically charged molecules (ions or electrolytes) between both sides of the membrane. The intracellular space is rich in potassium (K^+ = 150 mmol/l) and magnesium (Mg^{2+} = 12 mmol/l), whilst the extracellular space has a high concentration of sodium (Na^+ = 140 mmol/l), calcium (Ca^{2+} = 1 mmol/l), chloride (Cl^- = 110 mmol/l) and bicarbonate (HCO^{3-} = 30 mmol/l). Ion channels, exchangers, and pumps in the cell membrane make it possible for these ions to travel across the membrane.

Under normal conditions, the intracellular compartment is negatively charged in comparison to the extracellular space. This is due to different concentrations of Na^+ and K^+ on both sides of the cell membrane and the proportion of positive and negative charges. Numerous sodium-potassium pumps in the cell membrane constantly remove sodium from the cell (3 Na^+ molecules) in exchange for potassium (2 K^+ molecules) and this accounts for the accumulation of K^+ in the cell and of Na^+ in the extracellular space. It also accounts for the lower number of positive charges inside the cell combined with the fact that the membrane is semipermeable to K^+, allowing it to leak back into the extracellular space along its concentration gradient causing an even greater loss of positive charges. The resting membrane potential of the various cardiac cells varies between -50 to -95 mV.

Ion Channels, Exchangers, and Pumps

Before looking at cell depolarisation it is pertinent to mention the differences between the various types of ion carriers in the cell.

Ion Channels

Ion channels are pore-forming proteins in the cell membrane, which in their open state allow passage of ions along an electrical or concentration gradient. Each channel is guarded by one or more gates which open and close in response to different triggers. Most ion channels involved in cell depolarisation and repolarisation are voltage-gated, which open and close in response to differences in voltage across the membrane. Other triggers include ligands (e.g. acetylcholine) and stretching (detected by mechanoreceptors).

Ion Pumps

Ion pumps move ions against their concentration gradients by using energy in the form of ATP. They are responsible for maintaining the ion gradients across the cell membrane (e.g. 3 Na^+/2 K^+ pump).

Ion Exchangers

Ion exchangers are like ion pumps, but instead of using energy from ATP hydrolysis, they use the energy stored from the electrochemical gradient of one ion to move another ion against its electrochemical gradient. A classic example is the Na^+/Ca^{2+} exchanger that moves 3 Na^+ into the cell along its concentration gradient to remove 1 Ca^{2+} from inside the cell against its concentration gradient. The excess Na^+ entering the cell is later removed from the cell by the 3 Na^+/2 K^+ pump to restore the balance.

The Action Potential

As mentioned above, cardiac cells are interconnected so when one cell is depolarised, the wave of depolarisation sweeps through the entire myocardium from one cell to the next. The following paragraphs look at what happens once a cell is activated. To illustrate this, the example focuses on the depolarisation of a ventricular myocardial cell. The depolarisation of specialised pacemaker and conduction system cells is discussed later in this chapter.

The **process of cell depolarisation and repolarisation is termed the action potential**. It includes five different stages that are illustrated in Figure 4 and outlined below.

Stage 0 (rapid depolarisation stage)

In the resting state, the membrane potential of a ventricular cell sits at around -85 mV. Depolarisation of a neighbouring cell causes the potential to increase slightly due to flow of positive ionic charges via the gap junctions. When the membrane potential reaches -70 to -60 mV voltage-gated fast sodium channels are activated allowing an inward current of Na^+ (INa) that effectively causes depolarisation, causing the membrane potential to increase to above 0 mV. This inward current is brief as these channels are inactivated quickly (<4 msec). They remain inactive until the resting membrane potential has been restored at which point they enter a resting state and are ready to open again.

Stage 1 (rapid repolarisation)

As the membrane potential increases above 0 mV a different voltage-gated channel becomes active, which in turn allows rapid exit of K^+ from the cell (I_{to}). This coincides with inactivation of the fast-sodium channels causing the membrane potential to drop to approximately 0 mV.

Stage 2 (plateau phase)

During stage 0, as the membrane potential reaches -35 to -30 mV, L-type (long lasting) voltage-gated calcium channels become active allowing an inward flow of calcium into the cell (Ca-L). These channels open quickly (<1 msec) but only regain their inactive state slowly, accounting for the duration of stage 2. Simultaneously, different K^+ channels become active when the membrane potential reaches approximately -10 mV and are responsible for an outward K^+ current. The most important are the voltage-gated IKr (r for rapid) and IKs (s for slow) currents. The membrane potential during this stage changes minimally as the inward flow of positively charged Ca^{2+} is balanced by the outward loss of K^+. This is the plateau phase of the action potential. During this stage, the inward Ca^{2+} flow triggers release of Ca^{2+} from the sarcoplasmic reticulum causing muscle contraction in working myocardial cells.

Stage 3 (repolarisation)

With time the L-type calcium channels are inactivated and the inward Ca^{2+} current ceases. The outward K^+ currents continue until the membrane potential falls to its resting state and

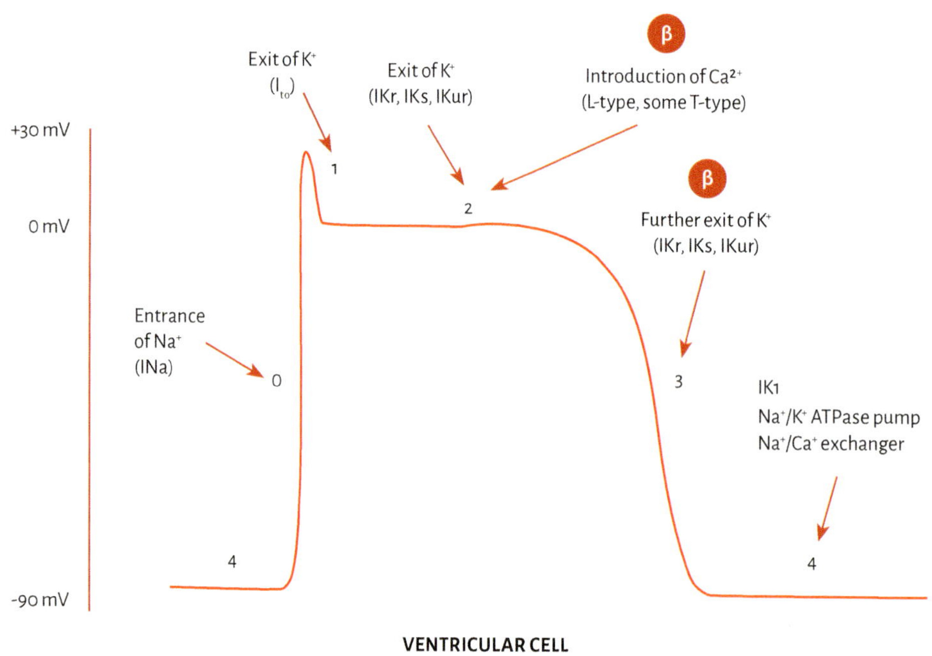

Figure 4. The action potential of a ventricular cardiomyocyte. The action potential is the process of depolarisation and repolarisation of a cell. In a working myocardial cell such as a ventricular cardiomyocyte it can be divided in five stages (0, 1, 2, 3, 4) (see text for explanation) (β = enhanced by sympathetic stimulation of β-adrenergic receptors).

repolarisation is complete. Many different outward potassium currents are involved, some of which may be influenced by drugs (e.g. amiodarone and sotalol) or the autonomous nervous system (e.g. IAch). In addition to the IKr and IKs currents mentioned above, a background K^+ current (IK1 or IKir) is also worth mentioning.

Stage 4 (resting state)

Stage 4 corresponds to the resting state during which the changes that occurred during depolarisation are rectified and the membrane potential is kept at -85 mV. Na^+/K^+ ATPase pumps remove excess Na+ from the cell whilst restoring K^+ levels. Excess Ca^{2+} is exchanged with Na^+ by the Na^+/Ca^{2+} exchanger. During this stage, the background K^+ current works to maintain the resting membrane potential (RMP) by allowing K^+ to exit the cell if the potential is above the RMP and to enter the cell if the membrane potential is below the RMP. During depolarisation, these channels are briefly shut and open again during repolarisation stages.

Excitation-contraction Coupling

Sarcomere contraction occurs in the presence of calcium in the cell's sarcoplasm. During stage 2 of the action potential a small increase in cellular calcium occurs, but this is not enough to account for contraction. The calcium necessary for sarcomere contraction is released from the sarcoplasmic reticulum (SR) in response to the transient increase in cellular calcium levels that occur during stage 2 of the action potential.

The SR is a specialised structure which forms a network around the myofibrils. It is limited by a membrane and its function is to store Ca^{2+} during diastole and release it during systole. Calcium release channels in the SR membrane, also called ryanodine receptors (RyR), are stimulated by calcium entering the cell via the L-type Ca^{2+} channels and open to release Ca^{2+} from the SR causing contraction to start. The sudden high concentration of Ca^{2+} in the cytoplasm of the cell stimulates Ca^{2+}ATPase pumps in the SR to re-uptake Ca^{2+} into the SR. As cellular calcium concentrations fall again, sarcomere contraction stops until the cells are next activated.

The concentration of calcium in the cells may be influenced by several drugs such as calcium-channel blockers (e.g. diltiazem, amlodipine) or phosphodiesterase inhibitors (e.g. pimobendan and sildenafil commonly known as Viagra®).

The Action Potential of Pacemaker Cells

Pacemaker cells in the sinus node and cells in the compact node of the atrioventricular junction display a different action potential in comparison to the working myocardium. The two striking differences are the slow increase in membrane potential during stage 0 and the spontaneous increase in membrane potential during stage 4, which accounts for the ability of these cells to spontaneously depolarize. These differences are summarised below and illustrated in Figure 5.

Pacemaker Currents During Stage 4

The resting membrane potential of pacemaker cells sits at around -65 mV in contrast to working myocardial cells (-85 mV). During stage 4, the membrane potential increases due to a combination of ion currents called the pacemaker currents, until the depolarisation threshold is reached at approximately -40 mV. These ion currents include:

Outward K^+ Current

The major K^+ current in pacemaker cells is the IK current (also called the delayed rectifier current). This current is activated by depolarisation and is time dependent. During depolarisation it becomes active, contributes to repolarisation of the cell during stage 3 but then stops working during stage 4, allowing membrane potential to increase again. The IKr, IKs and IK1 currents that help maintain the resting membrane potential in working myocardial cells do not exist in pacemaker cells.

Inward Na^+ Currents

Pacemaker cells possess channels that allow Na^+ and K^+ currents (If) depending on the membrane potential. They are called "funny" channels and are blocked by the drug ivabradine. During stage 4 of the action potential they become activated at approximately -40 to -45 mV and allow an inward flow of Na^+ and K^+ causing a progressive increase in membrane potential until the activation threshold is reached and the cell depolarises. Sympathetic stimulation optimizes this current causing an increase in heart rate. The involvement of another Na^+ current in the spontaneous depolarisation of pacemaker cells has been proposed. This current was named Ib for background or Ip for pacemaker.

Inward Ca^{2+} Currents

During stage 4 a transient calcium current occurs via T-type Ca^{2+} channels, which become activated when the membrane potential is approximately -60 to -50 mV. This current contributes to the spontaneous depolarisation of pacemaker cells with further entry of positive charges into the cell. In addition, activity of the Na^+/Ca^{2+} exchanger contributes to spontaneous depolarisation by exchanging 3 extracellular Na^+ ions for 1 intracellular Ca^{2+} ion, resulting in a net increase in positive intracellular charges.

Stage 0 (depolarisation)

The depolarisation of pacemaker cells occurs via inward Ca^{2+} currents (ICa) rather than fast sodium currents (INa) which explains the slow upstroke of the action potential during phase 0. This is an important characteristic of these cells as it allows slower conduction of the electrical impulse, which serves the purpose of slowing conduction in the atrioventricular node.

Stage 0 occurs due to activation of L-type channels when the membrane potential reaches approximately -40 mV.

Stage 3 (repolarisation)

With time, the L-type calcium channels are inactivated and the inward Ca^{2+} current stops. In the meantime, the IK current becomes active during depolarisation and contributes to outward movement of K^+ until the membrane potential falls to its resting state and repolarisation is complete.

Principles of Cardiovascular Function

The cardiac cycle, cardiovascular system organization, and how contraction occurs are covered in previous sections. What follows is a description of the principles of cardiovascular function, which are useful when understanding the pathophysiology of heart failure.

Important Terms and Concepts

With each heartbeat, the heart pumps a certain amount of blood into the pulmonary and systemic circulations. This amount of blood is called the **stroke volume** and depends on the following factors:

Preload

Preload is interpreted as the blood volume present in the ventricles at the end of diastole which was returned to the heart by the pulmonary and systemic veins. It actually refers to the pressure that a volume of blood exerts on the ventricular wall by stretching the sarcomeres. Preload is indirectly assessed with diagnostic imaging techniques such as echocardiography by simply measuring the size or volume of the cardiac chambers at the end of diastole (e.g. end-diastolic volume, etc.). Preload is variable and can be influenced by changes in autonomic tone or drugs by causing venodilation (e.g. more blood in the veins so less preload) or constriction (e.g.

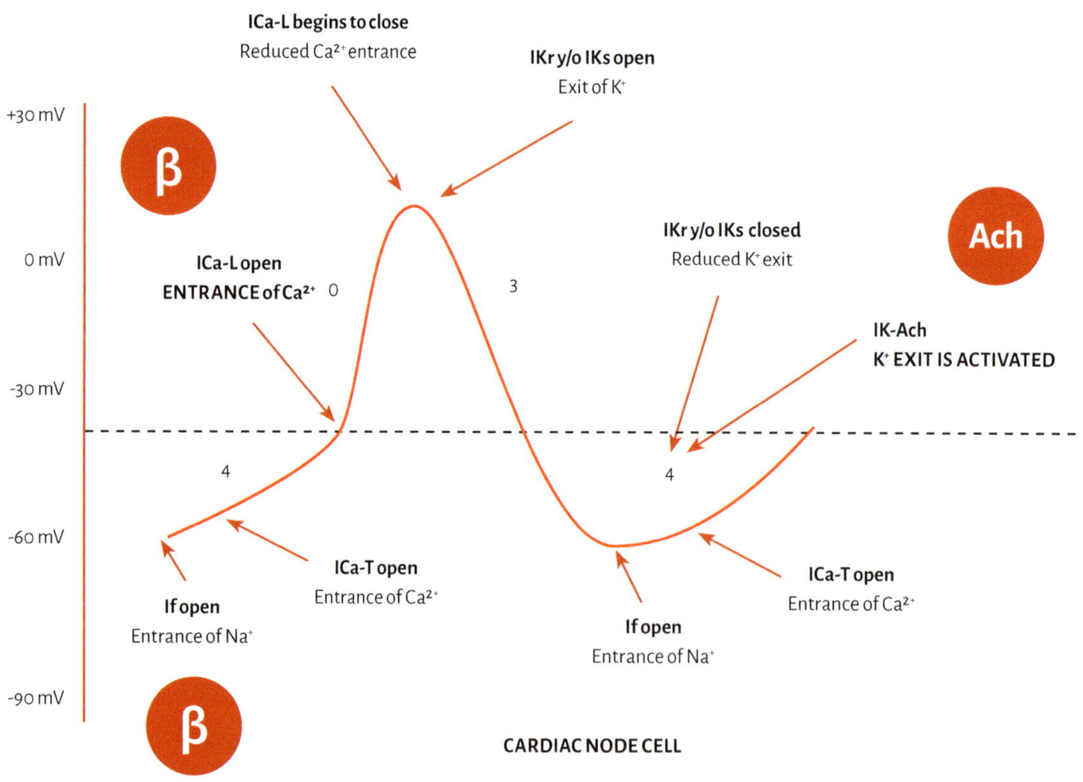

Figure 5. The action potential of a pacemaker cell. The action potential of pacemaker cells is composed of only three stages (0, 3, 4) (see text for explanation) (β = enhanced by sympathetic stimulation of β-adrenergic receptors; Ach = enhanced by parasympathetic stimulation via acetylcholine).

more blood is returned to the heart causing an increase in preload). It can also be influenced by heart rate by prolonging or reducing the time available for diastolic filling.

Afterload

Afterload can be described as the pressure that the heart needs to overcome to push blood through pulmonary and systemic arteries. As discussed above, the aortic valve only opens when the ventricular pressure is higher than the pressure inside the aorta which is approximately 80 mmHg during diastole. This is a result of peripheral vascular resistance that occurs mostly in the arterioles. Dilation or contraction of the arterial vessels can greatly influence afterload (e.g. vasodilating or vasoconstricting drugs). In the presence of obstructive disease such as pulmonic or aortic stenosis, afterload is increased by the obstruction in addition to peripheral vascular resistance. Pulmonary and systemic hypertension are other examples of increased afterload. The velocity of blood flow across the various valves with echocardiography is used in the clinical setting to assess afterload.

Contractility

Contractility is the innate ability of the cardiac muscle to generate contractile force. It is impossible to assess in a clinical setting and only indirect assessments are possible. The ability of the cardiac myocyte to generate contractile force depends on the amount of stretch the sarcomere is subjected to and the amount of calcium and energy available to generate actin and myosin interaction.

Sarcomere length is relevant as within certain limits, the more it is stretched, the more myosin heads will be able to interact with actin and cause more contractile force (Figure 6). This is a sophisticated characteristic of the heart that explains a property of heart muscle called the Frank-Starling mechanism. As preload increases, the sarcomeres are stretched, favouring more interactions between actin and myosin, which in turn lead to an increase in contractile force which ensures that blood is ejected efficiently. This means the presence of a larger amount of blood in the ventricle is met with a stronger contractile force to eject it. This concept will be revisited when discussing the pathophysiology of heart failure.

Cardiac Output

Another important determinant of cardiovascular function is **heart rate**. The heart beats a variable number of times every minute, ejecting a certain volume of blood. By **multiplying the stroke volume (ml) by the heart rate (beats/min), this volume can be calculated and is called the cardiac output (l/min)**. Stroke volume and cardiac output can be estimated via

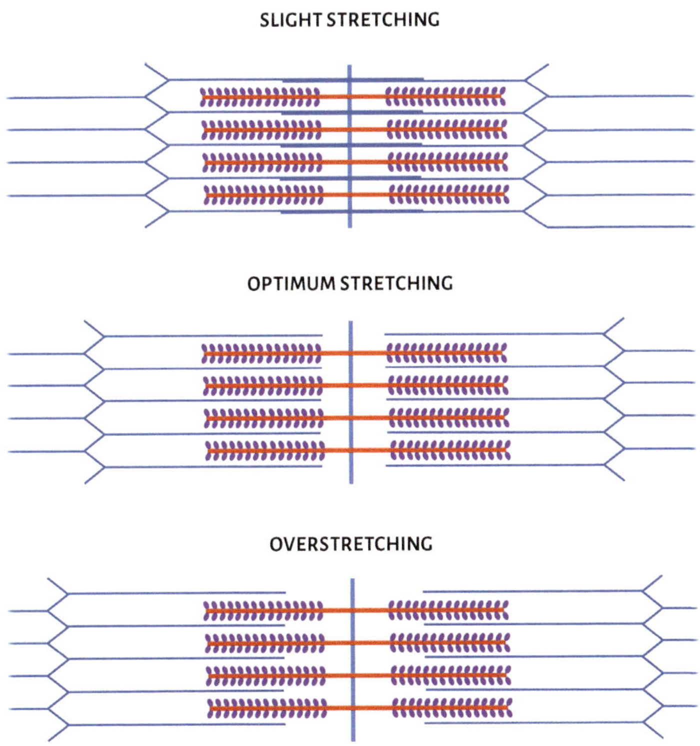

Figure 6. Sarcomere contraction and contractility. Depending on the amount of blood present in the ventricle immediately before contraction, the sarcomere is subjected to varying degrees of stretch and length change. Within limits, a greater degree of sarcomere stretch results in an increase in interactions between actin and myosin resulting in a greater contractile force. In a poorly stretched sarcomere (e.g. during hypovolaemia) the actin filaments overlap each other, preventing the myosin heads from interacting with the correct actin filament, therefore producing less contractile force. In an optimally stretched sarcomere, the maximum number of myosin heads interact with actin filaments. Overstretch (e.g. volume overload) prevents some of the myosin heads from interacting with actin at all, leading to a reduced force of contraction.

echocardiography. Heart rate is determined by the rate of depolarisation of the pacemaker cells in the sinus node, or other mechanisms in cases of cardiac arrhythmias. If heart rate is too low, a sufficient cardiac output is not possible and leads to signs of weakness, fainting, or even death. If heart rate is excessively high, the diastolic filling time may not be sufficient to ensure appropriate preload, leading to a low cardiac output. Additionally, the heart muscle may suffer damage causing a reduction in contractility. The heart rate is regulated by the following factors:

Parasympathetic Tone

Parasympathetic tone influences the sinus node via the right vagus nerve. Activation of the vagal centres in the medulla oblongata trigger acetylcholine (Ach) release which activates specific potassium channels in the pacemaker cells, promoting an outward K^+ current (IK-Ach) (Figure 5). This reduces the rate of spontaneous depolarization of pacemaker cells, effectively reducing heart rate. The conduction velocity of the cells in the compact node of the atrioventricular junction is also reduced and can lead to occasional atrioventricular block. Drugs which increase parasympathetic tone (e.g. opioids) can lower heart rate whilst parasympatholytics (e.g. atropine and glycopyrrolate) have the opposite effect.

Sympathetic Tone

Sympathetic activation causes an increase in heart rate by optimising the inward flow of Na^{2+} (If) during stage 4 and of Ca^{2+} (Ca-L) during stage 0 of the action potential in pacemaker cells in the sinus node (Figure 5). In working myocardial cells, sympathetic stimulation influences the inward Ca^{2+} current (Ca-L) during stage 2 and the outward K^+ currents (IKr, IKs, IKur) to increase the amount of calcium in the cell and accelerate repolarisation so the cells are prepared to depolarise again more quickly (Figure 4). The release and uptake of calcium from the SR is also optimised to increase contractility (inotropic effect) and relaxation (lusitropic effect).

Mean Arterial Blood Pressure

Baroreceptors present in the circulatory system (e.g. carotid sinus and aortic arch) sense variations in systemic blood pressure, and feedback to the vasomotor centre in the medulla oblongata in the brain via the vagus and glossopharyngeal nerves to influence parasympathetic and sympathetic tone. A reduction or increase in blood pressure triggers an increase or decrease in heart rate respectively. The main priority is to keep blood pressure at a normal level by adjusting heart rate, and therefore cardiac output. Arterial blood pressure is the product of cardiac output and total peripheral resistance (BP = CO x TPR).

Recommended Reading

- Section III: Cardiovascular physiology In B. G. Klein, ed. *Cunninghams Textbook of Veterinary Physiology*. 5th Edition, St Louis: Elsevier (2013).

Bibliography

- Hamlin R.L. (1999) Normal Cardiovascular Physiology. In: Fox, P.R., Sisson, D. & Moise, S. N. (eds) *Textbook of Canine and Feline Cardiology: Principles and Clinical Practice*. Philadelphia: WB Saunders Company, pp. 25–38.
- Kittleson, M.D. & Kienle, R.D. (1998). Normal Clinical Cardiovascular Physiology. In: Kittleson M.D. & Kienle R.D. (eds) *Small Animal Cardiovascular Medicine*. St. Louis: Mosby, Inc, pp. 11–35.
- Stephenson, R.B. (2013a) Electrical activity of the heart. In: Klein B.G. (ed) *Cunnighams Textbook of Veterinary Physiology*. St Louis: Elsevier, pp. 171–186.
- Stephenson, R.B. (2013b) Integrated cardiovascular responses. In: Klein B.G. (ed) *Cunnighams Textbook of Veterinary Physiology*. St Louis: Elsevier, pp. 252–262.
- Stephenson, R.B. (2013c) Overview of cardiovascular function. In: Klein B. G. (ed) *Cunnighams Textbook of Veterinary Physiology*. St Louis, pp. 158–168.
- Stephenson, R.B. (2013d) The heart as a pump. In: Klein B. G. (ed) *Cunnighams Textbook of Veterinary Physiology*. St Louis: Elsevier, pp. 200–210.

TEST

1. **During cardiac auscultation, a gallop sound can be heard during atrial contraction. What additional heart sound is heard during this process?**
   a. S1.
   b. S2.
   c. S3.
   d. S4.

2. **During the cardiac cycle, the period from the closure of the semilunar valves to the opening of the atrioventricular valves is defined as:**
   a. The ejection period.
   b. The isovolumetric relaxation period.
   c. The isovolumetric contraction period.
   d. The preejection period.

3. **The sarcomere is the contractile unit of the cardiomyocyte. Which of the following statements is correct regarding its structure?**
   a. It is made up of thin actin filaments.
   b. It is made up of fine myosin filaments.
   c. The thin filaments contain two regulatory proteins called tropomyosin and troponin.
   d. Troponin-I prevents calcium from binding to troponin-C.

4. **Cardiac cells are arranged in a syncytium with structures that hold them tightly together and others that allow free flow of ions from one cell to another. Which of the structures listed below is responsible for the strong mechanical bond between cardiac cells?**
   a. T tubules.
   b. Desmosomes.
   c. Gap junctions.
   d. Z lines.

ANSWERS ON PAGE 32

5. **The process of cell depolarization and repolarization is called the action potential. Which of the following statements is correct regarding this process?**
   a. Phase 0 of the action potential occurs in pacemaker cells due to the action of fast sodium channels.
   b. Action potential phase 1 occurs in pacemaker cells, but not in myocardial cells.
   c. During phase 2, the outward flow of Ca^{2+} triggers the release of Ca^{2+} from the sarcoplasmic reticulum, causing muscle contraction in myocardial cells.
   d. None of the above are correct.

6. **The autonomic nervous system plays a very important role in cardiovascular function. Which of the following statements is correct regarding the effects of sympathetic activation on cardiac cells?**
   a. In myocardial cells, sympathetic stimulation promotes the internal Ca^{2+} current (Ca-L) during action potential phase 2.
   b. Sympathetic stimulation reduces external K^+ currents (IKr, IKs, IKur) in myocardial cells.
   c. In pacemaker cells, sympathetic stimulation optimizes internal Na^{2+} flux during action potential phase 0.
   d. In pacemaker cells, sympathetic activation reduces internal Ca^{2+} flux during action potential phase 0.

Correct Answers:

1. d
2. b
3. c
4. b
5. d
6. a

Notes

Principles of Electrophysiology

Dolores Porteiro Vázquez

Action Potential

One function of myocardial cells is to transmit electrical impulses and transform them into a mechanical event; this is called **electromechanical coupling**.

Action potential is defined as *the difference in electrical charge between the intracellular and extracellular space, which is transmitted from cell to cell*. The electrical charge depends on the movement of ions through the cell membrane. The equilibrium between ions determines the resting potential of that cell or whether the cell initiates an action potential and consequent depolarization.

The action potential is different between cells depending on whether they are **slow response cells** (nodal structures or pacemakers) or **fast response cells** (atrial or ventricular myocardial cells, and conduction pathways):

- **slow-response** cells
  - are also known as sodium-dependent cells
  - present in nodal structures or pacemakers
- **fast-response** cells
  - are also known as calcium-dependent cells
  - atrial or ventricular myocardial cells and conduction pathways.

The main characteristic of slow response cells is that they are able to depolarize automatically spontaneously.

Fast Response Cells

The action potential is divided into five phases (Figure 1).

- **Phase 0 or depolarization phase**: The phase begins with the opening of voltage dependent Na^+ channels. The entry of Na^+ into the cell changes the resting potential from -90 mV to +40 mV.
- **Phase 1 or rapid repolarization phase**: Na^+ channels close and Cl^- channels open, allowing these ions to move into the intracellular space. The positive charge outside the cells is reduced slightly. I_{to} channels also activate, allowing the rapid passage of K^+ ions into the cell.
- **Phase 2 or plateau phase**: Ca^{2+} channels open, allowing these ions to pass into the cell. The passage of Ca^{2+} into the intracellular space facilitates the release of more Ca^{2+} and mechanical contraction of the myocardial cells occurs (mechanical excitation-contraction coupling). At the same time, K^+ ions leave the cell, which are equalised with the influx of calcium.
- **Phase 3 or repolarization phase**: increases the K^+ output from the cell by opening the K^+ channels (IKur, IKr, IKs), which means the inside of the cell becomes negative again.
- **Phase 4 or resting phase**: the sodium-potassium, sodium-calcium, and calcium ATPase pumps maintain a balance between K^+ and Ca^{2+} ions, maintaining the potential at -90 mV.

Slow Response Cells

The action potential in slow response cells consists of three phases (0, 3 and 4) (Figure 2).

- **Phase 4 or resting phase**: the resting potential is less negative with respect to the action potential of the rapid response cells, ranging between -40 mV and -70 mV. In this type of cell, the resting membrane potential is not completely stable, and a series of ionic

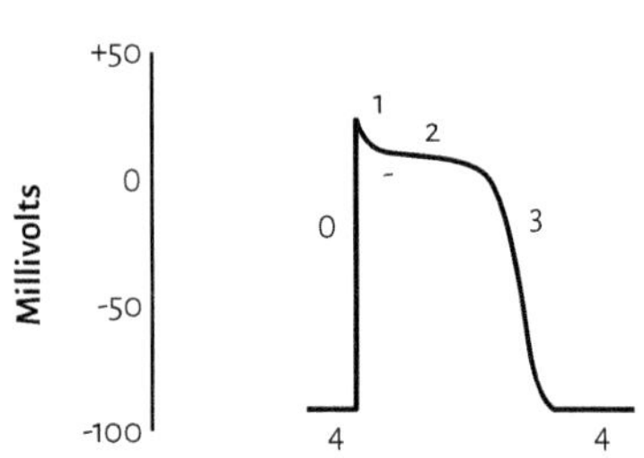

Figure 1. Five action potential phases of a rapid response cell.

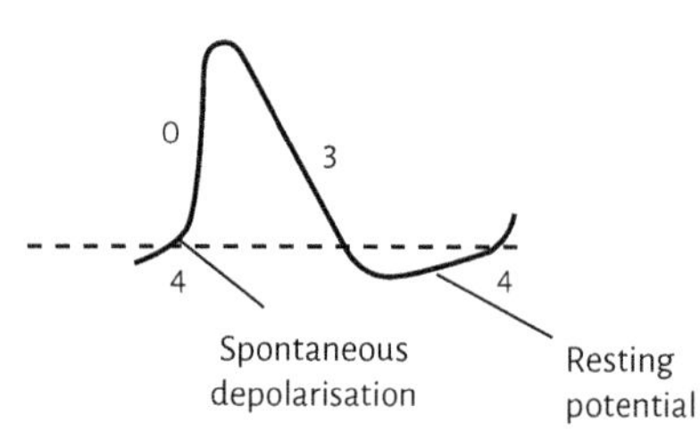

Figure 2. Action potential of a slow response cell.

currents prepare the action potential for the next phase of depolarization. The I(f) channels allow entry of Na^+ ions and the I(Ca,T) and I(Ca,L) channels of Ca^{2+} into the intracellular space.
- **Phase 0**: is slower than in fast response cells, mainly due to the absence of Na^+ channels and the predominance of I(Ca,L) channels that allow the passage of Ca^{2+} into the intracellular space.
- **Phase 3 or repolarization phase**: K^+ exits the cell by opening of the K^+ channels (IKr, IKs).

Anatomy of the Conduction System

Under physiological conditions, the electrical impulse generated by the sinus node travels through the specialised conduction system until it reaches the atrial and ventricular myocardium, where it produces the rhythmic contraction of heart muscle. The **electrical and mechanical activities are synchronised**, following the cardiac cycle.

The **conduction system (Figure 3) is made up of two tissue types: nodal structures and conduction tissue**.

Nodal structures are equipped with automatism because they possess **pacemaker cells** with the capacity to automatically depolarize (slow response cells). These structures are the:
- sinus node
- atrioventricular node
- Purkinje fibres.

The sinus node is the dominant pacemaker which regulates heart rate, whilst the atrioventricular node and Purkinje fibres are considered subsidiary pacemakers. Under normal conditions, the frequency of depolarization is:
- sinus node: 70–160 bpm
- atrioventricular node: 40–60 bpm
- Purkinje fibres: 15–40 bpm.

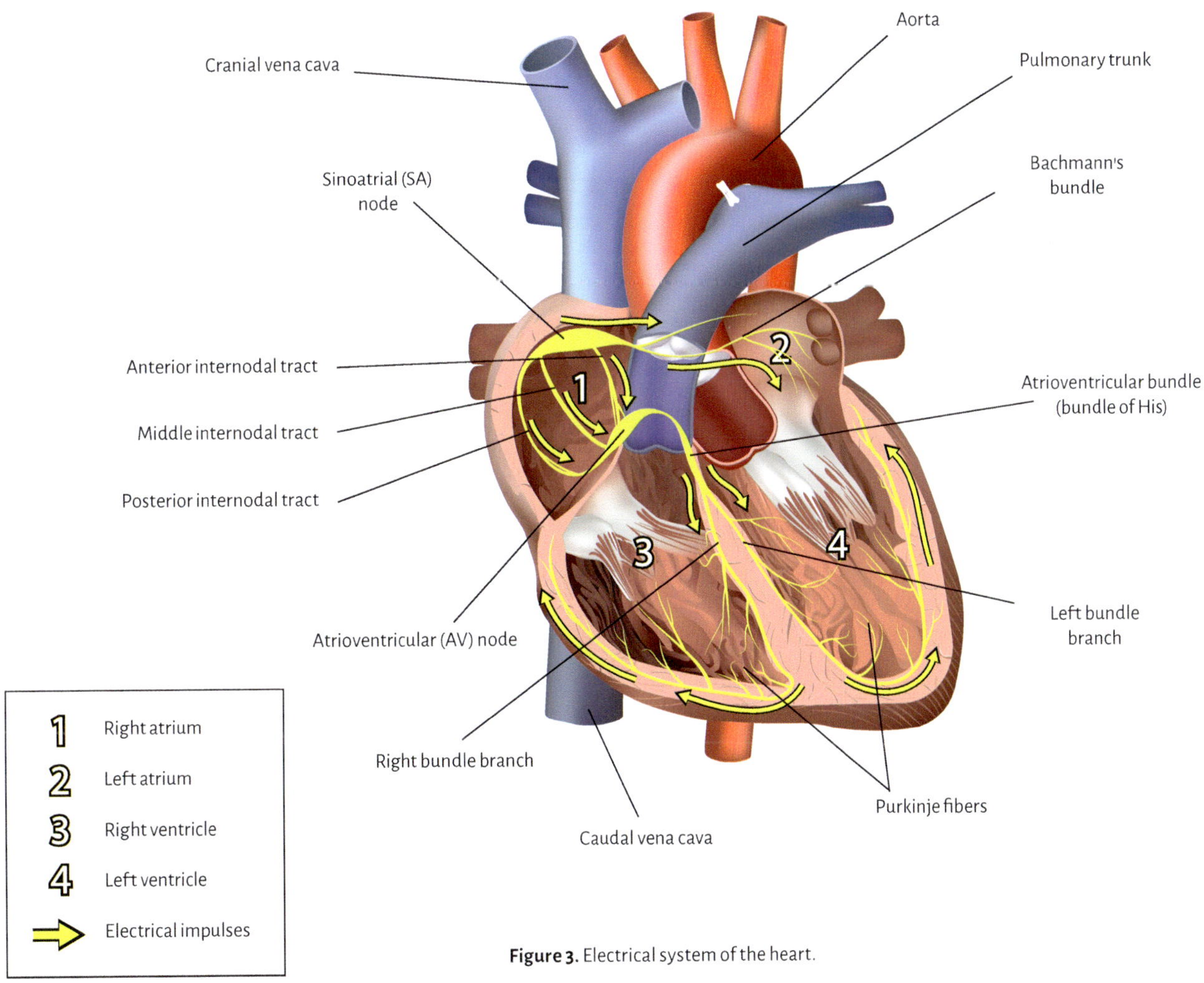

Figure 3. Electrical system of the heart.

Once the sinus node generates the impulse, it is transmitted through the **internodal** (anterior, middle, and posterior fascicle), **interatrial** (inferior fascicle and Bachmann's bundle), and **atrionodal** (superior, medial, and lateral fascicles that join to form the proximal atrioventricular bundle) fibres to the entire mass of the atrial myocardium, at a speed of between 0.8 and 1 m/s.

The impulse reaches the proximal portion of the atrioventricular node and slows down slightly (0.01–1 m/s). The velocity then increases again along the bundle of His.

The bundle of His is divided into a right and left branch. The left branch in turn divides into the **anterosuperior** (anterior fascicle) **and posteroinferior** (posterior fascicle) branches. In the most distal portion, the branches spread out forming the **Purkinje system**. Depolarization in the ventricle begins in the interventricular septum, continues through the right ventricle, and then finally the left ventricle. Activation of Purkinje fibres is at 15–23 m/s.

Principles of Electrocardiography

Equivalent Dipole Theory

The electrocardiogram **analyses the variations in electrical potential generated by the cardiac dipole on the body's surface**. That is, the sum of the different action potentials of myocardial cells can be registered by electrodes positioned on the surface of the body. Negative or positive charges move respectively to the positive or negative pole of the receiving electrode (Figure 4). In turn, this provides useful information about possible underlying cardiac conditions, and therefore influences the list of differential diagnoses.

In this way it is possible to establish a relationship between the action potential described above and the electrocardiographic waves (Figure 5).

- Phase 0 corresponds to the QRS complex.
- Phase 1 corresponds to the J point.
- Phase 2 corresponds to the ST segment.
- Phase 3 corresponds to the T wave.
- Phase 4 corresponds to electrical diastole.

The sum of all electrical charges generates a common vector with opposite direction and charge to the electrode positioned on the body surface. The magnitude and direction of the vector determines the amplitude and polarity of the electrocardiographic wave. If the vector is parallel to the receiving electrode, the recorded wave has a maximum amplitude. Conversely, if the vector is perpendicular the amplitude is minimal. The duration of the wave depends on the activation time of the myocardium and the myocardial mass to be depolarised.

Cardiac vectors move through the body along **three anatomical planes**:

1. the **frontal plane** (X axis in the Cartesian system)
2. the **sagittal plane** (Y axis of the Cartesian system)
3. the **transverse plane** (Z axis of the Cartesian system) (Figure 6).

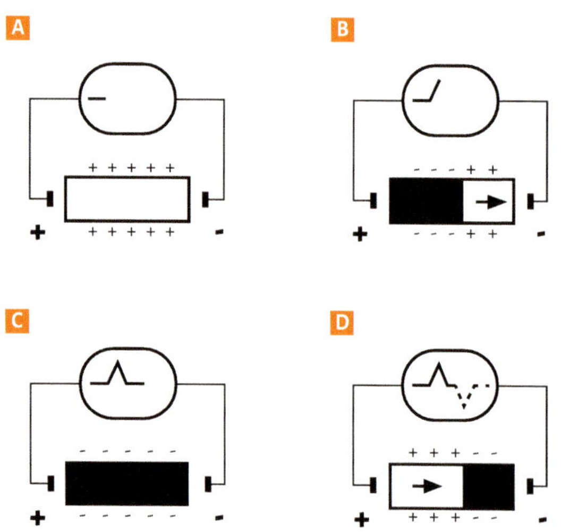

Figure 4. Rest phase (**A**), depolarisation phase (**B**), state of depolarisation (**C**), repolarisation phase (**D**).

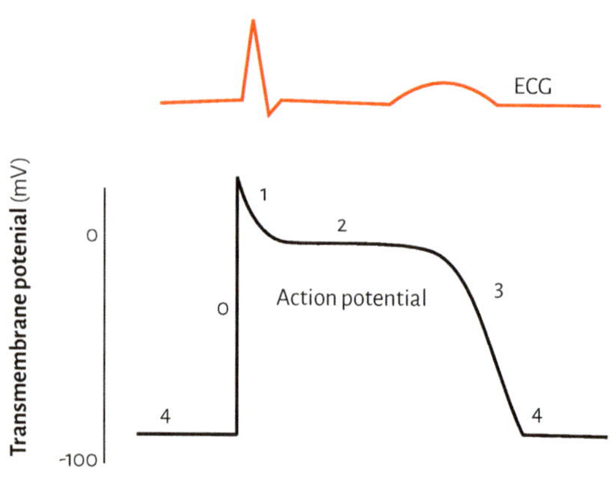

Figure 5. Relationship between the action potential and the surface electrocardiogram.

The different anatomical planes are considered with the animal in a bipedal position as in humans. Therefore, the **frontal plane** divides the body into a cranial and caudal half, the **sagittal plane** into a right and left half and the **transverse plane** into a ventral and dorsal half.

Derivation Systems

The position of the electrodes or leads influences the anatomical plane of the cardiac vector. These positions or systems are described below.

Bailey's Hexaxial System

Bailey's hexaxial system is used to calculate the **median electrical axis** in the frontal plane of the P wave and the QRS complex.

This system is based on positioning **three electrodes on the four extremities** following the diagram described by Einthoven in 1902. This system creates an equilateral triangle where the cardiac dipole is positioned at the centre (Figure 7).

Bipolar derivations:

- lead I: positive electrode on the left forelimb and negative electrode in the right forelimb
- lead II: negative electrode on the right forelimb and positive electrode on the left hindlimb
- lead III: negative electrode on the left forelimb and positive electrode on the left hindlimb.

Unipolar leads (the negative pole of the lead is the indifferent electrode for the electrocardiograph):

- aVR lead: positive electrode on the right forelimb
- aVL lead: positive electrode on the left forelimb
- aVF lead: positive electrode on the left hindlimb.

The direction of the activation vector as it encounters the various leads determines the morphology of those respective waves on the surface electrocardiogram. Under normal conditions, the depolarization front follows a right to left and top to bottom direction (from the base of the heart to the apex and from the right atrium to all cardiac chambers). Therefore, leads II, III and aVF have a similar morphology with maximum wave positivity, aVR and aVL leads have a similar morphology with maximum wave negativity, and lead I is positive with a lesser amplitude (Figure 8).

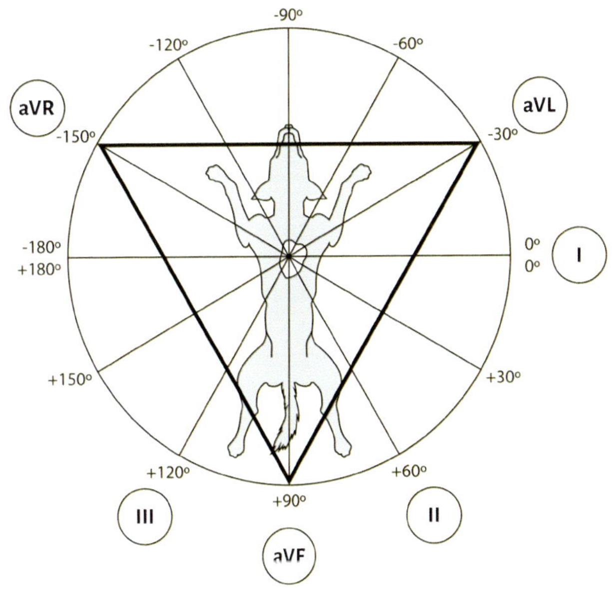

Figure 7. Bipolar leads (I, II, III) and unipolar leads (aVR, aVL, aVF).

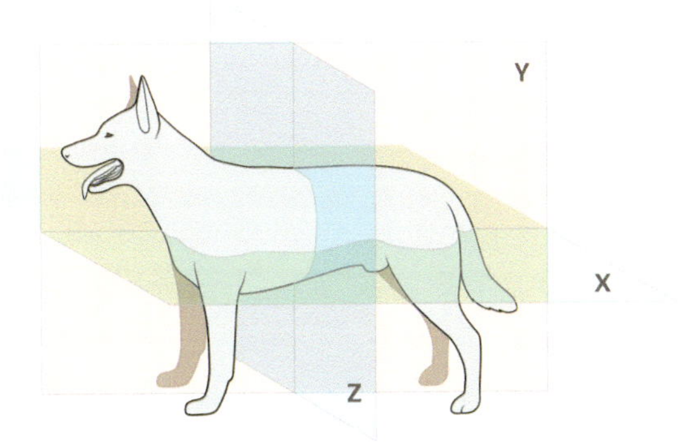

Figure 6. Frontal place (X), sagittal plane (Y) and transverse plane (Z).

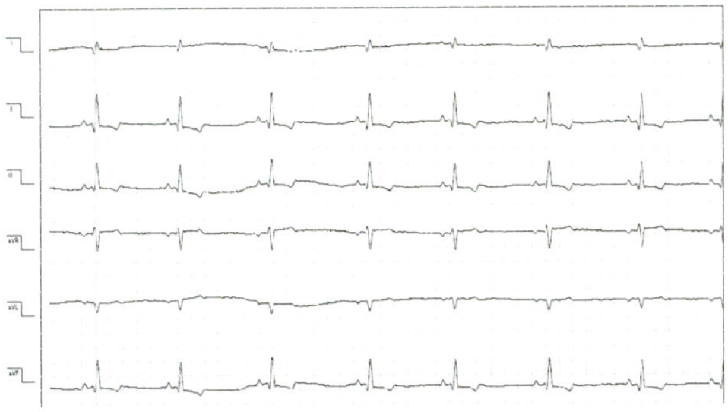

Figure 8. Dog electrocardiogram using standard leads.

Precordial System

The precordial system can be **useful for assessing the P wave and intraventricular conduction disorders**. However, in veterinary medicine, different thoracic conformations make the precordial system difficult to use since the intrathoracic position of the heart varies in different breeds.

The precordial system analyses the **electrical potential in the horizontal plane**. These are unipolar leads positioned at different points on the thorax. Different precordial systems are described in veterinary medicine, many adapted from human medicine. The most commonly used precordial system is the Wilson system modified by Kraus et al. in 2002 (Figure 9). However, often Lead V1 does not accurately assess the right ventricle due to different thoracic conformations. Therefore, the current recommendation is for Lead V1 to be positioned in the first intercostal space at the level of the costochondral junction.

Positioning:

- V1: fifth right intercostal space, level with the costosternal junction
- V2: sixth left intercostal space, level with the costosternal junction
- V3: sixth left intercostal space at an equidistant point between V2 and V4
- V4: sixth left intercostal space, level with the costochondral junction
- V5: sixth left intercostal space dorsal to V4
- V6: sixth left intercostal space dorsal to V5.

Lead V1 studies the right ventricle and, following ventricular depolarization vectors, the surface QRS complex presents a negative morphology similar to aVR. Leads V2 to V6 analyse the left ventricle and present a positive polarity with a morphology similar to lead II (Figure 10).

Orthogonal System

This system is widely used in the Holter technique and simultaneously records the resulting vector in three anatomical planes: frontal, sagittal, and transverse.

Electrocardiographic Trace

Electrocardiogram Recording

The **electrocardiogram must be performed in right lateral recumbence**, with the head resting on the table and the extremities placed parallel to each other (Figure 11). Other positions change the position of the heart relative to the frontal plane, and the vectors change direction relative to the examination electrodes.

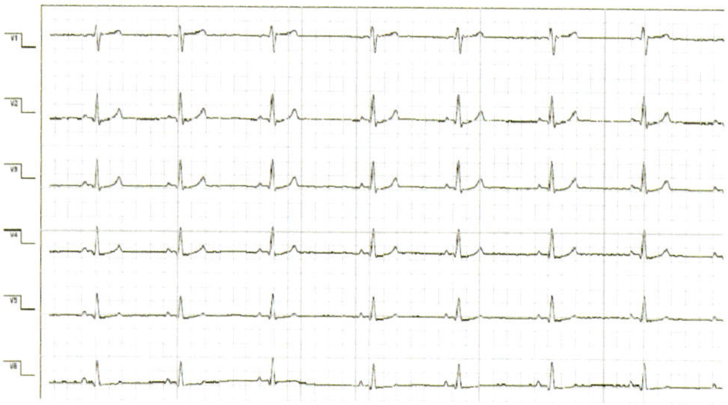

Figure 10. Electrocardiogram of a dog with precordial leads.

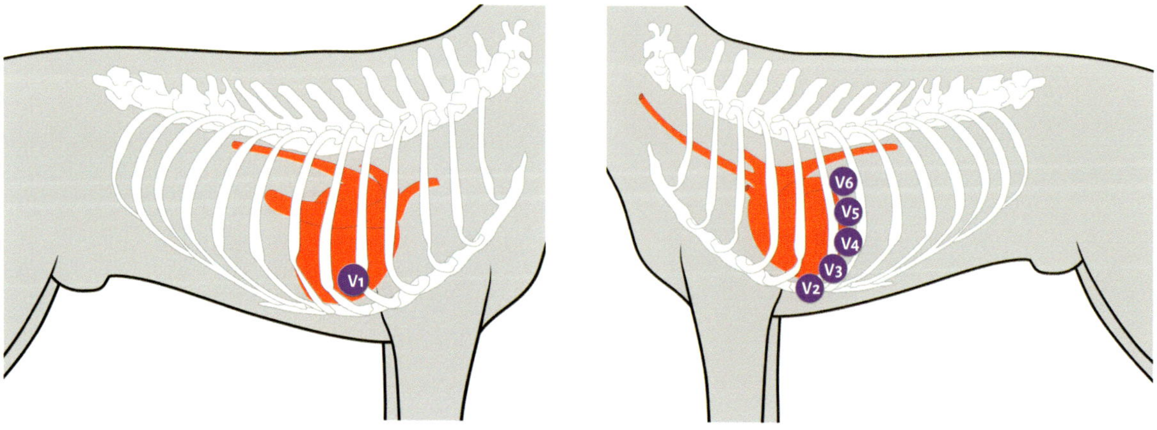

Figure 9. Wilson system modified by Kraus et al.

Following the standard colour system:

- **red electrode** is positioned on the right forelimb level with the elbow
- **yellow electrode** level with the elbow of the left forelimb
- **green electrode** level with the stifle of the left hindlimb
- **black electrode** level with the stifle of the right limb (Figure 11).

When performing an electrocardiographic trace, filters should be used to reduce base artefacts, plus calibration of the sensitivity and speed of the graph paper tracing:

- in the dog 50 Hz filters are used
- in the cat 150 Hz filters.

The **sensitivity determines the amplitude of the waves** in the trace. **Standard sensitivity is 1 mV**, which means that every millimetre that the wave is deflected vertically corresponds to 0.1 mV. Double sensitivity generates waves twice as high.

The paper speed is usually 25 or 50 mm/s. In the first instance, 25 squares measuring 1 mm pass under the needle every second. Each mm corresponds to 1/25 seconds or 0.04 s (40 ms). At 50 mm/s the number of ms is reduced by a mm and each is 20 ms/mm (Figure 12).

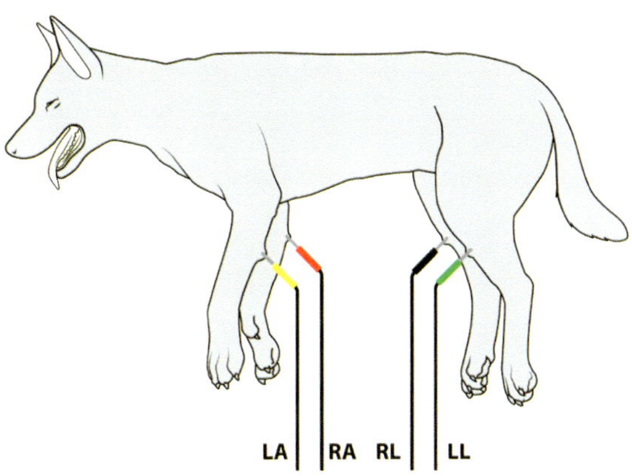

Figure 11. Surface electrocardiogram with the patient positioned in right lateral recumbence.

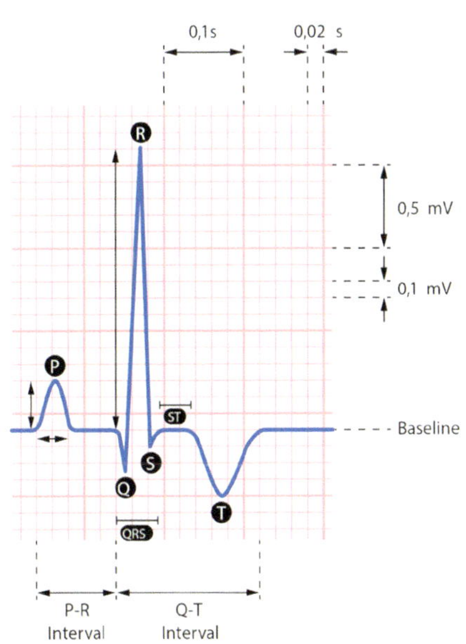

Figure 12. Paper speed of 50 mm/s and calibration 1 cm=1 mV.

Interpretation of Electrocardiographic Waves

The electrocardiographic trace is made up of (Figure 13):

- **waves**: a set of positive or negative deflections that separate from the isoelectric line
- **segments**: lines that join two waves and represent the equilibrium state of electrical charges
- **intervals**: distance between two consecutive cardiac events, measured in units of time (milliseconds).

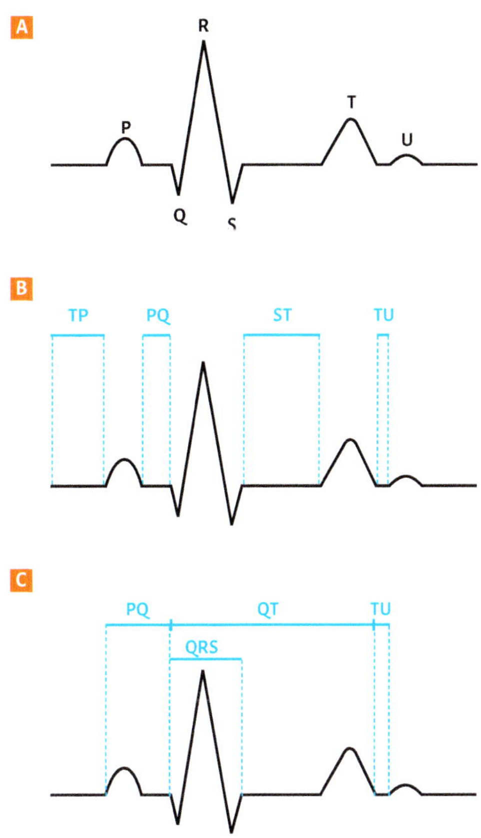

Figure 13. Waves (**A**), intervals (**B**) and segments (**C**) in an electrocardiographic trace.

The first wave is the **P wave or atrial depolarization wave and corresponds to the activation of the atrial myocardial mass**. Activation of the atrium follows a right-left, upper-lower, and anterior-posterior direction. The atrial activation vector generates a P wave on the electrocardiogram which is positive on leads II, III and aVF, negative on leads aVR and aVL and positive or isoelectric on lead I (Figure 14). The **duration of the P wave** is measured from the beginning to the end of the wave and the amplitude is assessed from the isoelectric line.

The P wave is followed by the **PQ segment** which joins the P wave to the next deflection (the QRS complex). The PQ interval represents the time taken by the electrical impulse generated in the sinus node to activate the atrial myocardium, traverse the atrioventricular and intraventricular conduction system, and initiate ventricular depolarization. The **PQ interval** is measured from the start of the P wave to the first wave of the QRS complex, either the Q wave or the R wave if the Q wave is not present.

The **QRS complex corresponds to the depolarization of the ventricular myocardium**. Depolarization begins in the interventricular septum and simultaneously activates the right and left ventricles, and is represented by three vectors. The ventricle activation sequence generates a succession of waves called the QRS complex, which can have different morphologies. Generally, depolarization of the ventricle generates a positive R wave on leads I, II, III, and aVF, a negative Q wave on leads I, II, III, and aVF, and a negative S wave on leads aVR and aVL (Figure 14).

- The **Q wave mainly corresponds to activation of the interventricular septum**.
- The **R wave** is the result of the activation of the left and right ventricles.
- The **S wave** represents the activation of the basal and posterior portion of the left ventricle.
- In the QRS complex:
  - the first positive wave is termed R
  - the negative wave preceding R is called Q
  - the negative wave following R is called S.

If the amplitude of the waves is greater than 0.5 mV it is named with capital letters and if it is less with lower case letters. If there are more waves, they are named taking their polarity into account and adding the superscript (').

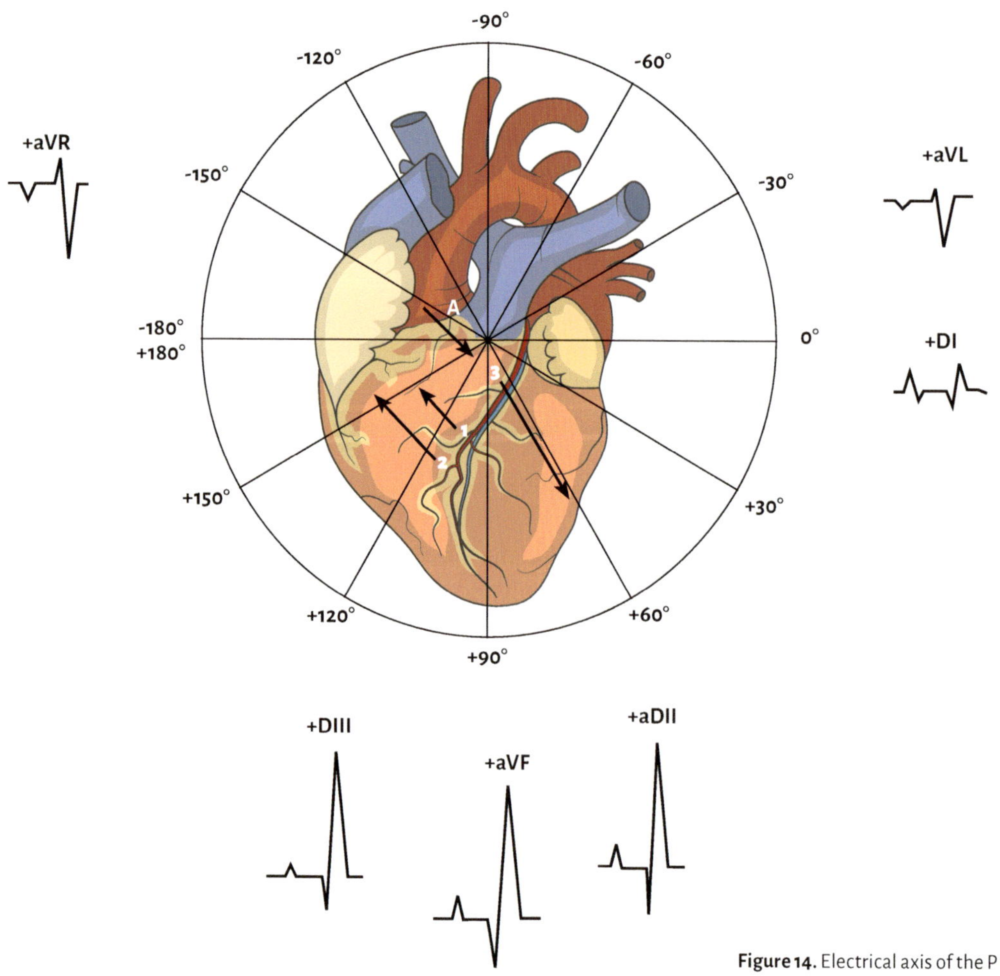

Figure 14. Electrical axis of the P wave and QRS complex.

The **duration of the QRS complex** is measured from the start of the Q wave to the end of the S wave. In the event that the Q wave is not present, the duration is measured from the beginning of the R wave to the end of the S wave. Similarly, if the S wave is absent the duration of the QRS complex is measured from the start of the Q wave to the end of the R wave. The measurement of the amplitude of each wave is taken from the isoelectric line to the maximum amplitude of each wave.

Repolarization of the atrial myocardium occurs during the PQ interval, which is identified by the Ta wave. The Ta wave has an opposite polarity to the P wave and is not visible under normal conditions because it is superimposed on the QRS complex.

The QRS complex is followed by the ST segment which extends to the T wave and corresponds to the plateau phase of the action potential. This segment has to be isoelectric. The T wave indicates the beginning of ventricular repolarization. The T wave can be positive, negative or biphasic (sum equal to 0) and should have an asymmetric morphology with a slow ascending phase and a fast descending phase, due to the difference in repolarization between the endocardium and the epicardium.

The **QT interval** represents the sum of the QRS complex, the ST segment, and the T wave. The QT interval varies slightly with the base heart rate. During tachycardia it decreases slightly and during bradycardia it increases.

The normal electrocardiographic measurements in the dog and cat are shown in Table 1. **Electrocardiographic measurements are made from lead II.**

Table 1. Reference ranges for electrocardiographic measurements in the dog and cat (Santilli, 2018).

Electrocardiographic measurements		Dog	Cat
Heart rate		· Adults 60–170 bpm · Puppies 60–220 bpm	0.5 (0.4–0.8)
P wave	Amplitude	<0.4 mV	<0.2 mV
	Duration	<40 ms (large breeds <50 ms)	<35 ms
	Electrical axis	-18° to +90°	0° to +90°
PQ interval		60–130 ms	50–90 ms
QRS complex	R wave amplitude	· >0.5 mV on DII, III and aVF · <0.5 mV on V1 · >1 mV between V2 and V6	<0.9 mV
	Duration	<70 ms	<40 ms
	Electrical axis	+40° to +100°	0° to +160°
ST segment		· Isoelectric · No more than 0.2 mV rise or fall in the hexaxial system	Isoelectric
QTc interval		150–240 ms	160–200 ms
T wave	Amplitude	<±0.05 to 1 mV on all leads	From ±0.03 mV
	Polarity	Variable	Variable
	Electrical axis	From -45° to -147°	

Calculation of Heart Rate

Heart rate is calculated as either **the average or an instantaneous heart rate**. When the **rhythm is regular the average heart rate is calculated**, but with irregular rhythms the minimum and maximum heart rate should be calculated.

- **Average heart rate**: the number of beats is counted in six seconds and multiplied by ten. If the electrocardiogram has been performed at a speed of 25 mm/s, 15 cm of paper is 6 seconds. Therefore, the number of QRS complexes is counted in 15 cm and multiplied by 10. If, on the other hand, the electrocardiogram has been carried out with a speed of 50 mm/s, 15 cm of paper is 3 seconds, and therefore must be multiplied by 20.
- **Instantaneous heart rate**: the milliseconds between one QRS complex and another should be counted. 60 000 ms (1 min) should be divided by the number of mm in the RR interval to obtain the heart rate bpm/min.

Electrical Axis Calculation

There are different methods for calculating the electrical axis.

- **Identification of the most positive or negative net wave of the QRS complex**. Net deviation is obtained by calculating the algebraic sum of the deviations of the QRS complexes.
- **Bailey's hexaxial system**. Firstly, the most isoelectric lead is measured, the perpendicular lead is sought, and the direction of the electrical axis established as a function of the polarity of this second lead. An adjustment of 150 is made taking into account the polarity of the most isoelectric lead.
- **Using leads I and aVF**. The algebraic sum of the QRS complex is measured on the two leads. The two vectors obtained are transferred to graph paper and a line is drawn that intersects the two vectors.

Electrocardiographic Abnormalities

The **duration and voltage of P waves and QRS complexes may vary slightly in some breeds** e.g. P waves and QRS complexes are slightly wider in giant breeds. This variation is less evident in cats.

The use of electrocardiography to determine the presence of cardiomegaly or enlargement of any cardiac chamber is limited. The amplitude of the waves on the surface electrocardiogram is influenced by the distance between the electrodes and the heart. The conformation of the chest (dolichomorphic, brachymorphic or mesomorphic) or degree of obesity have a physiological influence on the amplitude of the electrocardiographic waves. Patients with a **more rounded chest or obesity present waves with a lower voltage**. Pathological states such as pericardial effusion or pneumothorax also produce waves with a smaller amplitude.

P Wave

The P wave represents the depolarization of the atria. The activation sequence begins with the right atrium and continues with the left. The ascending branch of the P wave depends mainly on the depolarization of the right atrium and the descending branch on depolarization of the left. Generally, the amplitude of the P wave is influenced by the initial depolarization of the right atrium and the duration of the P wave mainly depends on the activation of the left atrium.

Dilation of the right atrium secondary to pathologies that occur with an increase in volume or pressure of this cardiac chamber, such as pulmonary pathologies, generate a P wave on the surface electrocardiogram characterised by a normal electrical axis, pointed morphology, and increased voltage.

Dilation of the left atrium (Figure 15) is present in cardiac pathologies that cause an increase of pressure or volume in this chamber, such as chronic degenerative mitral disease or cardiomyopathies. In this case, the P wave is characterised by a normal electrical axis, a forked appearance with an incision in the upper part and an increased duration.

In the case of biatrial dilation, there are changes in both the P wave duration and amplitude.

The amplitude of the P wave may also change during respiratory sinus arrhythmia. In this case, the amplitude of the P wave increases during inspiration, associated with an increase in sympathetic tone, and decreases during the exhalation phase with an increase in parasympathetic tone.

QRS Complex

The **QRS complex represents depolarization of the right and left ventricles**. The duration, voltage, and electrical axis of the QRS complex may be altered in case of single chamber or bicameral ventricular dilation, and pathologies with hypertrophy or ventricular dilation. The **surface electrocardiogram does not distinguish between hypertrophy or dilation** of the ventricle and, for this reason, echocardiography is necessary to determine the type of structural alteration.

The main electrocardiographic criteria for an increase in size of the right ventricle in the dog are:

- duration of the normal QRS complex (Figure 16);
- S waves present on leads I, II, III and aVF; and
- electrical axis deviation in the frontal plane between +100° and -80°.

In the cat it is difficult to differentiate an increase in the size of the right ventricle from a right bundle branch block on the surface electrocardiogram, and, for this reason, further tests are necessary to determine the cause of the electrical deviation.

The duration of the QRS complex may be increased in cases of increased left ventricle mass, both as a result of hypertrophy and dilation, but also due to delays in intraventricular conduction not associated with structural pathologies. In these cases, performing complementary tests such as echocardiography is required to exclude structural or systemic pathologies which may occur with cardiac remodelling.

The main electrocardiographic criteria for increases left ventricular size are:

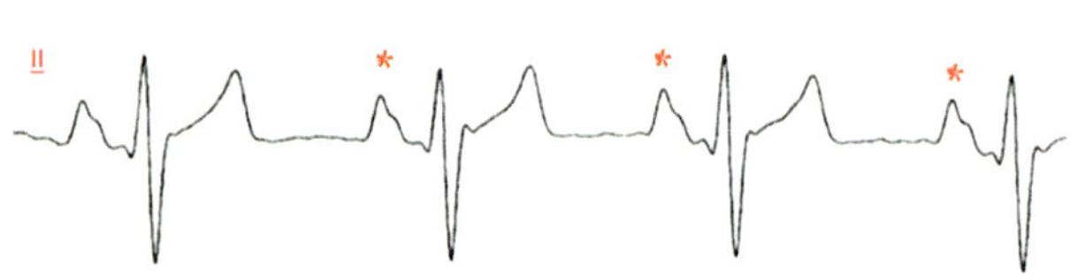

Figure 15. Electrocardiogram of a dog with degenerative mitral valve disease and severe left atrial dilatation (lead II). The asterisks mark the P waves which have an increased duration and amplitude with a forked morphology.

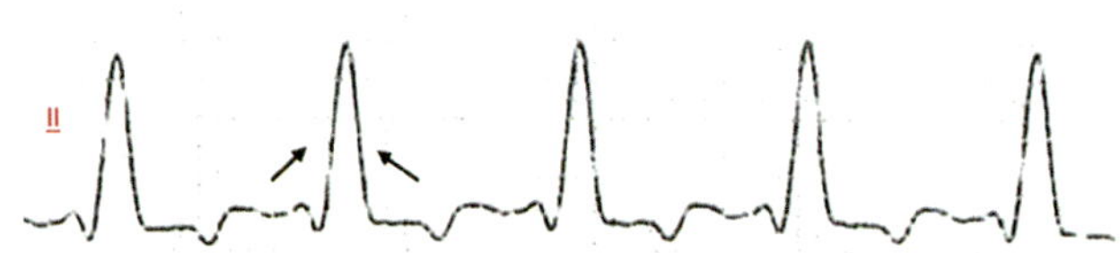

Figure 16. Electrocardiogram of a dog with idiopathic dilated cardiomyopathy (lead II). An increase in the duration of the QRS complex can be seen with a reduced angle to the ascending and descending part of the QRS complex (arrows).

– increased duration of the QRS complex;
– increased R wave amplitude;
– in the dog: >3 mV in lead II, aVF, V2 and V4 and >0.5 mV in lead I;
– in the cat: >0.9 mV in lead II, >1 mV in leads V2 and V4;
– left electrical axis deviation:
    ▪ in the dog: <40°
    ▪ in the cat: <0°
– increased duration of intrinsicoid deflection (ascending part of the R wave) and reduction of the slope of the descending portion of the R wave (slurring); and
– in the dog, a negative, deep T wave may be evident on leads I, II, III and aVF with deviation of the ST segment.

PQ Interval

The **duration of the PQ interval varies physiologically depending on heart rate**. It increases slightly during bradycardia and is slightly reduced during tachycardia.

The PQ range may be reduced pathologically in the case of accessory pathways, in so-called **preexcitation syndrome**. In this case, the conduction of the impulse to the ventricles occurs in part through bands of muscle tissue which are present at the time of birth. The accessory pathways quickly drive the impulse, and, for this reason, the PQ interval is reduced.

The duration of the PQ interval may be increased pathologically (Figure 17) in the case of degenerative pathologies of the conduction system, medications (such as beta-blockers), or electrolyte abnormalities (e.g. hyperkalaemia).

QT Interval

The **QT interval comprises the duration of the action potential, including both depolarization and repolarization**.

The duration of the QT interval, like the PQ interval, **varies with the heart rate**. The QT interval increases during bradycardia and is reduced during tachycardia. For this reason, different QT interval correction formulas described in human medicine are inaccurate for veterinary medicine. These formulas correct the duration of the QT interval based on the patient's heart rate.

The QT interval may be increased in cases of congenital pathologies in which mutations affect the genes that encode the channels involved in the repolarization phase (as in long QT syndrome), with certain drugs (such as procainamide), electrolyte abnormalities (e.g. hypokalaemia or hipocalcemia), or hypothermia. The QT interval may be shorter in cases of hypercalcaemia, digitalis toxicity and hyperkalaemia.

ST Segment

The ST segment may be elevated or depressed from the isoelectric line during an electrocardiogram. **Changes in the ST segment can be physiological** when associated with changes in heart rate **or pathological** indicating an abnormal repolarization. ST segment elevation is usually evident in cases of myocardial infarction, myocarditis, or myocardial hypoxia in general. It may also occur in cases where there are structural pathologies that occur with a marked hypertrophy of the ventricle.

It should be remembered that if depolarization is altered (e.g. bundle branch blocks or ventricular ectopic beats) repolarization is also abnormal and cause changes in both the ST and T wave.

T Wave

The T wave can change in amplitude, shape, or polarity. Changes may be present, but not specific, in cases of myocardial hypoxia (such as congestive heart failure, heart disease or heart attacks) or secondary to systemic disorders (e.g. anaemia, uraemia or fever). This means polarity can be affected, amplitude increased, and shape more aberrant. In cases of electrolyte abnormalities such as hyperkalaemia (Figure 18), the T wave is higher and more pointed. To the contrary, in cases of hypokalaemia, T waves are smaller and fork-shaped (two peaks).

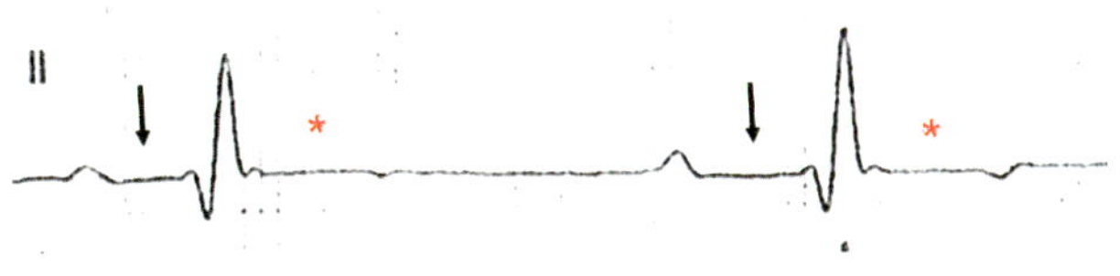

Figure 17. Electrocardiogram of a dog receiving procainamide treatment. An increase in the PQ interval is observed (black arrows) and also in the QT interval (asterisks).

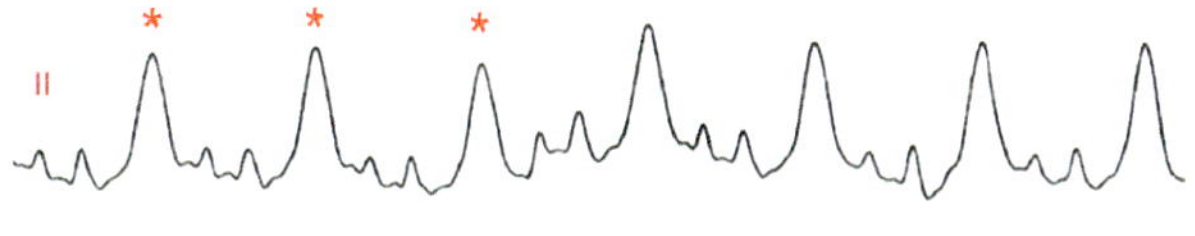

Figure 18. Electrocardiogram of a dog with hyperkalaemia (lead II). The asterisks mark the high T waves with a pointed morphology.

Bibliography

- Fox P., Sisson, D., Moise, N. (1988) *Canine and Feline Cardiology*. Philadelphia: Saunders.
- Kittleson, M, Kienle, R. (1998) *Medicina cardiovascular de pequeños animales*. St. Louis: Mosby.
- Santilli, R., Bussadori, C., Borgarelli, M. (2012) *Manuale di cardiología del cane e del gatto* (ed 1). Vaprio d'Adda, Milán: Elservier.
- Santilli, R.A., Perego, M. (2009) *Manuale di elettrocardiografia del cane e del gatto*. Elsevier, pp. 157–158.
- Tilley, L., Smith, F., Oyama, M., et al. (2008) *Manual de cardiología canina y felina*. Philadelphia: Saunders.
- Kraus, M.S., Moïse, N.S., Rishniw, M. et al. (2002) Morphology of ventricular arrhythmias in the Boxer as measured by 12-lead electrocardiography with pace-mapping comparison. *J Vet Intern Med*, 16, pp. 153–158.
- Santilli, R.A., Porteiro Vázquez, D.M., Gerou-Ferriani, M. et al. (2019) Development and assessment of a novel precordial lead system for accurate detection of right atrial and ventricular depolarization in dogs with various thoracic conformations. *Am J Vet Res*, 80, pp. 358-368.

TEST

ANSWERS ON PAGE 46

1. **Phase 3 of the action potential of rapid response cells is characterised by the entry of which ions into the cell:**
   a. Na^+.
   b. K^+.
   c. Ca^{2+}.
   d. Cl^-.

2. **Cells with pacemaker activity differ from those without automatism in the action potential because they lack:**
   a. Phase 1.
   b. Phase 2.
   c. Phase 3.
   d. Phase 0.

3. **What type of connection is the inferior fascicle?**
   a. Atrial-nodal connection.
   b. Internodal connection.
   c. Interatrial connection.
   d. Atrioventricular connection.

4. **The activation velocity is highest at:**
   a. Purkinje fibres.
   b. Atrioventricular node.
   c. Atrial myocardium.
   d. Ventricular myocardium.

5. **According to Bailey's hexaxial system, lead I records the potential difference between:**
   a. The left forelimb and right forelimb.
   b. The right forelimb and left hindlimb.
   c. The left forelimb and left hindlimb.
   d. The right forelimb and the right hindlimb.

6. **The Ta wave is the electrocardiographic representation of which phase:**
   a. Atrial depolarization.
   b. Atrial repolarization.
   c. Ventricular depolarization.
   d. Ventricular repolarization.

7. **Ischaemia can cause electrocardiographic disturbances such as:**
   a. Alterations to the PQ segment.
   b. Alterations to the ST segment.
   c. Alterations to the P wave.
   d. Alterations to the QRS complex.

Correct Answers:

1. b
2. a
3. c
4. a
5. a
6. b
7. b

Notes

Patients with Cardiovascular Disease: Prevalence, History, and Physical Examination

Mª Josefa Fernández-del Palacio

Cardiovascular conditions represent an important group of pathologies in dogs and cats. A **good clinical history and physical examination** are mandatory to detect and diagnose these conditions. **Epidemiological studies** also have a role to play in highlighting the prevalence of heart disease in the general pet population and groups within it.

Despite technological advances, the clinical history and physical examination remain fundamental to the detection of cardiovascular issues, utilizing techniques such as **observation, palpation, percussion, and auscultation**. Not only is this cost effective and beneficial, but the **non-invasive nature** of these investigations is particularly relevant for patients in a critical condition.

The particular characteristics of the cardiovascular system also **means routine physical examination can detect certain heart diseases at an early stage**. Likewise, data from the clinical history and physical examination provides valuable information as to which initial interventions (e.g. oxygen therapy) are necessary, determine additional procedures required to complete the examination (blood pressure, radiology, electrocardiography, echocardiography, laboratory analysis, etc.), and establish a diagnosis.

Prevalence

Factors that need to be considered when reviewing the prevalence of a specific heart condition in a population include:

- the proportion within the group of patients with cardiovascular disease, **in relation to healthy or sick animals** attending a clinic
- the proportion of heart disease in relation to the **clinical population for a given setting** (general consultation, referral hospital)
- the proportion of a certain heart disease **with respect to a group of heart diseases**
- predisposition of a **species, breed, sex and age** to a certain heart disease
- variability of the prevalence of different heart diseases in **different countries and over time**.

Most studies indicate cardiovascular conditions affect 2–5% of the clinical canine population and 3–4% of the feline population, (depending on the nature of the veterinary practice, be that first opinion or referral). Likewise, it is proven that **acquired heart diseases are more common than congenital disease**.

Numerous risk factors have been identified which predispose to cardiovascular disease in small animals. The most important of these are:

- **Species**. There are important differences between heart conditions affecting dogs and cats, both congenital and acquired.
- **Age**
  - Congenital conditions are more frequently detected in young animals.
  - Elderly animals have acquired conditions e.g chronic degenerative mitral disease in dogs or restrictive cardiomyopathy in cats. Mild congenital conditions may also be diagnosed in adulthood.
  - Certain conditions, such as cardiomyopathies, both in dogs (dilated cardiomyopathy) and in cats (hypertrophic cardiomyopathy), mainly occur in adult animals and can affect a wide age range.
- **Breed**
  - In dogs, both congenital and acquired diseases are more frequent in specific breeds.
  - A breed predisposition to hypertrophic cardiomyopathy has been demonstrated in cats.
- **Gender**
  - Dogs:
    - patent *ductus arteriosus* affects females to a greater extent than males;
    - males are especially predisposed to atrioventricular valve insufficiency (endocardiosis) and dilated cardiomyopathy.
  - Cats:
    - male cats appear more predisposed to hypertrophic cardiomyopathy than female cats.
- **Non-cardiac conditions**. Certain systemic conditions can have cardiac repercussions, for example:
  - arrhythmias (due to hypoadrenocorticism)
  - metastatic neoplasms
  - systemic arterial hypertension (due to chronic kidney disease, or hyperadrenocorticism).

- Geographic area
  - Some **parasitic heart diseases**, such as heartworm and leishmaniasis, are distributed throughout the warm areas of the planet, the former causing cor pulmonale, and the latter systemic arterial hypertension (secondary to chronic kidney failure).
  - Likewise, certain heart diseases may be more frequent in **specific lines** of dog breeds, depending on their distribution in different countries.

The Prevalence of Acquired Heart Disease in Dogs

Chronic, Degenerative, Mitral Valve Disease

This is the most common heart disease to affect **elderly, small breed dogs**, and accounts for **44% of all heart disease**.

The most commonly represented breeds include: Poodle, Maltese, Pekingese, Pomeranian, Miniature Schnauzer, Yorkshire Terrier, Dachshund, Chihuahua, Lhasa Apso and crossbreeds. Cavalier King Charles Spaniels are an exception in terms of age, since they can present with the disease from one year of age. Also, some medium and large breed dogs such as the Cocker Spaniel, Boxer and German Shepherd can also suffer from the condition. Males have a stronger predisposition than females.

Dilated Cardiomyopathy

This accounts for **15% of all heart diseases**.

The disease affects medium and large breeds of dogs of middle to old age including: American Cocker Spaniel, Dobermann, Boxer, Great Dane, Irish Wolfhound, German Shepherd, Spanish Mastiff, Neapolitan Mastiff, etc. Portuguese Spaniels are an exception in terms of age, as they present a juvenile form of dilated cardiomyopathy. In general, males have a stronger predisposition than females (2:1).

Pericardial Effusion and Cardiac Tumours

These account for **10% of all cardiac conditions. Idiopathic pericarditis** is the most common condition to affect the pericardium. The most commonly affected breeds are the Golden Retriever, German Shepherd, Labrador Retriever, German Pointer and Akita.

Neoplasms are the cause of effusion in 35–50% of cases. The most frequent primary neoplasms are haemangiosarcoma of the right atrium in German Shepherds and Golden Retrievers and heart-based chemodectomas in brachycephalic breeds.

Arrhythmias

Arrhythmias constitute **approximately 8% of all heart diseases**. They can appear secondary to structural heart diseases or primary as associated with specific breeds.

The most frequent primary arrhythmias are:

- **sick sinus syndrome**. With a high incidence in Miniature Schnauzer dogs with a female to male ratio of 3:1. Breed predisposition has also been described in the Pomeranian, Boxer, Cocker Spaniel and West Highland White Terrier;
- **persistent atrial standstill**. Springer Spaniel's and Labradors as well as Siamese cats seem to show a particular breed predisposition;
- **hereditary ventricular arrhythmias**. Characteristic of juvenile German Shepherd dogs.

Other Conditions

Endocarditis, systemic arterial hypertension and dirofilariasis are less common and account for 3–5% of all cardiopathies.

Prevalence of Congenital Cardiopathies in Dogs

These account for 0.5% to 1.5% of the clinical canine population and 18% of all cardiopathies (Table 1).

Prevalence of Acquired Cardiopathies in Cats

These account for 80% of all feline cardiopathies. The most common forms are the following.

Cardiomyopathies

Hypertrophic (the most common), restrictive, dilated, unclassified, and right ventricular arrhythmogenic. They account for 70% of feline heart disease. Although they can occur in any breed, the most commonly affected breeds are Maine coon, Persian, Norwegian Forest, Sphynx, American and British Short Hair, and Ragdoll.

Table 1. Dog breeds with a predisposition to congenital cardiopathies.

Congenital cardiopathy	Predisposed dog breeds
Patent *ductus arteriosus* (PDA)	Maltese, Poodle, Keeshond, Bichon Frise, Pomeranian, Yorkshire Terrier, English Springer Spaniel, Alsatian, Cocker Spaniel, Chihuahua, Miniature Schnauzer, German Shepherd, Collie, Golden Retriever, Labrador Retriever. (The proportion of females/males is 3:1)
Pulmonary stenosis	Bulldog, Scottish Terrier, Miniature Schnauzer, West Highland White Terrier, Chihuahua, Samoyed, Yorkshire Terrier, Cocker Spaniel, German Shepherd, Collie, Golden Retriever, Labrador Retriever and Beagle
Aortic/subaortic stenosis	Terranova, Boxer, Golden Retriever, Rottweiler, German Shepherd. Some authors have also mentioned the Samoyed, Great Dane and English Bulldog
Ventricular septal defect	West Highland White Terrier, English Springer Spaniel, Basset Hound, English Bulldog, Akita, Shih Tzu, Poodle, Husky, Chow Chow, Beagle, Labrador Retriever
Tricuspid dysplasia	Labrador and Golden Retriever, German Shepherd, English Sheepdog
Mitral dysplasia	Great Dane, German Shepherd, Bull Terrier, Terranova
Tetralogy of Fallot	Breeds which frequently suffer from pulmonary stenosis and ventricular septal defects are at risk: West Highland White Terrier, Wirehaired Fox Terrier and Keeshond above all
Atrial septal defect	Boxer and Terranova. Some authors have noted a predisposition in the Dobermann and Samoyed

Other Conditions

Pericardial effusion, neoplasia, arrhythmias and systemic arterial hypertension account for 8% of diseases.

Prevalence of Congenital Cardiopathies in Cats

These account for approximately 12% of all feline cardiopathies.

The most common are septal defects, followed by atrioventricular valve dysplasia, tetralogy of Fallot and, less frequently, pulmonary stenosis, aortic stenosis, and patent *ductus arteriosus*.

Clinical History

The purpose of the clinical history is to **identify if the patient may have cardiovascular disease** and then differentiate between cardiac, respiratory or systemic conditions; and determine the course of the disease and response to treatment. Likewise, taking an extensive history establishes a connection or link with the owner that can become valuable to achieve their collaboration with complicated diagnostic procedures and treatments, including the most complex ones.

The first phase of the history includes the collection of data from **the animal's signalment** (species, age, breed and sex), the patient's clinical history, and the reason for the consultation (current clinical signs). The signalment is important in the context of the clinical case. As indicated previously, most heart diseases are more prevalent in a specific species, age group, breed, or sex.

The questions posed to the owner about the background and reason for the consultation can be grouped into three sections:

1. **general** questions
2. questions about signs related to **other body systems** or organs
3. questions about **symptoms** frequently associated with heart conditions.

General Questions

These should include: reason for consultation, beginning and duration of clinical signs (acute or chronic condition), exposure to infectious diseases, vaccination status, medications received and response to treatment, attitude of the animal and degree of exercise tolerance.

Questions About Signs Related to Other Body Systems or Organs

These should include: appetite, water consumption, urinary habits, defaecation, vomiting or regurgitation, seizures, syncope episodes, reproductive status, lameness (possible endocarditis) or paresis, previous conditions or trauma, geographical area in which the dog lives or has been living (heartworm).

Questions About Symptoms Frequently Associated with Heart Conditions

There are important differences between dogs and cats in terms of the clinical manifestations related to the cardiovascular system and the course of cardiac pathology.

- In dogs, the evolution of heart disease is usually progressive.
- In cats, owners rarely observe early clinical signs related to heart disease. The most typical presentation is of acute, progressive onset (24–48 hours) with respiratory distress and/or paralysis (aortic thromboembolism). Signs such as lethargy and decreased appetite can appear previously, at variable times beforehand.

Signs Most Commonly Associated with Heart Disease

Exercise Intolerance and Weakness

These signs can appear in patients with significant heart disease due to arrhythmias, pulmonary oedema (chronic degenerative mitral disease, pericardial tamponade, poor tissue perfusion, and right-to-left sided shunts). However, differential diagnoses of respiratory diseases, significant anaemia, systemic, metabolic, and toxic conditions must be ruled out.

Respiratory Signs

Differential diagnoses should include those of both cardiac or respiratory origin. One of the most typical signs is a cough. This reflex is stimulated by mechanical or chemical agents that mainly affect the pharynx, larynx, trachea, and large diameter bronchi.

- In cats, coughing is associated with bronchial disease and only in some cats with heart disease.
- **In dogs, coughing occurs both due to tracheal and bronchial problems** (tracheobronchitis, tracheal collapse, neoplasms), **as well as heart disease** that causes dilation of the left atrium by compressing the left main bronchi, as occurs in small breed dogs with chronic degenerative mitral disease. In these cases, the cough may result from the coexistence of both conditions (heart disease and tracheobronchial disorders).

The **nature of the cough and the time of day** it occurs can help in differentiating the conditions responsible. Tracheal collapse produces a characteristic "goose squawk" cough, stimulated by nervousness, pressure from the collar, or drinking water. Coughing in patients with heart disease tends to be worse at night, except in advanced stages where it also occurs during the day.

Syncope

Syncope is defined as a sudden and transient loss of consciousness and postural tone, of short duration and with spontaneous recovery. It is due to an abrupt interruption of blood supply to the brain. It can be secondary to heart disease (arrhythmias, heart failure) or of a vasovagal nature (neurocardiogenic), but in more than 50% of patients the causes are not established due to the complexity of its aetiology.

Syncope must be distinguished from loss of consciousness caused by hypoglycaemia, hypoxia, or sympathetic inhibition (normal brain flow).

The history of events is extremely important in determining the aetiology of syncope, the precipitating factors, premonitory symptoms, the presence or absence of seizures and symptoms after the episode. The clinical signs do not always present in the same way, so when there is partial reduction in blood flow, the signs are characterised by weakness, collapse and ataxia, without reaching syncope, and are called "near syncope". Likewise, when cerebral hypoxia is prolonged, seizure activity may occur, specifically in severe bradyarrhythmias.

In cats, syncope of cardiovascular origin sometimes manifests with neurological signs, so it is important to differentiate them. In general, neural syncope has a better prognosis than those associated with heart disease.

Increased Abdominal Size

Due to organomegaly and/or ascites, secondary to right-sided congestive heart failure (see the "Abdominal Examination" section).

Other Signs Related to Cardiovascular Disease

Depending on which congenital heart disease the animal is suffering from, different clinical signs are observed.

- In dogs:
  - reduced growth (PDA in large dog breeds, tetralogy of Fallot);
  - weight loss (advanced congestive heart failure);
  - vomiting and diarrhoea (right-sided heart failure);

  - oliguria (decreased renal perfusion due to left-sided heart failure);
  - hyperthermia: endocarditis; and
  - subcutaneous oedema: may appear in the lowest part of the thorax and abdomen in large breed dogs with significant right-sided congestive heart failure. The extremities are not usually affected. When present, the most common cause is hypalbuminaemia (protein loss, severe liver disease).
- In cats:
  - paralysis of the posterior third (aortic thromboembolism secondary to cardiomyopathies).

Physical Examination

The *physical examination of the patient begins whilst taking the history* by watching their demeanour and attitude, mental state, posture, respiratory pattern and body condition.

The information obtained from the physical examination can indicate whether the clinical signs may be due to a cardiac condition or be symptoms of one, and how relevant these are to the differential diagnosis list.

A **systematic physical examination** is essential in order not to miss anything. Since non-cardiac conditions may affect the functionality of the cardiovascular system and certain signs are common to different systems, the examination should include all the organs and body systems.

General Observation of the Patient

The first thing to consider is the animal's posture, respiratory rate and pattern, and respiratory duration and effort, in order to determine whether urgent intervention (oxygen therapy) is required. Likewise, the patient's body condition and attitude are important.

Posture

Dogs refuse to lie down when they have pulmonary oedema or pleural effusion. In the case of alveolar pulmonary oedema, they present with an orthopnoeic position (elbows abducted, neck extended, and open mouth breathing).

Cats in respiratory distress frequently position themselves in sternal recumbency.

Respiratory Rate and Rhythm

In dogs, the normal respiratory rate is between 10–30 breaths per minute (bpm) and in cats between 20–30 bpm, although if it is hot or the animal has just been exercising or playing the frequency may be higher.

Tachypnoea and panting, which is common in dogs, can be due to the animal's excitement in the consult, but can also be signs of respiratory failure.

In cats, it is advisable to evaluate the respiratory rate while they are still in the cage or carrier, in order to avoid stress.

Respiratory Pattern/Dyspnoea

Etymologically, dyspnoea means gasping for breath. Establishing the phase of respiration in which it occurs (inspiratory, expiratory, restrictive, paradoxical) and the degree of respiratory distress are important.

- **Inspiratory dyspnoea** is characterised by a prolonged and difficult inspiratory phase. It is a **sign of upper airway obstruction** when it is audible (brachycephalic syndrome in dogs, upper respiratory tract infection in cats, and laryngeal conditions in dogs), or of difficulty in expanding the lungs (pleural effusion, diaphragmatic dysfunction or large peritoneal effusions).
- **Expiratory dyspnoea** is characterised by **difficulty in removing air from the lungs** due to a decrease in lung elasticity (pulmonary oedema, pneumonia) or narrowing of small airways (feline bronchial disease).
- **Restrictive dyspnoea** is characterised by rapid, short, and laboured breaths characteristic of **pleural effusion, pneumonia, and pulmonary oedema**.
- The **paradoxical breathing pattern** is characteristic of **rib fractures** and diaphragmatic dysfunction.

Likewise, the way dyspnoea presents can guide towards its aetiology.

- **Acute dyspnoea**: includes foreign bodies, laryngeal oedema, massive pulmonary embolism and pneumothorax. In cats, congestive heart failure with pulmonary oedema and pleural effusion can be detected by owners in the acute form.
- **Chronic dyspnoea**: is usually due to bronchial conditions (feline asthma), interstitial lung conditions, and heart disease.

Body Condition

Patients with congestive heart failure may **appear weak and cachectic** (loss of muscle mass) due, among other reasons, to poor tissue perfusion and the release of cytokines.

In contrast, many dogs with chronic airway conditions (bronchitis, fibrosis, tracheal collapse) are often obese.

Systematic Examination

The physical examination should include:

- head: mucous membranes
- neck: jugular veins
- thorax: palpation of the precordial area, auscultation
- abdomen: presence of effusion, organomegaly
- extremities: temperature, femoral pulse.

Examination of the Head

This should include the colour of the mucous membranes (pink, pale, dark red, cyanotic) and capillary refill time (in addition to possible oral conditions):

- **pale mucous membranes** may be due to anaemia, poor cardiac output, or high sympathetic tone (stress in the consult);
- **a dark red colour** can be a sign of polycythaemia, sepsis, and nervousness;
- **cyanosis (bluish colour of mucous membranes)** (Figure 1) can be a sign of airway obstruction, conditions affecting the lung parenchyma and pleural space, pulmonary oedema, right-to-left shunt, congenital heart defects, hypoventilation, or shock. When cyanosis predominates in the caudal mucous membranes (differential cyanosis), it indicates the existence of a reverse shunt (pulmonary artery to the descending aorta) through a patent *ductus arteriosus* (although no obvious murmur is detected).

Increased capillary filling time (>2 s) may suggest low cardiac output (subaortic and pulmonary stenosis), but also dehydration, elevated sympathetic tone, and vasoconstriction.

In cats with heart disease the colour of mucous membranes and capillary filling time may be normal.

Examination of the Neck

Examination of the neck can reveal primary and secondary conditions which may affect the heart. It should include observation of the jugular veins and palpation of the trachea, lymph nodes, and thyroid area. Examination of the jugular veins provides valuable information on central venous pressure (right-sided chambers).

In the standing animal with the neck and head in a normal position, the jugular veins should not be distended. Jugular distention occurs when there is an increase in the filling pressure of the right side of the heart (tricuspid stenosis, pericardial effusion/tamponade) or obstruction of the cranial vena cava that hinders venous return (Figure 2).

In dogs with mediastinal or cardiac base neoplasms that compress the cranial vena cava, varying degrees of enlargement of the neck up to the entrance to the thorax are observed (cranial vena cava syndrome) (Figure 3).

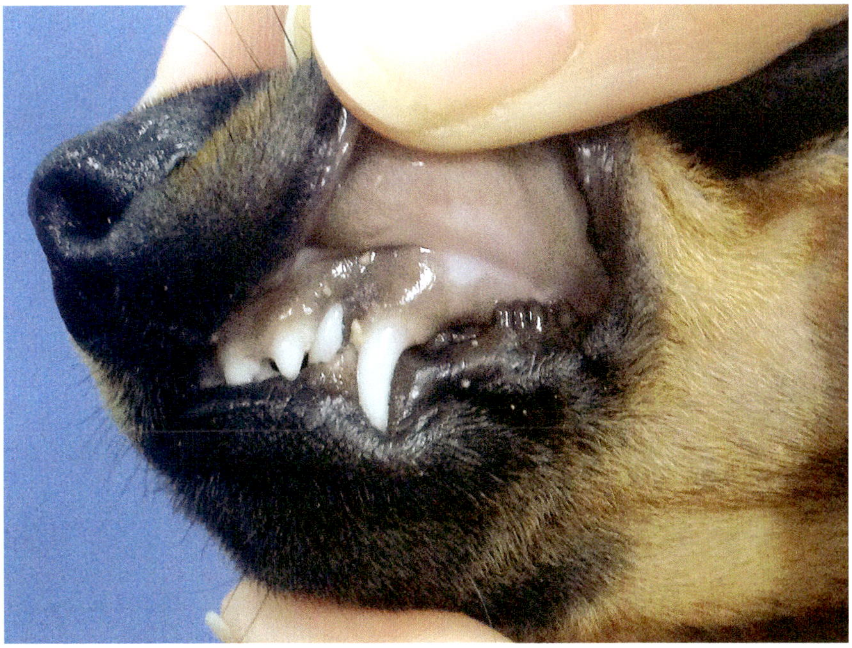

Figure 1. Cyanotic oral mucous membranes in a dog with severe pulmonary oedema.

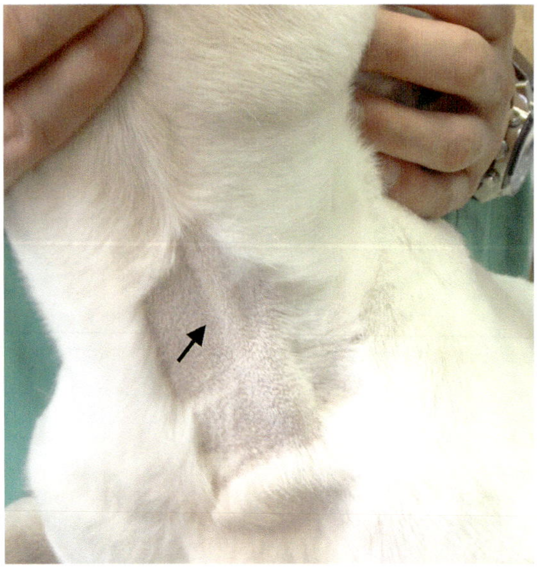

Figure 2. The neck of a dog with congenital pulmonary stenosis and significant tricuspid insufficiency, showing jugular vein distension (arrow).

Distention plus pulsation (up to the level of the scapula) is observed in the course of various right heart diseases with decreased compliance (ventricular hypertrophy, severe tricuspid regurgitation) or atrioventricular dissociation (complete AV block).

As a general rule, **distension of the jugular veins in a dog with ascites suggests cardiac aetiology**. Jugular vein distention can be accentuated by pressing on the abdomen (liver) with both hands (hepatojugular reflux) just behind the xiphoid process of the sternum.

Palpation of the trachea may reveal increased sensitivity in patients with inflammatory conditions, but also tracheal collapse or masses. The thyroid may be enlarged in cats with hyperthyroidism or older dogs with thyroid carcinoma.

Thoracic Examination

Evaluation of the thorax includes observation of respiratory movements (previously described), palpation of the precordial area, percussion, and auscultation.

Palpation and Percussion

The thorax should be carefully palpated to detect **bony abnormalities** such as pectum excavatum, **changes in the intensity of the heartbeat, or precordial thrill**. An increase in the intensity of the heartbeat (pressure of the ventricular chamber x ventricular diameter) against the thoracic wall can be interpreted as an increase in the force of contraction, but also as a ventricular dilation.

The **intensity of the heartbeat** also appears increased in very lean animals and in those in hyperdynamic states (anaemia, fever, hyperthyroidism). The reduction or absence on palpation of the heartbeat may appear in obese animals, but it is also indicative of fluid (pleural, pericardial effusion) or a mass interposed between the heart and the thoracic wall. Detection of a **precordial thrill** (a sensation of vibration transmitted to the thoracic wall by turbulent flows in the heart or great vessels) is indicative of a severe heart murmur (5/6 and 6/6).

Thoracic percussion can be useful in animals with dyspnoea to assess the existence of pleural effusion or pneumothorax without risk to the patient. It is performed by placing the fingers of one hand over the intercostal spaces and tapping with

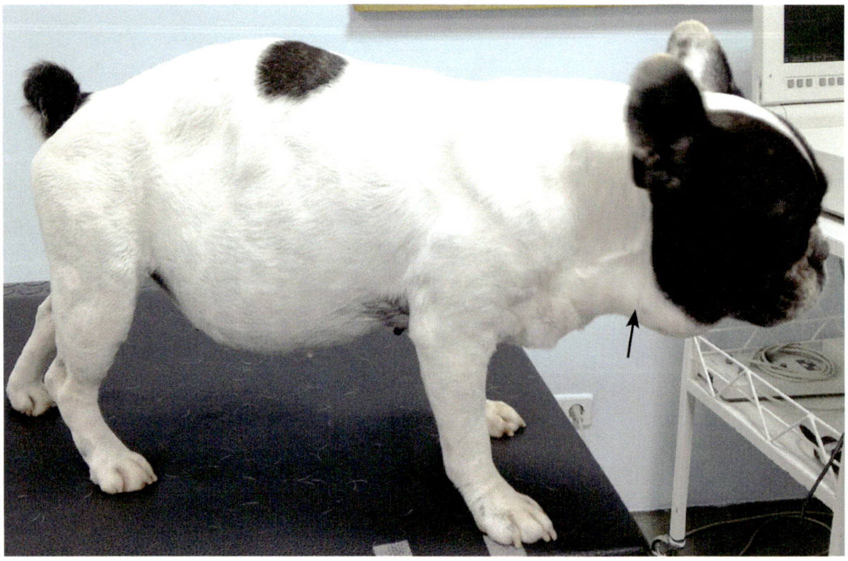

Figure 3. French Bulldog with right-sided congestive heart failure due to cardiac blockage and neoplasia in the heart base. An increase in abdominal size due to ascites is seen, along with poor body condition and subcutaneous oedema in the lower part of the thorax and neck (arrow).

the fingers of the other hand on them, in a dorsal ventral direction. Thus, a high-pitched (dorsal) sound is characteristic of pneumothorax and a low-pitched or dull (ventral) sound suggests the presence of fluid.

Auscultation

Thoracic auscultation is safe for the critically ill patient and accessible to all clinicians, and so despite advances in diagnostic techniques it continues to be a key piece of cardiac semiology. It should be performed in a **quiet room**, with the patient as calm as possible and with a stethoscope that is appropriate for the size of the animal. It should be carried out systematically, listening to the respiratory system and the heart separately since it is impossible to concentrate on both at the same time.

Auscultation of the Respiratory System

The normal sounds heard are the so-called **bronchovesicular sounds**: soft sounds produced by the passage of air through the airways. They are more audible in the trachea and bifurcation and they diminish in intensity towards the distal parts of the lung. They can be accentuated in cases of tachypnoea, nervousness or stress and decrease in intensity when there is fluid or pneumothorax.

The main pathological sounds audible by auscultation are:

- **attenuation of the normal bronchovesicular sounds**: mainly due to the presence of thoracic masses, pleural effusion, pneumothorax, pneumonia, or obesity;
- **crepitations**: sounds similar to those produced when detaching Velcro. They are of two types:
    - **soft and inspiratory**, generated by the movement of air through a fluid. They are associated with pulmonary oedema, pneumonia, and pulmonary haemorrhage;
    - **strong and discontinuous**, generated by the sudden equalization of pressures between open and closed airways. Typical of fibrosis and chronic bronchitis.
- **wheezes**: musical sounds, generally continuous, of low frequency, caused by the movement of air through narrow airways. They are heard in patients with primary bronchial conditions (bronchitis and feline asthma);
- **rhonchus**: the sound is similar to a gurgling, loud and intense, like a low-pitched snoring, which is more intense during inspiration. They are caused by the passage of air through partially obstructed airways (bronchioles with mucous, spasm). They can be modified by coughing. Rhonchi are heard in patients with pneumonia, asthma, bronchiectasis, and bronchopulmonary neoplasms;
- **pleural friction**: sounds that are heard both during inspiration and expiration produced by the friction of the two dry, rough pleural sheets against each other. They are not modified by coughing;
- **pericardial friction**: short, harsh sounds produced by pericarditis and heart movement. They should not be confused with the so-called "pericardial knocks", diastolic sounds that occur in animals with constrictive pericarditis.

Cardiac Auscultation

Includes evaluation of heart rate, rhythm, and sounds.

The use of **an appropriate stethoscope** is essential for detailed auscultation. In small breed dogs and cats, paediatric stethoscopes are advisable, with a small diaphragm, so they do not exceed the cardiac projection area. Using the diaphragm or membrane, most of the higher frequency heart sounds (first and second heart sounds and systolic murmurs) and respiratory sounds can be assessed, the bell transmits low frequency sounds better (galloping sounds and some diastolic murmurs). Sufficient time (at least one or two minutes) should be dedicated to auscultation in order to detect low intensity murmurs and transient arrhythmias.

Sometimes momentarily stopping the animal's breathing is necessary to **distinguish between heart and breath sounds**. Likewise, auscultation should be considered a dynamic examination, **encompassing the entire thorax** and systematically exploring the focus of each valve, the entrance to the thorax, and the carotids (to detect normal sounds and their spread).

Simultaneous auscultation and palpation of the pulse is essential for a good cardiovascular examination. The two main areas of auscultation include the apex and the cardiac base of both hemi thoraces. The first heart sound is best heard towards the apex, over the mitral focus, and the second heart sound over the left heart base (pulmonary and aortic foci).

Heart sounds can be more pronounced in cases of cardiomegaly, but also in hyperdynamic states (fever, anaemia, hyperthyroidism, etc.) and are muffled in obese patients and in cases of pericardial and pleural effusions. Displacement of sounds may indicate the presence of thoracic masses or a peritoneal-pericardial diaphragmatic hernia.

Heart Rate

The heart rate is highly variable depending on the species, age, breed and nervous state of the animal. The normal range includes **70–140 beats/minute in dogs and 140–200 beats/minute in cats**. This may be higher in patients with heart failure, but also in hyperdynamic states.

Heart Rhythm

In dogs, the rhythms which are considered normal are regular sinus rhythm and sinus arrhythmia.

Sinus arrhythmia (SA) is associated with elevated vagal tone and common in brachycephalic breeds. Generally, SA coincides with the phases of respiration:

- during inspiration the heart accelerates;
- during expiration it slows down.

In these cases, the intensity of normal heart sounds can be variable. **In patients with heart failure, SA disappears** and may be accentuated in patients with severe lung disease.

In cats, only regular sinus rhythm is considered normal in the consult room. When the femoral pulse does not coincide with the heartbeat, it is indicative of premature beats or atrial fibrillation. In the latter case, the existence of a pulse of 100 beats/minute with a heart rate of 180–220 beats/minute is typical.

Other clinically significant arrhythmias, such as ventricular tachycardia, cause a sudden change in heart rate and intensity of heart sounds. Within the bradyarrhythmias, complete block (third degree) causes bradycardia with a marked increase in pulse strength.

Heart Sounds

The normal heart sounds heard in healthy dogs and cats include:

- **first heart sound (S1)**. Generated by the vibrations and tension of the closure of the atrioventricular valves at the beginning of ventricular systole. It is heard with greater intensity towards the cardiac apex on the left sternal border;
- **second heart sound (S2)**. Generated by the closure of the aortic and pulmonary valves. It is heard with greater intensity towards the left heart base.

Sounds considered abnormal, generally associated with heart disease, include gallop sounds, systolic clicks, doubling of normal sounds, and murmurs.

Gallop Sounds

Gallop sounds include **the combination of S1 and S2 along with S3 or S4 sounds**. The latter are generally not audible in small animals, and occur during diastole and are of a low frequency. S3 and S4 are best heard using the bell of the stethoscope:

- **S3** is a sound generated by rapid ventricular filling in patients with ventricular dilatation and systolic dysfunction (dilated cardiomyopathy);
- **S4** is a sound caused by atrial contraction by forcing the ejection of blood flow into a ventricle with reduced compliance (cats with restrictive or hypertrophic cardiomyopathy).

If the heart rate is high, differentiating between an S3 and an S4 can be difficult, and it is called a "summation gallop".

Systolic Clicks

Systolic clicks are a different type of third heart sound added to the S1 and S2, sounds, with a different mechanism and character to a gallop rhythm. They are short, mesosystolic sounds with a higher frequency than a gallop rhythm and, therefore, better audible with the membrane of the stethoscope. These systolic clicks are characteristic of atrioventricular valve abnormalities, specifically **mitral valve prolapse**.

Repetition of Normal Sounds

Repetition of the normal sounds constitutes a type of triple rhythm. These occur when there is an asynchronism in the closure of the atrioventricular valves (S1) or the aortic and pulmonary sigmoid valves (S2). In dogs, the latter is highly suggestive of the presence of **pulmonary hypertension**.

Heart Murmurs

Murmurs are longer than normal S1 and S2 heart sounds. They are produced by vibrations within the cardiovascular system due to turbulent blood flow. Not all murmurs indicate structural heart disease.

These are classified as follows.

- **Pathological**. Secondary to structural heart diseases such as ventricular outflow tract obstruction (pulmonary and aortic stenosis), valve insufficiencies and communications between chambers and great vessels (septal defects, patent *ductus arteriosus*).
- **Physiological**. Associated with hyperdynamic states (fever, hyperthyroidism and anaemia) or exercise.
- **Innocent**. Characteristic of puppies and usually disappear after 4–5 months of age.

Characterization of the murmurs, that is, the time of the cardiac cycle at which they are heard, the intensity and timbre and the area of maximum intensity can help in their interpretation. Both innocent and physiological murmurs occur during systole, are low intensity, best heard on the cardiac base, and can change with heart rate, from day to day, and with body position.

Classification is according to the duration and timing of the murmurs in the cardiac cycle.

- **Systolic murmurs**: the most frequent murmur in small animals. They appear during systole (between S1 and S2). They are classed as one of three types:
  - **protosystolic**: heard at the beginning of systole and have a decrescendo configuration. They are characteristic of acute mitral insufficiency (tendinous cord rupture) due to the progressive attenuation of the pressure gradient between the ventricle and the left atrium with poor compliance;
  - **mesosystolic**: start after S1 and end before S2. Their configuration is crescendo-decrescendo. They are characteristic of ventricular outflow tract obstructions, pulmonary stenosis related to volume increase due to a wide atrial septum defect, obstructive hypertrophic cardiomyopathy (cats), hyperdynamic states (anaemia, stress, fever, exercise, etc.);
  - **holosystolic**: occupy the whole of systole, they have a plateau configuration. They are characteristic

of heart diseases that present with a wide and continuous pressure gradient between two chambers, as occurs in dogs with chronic degenerative mitral disease, tricuspid regurgitation (pulmonary hypertension, valvular dysplasia) and left to right sided ventricular septum defects.

- **Diastolic murmurs**: less common in small animals than systolic murmurs. They occur during diastole (the filling phase of the ventricles), that is, in the S2–S1 interval. The most frequent are divided into two types:
  - **protodiastolic**: characteristic of aortic and pulmonary regurgitation
  - **mesodiastolic**: characteristic of mitral and tricuspid stenosis.
- **Continuous murmurs**: begin in systole, with the peak near S2, and continue in diastole. They are due to the presence of a pressure gradient between two chambers or vessels in both phases of the cardiac cycle. These murmurs are characteristic of patent *ductus arteriosus*, pulmonary arteriovenous fistula, and aortic-pulmonary defects.
- **To-and-fro murmurs**: coexistence of a systolic and a diastolic murmur. They are characteristic of dogs with aortic regurgitation associated with subaortic stenosis or interventricular septal defect (prolapse of one of the sigmoids through the defect). They can be difficult to differentiate from continuous murmurs.

According to intensity, murmurs are classified by grades from I to VI out of VI (Table 2).

In dogs, there is a positive correlation between murmur intensity and the severity of pulmonary and aortic stenosis, as well as the clinical stage of chronic degenerative mitral disease.

The **area of maximum intensity** corresponds to the area in which the murmurs are most intense and easiest to hear (Figure 4).

Table 2. Classification of heart murmurs according to their intensity.

Murmur intensity	Characteristics
Grade I/VI	Very soft and only detected in a quiet room after several seconds of auscultation
Grade II/VI	Also, a soft murmur, but easily auscultated
Grade III/VI	Moderately intense murmur
Grade IV/VI	Intense murmur which is not accompanied by fremitus
Grade V/VI	Very intense murmur accompanied by fremitus
Grade VI/VI	Very intense murmur which can even be heard when the stethoscope is taken away from the thoracic wall

- **Mitral valve area**: located on the left ventricular apex (5th intercostal space towards the sternum), although sometimes these murmurs radiate towards the base and the right hemithorax.
- **Aortic valve area**: located on the left cardiac base, at the level of the 3rd–4th intercostal spaces. Over this area, murmurs due to aortic stenosis can be heard, which are also heard in the right cranial hemithorax, and radiate towards the ventricular apex.
- **Pulmonary valve area**: located on the left cardiac base, somewhat more cranial than the aortic area and towards the sternum. It is the point of maximum intensity of murmurs due to stenosis and pulmonary insufficiency, which are also heard over the right cranial hemithorax.
- **Tricuspid valve area**: located over the 4th intercostal space in the right hemithorax, on the costochondral junction. Murmurs due to tricuspid regurgitation are heard more intensely here.

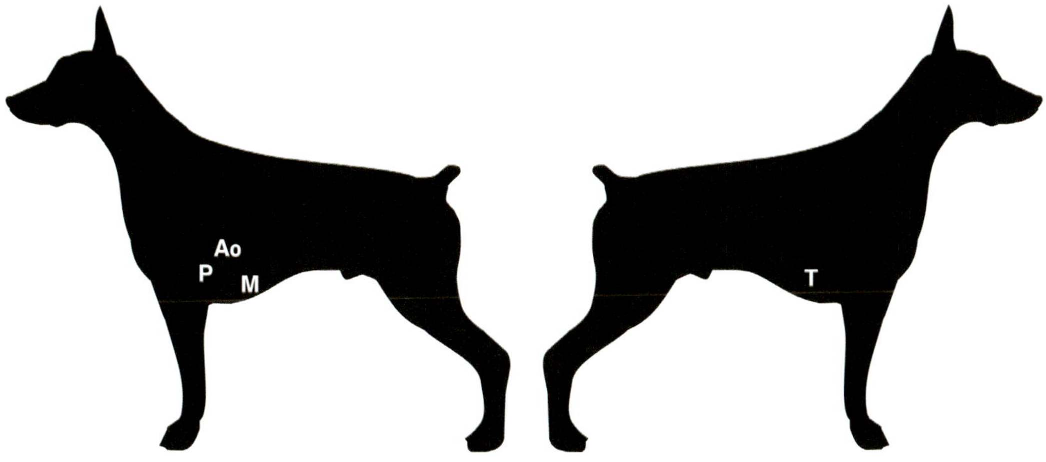

Figure 4. Diagrams which show the areas for cardiac auscultation in the dog: M: mitral, P: pulmonary, Ao: aortic, T: tricuspid.

Others:

- murmurs corresponding to peri- or paramembranous **ventricular septal defects** are heard with greater intensity over the right hemithorax, towards the sternum, and cranially;
- a murmur due to a **patent *ductus arteriosus*** is heard with greater intensity over the cardiac base of both hemi thoraces, radiating towards the entrance of the thorax.

Abdominal Examination

The abdomen should be examined to detect the presence of ascites (Figure 3) or organomegaly, secondary to right-sided congestive heart failure caused by dilated cardiomyopathy, tricuspid regurgitation, heartworm, pericardial or congenital conditions. However, differential diagnoses should also include **conditions that induce protein losses**, neoplasms, and liver conditions. Ascitic fluid secondary to right congestive heart failure generally presents with the characteristics of a modified transudate, although it can be chylous in nature, especially in cats.

In cats, ascites secondary to right-sided congestive heart failure is usually accompanied by pleural effusion and sometimes pericardial effusion.

Rectal Temperature

Persistent feverish signs may suggest infective endocarditis. Conversely, hypothermia can be a sign of cardiogenic shock and low cardiac output.

Examination of the Limbs

The limbs should be examined for temperature and muscle tone, the presence or absence of peripheral oedema, and the characteristics of the femoral pulse. Animals with low cardiac output or cats with thromboembolism may have cold hindlimbs and purplish pads when compared to the forelimbs (Figure 5).

Thromboembolism is characterised by acute paresis of the hindlimbs or one of the forelimbs. The thrombus is generated in the left atrium, which is significantly dilated in cases of cardiomyopathies, part of it breaks off and travels through the arterial system to the trifurcation of the iliac or other arteries (renal, forelimbs, etc.).

Femoral Pulse

The femoral pulse provides information about the **rate, quality, rhythm, synchrony** with the heartbeat, and symmetry in both extremities. It must be evaluated with the animal standing up, comparing it with both limbs and with the heartbeat, since they should coincide.

The pressure detected by palpating the pulse, or quality, corresponds to the systolic minus the diastolic blood pressure. It can vary depending on the conformation of the animal, age, hydration, heart rate, heart function and level of activity and nervous state.

In cats, palpation of the pulse can be difficult, so its absence should not be confused with arterial obstruction.

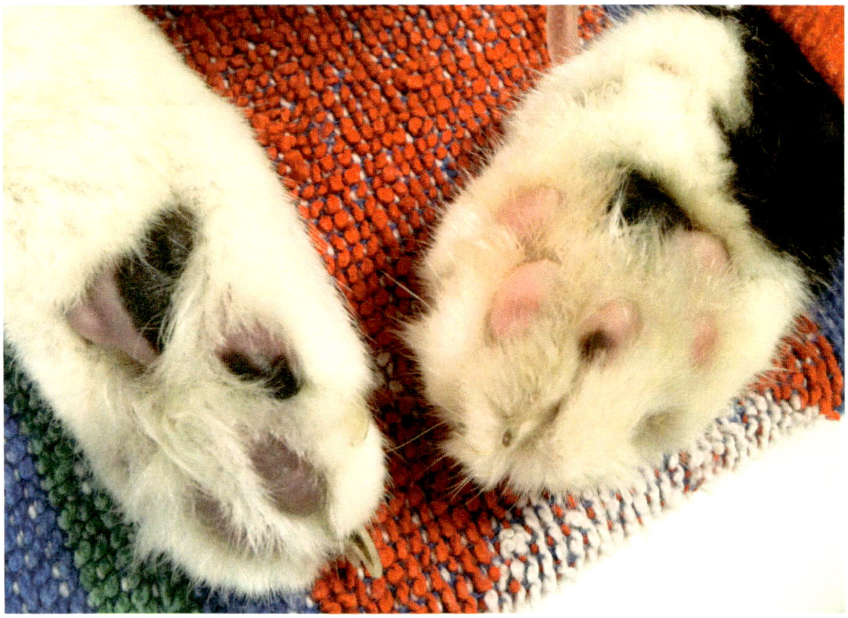

Figure 5. Image showing a comparison of the pad colour of a hindlimb (left) with the pad colour of a forelimb in a cat with aortic thromboembolism. The hindlimb affected by ischaemia (left) shows a purple colour in comparison the normal pink colour of the forelimb (right).

The characteristics of the femoral pulse include:

- **weak pulse**: decreased pulse pressure can occur when systolic stroke volume is reduced, as occurs in patients with heart failure, severe aortic or pulmonary stenosis, or decreased peripheral resistance;
- **bounding or hyperkinetic pulse**: the increase in pulse pressure can appear in cases of systemic systolic arterial hypertension, decrease in diastolic pressure (aortic insufficiency) or a combination of both (patent *ductus arteriosus*);
- **pulse deficits**: can be secondary to tachyarrhythmias, due to the ventricles not filling adequately because diastole is very short;
- **paradoxical pulse**: characterised by a decrease in pulse pressure during inspiration and an increase during expiration, and considered characteristic of patients with pericardial tamponade;
- **alternating pulse**: characterised by an alternation in the intensity of the pulse (strong and weak). It can appear in cases of myocardial failure and some tachy-arrhythmias.

Bibliography

■ Buchanan, J.W. (1992) Causes and prevalence of cardiovascular disease. In: KirK, R.W., Bonagura, J.D. (eds) *Current Veterinary Therapy XI*. Philadelphia: WB Saunders, pp. 647–651.

■ Coté E., MacDonald K.A., Meurs, K.M., et al. (2011) *Feline cardiology*. Ames (USA): Wiley-Blackwell.

■ Darke, P.G., Bonagura, J.D., Kelly, D.F. (1996) *Color atlas of veterinary cardiology*. London: Mosby-Wolfe.

■ Gompf, R.E. History and Physical examination (2016) In: Smith, F.W.K., Tilley L.P., Oyama, M.A., et al. (eds.) *Manual of Canine and Feline Cardiology*. 5th Ed. St Louis: Elsevier, pp. 3–24.

■ Keene, B., Smith F., Tilley, L. et al. (2015) *Rapid interpretation of heart sounds, murmurs, arrhythmias and lung sounds: a guide to cardiac auscultation in dogs and cats.* 3rd ed. Philadelphia: Elsevier.

■ Schrope, D.P. (2015) Prevalence of congenital heart disease in 76,301 mixed-breed dogs and 57,025 mixed-breed cats. *J Vet Cardiol*, 17, 192–202.

Test

Answers on Page 62

1. **Which of the following is true regarding the prevalence of heart disease:**
   a. Primary dilated cardiomyopathy is the most. common heart disease in large breed dogs.
   b. Subaortic stenosis is very prevalent in French Bulldogs.
   c. In cats the most common congenital heart disease is pulmonary stenosis.
   d. None of the above.

2. **6-month-old West Highland White Terrier with grade IV/VI systolic murmur and point of maximum intensity on the left heart base. He is asymptomatic and there are no other abnormalities on physical examination. What would be the most likely cardiopathy?**
   a. Pulmonary stenosis.
   b. Tetralogy of Fallot.
   c. Subaortic stenosis.
   d. Mitral dysplasia.

3. **Jugular distension without pulsation may suggest:**
   a. Severe pulmonary stenosis.
   b. Pericardial tamponade.
   c. Mitral dysplasia.
   d. Pulmonary hypertension.

4. **Which of the following clinical signs are not common in cats with hypertrophic cardiomyopathy:**
   a. Cough.
   b. Exercise intolerance.
   c. Respiratory distress.
   d. Orthopnoeic posture.

5. **Pulmonary crepitations suggest the presence of which of the following:**
   a. Pleural effusion.
   b. Tracheal collapse.
   c. Pulmonary fibrosis.
   d. Pneumomediastinum.

6. **A dog with a lower pulse than heart rate suggests:**
   a. Presence of symptomatic bradycardia.
   b. Wandering pacemaker.
   c. Pulmonary thromboembolism.
   d. Atrial fibrillation.

Notes

Correct Answers:

1. a
2. a
3. b
4. a
5. c
6. d

Notes

Introduction to Thoracic Radiography

Gemma Fraga Veloso

Radiography is a very helpful tool which can be used to assess thoracic structures. Its main advantages include its **wide availability** in veterinary clinics, **low cost**, the ease with which radiographs can be obtained, due to the fact it is a **non-invasive** technique and, that in most patients, it does not require anaesthesia.

Although obtaining radiographs is relatively simple, in order to achieve high quality results (diagnostic quality), using an optimised technique to provide the maximum information possible is necessary. **Poor quality radiographs limit interpretation** and, in many cases, mean a diagnosis cannot be reached and can even lead to an incorrect diagnosis.

Obtaining Good Quality Thoracic Radiographs

Preparation and Positioning of the Patient

Correct positioning of the patient and keeping them still is key in order to obtain **good quality** radiographs. Radiographs can be attempted while the patient is conscious, using materials such as sandbags to hold them in position. However, sedation or even anaesthesia is sometimes necessary, since even slight movement can affect the quality of radiographs. In addition, the use of sedation **decreases the operator's exposure to radiation**. In situations where one or more operators have to restrain a patient because the patient is not keeping still and/or sedation is not possible, they should always be protected from radiation with the **appropriate protective equipment** (lead aprons, gloves and thyroid protectors).

Materials such as sandbags, wedges, and ropes can be used to achieve correct patient positioning. When taking lateral projections, the animal is placed in lateral recumbency and sandbags are used to support the neck. The front limbs should be stretched forward, and these can be secured with sandbags or tied with ropes to keep them extended, **avoiding overlap on the cranial part of the thorax**. To prevent the animal from getting up, putting weight on the back third of the patient is necessary; sandbags can also be used for this purpose. The head and neck should be extended. The **sternum and thoracic vertebrae should be level**, for this, wedges can be used under the sternum that will level the sternum with the vertebrae in most thoracic conformations found in dogs and cats.

Dorsoventral (DV) projections are preferred over ventrodorsal (VD) projections in most situations. When DV projections are performed, the patient is positioned sternally, with the elbows to the sides of the thorax stretching the front legs forward with the hindlegs flexed under the patient or stretched backwards. The spine and sternum should be aligned/overlapping, and the neck extended (wedges or pads can be used under the patient's head to make it more comfortable). To restrain the patient, a sandbag can be placed over the neck.

Technique for Obtaining Thoracic Radiographs

The exposure parameters necessary to obtain quality thoracic radiographs include a **high kilovoltage (kV) and a low milliamperage per second (mAs)**. To obtain a low mAs a high milliamperage (mA) and a short exposure time can be used. The main reason for using a lower mAs is to limit the exposure time and **avoid motion artefacts** caused by respiration.

It is very important to **centre and collimate the field to be radiographed**, in this way scattered radiation can be limited. In addition, **grids** should be used in patients with a thoracic thickness greater than 10 cm to reduce the effects of scattered radiation. The collimated area should include the entrance to the thorax and the entire diaphragm. Lateral projections should include the spine dorsally and the sternum ventrally, and the radiation beam should be centred on the caudal borders of the scapulae. VD or DV views should include the lateral borders of the thorax, that is, the ribs and thoracic wall, and the beam should be centred between the shoulders. A **radiopaque marker should always be used to indicate right or left** within the collimated area.

Whenever possible, thoracic radiographs **should be performed at the end of inspiration** as this is when the lung is well ventilated. When radiographs are obtained during the expiratory phase, the lung is not fully inflated, and pulmonary opacities that can be mistaken for pathological infiltrations may be seen. On the other hand, in certain studies, the combined use of inspiratory and expiratory views can help to assess dynamic changes in the lung and/or trachea.

Radiographic Views

A complete thoracic study **ideally includes three projections (two lateral and one VD or DV)**, although there are situations in which two orthogonal views may be sufficient (to evaluate most cardiac pathologies, for example).

A single view is insufficient to evaluate the thorax and can lead to incomplete or misdiagnosis.

Introduction to the Interpretation of Thoracic Radiographs

When interpreting thoracic radiographs, it is important to **follow a specific order**, to perform a systematic evaluation. The chosen order does not matter, but it is important to always follow the same order so as not to forget to evaluate any structures.

An adequate interpretation of the thorax should include assessment of the following structures:

- surrounding soft tissues
- bones (ribs, vertebrae, sternum)
- cranial abdomen and diaphragm
- neck
- pleural space
- mediastinum
- trachea including the carina
- bronchi
- cardiac silhouette
- aorta
- caudal vena cava
- pulmonary vasculature
- lung field.

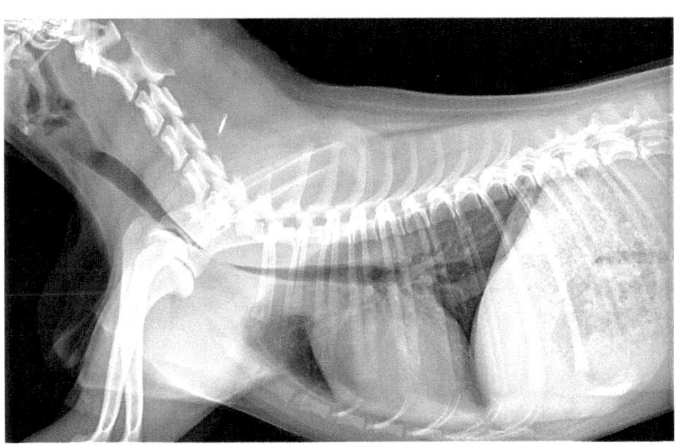

Figure 1. Left lateral thoracic radiograph of a dog which shows cervical tracheal collapse at the entrance to the thorax.

Evaluation of the Airways, Lung Field, Pleural Space and Mediastinum

Trachea

The trachea is a **semi-rigid** air-filled tube that connects the larynx to the bronchi. Caudally, the trachea ends with its bifurcation at the carina. In dogs and cats, the carina should be level with the fourth or fifth intercostal space. The trachea is made up of cartilaginous rings that are open dorsally and are connected by the *trachealis* muscle and connective tissue.

The normal diameter of the trachea varies depending on the species and breed. The **ratio between the diameter of the trachea and the entrance to the thorax** is considered an objective method to evaluate its size. Normal values are:

- brachiocephalic breeds: 0.16 ± 0.03 (0.11 ± 0.03 in Bulldogs)
- non-brachiocephalic breeds: 0.21 ± 0.03.

Under normal conditions, the **diameter of the trachea should not vary significantly during the different respiratory phases**. However, its diameter can vary between expiration and inspiration in patients with tracheal collapse (Figure 1). It is important to remember that dynamic collapses of the trachea and bronchi may not be detected on thoracic radiography (for this, the use of fluoroscopy and/or bronchoscopy is recommended).

When there is persistence of the fourth right aortic arch, ventral and left deviation of the trachea has been described. Assessing for abnormal tracheal deviations, intratracheal masses, foreign bodies, or tracheal lacerations/rupture is also important.

Bronchial Tree

The bronchial tree begins after the bifurcation of the trachea into the left and right main bronchi and continues to branch into the lobar bronchi, segmental bronchi, and bronchioles.

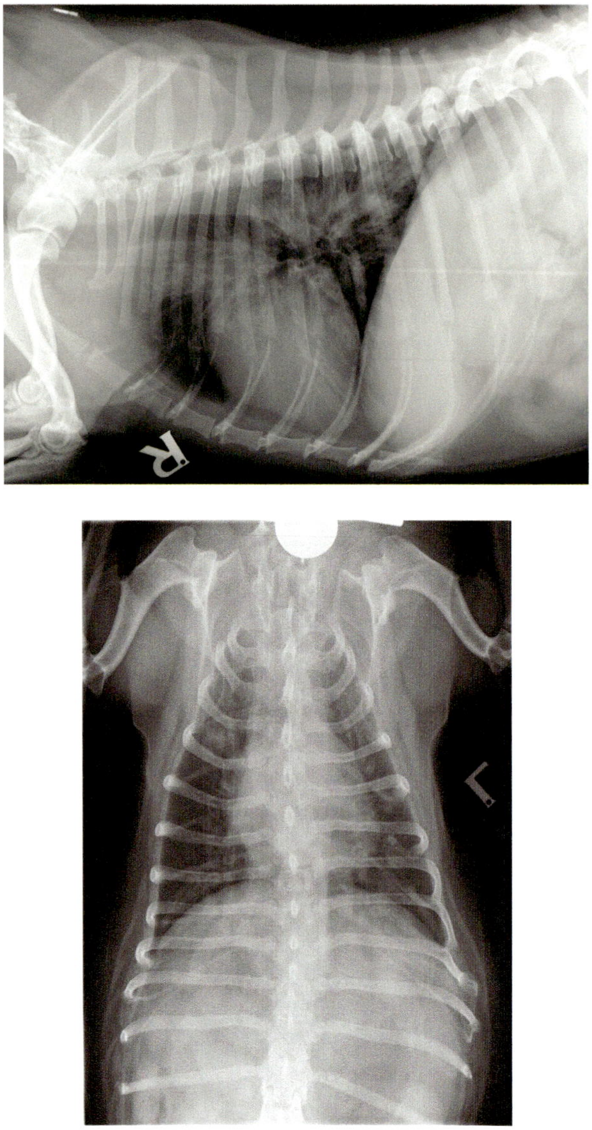

Figure 2. Right lateral and dorsoventral thoracic radiographs of a dog showing a bronchial pattern.

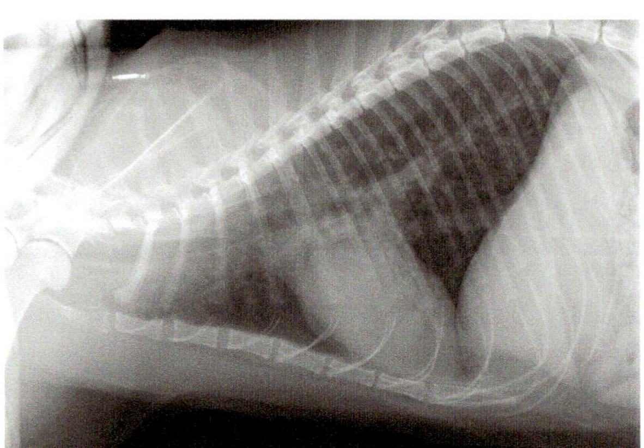

Figure 3. Right lateral thoracic radiograph of a cat with feline asthma where a diffuse bronchial pattern can be seen.

Under normal conditions, the walls of the bronchi are not usually seen radiographically (only the large bronchi in the hilar region). However, these become visible when their walls are thickened or calcified, giving rise to a bronchial pattern. When there is a **bronchial pattern**, the bronchi are seen as "train rails" on a longitudinal axis or "donuts" when they are transected on a transverse axis (Figures 2 and 3). The causes of a bronchial pattern include thickening of the walls of the bronchi, excessive mineralization of these and/or bronchiectasis. It can be seen in **inflammatory conditions** such as chronic bronchitis in dogs and asthma in cats (Figure 3), **infectious conditions** (bacterial, viral, parasitic bronchitis) or **neoplastic ones** (such as bronchogenic carcinoma).

It is important to note that the **severity of clinical signs in animals with chronic bronchitis does not always correlate with radiographic signs**, radiographs can even be normal in dogs with chronic bronchitis.

Pulmonary Parenchyma

Cats and dogs have two lungs (right and left) that are neither symmetrical in size nor in their division into pulmonary lobes. The left lung has two lobes: cranial and caudal. In turn, the left cranial lobe is subdivided into cranial and caudal segments. The right lung has four lobes: cranial, middle, caudal, and accessory.

The lung field is one of the most difficult areas to interpret radiographically. The following steps should be taken when radiographic abnormalities in the lung field are identified and a list of differential diagnoses is generated:

- location and extent of the lesion/s
- identification of the pulmonary pattern present
- correlation of changes in lung opacity and volume with the phase of respiration
- consider the species, age, breed, and clinical signs in the patient.

Lung Patterns

Alveolar Pattern

Increased opacity in the alveolar space occurs when the alveoli are completely collapsed or when they are filled with fluid (blood, oedema) or soft tissue material (inflammatory, neoplastic cells).

Radiographic characteristics of an alveolar pattern include (Figure 4):

- homogeneous soft tissue opacity
- inability to differentiate (obliteration) other adjacent soft tissue structures or fluid
- possible presence of air bronchograms when the bronchi are filled with air.

The most common causes of the alveolar pattern include pathologies such as cardiogenic and non-cardiogenic pulmonary oedema, pneumonia, pulmonary haemorrhage, and neoplasms.

Bronchial Pattern

See previous "Bronchial tree" section.

Vascular Pattern

When a vascular pattern is present, the **vessels** are seen as radiopaque bands on a longitudinal axis, however, when they appear on a transverse axis they can be seen as circular or nodular structures. This pattern occurs when there is **distention of the pulmonary vessels** (arteries, veins, or both).

Interstitial Pattern

This pattern is seen when there is an increase in lung opacity caused by **changes in the pulmonary interstitium**. It can be classified as either:

- **structured interstitial pattern (nodular or miliary)** (Figures 5 and 6), caused by well-differentiated interstitial lesions (metastatic neoplasia, granulomatous disease, primary miliary neoplasia). In the nodular interstitial pattern, nodules of soft tissue density are observed in the lung field (Figure 6). Radiographic visualization of soft tissue nodules depends on their size: the minimum diameter that allows a single nodule to be visualised is 3–5 mm, so nodules smaller than this cannot be detected radiographically;
- **unstructured interstitial pattern** (Figure 7), caused by diffuse inflammation of the interstitial tissue (interstitial oedema, fibrosis, diffuse infiltrative neoplasia, mineralization) and may also be visible when the lungs are not fully inflated (expiratory radiographs). An unstructured interstitial pattern is seen as a diffuse increase in lung opacity. The pulmonary vessels are still visible when there is an interstitial pattern. It is common for an interstitial component to exist along with other patterns (mixed patterns).

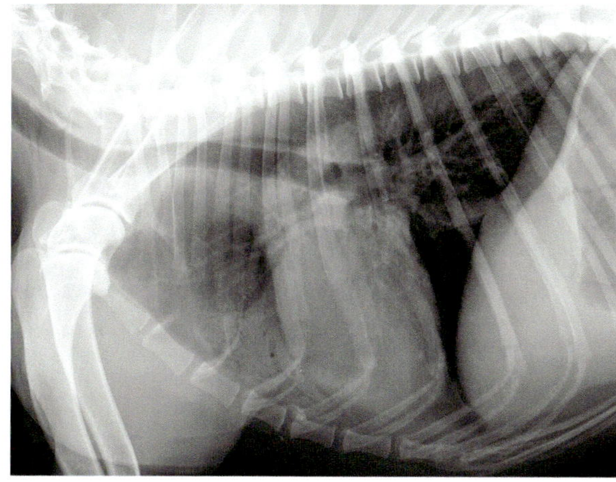

Figure 4. Right lateral thoracic radiograph: air bronchograms (alveolar pattern) in the cranial ventral lung field can be seen in a dog with aspiration pneumonia.

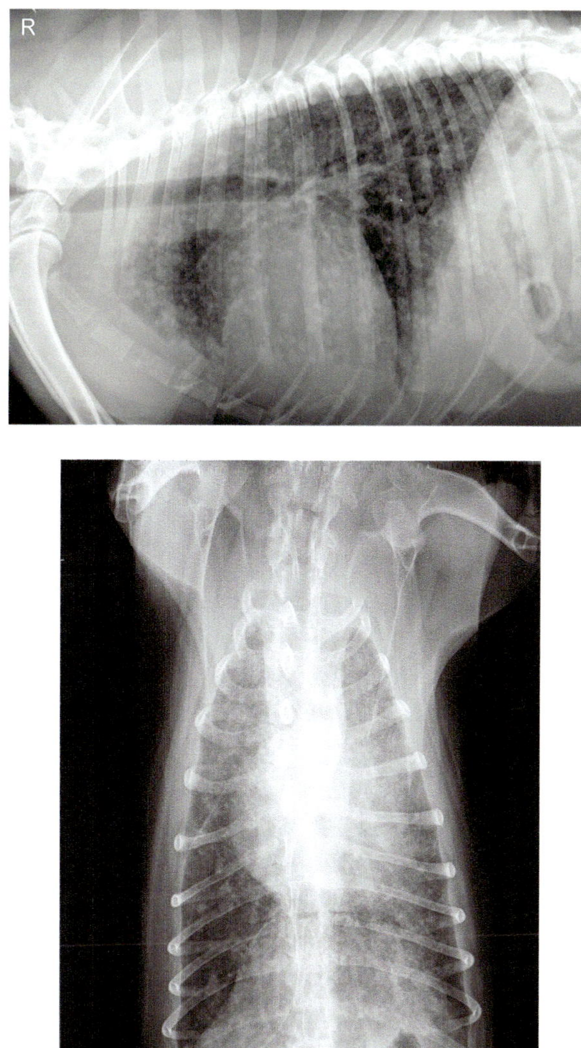

Figure 5. Right lateral and dorso-ventral thoracic radiographs which show a miliary interstitial pattern in a dog with pulmonary metastasis.

Pleural Space

The pleural membrane is made up of a layer of mesothelial cells located on a layer of connective tissue that contains blood and lymphatic vessels. It can be divided into a **parietal pleura** (lining the inner part of the thoracic wall and the diaphragm, including the great vessels, heart and oesophagus to form the mediastinum) and a **visceral pleura** (lining the lungs), leaving a space between them (pleural space) which normally contains a small amount of fluid (2–3 ml). This fluid has a lubricating function, reducing the friction that exists during breathing. The **pleural space has a negative pressure** that allows the lungs and minor airways to expand during breathing. Production of pleural fluid is continuous, and its drainage system is essential to prevent it from accumulating.

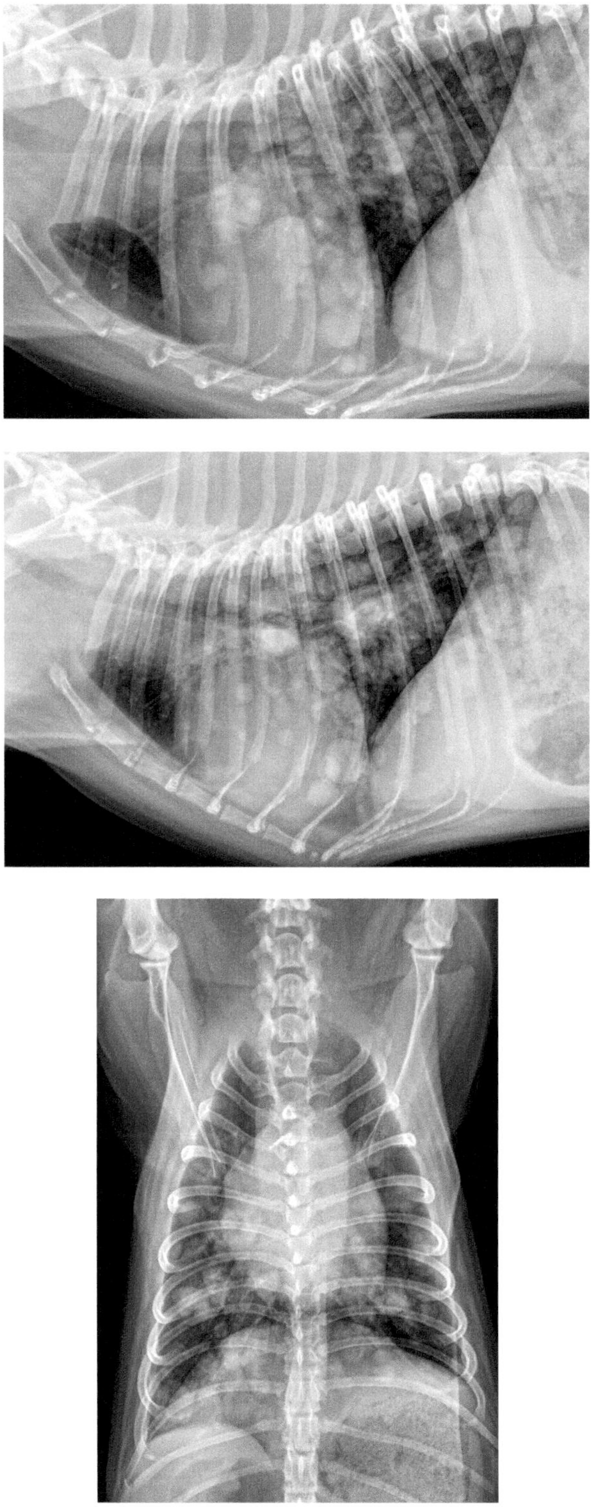

Figure 6. Right and left lateral and ventrodorsal thoracic radiographs of a dog where a nodular lung pattern caused by pulmonary metastasis can be seen.

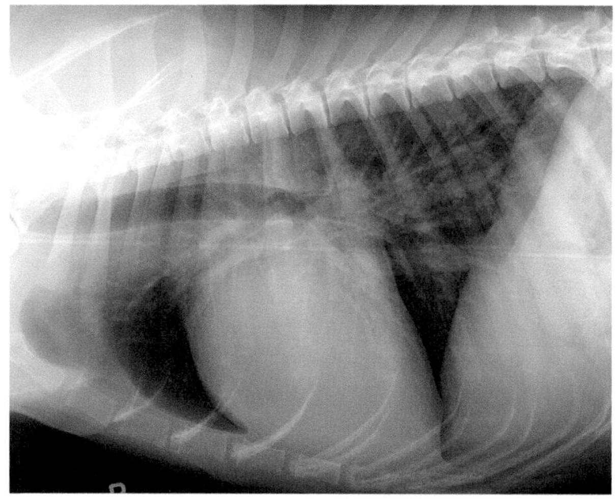

Figure 7. Right lateral thoracic radiograph of a dog where an interstitial pattern can be seen in the dorso-caudal field.

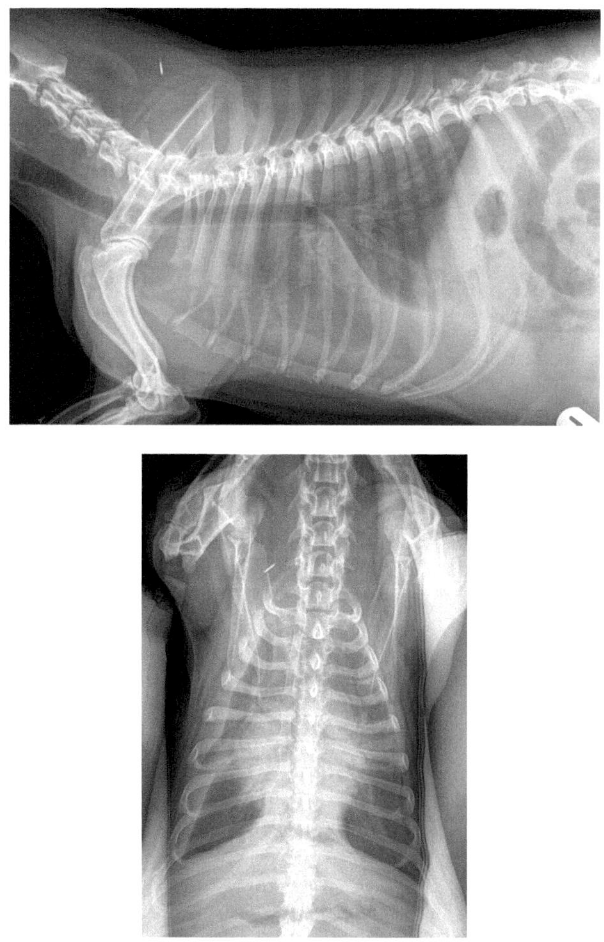

Figure 8. Right lateral and ventrodorsal thoracic radiographs of a dog with pleural effusion. An increase in the opacity of the pleural space (soft tissue/fluid density) can be appreciated, as well as the presence of interlobar fissures with retraction of the lung from the costal wall and obscuring of the cardiac silhouette.

In small animals, the **parietal pleura receives blood from the systemic circulation** (left heart), while the **visceral pleura receives it from the pulmonary circulation** (right heart). Pleural fluid moves from the capillaries of the parietal pleura to the pleural space and from here it is absorbed by the capillaries of the visceral pleura and by the lymphatic vessels of the visceral and diaphragmatic pleura. Cats have a different pleural drainage system to dogs and humans, which predisposes them to pleural effusions when they suffer from left-sided heart failure.

Certain pathological conditions may cause an **accumulation of fluid (pleural effusion) or air (pneumothorax) in the pleural space**. Depending on the volume accumulated, the clinical signs can vary from an asymptomatic condition to severe respiratory distress, manifesting with a restrictive respiratory pattern.

Pleural fluid can be classified as **transudate (pure or modified) or exudate (septic, aseptic, blood, chyle, pseudochyle)**. This classification is very important as it allows a list of differential diagnoses to be formulated for each type of fluid, thus guiding the clinician towards the most appropriate diagnostic tests in order to reach a diagnosis (Table 1).

Table 1. Types of pleural effusion and most common differential diagnoses.

Type of effusion	Most common differential diagnoses
Air (pneumothorax)	· trauma · iatrogenic · spontaneous (pulmonary bullae or vesicle rupture, with or without underlying pulmonary disease)
Pure transudate	· hypalbuminaemia
Modified transudate	· right-sided heart failure (pericardial effusion, restrictive pericarditis, tricuspid regurgitation, dilated cardiomyopathy, pulmonary hypertension...) or left-sided (cats) · diaphragmatic hernia · neoplasia · lung lobe torsion
Aseptic exudate	· neoplasia · FIP · chronic lung lobe torsion · chronic chylothorax · fungal infection (USA) · pneumonia
Septic exudate (pyothorax)	· penetrating thoracic wounds · respiratory or migratory foreign body · oesophageal perforation · pneumonia/pulmonary abscess rupture · systemic bacterial infection · iatrogenic (surgery or thoracocentesis)
Blood (haemothorax)	· trauma · neoplasia · coagulopathy · lung lobe torsion
Chyle (chylothorax)	· right-sided heart failure (see modified transudate) or left-sided (cats) · neoplasia · lung lobe torsion · diaphragmatic hernia · dirofilariasis · fungal infection (USA) · thoracic duct lesions (rare) · idiopathic
Pseudochyle (psuedochylothorax)	· uncommon. Has been described associated with tuberculosis, although may also be caused by other conditions such as intrathoracic neoplasms.

Radiographic Signs of Pleural Effusion

Radiographic findings of pleural effusions include (Figure 8):
- increased opacity in the pleural space (soft tissue/fluid density)
- presence of interlobar fissures
- retraction of the lung from the costal wall
- blunting of the pulmonary margins around the costophrenic angle
- increased opacity in the lung field secondary to underinflation of the lungs and the effusion
- obscuring of the cardiac silhouette
- sometimes an elevation of the cardiac silhouette (± trachea) relative to the sternum (soft tissue density) can be seen in lateral projections.

Radiographic Signs of Pneumothorax

Radiographic findings include (Figure 9):
- reduced opacity surrounding the lungs, in this radiolucent space **no vessels or lung tissue are observed**
- elevation of the cardiac silhouette relative to the sternum in lateral projections (radiolucent density without vessels or lung tissue)
- retraction of the lung from the costal wall, diaphragm and spine
- collapsed pulmonary lobes
- additional radiographic signs of **tension pneumothorax** include:
  - rapid worsening of radiographic signs
  - severe collapse of the pulmonary lobe(s)
  - flattening of the diaphragm
  - overdistention of the thorax with widening of the intercostal spaces
  - contralateral displacement of the mediastinal structures in the case of unilateral tension pneumothorax.

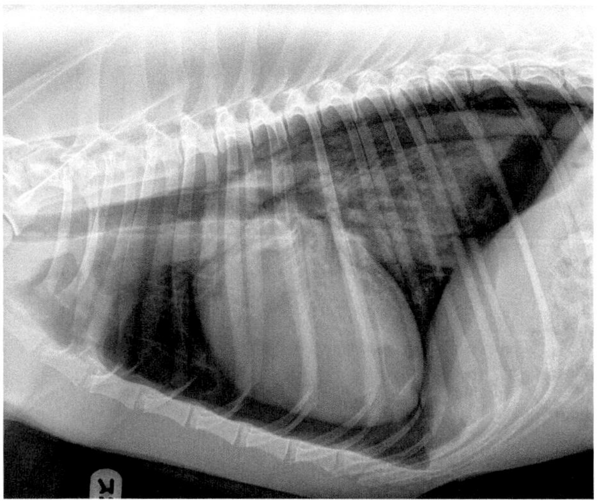

Figure 9. Right lateral thoracic radiograph of a dog with pneumothorax. Elevation of the cardiac silhouette relative to the sternum can be seen with a radiolucent space without vessels or pulmonary tissue ventral to the heart, retraction of the lung from the costal wall, diaphragm and spine, as well as collapse of the lung lobes.

Mediastinum

The mediastinum is the **space between the left and right pleural cavities** and contains all the structures located in the thoracic midline. The mediastinum continues cranially with the fasciae of the neck and caudally with the retroperitoneal space via the aortic hiatus.

The structures found in the mediastinum are the heart and great vessels, trachea, oesophagus, thoracic duct, nerves, lymph nodes, and thymus. All these structures which are found in the mediastinum (with the exception of the trachea and sometimes the oesophagus filled with air) are of soft tissue opacity, so under normal conditions the mediastinum appears as a **homogeneous structure** of soft tissue density and little contrast between adjacent structures.

In the **transverse plane** the mediastinum is divided into **cranial, middle** (contains the heart) and **caudal**, using the heart as a reference point. It is also divided dorsally and ventrally, using the carina as a reference point.

The **maximum thickness of the cranial mediastinum in dogs** in VD/DV views should not exceed **twice the width of the spine** at the same level. However, obese and brachiocephalic dogs tend to have more fat accumulation in this area and the thickness of the cranial mediastinum in these views can exceed twice the width of the spine even when mediastinal disease is not present. In **cats, the cranial mediastinum in VD/DV views should not exceed the width of the overlapping thoracic spine**.

To correctly evaluate the mediastinum, **two orthogonal projections of the thorax** are required. Lateral views allow evaluation of many of its structures, but mediastinal deviation cannot be assessed, VD/DV views allow evaluation of the position of the mediastinum and are more sensitive for detection of the presence of effusions and/or mediastinal masses.

There are mediastinal structures that are **not usually visible under normal conditions**. These include the cranial vena cava, brachiocephalic trunk, left subclavian artery, azygos vein, main pulmonary artery, vagus nerve, recurrent laryngeal nerve, phrenic nerve, thoracic duct, and tracheobronchial, cranial and sternal mediastinal lymph nodes. The sternal lymph node is located cranially and ventral to the heart and is responsible for draining the abdomen and thoracic wall. The mediastinal structures that are usually observed include the trachea and its bifurcation, heart, aorta, caudal vena cava, thymus in young animals and oesophagus, although the latter is not usually visible unless there is megaoesophagus (secondary to anaesthesia or pathological), aerophagia or an oesophageal foreign body.

Pneumomediastinum

Refers to the presence of **free gas in the mediastinum**. Depending on its cause, it can be accompanied by pneumothorax, subcutaneous emphysema and/or pneumoperitoneum. When pneumomediastinum and pneumothorax are present simultaneously, pneumomediastinum can be suspected as being the origin of the pneumothorax. However, the opposite is not possible.

Under normal conditions, most mediastinal structures are not distinguishable because they are all of soft tissue density. However, when there is a pneumomediastinum, the gas, which is observed as an increase in radiolucency, enhances the edges and mediastinal structures become visible (especially the aorta, oesophagus, cranial vessels and the wall of the trachea become visible) (Figure 10).

Mediastinal Masses

The most common mediastinal masses are located in the **cranial and perihilar mediastinum**. Radiographically, their appearance will depend on location and size.

If a mass is small, it may not be visible, since it is often obscured due to overlap with other structures of a similar opacity, although it may be suspected if widening of the cranial mediastinum is present. Larger masses can displace nearby or associated structures.

Border effacement of the cardiac silhouette can be present with cranial mediastinal masses (Figures 11 and 12),

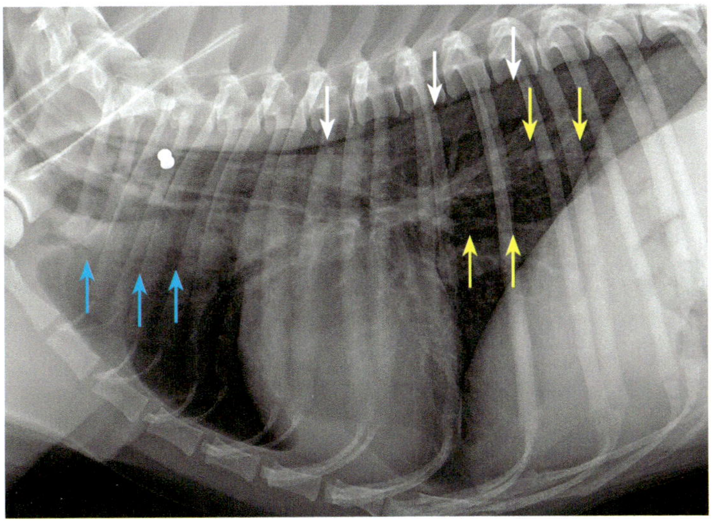

Figure 10. Left lateral thoracic radiograph of a dog with pneumomediastinum. Free gas can be seen in the mediastinum, which enhances the edges of the mediastinal structures making the wall of the trachea and cranial vena cava visible (blue arrows), as well as facilitating visualisation of the aorta (white arrows). An oesophagus which is mildly distended with air can also be appreciated (yellow arrows) and a metallic structure, which corresponds to a pellet at the level of the second rib (incidental finding).

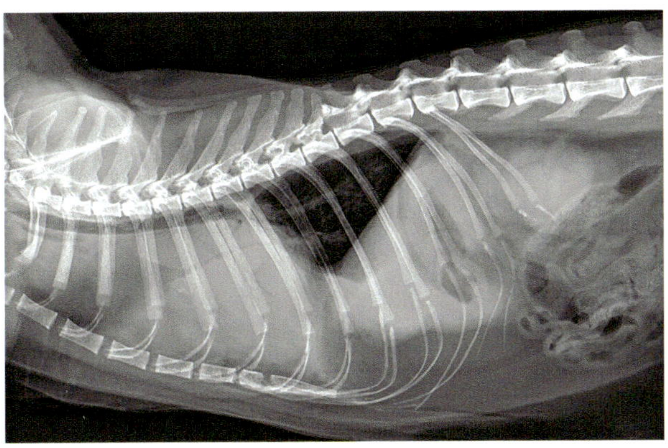

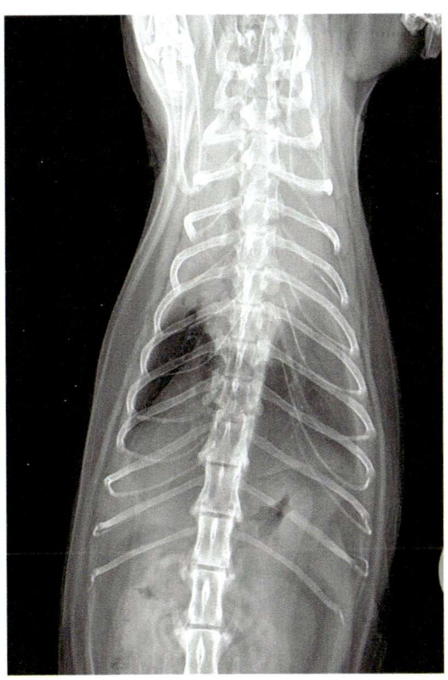

Figure 11. Lateral and dorsoventral thoracic radiographs showing a cranial mediastinal mass in a cat with lymphoma.

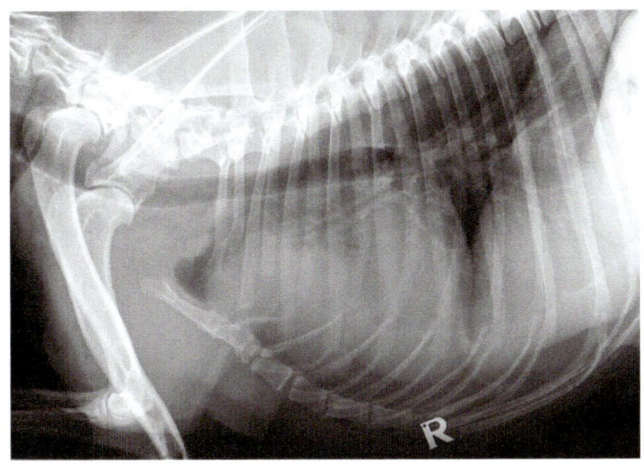

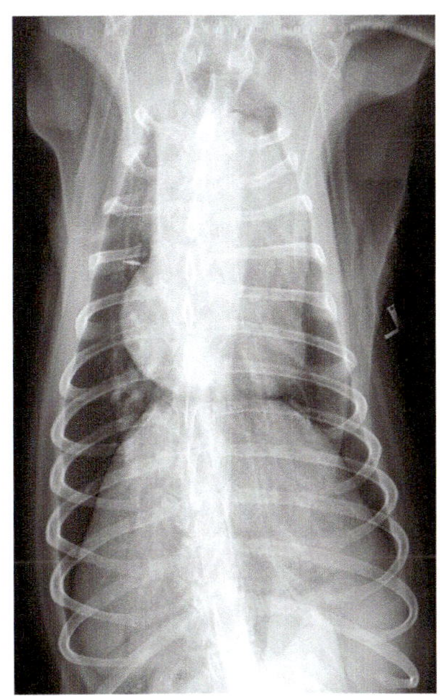

Figure 12. Right lateral and dorsoventral thoracic radiographs of a dog where a cranial mediastinal mass can be seen.

making it difficult to assess the heart. Occasionally, large masses can displace the trachea and push the heart caudally. The **location of the carina caudal to the sixth intercostal space in lateral views suggests the presence of a cranial mediastinal mass.**

DV views are most useful for differentiation of a mediastinal mass from a mass in the cranial lung lobes. Mediastinal masses can be associated with mediastinal and/or pleural effusion.

Mediastinal Cysts

Seen in cats and **less frequently in dogs**. Cysts can be pleural, thymic, lymphatic, bronchogenic, or neoplastic. They are usually a benign, incidental finding.

Idiopathic mediastinal cysts are **relatively common in cats**. They usually present as solitary cysts in the cranioventral mediastinum. If they are not very large and do not compress structures, they are **usually benign and asymptomatic**. Ultrasound is a very useful technique for differentiation of cysts from solid mediastinal masses.

Bony Structures and Thoracic Conformation

Thoracic radiography also allows us to evaluate bony structures and thoracic conformation. Pathologies worth highlighting include:

- rib fractures
- presence of spondylosis
- hemivertebrae (especially in Bulldogs)
- *pectus excavatum/pectus carinatum*.

Evaluation of the Cardiovascular System and Interpretation of Thoracic Radiography in Cardiac Pathologies

Thoracic radiography is a **very useful** instrument for the **diagnosis and monitoring of heart diseases**. It allows position and size of the cardiac silhouette, as well as the great vessels, vasculature and pulmonary parenchyma to be assessed. Knowledge and understanding of thoracic anatomy is essential to be able to interpret radiographs correctly and to get the most out of this diagnostic technique.

The main points to consider when interpreting thoracic radiographs are:

- recognition and observation of all the thoracic structures and surrounding tissues
- detection of anomalies (if they exist) in these structures
- interpretation of the radiological data obtained, together with the clinical history and physical examination, in order to reach a diagnosis.

Evaluation of Heart Size

There are several factors that can alter the radiographical appearance of the heart:

- positioning of the animal
- breed (mainly in dogs)
- age
- pericardial fat
- respiratory phase
- phase of the cardiac cycle.

Therefore, it is essential that the clinician is aware of them to avoid making mistakes when interpreting radiographs. The appearance of the **cardiac silhouette can vary** between right and left lateral views, as well as between DV and VD views, and this should be taken into account when interpreting a thoracic radiograph.

When it comes to assessing the size of the heart, there are differences between species. Below, some general rules are described that allow the size of the cardiac silhouette in dogs and cats to be assessed.

Evaluation of Heart Size in the Dog

It is important to note that the cardiac silhouette will **vary significantly in shape and size between different breeds of dog**, and this should always be taken into account when interpreting a thoracic radiograph. For example, breeds such as the Bulldog and Dachshund have larger hearts in lateral views, but this should not be confused with the presence of cardiomegaly.

In the **lateral view, the heart should be less than 2.5–3.5 intercostal spaces (wide) and two thirds the height of the thorax (long)**.

Another way to assess cardiac size in lateral views is by calculating the **Buchanan index, vertebral cardiac index, or vertebral heart score (VHS)**. The VHS is calculated taking into account the **length and width of the cardiac silhouette**, using the thoracic spine from the T4 vertebra to obtain a measurement that estimates global cardiac size. To obtain this index, the following steps should be followed (Figure 13).

- Measure the length of the heart: to do this, take the distance from the ventral aspect of the carina to the cardiac apex.
- Measure the width of the heart: draw a line perpendicular to the one drawn to obtain the length of the heart at the point of maximum width of the cardiac silhouette.
- Draw these 2 lines parallel to the vertebral column, taking the cranial edge of the fourth thoracic vertebra (T4) as a starting point, and count the vertebral bodies that each of these lines occupy.
- To obtain the VHS, the vertebral bodies that occupy each of these two lines must be added together.

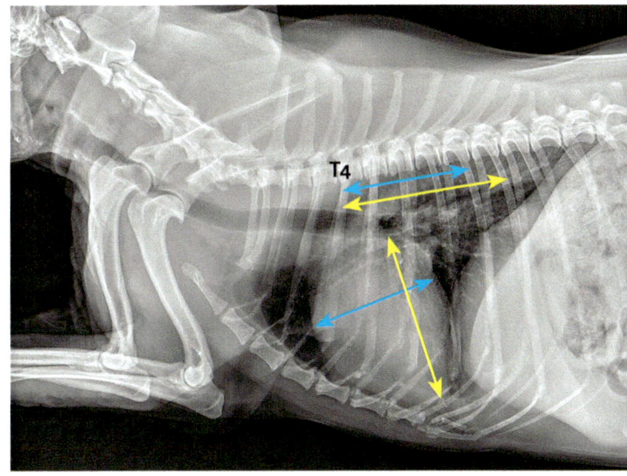

Figure 13. Right lateral thoracic radiograph of a normal dog showing how the VHS can be measured. The yellow line represents the length of the cardiac silhouette and the blue line its width. T4: fourth thoracic vertebra.

In **dogs, the VHS has a normal mean value of 9.7 ± 0.5 vertebrae (v) with a reference range of 8.5–10.5 v**, although this value varies between breeds (Table 2). Therefore, in the event that there is a specific reference value for a breed, this is the one that should be used to assess the size of the cardiac silhouette.

In the DV view the cardiac silhouette should not exceed 60–65% of the width of the rib cage and in the VD view the maximum width of the cardiac silhouette should not exceed two thirds of the width of the thorax.

Table 2. VHS values specific to some dog breeds.

Breed	VHS
Boxer	11.6 ± 0.8 v
Cavalier King Charles Spaniel	10.6 ± 0.5 v
Doberman	10.0 ± 0.6 v
German Shepherd	9.7 ± 0.7 v
Labrador Retriever	10.8 ± 0.6 v
Yorkshire Terrier	9.7 ± 0.5 v
Whippet	11.0 ± 0.5 v
Beagle	9.9–10.7 v
Greyhound	10.4–10.6 v
Kangal (Turkish Shepherd)	9.03–10.37 v

Evaluation of Heart Size in the Cat

In the lateral view, the cardiac silhouette should be **less than 2.0–2.5 intercostal spaces wide**. As in dogs, cardiac size can also be assessed by calculating the VHS in the lateral view, following the same methodology described in dogs. In cats, the **VHS reference range which is considered normal is 7.5 ± 0.3 v** and when there is a VHS greater than 8.0 v it is considered compatible with the presence of cardiomegaly.

Evaluation and Identification of the Cardiac Chambers

Thoracic radiographs can only assess the contours of the heart and great vessels, but not their contents or function. By using the **clock analogy**, it is possible to locate the projection areas of the cardiac chambers and great vessels. This analogy can be used in both lateral and DV views. Below is a description of the clock analogy in the various cardiac views:

- **lateral view** (Figure 14):
  - 12–2 o'clock: left atrium (LA)
  - 2–5 o'clock: left ventricle (LV)
  - 5–9 o'clock: right ventricle (RV)
  - 9–10 o'clock: pulmonary trunk and right atrium
  - 10–11 o'clock: aortic arch
- **DV view** (Figure 15):
  - 11–1 o'clock: aortic arch
  - 1–2 o'clock: pulmonary trunk
  - 2–3 o'clock: left atrial appendage (LAA)
  - 3–5 o'clock: left ventricle (LV)
  - 5–9 o'clock: right ventricle (RV)
  - 9–11 o'clock: right atrium (RA).

It is important to note that in the DV view, the body of the left atrium (LA) is located caudal to the carina, between the left and right main bronchus (Figure 16).

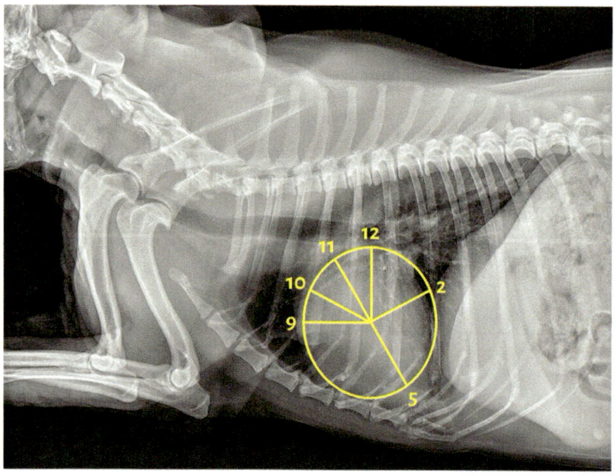

Figure 14. Right lateral view of a normal canine thorax with the clock analogy superimposed for the localisation of cardiac chambers and great vessels.

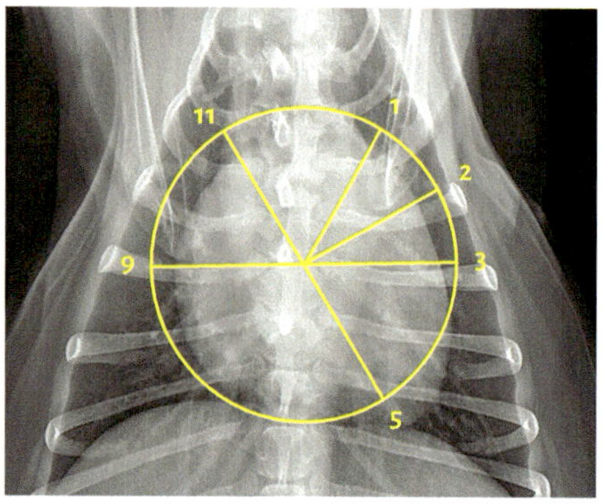

Figure 15. Dorsoventral view of a normal canine thorax with the clock analogy superimposed for the localisation of cardiac chambers and great vessels.

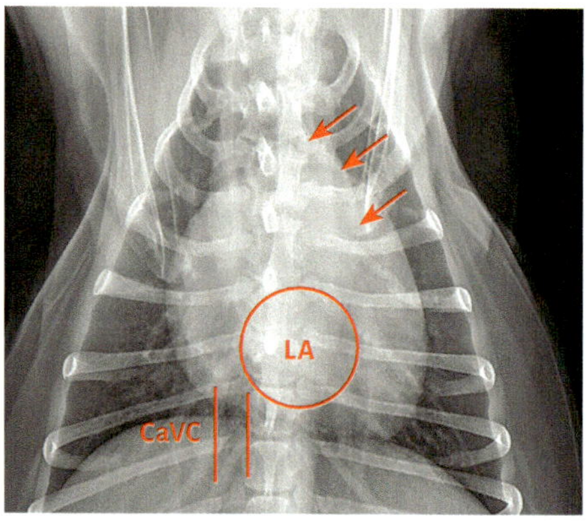

Figure 16. Dorsoventral view of a normal canine thorax. The red arrows indicate the location of the aortic arch and descending aorta. LA: left atrium. CaVC: caudal vena cava.

Evaluation of the Great Vessels

Aorta

The aorta is divided into three sections:

- **ascending aorta** (exits the LV)
- **aortic arch** (exits the brachiocephalic trunk, left subclavian artery)
- **descending aorta** (thoracic and abdominal portion).

In lateral views of the thorax, the ascending aorta overlaps the RA and the heart base, making it difficult to distinguish radiographically. In the DV view, it is at the 11–1 o'clock position, and it is often easier to identify radiographic changes (Figure 16).

The diameter of the aorta must be compared with the height of the vertebral bodies and is not affected by changes in systemic pressure or intravascular volume.

The **most common pathologies that produce radiographically visible changes** are aortic/subaortic stenosis (poststenotic dilation), patent *ductus arteriosus*, aneurysms, systemic hypertension, coarctation of the aorta and redundant aorta (dilatation of the aortic outlet, not considered pathological in old cats).

Caudal Vena Cava

Receives blood from the abdomen, pelvic area, and hindlimbs. It enters the thorax through the diaphragm on the right side and enters the RA dorsal to the coronary sinus (Figures 16

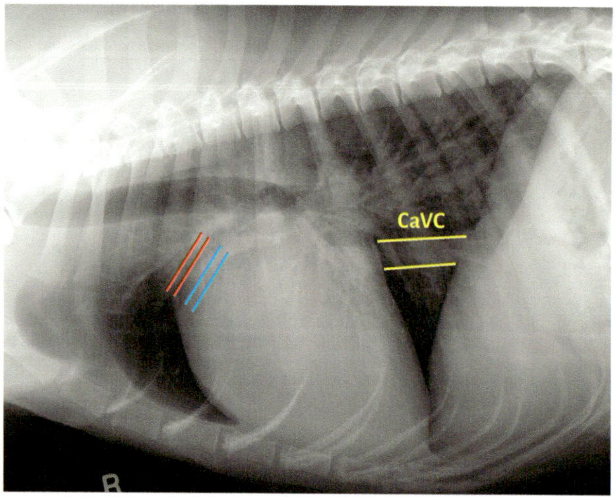

Figure 17. Right lateral thoracic view in a dog. The red lines delineate the cranial pulmonary lobar artery and the blue lines the cranial pulmonary lobar vein. The yellow lines delineate the contour of the caudal vena cava. CaVC: caudal vena cava.

and 17). Its **diameter varies in non-pathological conditions** with intrathoracic pressure changes that occur during respiration and this depends on the timing in the cardiac cycle.

Pathological conditions that can produce a change in its diameter include: right-sided heart failure, hypovolaemia (dehydration, *shock*, hypoadrenocorticism) and obstructive lesions (thrombi, masses, stenosis).

When the diameter of the caudal vena cava **exceeds 1.5 times that of the descending aorta**, it is highly suggestive of a pathological dilation of this vessel.

Cranial Vena Cava

This vessel receives blood from the head, neck, thoracic wall, and forelimbs. It crosses the cranial mediastinum and receives blood from the costocervical, internal thoracic, and azygos veins, before entering the RA. Under normal conditions it is not visible and **can only be visualised when there is pneumomediastinum**.

Main Pulmonary Artery (pulmonary trunk)

The pulmonary artery originates from the RV, running caudally and bifurcating into the left and right main branches at the root of the aorta. In lateral views it is difficult to visualize due to its superposition over the heart, although in the DV view, at the 1–2 o'clock position using the clock analogy, its outflow tract and ramifications can be assessed (Figures 18 and 19).

The most common cardiac **pathologies** that produce radiologically visible changes at this level are pulmonary stenosis (poststenotic dilation), patent *ductus arteriosus*, pulmonary hypertension, and parasitic diseases caused by *Dirofilaria* or *Angiostrongylus*.

Radiological Signs of Cardiomegaly and Enlargement of the Great Vessels

Enlargement of one or more chambers of the heart, or of the great vessels, may be suspected when thoracic radiographs show an enlarged heart or bulges in the cardiac silhouette.

Overall Cardiomegaly

As mentioned in previous sections, the appearance of an enlarged cardiac silhouette can be normal in certain breeds of dogs and, therefore, it is important that this factor be taken into account when assessing for cardiomegaly. In addition, the presence of **excess pericardial fat can also cause the size of the cardiac silhouette to be overestimated**. Radiographically, overall cardiomegaly is observed as a **general increase in the size of the cardiac silhouette**. It is usually due to the simultaneous enlargement of several cardiac chambers or the presence of pericardial effusion.

There are certain findings that can help differentiate between cardiomegaly caused by dilation of the cardiac chambers or the presence of a pericardial effusion. Firstly, in the event of an **enlarged cardiac chamber**, bulges can normally be identified in the cardiac silhouette in the area of projection of

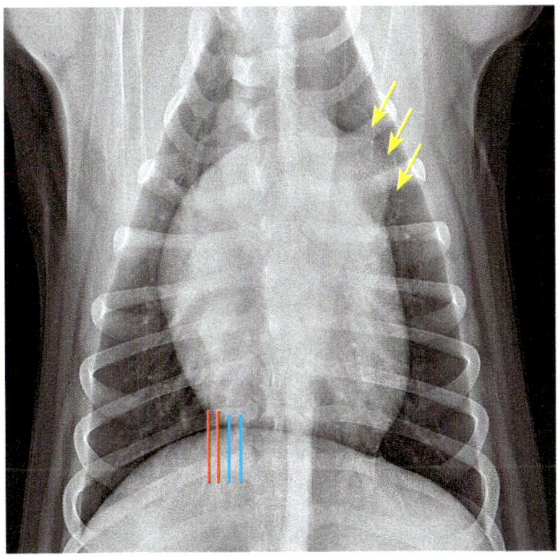

Figure 18. Dorsoventral thoracic radiograph of a dog where a bulge is seen in the projection area of the pulmonary artery (yellow arrows). The red and blue lines delineate the right caudal pulmonary lobar artery and vein respectively.

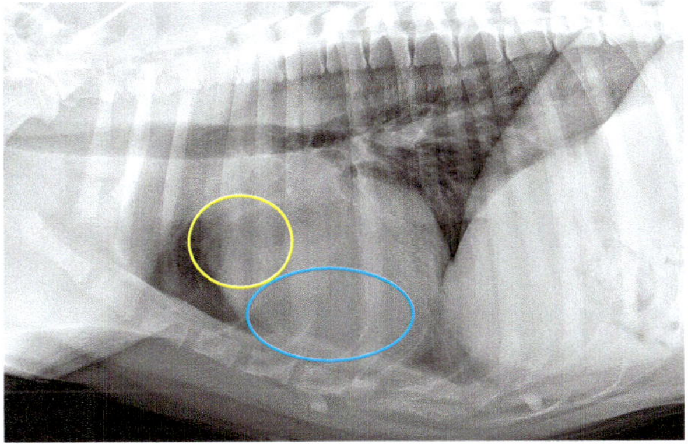

Figure 19. Left lateral thoracic radiograph of a dog with severe pulmonic stenosis. The yellow circle shows a bulge in the area of projection of the main pulmonary artery. The blue circle shows enlargement of the right ventricle with a bulge in its area of projection and increased sternal contact of the cardiac silhouette.

these chambers (clock analogy), while **pericardial effusion** usually causes a widespread enlargement of the cardiac silhouette, resulting in a globoid heart shape without bulges which can be identified in any particular area of the silhouette (Figure 20).

In addition, evaluation of the size of the pulmonary lobar vessels can also help differentiate between these two conditions, since in the case of a pericardial effusion with cardiac tamponade, they are usually small in size (hypoperfusion of the lung) due to the reduction in cardiac output, while when cardiomegaly is due to the enlargement of cardiac chambers and there is an elevation of pressures on the left side of the heart, these vessels may be congested and appear dilated on thoracic X-rays.

Left Atrial Dilation

The **most common causes** of enlargement of this chamber include:

- mitral valve regurgitation (degenerative mitral valve disease, dilated cardiomyopathy, mitral valve dysplasia, endocarditis)
- left to right shunts (patent *ductus arteriosus*, ventricular septal defect, aortopulmonary window)
- left ventricular pressure overload (systemic hypertension, aortic/subaortic stenosis)
- dilated cardiomyopathy
- feline cardiomyopathies.

The **radiographic signs** that indicate the presence of left atrial enlargement on the different projections are as follows:

- lateral projection (Figure 21):
    - bulging at the 12–2 o'clock position (clock analogy) of the cardiac silhouette
    - loss of the curvature of the caudodorsal margin of the cardiac silhouette
    - loss of the caudal "cardiac waist"
    - elevation of the caudal part of the trachea, which appears parallel to the spine
    - elevation of the left main bronchus
- DV projection (Figure 22):
    - bulging of the cardiac silhouette at the 2–3 o'clock position of the clock analogy (enlarged LAA)
    - lateral displacement of the main bronchi caudal to the carina ("cowboy sign").

Left Ventricular Enlargement

The most common causes of enlargement in this chamber are similar to those that cause left atrial dilation. In addition, left ventricular dilation is usually accompanied by an enlarged left atrium.

Radiographic findings suggestive of left ventricular enlargement in different views of the thorax include:

- lateral projection (Figure 21):
    - rounding of the caudal border of the heart (bulging of the cardiac silhouette at the 2–5 o'clock position) with an increase in contact with the diaphragm
    - elevation of the trachea and displacement of the normal position of the carina
    - increased angle formed by the caudal vena cava and the heart, appearing horizontal or even elevated

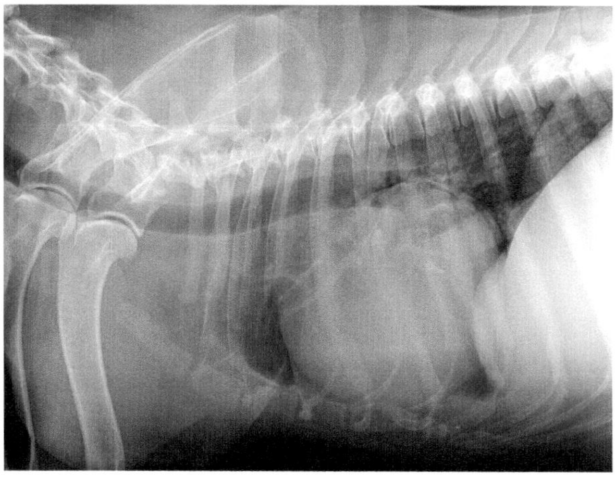

Figure 20. Left lateral thoracic radiograph of a dog with pericardial effusion. The heart has a rounded shape, with no appreciable bulges in the cardiac silhouette, which could suggest the presence of swelling in a particular cardiac chamber. In addition, the cranial pulmonary lobar vessels show a reduction in diameter.

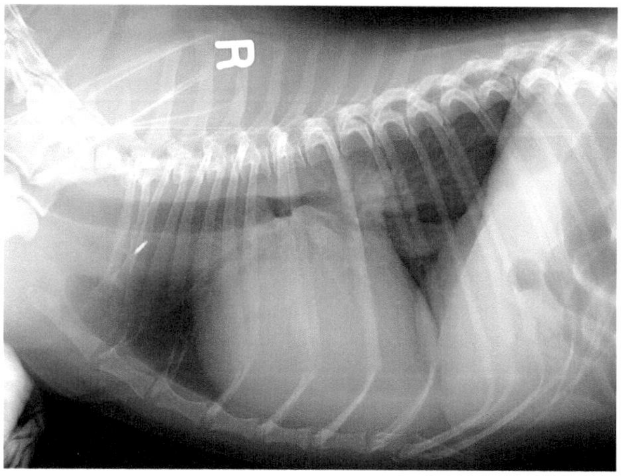

Figure 21. Right lateral thoracic radiograph of a dog with degenerative mitral valve disease where left atrial and ventricular enlargement can be seen. Elevation of the trachea can be appreciated, with a bulge in the area of projection of the left atrium, loss of the caudal cardiac waist and elevation of the main left bronchus.

- DV projection (Figure 22):
    - bulging of the cardiac silhouette at the 3–5 o'clock position of the clock analogy
    - displacement of the apex towards the midline or even to the right side in severe cases.

Dilation of the Aortic Arch or Descending Aorta

The most common causes of dilation in this area have already been mentioned in previous sections.

Radiographic findings suggesting dilation in this area in different thoracic views include:

- lateral projection:
    - bulging of the cardiac silhouette towards the cranial mediastinum (10–11 o'clock position of the clock analogy)
- DV Projection:
    - bulging at the 11–1 o'clock position.

Right Atrial Enlargement

The **most common causes** of enlargement in this chamber are:

- tricuspid valve failure (degenerative valvular disease, tricuspid valve dysplasia)
- right ventricular pressure overload (pulmonary hypertension, pulmonary stenosis)
- tetralogy of Fallot
- right atrial aneurysm caused by a pericardial sac defect.

Radiographic findings that suggest an enlarged right atrium include:

- lateral projection:
    - bulging of the cardiac silhouette in the 9–10 o'clock position of the clock analogy
    - displacement of the trachea, just cranial to the carina
    - loss of the cranial "cardiac waist"
- DV projection:
    - bulging at the 9–11 o'clock position.

Right Ventricular Dilation

The **most common causes** of enlargement in this chamber are:

- tricuspid valve insufficiency
- pulmonary valve insufficiency
- interventricular septal defects
- interatrial septal defects
- persistent atrioventricular canal
- right ventricular pressure overload (pulmonary hypertension, pulmonary stenosis, tetralogy of Fallot)
- dilated cardiomyopathy (accompanied by dilation of the left side of the heart causing generalised cardiomegaly)
- arrhythmogenic right ventricular cardiomyopathy (ARVC).

Radiographic findings that suggest an enlargement in this area include:

- lateral projection (Figures 19 and 23):
    - bulging of the cardiac silhouette in the 5–9 o'clock position of the clock analogy
    - elevation of the cardiac apex from the sternum
    - increased sternal contact of the cardiac silhouette. The level of contact between the sternum and the cardiac silhouette depends to a great extent on the thoracic conformation and breed of the animal, so it is not a very specific sign of right ventricular enlargement and should be interpreted with caution.
- DV projection:
    - bulging or rounding of the right border of the heart at the 5–9 o'clock position, resulting in an inverted "D" shape
    - displacement of the cardiac apex to the left.

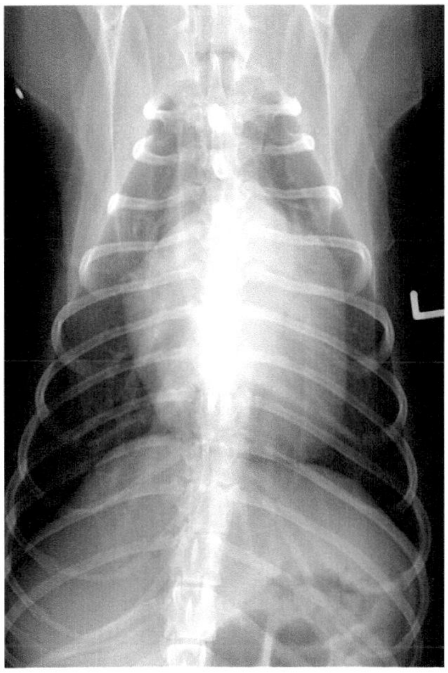

Figure 22. Dorsoventral thoracic radiograph of a dog with degenerative mitral valve disease where the left atrium and ventricle can be seen to be enlarged. Swelling of the cardiac silhouette in the projection area of the left atrial appendage and ventricle. In addition, a lateral displacement of the main bronchi is seen, caused by the bulging of the left atrium (cowboy sign).

Pulmonary Artery Dilatation

The most common causes of dilation in this area have already been mentioned in previous sections.

Radiographic findings **suggesting dilation in this area in different thoracic views include**:

- lateral projection (Figure 19):
  - bulging in the 9–10 o'clock position
  - dilation of the craniodorsal cardiac border towards the cranial mediastinum
- DV projection (Figure 18):
  - bulging in the 1–2 o'clock position
  - possible displacement of the trachea cranial to the heart (mass effect).

Evaluation of the Pulmonary Vessels

The pulmonary veins are seen ventrally in lateral views and medially in DV/VD views, and the pulmonary arteries are seen dorsally and laterally. On lateral radiographs, the cranial triad (cranial lobar arteries and veins) can be seen (Figure 17) and in the DV/VD view the caudal triad (caudal lobar arteries and veins) (Figure 18). In the pulmonary triads, the bronchi are positioned centrally and are delimited by veins and arteries.

Under normal conditions, the **size of the arteries and veins is very similar**. In lateral views, the diameter of the vessels of the cranial triad at their intersection with the fourth rib should not exceed the diameter of the proximal third of the fourth rib. In DV/VD views, the diameter of the vessels of the caudal triad should not exceed the width of the ninth rib where intersection occurs.

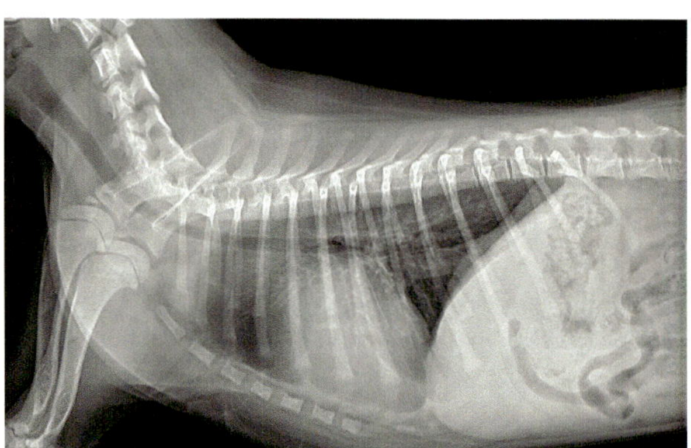

Figure 23. Right lateral thoracic radiograph of a dog showing enlargement of the right ventricle. Bulging in the projection area of the right ventricle can be seen, as well as an increase in the amount of sternal contact of the heart.

Vascular patterns are characterised by changes in the number, size, shape, and radiopacity of the pulmonary vessels.

Different vascular patterns that can be found and their most common causes are described below.

- **Dilation of the pulmonary arteries**: pulmonary hypertension, dirofilariasis, pulmonary parasites (*Angiostrongylus vasorum* in dogs or *Aelurostrongylus abstrusus* in cats), pulmonary thromboembolism and left-to-right shunts (patent *ductus arteriosus*, interventricular or interatrial septal defects, aortopulmonary shunts).
- **Pulmonary vein dilation**: venous congestion (left-sided congestive heart failure) (Figure 24).
- **Dilation of the pulmonary veins and arteries**:
  - pulmonary overcirculation caused by left to right shunts:

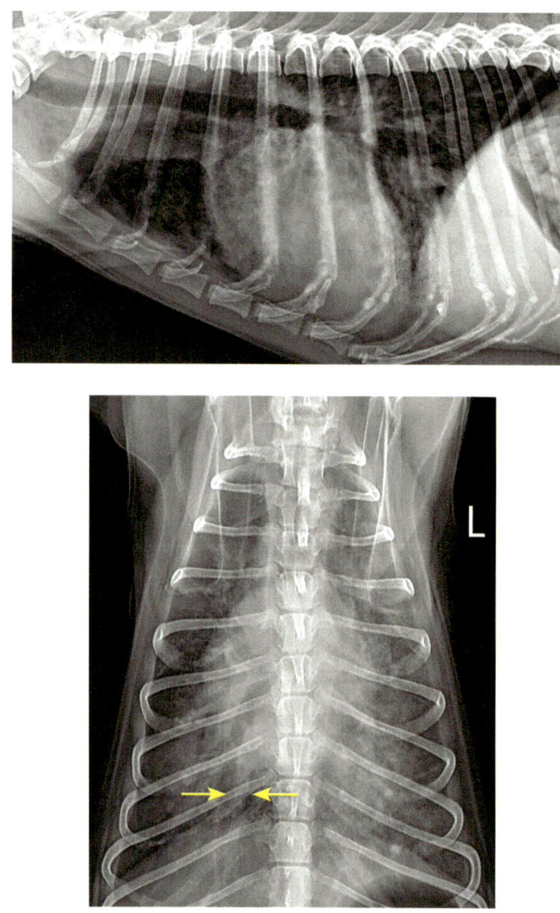

Figure 24. Right lateral and dorsoventral thoracic radiographs of a dog with degenerative mitral valve disease and left-sided congestive heart failure. An enlarged left atrium can be appreciated, alveolar patter in the caudal pulmonary lobes and perihilar area as well as dilation of the caudal lobar veins (yellow arrows).

- extracardiac: patent *ductus arteriosus*, aortopulmonary window, aortopulmonary shunt
- intracardiac: interventricular septal defects, interatrial septal defects

- left-sided congestive heart failure
- hypervolaemia (excessive administration of fluids)

– **Reduction in the diameter of pulmonary veins and arteries**: pulmonary hypoperfusion that may be accompanied by microcardia and reduction in the diameter of the caudal vena cava (*shock*, severe dehydration, blood loss, hypoadrenocorticism), pericardial diseases (pericardial effusion with cardiac tamponade, restrictive pericarditis), right-to-left cardiac shunts (tetralogy of Fallot, reverse patent *ductus arteriosus*, reverse interventricular or interatrial septal defects), and severe pulmonary stenosis.

Evaluation of Lung Parenchyma and the Pleural Space in Patients with Heart Disease

Previous sections of this chapter have described the different pulmonary patterns that can be seen, and the radiographic findings present in patients with pleural effusions. This section aims to provide a brief description of the changes in the lung parenchyma and pleural space that can be found in patients with heart failure.

Dogs that develop left-sided congestive heart failure with cardiogenic pulmonary oedema usually present with pulmonary changes with a typical distribution pattern. These changes consist of the presence of an interstitial and/or alveolar pattern which is typically located in the perihilar area and/or caudal lung lobes (Figures 24 and 25). However, **in cats, patterns caused by pulmonary oedema can vary in location and appearance**, making diagnosis of heart failure difficult.

Additionally, **dogs with left-sided congestive heart failure** often present with pulmonary venous congestion, seen as dilated lobar pulmonary veins on thoracic radiographs (Figure 24). **Cats with left-sided congestive heart failure** usually present with pulmonary venous congestion (dilation of pulmonary lobar veins) or pulmonary venous and arterial congestion (dilation of both pulmonary lobar veins and arteries).

The presence of pleural effusion may be due to the existence of **right-sided congestive heart failure in dogs and cats or left-sided heart failure in cats** (Figure 8). These signs include loss of visualization of the cardiac silhouette, visualization of pleural fissures, elevation of the trachea, and the presence of radiopaque soft tissue/fluid contents in the pleural space.

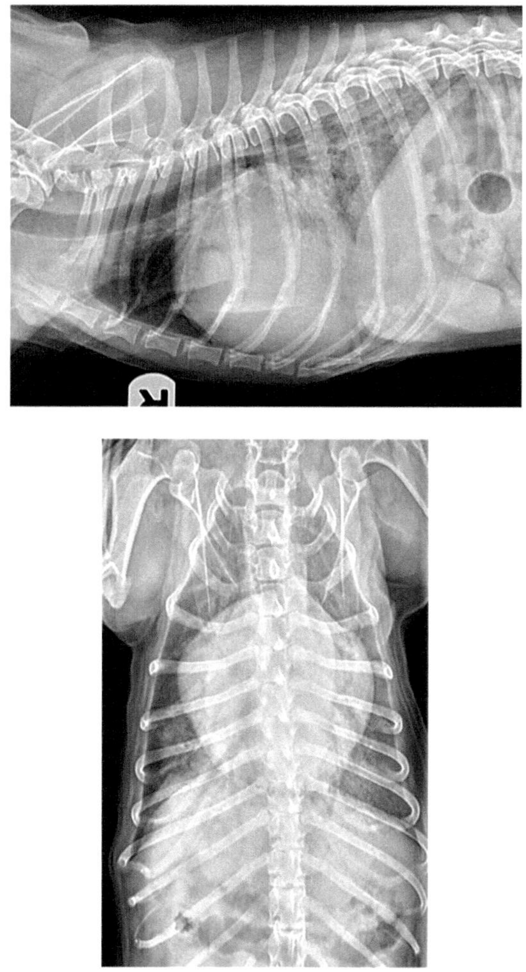

Figure 25. Right lateral and dorsoventral thoracic radiographs of a dog with degenerative mitral valve disease and left-sided congestive heart failure. Enlargement of the left atrium (bulging in the projection area of the left atrium with loss of the caudal cardiac waist) with elevation of the trachea and left main bronchi, and a bilateral alveolar patter in the caudal pulmonary lobes.

Bibliography

- Thrall, D.E. (2013) *Textbook of Veterinary Diagnostic Radiology*. 6th edition. Elsevier.
- King, L.G. (2004) *Textbook of Respiratory Disease in Dogs and Cats*. Saunders.
- Martin, M., Corcoran, B. (2006) *Notes on Cardiorespiratory Diseases of the Dog and Cat*. Blackwell Publishing.
- Dennis, R., Kirberger, R.M., Barr, F., et al. (2010) *Handbook of Small Animal Radiology and Ultrasound*. 2nd edition. Elsevier.
- Schwarz, T., Johnson, V. (2008) *BSAVA Manual of Canine and Feline Thoracic Imaging*. BSAVA.
- Fuentes, V.L., Johnson, L.R., Dennis, S. (2010) BSAVA *Manual of Canine and Feline Cardiorespiratory Medicine*. BSAVA.

Test

Answers on Page 82

1. **Please indicate which of the following statements regarding thoracic radiographs is true:**
   a. The exposure parameters necessary to obtain quality thoracic radiographs include a high kilovoltage (kV) and a low milliampere-seconds (mAs).
   b. To obtain a low mAs a low milliamperage (mA) and a long exposure time should be used.
   c. Centering and collimating the field to be radiographed well will not influence the amount of scattered radiation generated.
   d. To collimate a thoracic radiograph the patient's head should be included in the radiograph.

2. **Indicate which of the following statements is true:**
   a. Thoracic radiographs are the test of choice to diagnose pulmonary stenosis.
   b. Thoracic radiographs are the test of choice to diagnose aortic stenosis.
   c. Echocardiography is the test of choice for diagnosis of congenital diseases.
   d. Thoracic radiographs allow evaluation of the size and functionality of the cardiac chambers.

3. **Please indicate which of the following statements regarding the interpretation of thoracic radiographs is false:**
   a. When interpreting thoracic radiographs, it is important to follow an order to perform a systematic evaluation.
   b. The chosen order does not matter, but it is important to always follow the same order so as not to forget to evaluate any structure.
   c. An adequate assessment of the thorax should only evaluate the following structures: cardiac silhouette, aorta, caudal vena cava, pulmonary vasculature and pulmonary field.
   d. An adequate assessment of the thorax should evaluate the following structures: surrounding soft tissues, bones (ribs, vertebrae, sternum ...), cranial abdomen and diaphragm, neck, pleural space, mediastinum, trachea including the carina, bronchi, cardiac silhouette, aorta, caudal vena cava, pulmonary vasculature and pulmonary field.

4. **Indicate which of the following statements is true:**
   a. The normal diameter of the trachea is the same in all dog breeds.
   b. Brachiocephalic dogs usually have a trachea with a larger diameter.
   c. The ratio between the diameter of the trachea and the entrance to the thorax is considered an objective method for evaluation of the diameter of the trachea.
   d. Under normal conditions the diameter of the trachea should vary significantly during respiratory phases.

5. **Indicate which of the following statements is true:**
   a. Patients with chronic degenerative mitral disease present with increased sternal contact.
   b. Increased sternal contact is very specific to left ventricular enlargement.
   c. Increased sternal contact is very specific to right ventricular enlargement.
   d. Increased sternal contact is a nonspecific sign for right ventricular enlargement.

6. **Indicate which of the following is true regarding evaluation of cardiac size on lateral thoracic radiographs:**
   a. The vertebral heart score measurement system is based on comparing the size of the heart with the size of the first thoracic vertebra.
   b. The cardiac size obtained by the vertebral heart score measurement system is greater in cats than in dogs.
   c. A prominent aortic arch on lateral radiographs in cats is always indicative of congenital pathology.
   d. Dogs with patent *ductus arteriosus* show an increased silhouette size of the left-sided chambers, aortic arch, and main pulmonary artery.

7. **Which statement is correct regarding patients with a cranial mediastinal mass?**
   a. There is cranial displacement of the carina.
   b. There may be caudal displacement of the carina.
   c. Cranial mediastinal masses are not usually detected on thoracic radiographs.
   d. A single lateral view is sufficient to diagnose a cranial mediastinal mass.

8. The most likely cause of a dyspnoeic dog with a grade IV/VI murmur with a PMI over the left apex, cardiomegaly, and a severe interstitial pattern in the dorsocaudal lung field is:

a. Left-sided heart failure.
b. Right-sided heart failure.
c. Bilateral heart failure.
d. Respiratory disease.

9. Indicate which statement is correct regarding cats with left-sided heart failure:

a. They present a typical distribution of pulmonary oedema in the perihilar area.
b. They may have ascites.
c. They may present with pleural effusion.
d. In cats, bilateral heart failure with ascites, pleural effusion, and subcutaneous oedema is common.

10. Indicate which vascular pattern is usually present in dogs with left-sided heart failure:

a. Dilation of the pulmonary veins.
b. Dilation of the pulmonary arteries.
c. There is not usually a vascular pattern in dogs with left-sided heart failure.
d. Reduction in the size of the pulmonary veins.

11. Indicate which of the following statements about pneumomediastinum is true:

a. Pneumomediastinum is common in patients with pleural effusion.
b. The most common cause of pneumomediastinum is trauma.
c. When there is pneumomediastinum, it is very difficult to see the structures contained in the mediastinum.
d. It is a common finding in patients with heart failure.

12. A 4-month-old dog with cardiomegaly and marked dorsal displacement of the trachea on lateral radiography suggests:

a. Mitral valve dysplasia.
b. Congenital pulmonary stenosis.
c. Severe aortic stenosis.
d. Restrictive interventricular septal defect.

13. Please indicate which of the following statements regarding thoracic radiographs of a dog with chronic bronchitis is true:

a. The typical pattern in these animals is a vascular pattern.
b. The typical pattern in these animals is an interstitial pattern.
c. The typical pattern in these animals is an alveolar pattern.
d. Thoracic radiographs do not always show changes in the lung field.

14. What is the most likely diagnosis in an 8-year-old Dachshund with a grade V/VI systolic murmur with PMI over the left apex and radiographic signs of cardiomegaly on the left side of the heart?

a. Mitral valve dysplasia.
b. Degenerative mitral valve disease.
c. Dilated cardiomyopathy.
d. Pulmonary hypertension.

15. What is the most likely diagnosis in a 7-year-old Dobermann dog with a grade II/VI systolic murmur with PMI over the left apex and radiographic signs of generalised cardiomegaly?

a. Mitral valve dysplasia.
b. Degenerative mitral valve disease.
c. Dilated cardiomyopathy.
d. Pulmonary hypertension.

Correct Answers:

1. a
2. c
3. c
4. c
5. d
6. d
7. b
8. a
9. c
10. a
11. b
12. a
13. d
14. b
15. c

Notes

Echocardiography: Imaging Modalities and Echocardiographic Examination Protocol

Mª Josefa Fernández-del Palacio

Echocardiography is the **main non-invasive imaging technique** with no known side effects used to **evaluate the heart and great vessels**. It uses ultrasound to form images of the heart in motion, providing information on both cardiac anatomy and functionality. It is, in most cases, the definitive diagnostic tool.

The development of echocardiographic technology and portable equipment means this technique is now widely used in veterinary medicine, both in first opinion practice and referral hospitals, and on an outpatient basis. Furthermore, its use in emergency situations ("echo FAST") allows the cardiac or respiratory origin of respiratory distress to be determined quickly, with minimal stress to the animal.

The optimal application of echocardiography and the interpretation of its results requires an appropriate technical and theoretical understanding of both the technique and the anatomy, physiology and pathologies affecting the cardiovascular system. It is a **highly operator-dependent technique**, which is more efficient when carried out and interpreted by the clinician responsible for the patient.

Box 1. Guidelines for Echocardiographic Examination

Echocardiographic examination has been shown to be useful in the following situations:

- **examination of patients with symptoms potentially of cardiac aetiology;**
- **evaluation of congenital cardiopathies;**
- **initial examination of an animal with a murmur when there is a reasonable suspicion of a valvulopathy or structural cardiac disease;**
- **initial examination of patients where endocarditis or a new murmur are suspected;**
- **examination of the heart mass (suspicion of tumour or thrombus);**
- **evaluation of pericardial pathologies: pericardial effusion and constrictive pericarditis;**
- **initial evaluation of a known or suspected cardiomyopathy;**
- **examination of patients with arrythmias; and**
- **monitoring of patients after diagnosis or treatment of a cardiopathy.**

Echocardiography should be performed for definitive diagnostic purposes rather than screening and should be guided by the history and physical examination (Box 1). **Results of the echocardiographic examination must be considered in the clinical context of the patient**, together with the clinical history, physical examination, and other diagnostic techniques such as thoracic radiographs, electrocardiogram, laboratory tests, and systemic blood pressure.

Development of Echocardiography and Echocardiographic Imaging Modes

Echocardiography uses ultrasound at frequencies between 1 and 12 MHz for structural, functional and haemodynamic evaluation of the cardiovascular system. Ultrasound waves are reflected by tissues as they progress through them, so that some of the ultrasound is reflected and some is refracted, reaching deeper tissues. Afterwards, through specialised processing of the signals that return to the transducer (reflected), these are transformed and reproduced in visual or audible formats on the ultrasound monitor.

In the 1950's, Edler and Hertz recorded the movements of cardiac structures for the first-time using ultrasound in human patients, specifically the mitral valve, and were able to differentiate normal patients from those with valvular stenosis using M-mode. Given the limitations of M-mode, echocardiographic technology continued to develop, and in the late 1970's, the two-dimensional mode was first used to obtain real-time images of cardiac morphology and functionality. In the late 1970's and early 1980's, spectral Doppler and colour Doppler, respectively, were subsequently employed in the study of cardiovascular haemodynamics.

In veterinary medicine, the first publications on the clinical use of M-mode ultrasound date from the early 80's. At the end of the 80's, the first ultrasound equipment, which included M and 2D modes, was used in institutions and large hospitals for cardiological diagnosis. In the mid-90's, Doppler technology was first applied in companion animal and equine practice. Subsequently, transoesophageal echocardiography, tissue Doppler, three-dimensional echocardiography and strain and strain rate studies, developed in human patients, have been adapted for use in animals.

In this chapter, the main modes used in small animal practice will be discussed:

- two-dimensional, BD, or 2D echocardiography
- time-motion, M or TM echocardiography
- Doppler echocardiography:
    - pulsed
    - continuous
    - colour
- tissue Doppler echocardiography.

Two-dimensional, BD, or 2D Echocardiography

Allows examination of the heart in a plane, obtaining a two-dimensional image (Figure 1). The 2D sector transducer sequentially emits multiple arc-shaped ultrasound lines or pulses. The ultrasound waves returning from the field within the sector produce an **image in two dimensions: depth or distance from the transducer and a perpendicular or lateral dimension**. The 2D image is rapidly updated with a high frame rate/second (>150 images/sec on digital ultrasound machines), providing a time sequence of heart movement.

This echocardiographic modality allows **evaluation of the anatomy and movement of cardiac structures as well as specific measurements used in the study of cardiac functionality** (areas, volumes, chambers and great vessels, etc.) to be obtained. Furthermore, it constitutes a guide for obtaining adequate information in other echocardiographic modes (M-mode and Doppler).

Time-motion Echocardiography, M or TM

Allows examination of the heart by means of a linear ultrasound beam, obtaining a one-dimensional image. The ordinate axis shows the **depth of the cardiac structures** and the abscissa axis, the time, that is, their **movement, during the cardiac cycle** (Figure 2).

The main use of M-mode is to obtain **quantitative data on the size of the cardiac chambers, walls and great vessels and qualitative data on the movement of cardiac structures**.

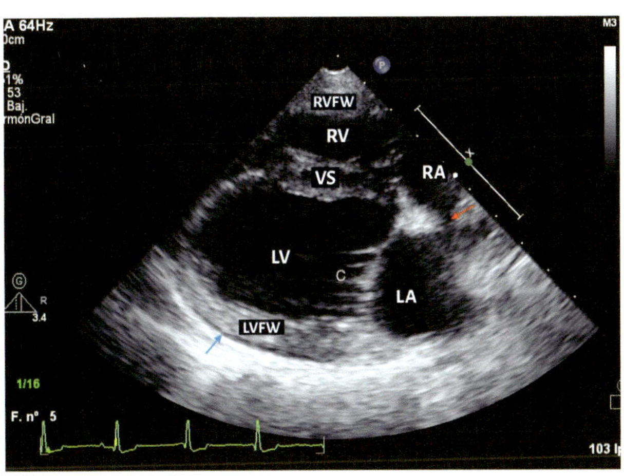

Figure 1. 2D echocardiogram of a normal dog, right-sided long axis four chamber parasternal view: the left-sided chambers appear larger in size than the right-sided ones and the atrioventricular valves are situated between the atria and ventricles. The *fossa ovalis* is seen as a poor quality area on the ultrasound in the interatrial septum (red arrow). LA: left atrium, LV: left ventricle, RV: right ventricle, RA: right atrium, RVFW: right ventricular free wall, LVFW: left ventricular free wall, blue arrow: pericardium.

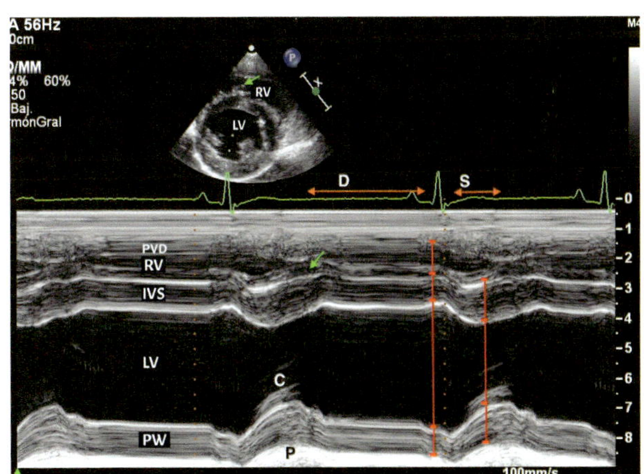

Figure 2. M-mode echocardiogram at the level of the left ventricle, obtained using a right-sided short axis parasternal view in a normal dog. In the upper part of the image the short axis of the left ventricle (LV) can be seen using 2D ultrasound, which serves as a guide to position the cursor and obtain the corresponding M-mode image. The phases of the cardiac cycle can be easily identified on the ECG: systole (S) and diastole (D). Note that the interventricular septum (IVS) and the posterior wall (PW) of the left ventricle (LV) near each other in systole and separate in diastole. Diastolic measurements are taken at the level of the Q wave on the ECG and the systolic ones where the IVS is lowest; in both cases from the upper border to the upper border (red lines).

Doppler Echocardiography

Doppler echocardiography is specialised processing of cardiac ultrasonography, characterised by a continuous update of **blood flow velocity during the cardiac cycle**.

It allows the following to be assessed:

- **normal flow** within cardiac and vascular structures
- detection of the presence of **abnormal flow** due to changes in direction and speed
- information on the presence of **valvular lesions** (stenosis or insufficiency) and **abnormal cardiac communications**.

86

Doppler technology is based on the frequency changes that sound waves experience when reflected by a moving object. When an object moves towards the observer, the frequency increases with respect to the original, while when it moves away, it decreases. In the case of echocardiography, the frequency change of the ultrasound occurs on the blood cells, which are the moving object (Figure 3).

Ultrasounds are emitted with a certain frequency, so that, when coming into contact with the moving red blood cells, the return frequency varies with respect to the original emission. The difference that exists between the emitted and the reflected frequency is proportional to the speed of the object against which it has "collided", in this case, the blood. This phenomenon is known as ultrasound Doppler shift (described by the Austrian physician and astronomer Johann Christian Doppler, 1803–1853).

The scan angle is critical as the **ultrasound beam must be aligned as closely as possible with the flow** to obtain maximum velocity data. As the angle is increased, the velocity value decreases. This is because the equation uses the cosine of the angle between the Doppler cursor and the flow, and as the angle increases, the cosine value decreases and gets closer to zero.

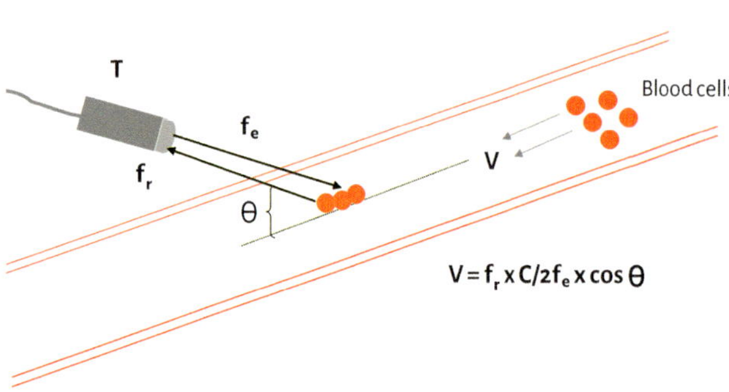

Figure 3. Diagram showing calculation for blood flow velocity using the Doppler effect on ultrasounds. T: transducer, V: blood cell velocity, f_e: frequency emitted by the transducer, f_r: change in frequency, θ: angle of incidence (<20°), C: ultrasound velocity in blood.

A haemodynamic study can be carried out using measurements of blood flow velocities (V), calculating the pressure gradient (PG) through the **simplified Bernoulli equation**:

$$\textbf{Doppler PG (mmHg)} = 4 \times V^2$$

Under normal conditions, blood flows through the cardiovascular structures forming laminar flow, that is, forming layers of ordered red blood cells, going in the same direction, and at very similar speed (Figure 4 A). However, when there is abnormal flow (valve insufficiencies and stenosis or communications between chambers and great vessels), the layers of red blood cells tend to become disordered, forming eddies and therefore changing direction and speed abruptly, causing the appearance of turbulent flow patterns (Figure 4 B).

The utility of Doppler in the echocardiographic examination is for the detection of flow, its classification as normal or turbulent, and quantification of the velocity and pressure gradient.

Within Doppler echocardiography, the following formats are of particular interest:

- spectral Doppler, which in turn can be:
  - pulsed Doppler
  - continuous Doppler
- colour Doppler, colour flow Doppler or colour Doppler imaging
- tissue Doppler.

Spectral Doppler

With spectral Doppler, the signal or Doppler spectrum collected by the transducer is arranged along an axis in which time is represented horizontally, while speed (cm/s or m/s) is located on the vertical axis. Therefore, the baseline is 0 m/s, above the "positive" velocities of the flow that approaches the transducer and below the "negative" ones, that is, those that move away from the transducer.

Examination of blood flow using **ECO Doppler requires a synchronous ECG** with echocardiographic images, which allows the phase of the cardiac cycle in which the different Doppler spectra are obtained, as well as the presence of arrhythmias to be evaluated.

Pulsed Doppler

Uses a single crystal that acts as both an ultrasound emitter and a receiver. The transducer emits a pulse with a certain

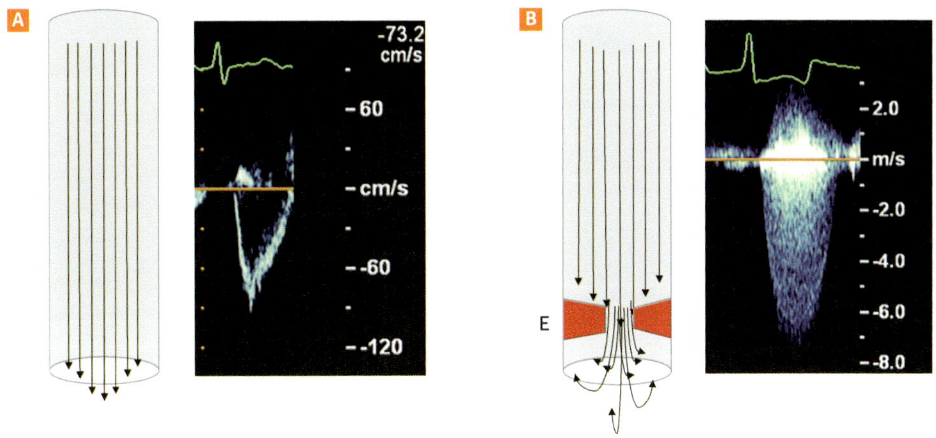

Laminar flow: pulsed Doppler 0.9 m/sg

Turbulent flow: continuos Doppler 7 m/sg

Figure 4. A. Diagram showing laminar flow inside a vessel (the blood cells circulate in layers of similar velocities with slight contact near to the walls) and corresponding flow shown using pulsed Doppler (pulmonary artery). The inner part of the spectrum is seen as being "empty". **B**. Diagram showing what occurs in the case of valvular stenosis. In this case blood flow forms eddies (turbulent flow) and the velocity increases when passing the stenosed area E, consistent with the pressure gradient between the chamber situated before and after the stenosis. The flow spectrum for continuous Doppler corresponds to aortic stenosis and appears "full" with a high velocity.

interval and the next one is not sent until the response to the previous one has returned. This type of Doppler has the **advantage that it allows blood flow measurements to be made in a specific area**, called "sample volume". The sample volume size and location are selected by the operator and the region of interest guided by 2D mode or colour Doppler, if previously used to determine abnormal flow (Figure 5).

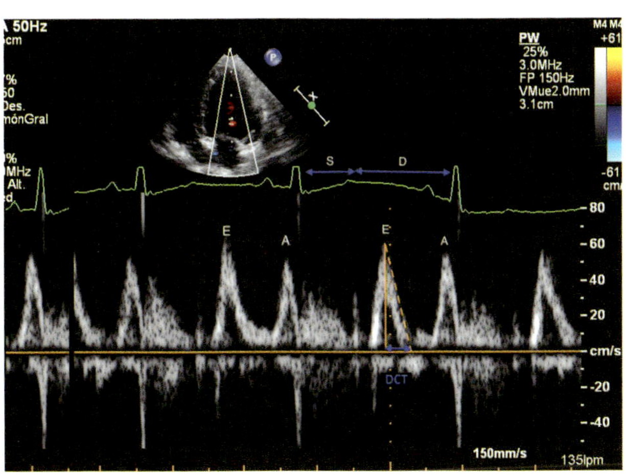

Figure 5. Pulsed Doppler echocardiogram with transmitral flow in a normal dog, obtained using a left apical parasternal view. At the edge of the image (ordinate axis) a scale corresponding to the range of velocities can be seen and horizontally (abscissa axis) the time in the cardiac cycle, which correlates with the electrocardiogram. Spectral Doppler consists of two peaks: E at the start of diastole (D) and A at the end, after atrial contraction (P wave on the ECG). This is shown where the deceleration time (DCT) is shown for peak E.

However, the maximum speed that can be recorded with this mode is limited by the transducer frequency, the distance between the sample volume and the transducer, and the pulse repetition rate:

- the greater the distance to the measurement point, the lower the maximum speed which can be measured;
- low transducer frequencies allow higher velocities to be measured.

In other words, the **main limitation of pulsed Doppler is that it cannot measure high blood flow velocities** because it cannot detect large changes in frequency, such as those that occur when there are high velocities. When the return Doppler frequency deviation is greater than twice the pulse repetition frequency (Nyquist limit) the velocity spectrum appears "wrapped" around the baseline, appearing in the opposite direction to the flow. That is, artefacts and errors in the speed and direction of blood flow are measured (Figure 6). This phenomenon is called *aliasing*.

Continuous Doppler can be used to measure abnormally high velocities.

Continuous Doppler

This technology uses two piezoelectric crystals in the transducer, one to emit the ultrasound beam and the other to receive the ultrasounds that are reflected, **allowing high blood flow rates to be measured** and complementing pulsed Doppler.

Continuous Doppler is guided with a cursor, not with a sample volume, and therefore does not allow a small study area to be chosen, but rather the **flow is evaluated throughout the entire ultrasound beam** (Figure 7). As it does not depend on a repetition pulse, it is not affected by the Nyquist limit and therefore the *aliasing* artefact does not occur.

Colour Doppler

This mode uses the two echocardiography applications in combination, that is, 2D imaging and blood flow movement (Figure 8). It shares the same technology as pulsed Doppler but differs in that it **uses multiple sample volumes across multiple ultrasound beams that scan a given area**, so that the operator can select the area to be examined. The larger the size of the window, the more likely it is that errors will be observed, so it is advisable to focus on the area to be evaluated.

Differences in flow speed and direction are colour coded:
- red corresponds to the flow approaching the transducer;
- blue to the flow moving away from it.

The brighter the colour, the faster the flow speed. As it is pulsed Doppler, when turbulence and high velocities appear, the *aliasing* effect occurs, in the form of colour inversions (colour mosaic) (Figure 9).

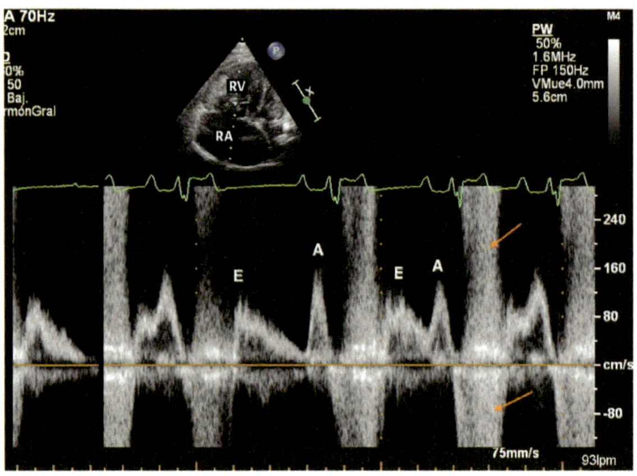

Figure 6. Pulsed Doppler echocardiogram of the flow through the tricuspid valve in a dog with valvular dysplasia, obtained using a left apical parasternal view. During diastole the two peaks in flow entering the right ventricle (RV) from the atrium (RA) can be seen. In systole a band at both sides of the base line (arrows) which corresponds to tricuspid insufficiency can be seen and cannot be measured using pulsed Doppler: selection of continuous Doppler is necessary.

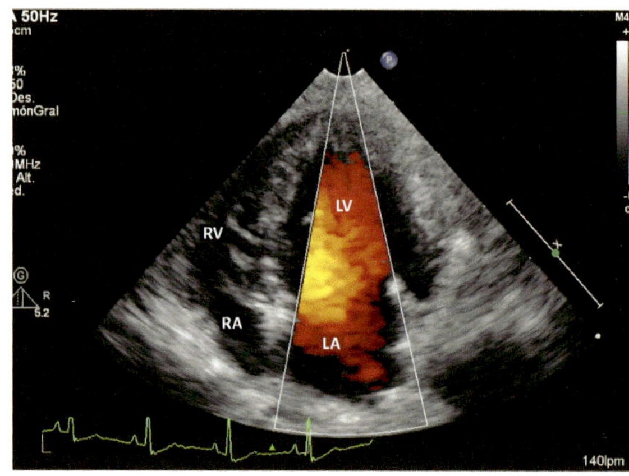

Figure 8. Colour Doppler echocardiogram of mitral flow in a normal dog, obtained using left apical parasternal view. Flow which is red in colour can be seen as it approaches the transducer (from the left atrium – LA – to the left ventricle – LV –). On the right side of the image the colour scale can be seen with numbering corresponding to the pulse repetition frequency which represents the flow velocity to be measured. RA: right atrium, RV: right ventricle.

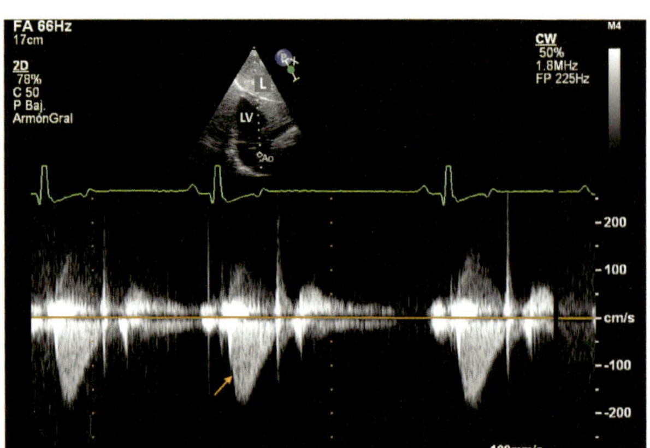

Figure 7. Continuous Doppler echocardiogram of aortic flow (arrow) in a normal dog, obtained using a subcostal view. The liver (L) acts as a window for the ultrasound waves. LV: left ventricle, Ao: ascending aorta.

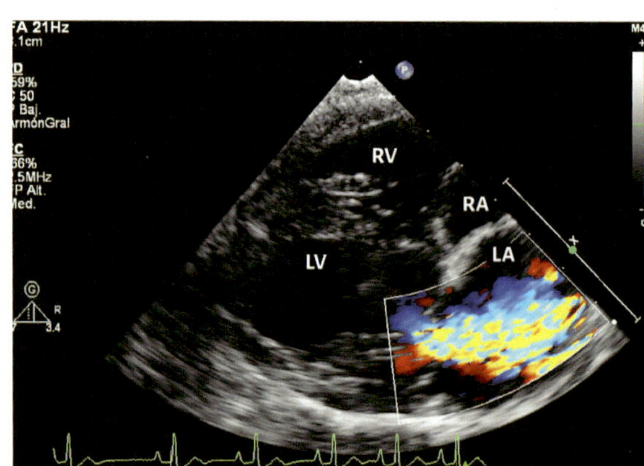

Figure 9. Colour Doppler echocardiogram in a dog with chronic degenerative mitral disease obtained using a right-sided parasternal view showing a long axis four chamber image which demonstrates turbulent flow in the left atrium (LA) during systole due to mitral valve insufficiency. LV: left ventricle, RV: right ventricle, RA: right atrium.

When examining transvalvular or orifice flow, the use of colour Doppler is recommended as first option and when an abnormal flow is observed, it should be studied and quantified using spectral Doppler.

Tissue Doppler (TD)

TD uses the same principles as conventional Doppler, except that the **moving object is not blood cells, but myocardial tissue**.

Since myocardial tissue has higher reflectivity and lower velocity, TD focuses on high-amplitude, low-frequency Doppler deviations obtained from **tissue movement** and, therefore, filters are selected to exclude high velocities and low intensity reflections. This requires a high frame rate. In this way, the movement of both the myocardium and the fibrous tissue of the myocardial skeleton can be examined.

Both **pulsed Doppler and colour Doppler are used in TD**. From 2D mode, colour tissue Doppler is selected first and then pulsed wave Doppler. As in conventional pulsed Doppler, in TD the area to be evaluated is also selected by positioning the sample volume (Figure 10). This can be located on the myocardium or on the mitral (lateral and medial) or tricuspid (lateral) *annulus* so that a spectrum of tissue movement is obtained in systole and diastole. This modality allows evaluation of both systolic and diastolic ventricular function. As in conventional Doppler, measurement of tissue velocity depends on the angle between the incident ultrasound beam and the tissue line to be evaluated and, therefore, in the examination protocol the operator must focus on minimizing this angle.

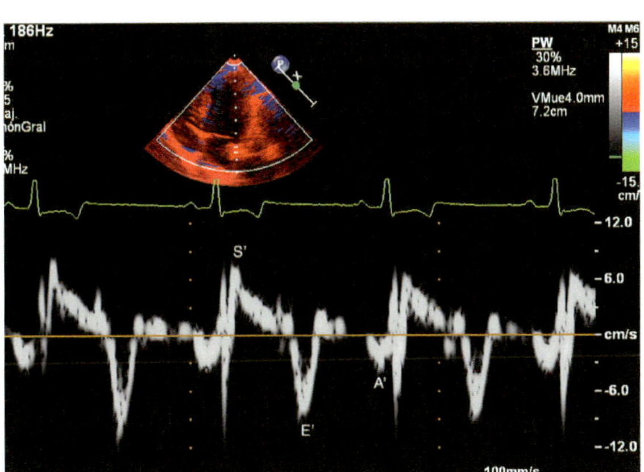

Figure 10. Tissue Doppler echocardiogram in a normal dog obtained using a left apical parasternal view, positioning the volume of the sample on the lateral mitral *annulus*, showing a systolic (S') wave and two diastolic (E' and A') waves.

Another type of tissue Doppler is the evaluation of deformation and deformation speed (strain and strain rate, respectively) of one or more myocardial segments, using specific software from the ultrasound equipment company. This format is also subject to the limitation of the interrogation angle. To solve this problem, more recently, ultrasound companies have developed their own software that calculates myocardial deformation and deformation speed based on images obtained in 2D mode, thus eliminating the problem of the interrogation angle. This technology is called **two-dimensional speckle echocardiography,** more commonly known as **"speckle tracking echocardiography"**.

This chapter will focus on 2D, M, spectral Doppler, colour Doppler, and tissue Doppler modes.

Echocardiographic Examination Protocol

The echocardiographic examination is an interactive procedure that involves the operator (veterinarian), the ultrasound equipment and the animal. The perfect interaction between these three components is the key to obtaining echocardiographic images and signals that can be useful in the diagnosis and monitoring of heart disease.

The **operator** conducting the examination must know how to:

- use the equipment and the basic aspects of the physics of ultrasound
- be aware of the anatomy and physiology of the cardiovascular system
- understand the haemodynamic effects of different heart diseases.

The list below shows what an ultrasound equipment should include.

- 2D, M and spectral Doppler modes (pulsed and continuous), colour flow Doppler and tissue Doppler (if possible).
- Digital video and an image recording system.
- *Specific software* for measurements of cardiac structures and blood flow velocities.
- Sectorial *phased array* transducers with an appropriate frequency for the size of the animal and echocardiographic mode (Figure 11). **Typically, high frequency transducers are used for small dogs and cats and lower frequencies for medium and large dogs**. The frequency affects the depth of ultrasound penetration and the resolution of the image (higher frequency, lower penetration and better resolution, and vice versa). Body condition must also be taken into account, low frequency

transducers are needed in obese animals, as well as for left apical and subcostal echocardiographic views, even in the same animal. Likewise, for Doppler examination, transducers with frequencies between 2.5 and 3.5 MHz are more suitable since the Doppler spectra are of better quality and *aliasing* is reduced.

– Synchronous electrocardiogram, in order to obtain the electrocardiographic record simultaneously alongside the echocardiographic image (Figure 2). This will allow the phase of the cardiac cycle to which each image corresponds to be established (especially important for taking measurements or evaluating Doppler spectra). For this, three electrodes are connected by paediatric adhesive discs or clamps on the extremities, held with a cohesive bandage or tape. The author prefers the discs since they do not disturb the animal and maintain a good quality ECG recording throughout the examination (Figure 12).

– The table where patients are positioned for the examination should have a recess and be comfortable (preferably padded) since a full echocardiographic examination can take between 15 and 30 minutes (even when performed by experienced operators), a length of time that some animals find difficult to tolerate without moving. There are several types of tables, depending on the position of the lateral or central notch, so as to facilitate the positioning of the transducer on the thoracic wall below. The author prefers tables with a double lateral groove as these adapt better to different sizes of dogs and cats (Figure 11).

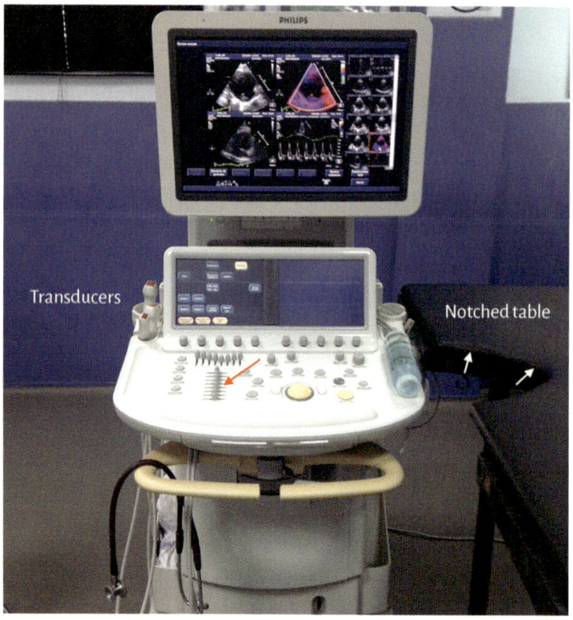

Figure 11. Ultrasound equipment used by the author where three sectorial transducers of varying frequencies can be seen, in addition to the keys for modification of the time-gain compensation (red arrow). In the image the table used to support the animals with two notches can be seen.

Preparation and Positioning of Animals

Preparation

Echocardiographic examination is **generally well tolerated by most animals**. However, in puppies, some unruly animals, or stressed animals, **sedation may be necessary**. Although there is no sedative or combination of drugs that acts without causing side effects on the cardiovascular system (modifying sympathetic tone, changing blood pressure or altering ventricular function) the **most commonly used sedatives are**:

- **in dogs**: the combination of acepromazine (0.03 mg/kg) and buprenorphine (0.005–0.0075 mg/kg) IM or IV
- **in cats**: the combination of acepromazine (0.1 mg/kg) and butorphanol (0.25 mg/kg) IM
- when acepromazine is contraindicated (patients with right to left shunts, hypotensive animals etc.) or in critical patients, **butorphanol can be used alone**, to reduce anxiety.

Given that ultrasound equipment currently allows echocardiographic measurements to be performed *offline*, sedation with butorphanol alone is usually sufficient to perform the examination in less than 30 minutes. In order to improve the quality of the images, clipping the hair from the heart area is recommended (from the 3rd to the 6th intercostal spaces), bilaterally. The area should be cleaned with an alcoholic solution.

Position

To begin the examination, the animal is placed in lateral recumbency (right and left) (Figure 12), ensuring the cardiac area coincides with the notch in the table, in order to apply the transducer underneath and widen the access window to the heart. When this position is not well tolerated (particularly in dyspnoeic animals), an **emergency echocardiographic**

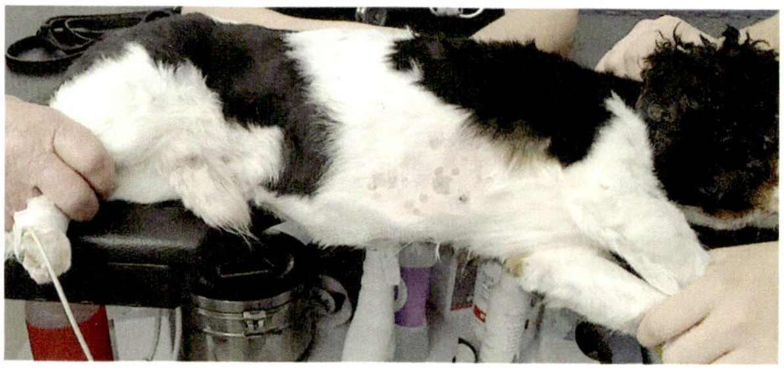

Figure 12. Position of a dog in left lateral recumbency showing the electrodes on the pads for the simultaneous ECG recording alongside the echocardiographic images.

examination can be performed with the animal standing up (dog) or in sternal recumbency (cat), in order to determine the presence of pleural effusion (frequent in cats with hypertrophic cardiomyopathy), pericardial effusion with cardiac tamponade, dilated cardiomyopathy, severe atrial dilation in dogs with chronic degenerative mitral disease etc. quickly and with minimal stress for the animal. It may be difficult to obtain some standard images in the standing or sternal position.

Basic Ultrasound Equipment Controls

2D Mode Controls

Once the animal is ready and the ultrasound machine is turned on, **adjusting some basic settings** on the equipment to obtain an adequate image in 2D mode is necessary (it is the first echocardiographic mode selected).

- **Field depth**: the image of the cardiac structures to be visualised should occupy most of the two-dimensional image sector. A scale will appear on the sides of the sector indicating the depth, so that the distance between two points corresponds to 1 cm.
- **Gain**: used to control the signal strength of the transducer, throughout the sector. Very high gains produce a very white image, while very low gains cause a weak signal and an inconspicuous image. The ideal gain will allow the cardiac structures to be clearly observed without overlapping echoes.
- **Time-gain compensation**: consists of modifying the gain at different depths, so that the image is of good quality without losing information in superficial or deep fields (Figure 11).
- **Sector size**: the width of the sector can be adjusted from approximately 120° to 45°, shrinking leads to better image resolution. Reducing it when using Doppler mode is recommended.

M-mode Controls

- **Cursor position**: the cursor moves with the trackball over the 2D image until it is in the appropriate position. Subsequently, the specific key should be pressed and the trace will be obtained in M-mode.
- **Trace speed**: the speeds that can be used are 25, 50, 100, 150 and 200 mm/s, the lower the speed, the more cardiac cycles will be observed on the trace and vice versa. High speeds are recommended for patients with high heart rates, in order to better separate events during the cardiac cycle.

Colour Doppler Controls

- **Position of the colour sector on the area of interest**, reducing the angle between the sector and the direction of blood flow.
- **Sector width**: reducing the width of the sector increases the frequency of images and improves the colour information on blood flow.
- **Baseline**: by adjusting the baseline of the colour bar, higher speeds can be obtained in a given direction. The number at the top of it represents the maximum detectable speed before *aliasing* appears.

It should be taken into account that *aliasing* is more frequent in colour flow Doppler processing than in spectral Doppler because some of the pulses are destined to obtain 2D images, to the detriment of the colour.

Spectral Doppler Controls

- **Cursor**: moves with the trackball until it is placed in the area of interest.
- **Sample volume and size**: a mark located on the cursor line corresponding to the area to be examined. The smallest size is recommended except to obtain mild regurgitation flows or pulmonary vein flow.
- **Baseline**: moved up or down depending on the direction of blood flow.
- **Velocity scale**: selected according to the velocity of blood flow.
- **Doppler gain**: adjusted to regulate the intensity of the signals or Doppler tracing.
- **Wall filter**: decreases the amount of low-frequency noise produced by the heart walls.
- **Trace speed**: the same concept as above for M-mode; when measuring times in spectral Doppler, as well as at high heart rates, using high scanning speeds is preferable so that the Doppler spectra can be properly studied.

Interpretation of Echocardiograms

Once the optimal echocardiographic images have been obtained, their interpretation should be performed both qualitatively and quantitatively. **Qualitative analysis** should evaluate and draw conclusions on the normality of the appearance, shape and movement of cardiac structures, characteristics of blood flow (using colour Doppler) and Doppler spectra. **Quantitative analysis** will include direct measurements of cardiac walls and chambers, volumes, blood flow velocities, ejection times, acceleration, deceleration, pressure gradients, etc. and will compare them with those established for the species and breed, if applicable. From the direct measurements, the indirect or echocardiographic indices are obtained, through the corresponding formulas or directly through the ultrasound *software*.

Obtaining Standard Echocardiographic Images

The terminology and image orientation that will be discussed in this chapter are those recommended by the Echocardiography Committee of the Specialty of Cardiology of the American College of Veterinary Internal Medicine (Thomas et al., 1993). Likewise, in the article by Gómez *et al.* (2011) 2D images are shown with the corresponding anatomical image and the orientation of the ultrasound beam.

Animal Position: Right Lateral Recumbency

In this position, the transducer is applied underneath (facilitated by the notch in the table) over the 4 intercostal spaces and 1–5 cm from the sternal border, applying abundant ultrasonic gel, in order to optimize the passage of the ultrasounds through the skin.

The transducer is placed almost perpendicular to the thorax, with the mark away from the operator, that is, towards the spine of the animal and the reference point on the screen to the right of the sector. Once the cardiac structures have been located, the transducer should be oriented to obtain standardised images from the different projections.

Right-sided Long Axis Parasternal View

Two main cross-sectional planes are obtained.

Four Chamber View (atria and ventricles)

Obtained with the mark on the transducer facing the spine (Figure 1). The left ventricular apex is on the left of the image and the cardiac base with the atria on the right.

Qualitative Analysis

The following should be considered and evaluated in this plane.

- The appearance, movement and size of the set of cardiac structures: walls, chambers, valves, cardiac septa, right pulmonary artery and vein and pericardium.
- The right-sided chambers are located closest to the transducer and are smaller in size than the left-sided ones. A papillary muscle and the tricuspid valve are usually seen separating the right atrium and right ventricle.
- The free wall of the right ventricle (RV) is thin, approximately one third of the thickness of the free wall of the LV.
- The left ventricle in normal cats and dogs is ellipse shaped.
- The cardiac apex corresponds only to the LV.
- The ventricular septum should appear as a continuous structure from apex to base. Although rare in dogs and cats, ventricular defects can also be located in the muscular septal part.
- The mitral valve closes in a slight arc towards the LV. The leaves and the valvular *chordae tendineae* are thin.
- The left atrium (LA) is square in shape when the mitral valve is closed.
- The *fossa ovalis* is visualised in the centre of the atrial septum as a hypoechoic area or without echoes, simulating a septal defect (Figure 13).
- The pulmonary vein located next to the atrial septum and the right pulmonary artery appear first on the longitudinal axis and second on the transverse axis (Figure 13).
- The coronary sinus is located at the atrioventricular junction. Generally, it is not visible in normal cats and dogs or appears as a hypoechogenic spot. In patients with pressure or volume overload of the right atrium or with abnormal venous drainage (left cranial vena cava or azygos vein), the coronary sinus dilates and is observed as a circular or slightly oval structure (hypo or anechoic), in the ventral part of the left atrium, adjacent to the left atrioventricular junction (Figure 14).
- The pericardium is visualised as a hyperechogenic line (due to the connective tissue of the parietal layer) that

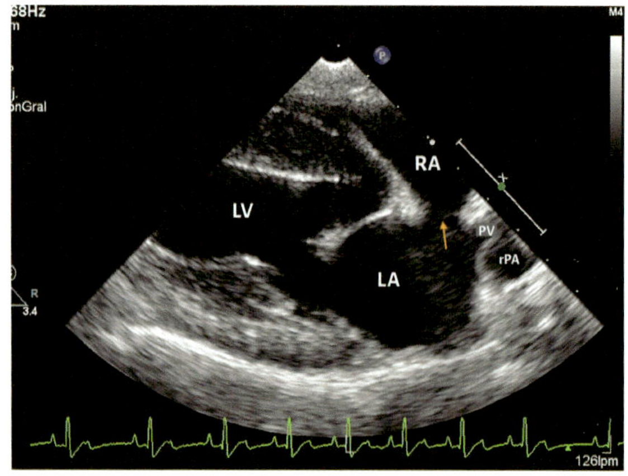

Figure 13. 2D echocardiogram in a normal dog, right-sided long axis four chamber parasternal view, optimised for visualisation of the structures at the base of the heart. The *fossa ovalis* is seen as an area without echoes simulating a defect in the atrial septum (arrow). The pulmonary vein (PV) and right pulmonary artery (rPA) can also be seen. LA: left atrium, LV: left ventricle, RV: right ventricle, RA: right atrium.

surrounds the heart and the great vessels. Between the visceral and parietal layers, a virtual space is created that can contain a small amount of fluid. It functions as a lubricant to facilitate the displacement of the layers during the different phases of the cardiac cycle, but it is not observed through echocardiography in healthy animals.

On the 2D image of this four-chamber plane, the **colour Doppler** function must be selected to qualitatively evaluate:

- atrial and ventricular septa (when 2D-mode examination or physical examination suggests it is necessary) in order to determine possible very small septal defects, which are better detected by colour Doppler. Near the *fossa ovalis*, in the right atrium, flow corresponding to the entrance to the vena cava can be seen and should not be confused with a left-right deviation corresponding to an atrial septum defect;
- both ventricular inlet tracts, in order to assess atrioventricular flow and determine possible valvular stenosis and/or insufficiency. This plane is not suitable for determining mitral and tricuspid flow velocities using spectral Doppler because the angle between the ultrasound beam and the direction of blood flow is very wide and velocity would be underestimated.

Quantitative Analysis

In this cross-sectional plane, the following should be measured.

- The diameter of the LA, from the interatrial septum to the wall of the left atrium (parallel to the mitral *annulus*) (Figure 15 A).
- LV diastolic (LVd) and systolic (LVs) volumes using the modified Simpson disk formula (Figure 15 A and B). From them, the ejection fraction (EF) is calculated using the formula:

$$\textbf{EF (\%) = LVd - LVs/Vid}$$

Generally, EF is measured directly by the ultrasound software from measurement of the ventricular volumes. To measure ventricular volumes, in systole and diastole (modified Simpson disc technique or area-length technique), visualization of the left ventricular endocardium should be optimised, also including the apex (Figures 15 A and B).
- Measurement of the diastolic length of the left ventricle (Ld), from the diastolic volumetric image can be used to calculate the sphericity index (SI), together with the ventricular diastolic dimension (Sd) obtained in M-mode, using the formula:

$$\textbf{SI = Ld/Sd}$$

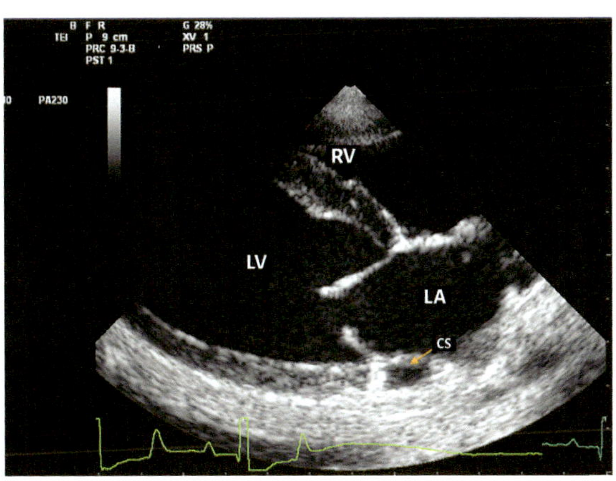

Figure 14. 2D echocardiogram in a dog with a persistent left cranial vena cava (plCrVC), obtained using a right-sided long axis four chamber parasternal view. The coronary sinus (CS) (arrow) can be seen to be dilated due to the connection with the (plCrVC). LA: left atrium, LV: left ventricle, RV: right ventricle, RA: right atrium.

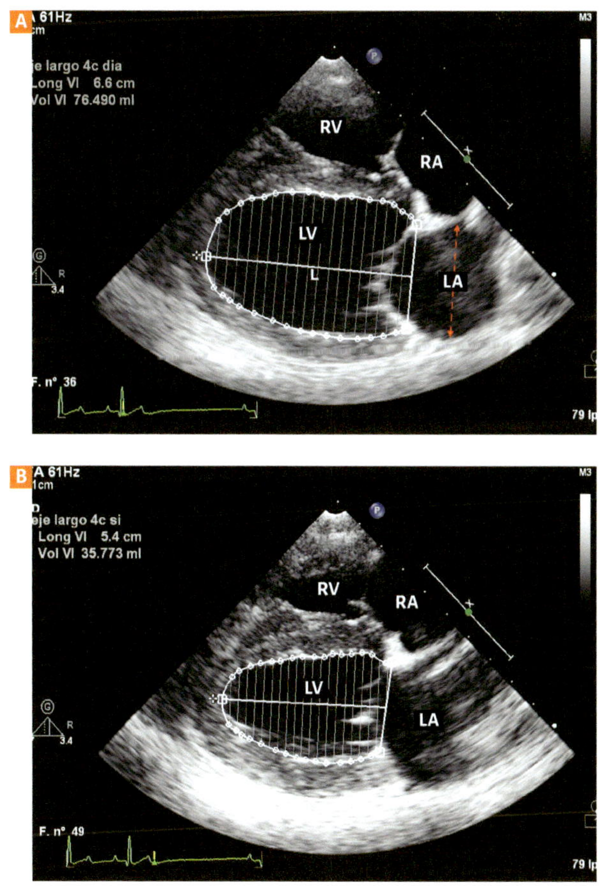

Figure 15. 2D echocardiogram in a normal dog, right-sided long axis four chamber parasternal view, showing measurement of the left ventricular (LV) volume in diastole (**A**) and systole (**B**), using the modified Simpson method. In A measurement of the left atrium is also shown. L: LV length, LA: left atrium, LV: left ventricle, RV: right ventricle, RA: right atrium.

- Pulmonary vein/right pulmonary artery ratio, both in 2D and M-mode. In normal dogs they are of similar sizes (Figures 13 and 16).

Left Ventricular Outflow Tract View with the Ascending Aorta

Obtained by rotating and slightly tilting the transducer from the previous position (four-chamber projection) towards the head of the animal (Figure 17). This step varies with each animal, since the orientation of the heart in the thorax varies with different thoracic conformations.

Qualitative Analysis

In this image the following should be evaluated.

- Shape and size of the LV outflow tract to identify a possible congenital subvalvular stenosis, which is especially common in large breed dogs.
- Shape of the ascending aorta and aortic arch.
- Appearance and movement of the aortic valve in order to rule out congenital valvular anomalies or vegetations due to endocarditis. Normal aortic sigmoids appear as thin curved lines.
- Continuity between the upper (membranous) part of the ventricular septum and the anterior wall of the aorta. Most ventricular septal defects have a subaortic location.
- Movement of the anterior leaflet of the mitral valve. This is especially important in cats with obstructive hypertrophic cardiomyopathy, where anterior systolic movement of the mitral valve is observed.
- In dogs the whole left atrium is not in the same plane as the ascending aorta, so it is partially visualised. It is next to the right pulmonary artery.

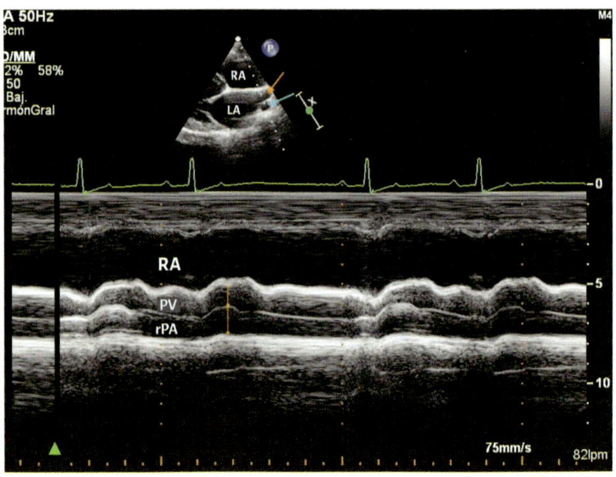

Figure 16. M-mode echocardiogram in a normal dog, placing the cursor over the pulmonary vein (PV) (red arrow) and the right pulmonary artery (rPA) (blue arrow), showing the location for their measurement and calculation of the PV/rPA ratio. It can be seen that they are equal in size. LA: left atrium, RA: right atrium.

In the 2D image of the LV outflow tract projection, **colour Doppler** mode should be selected (Figure 18), adjusting the colour scale to the aortic velocity (1–1.5 m/s) to qualitatively evaluate the subvalvular, valvular and supravalvular blood flow characteristics, determining whether it is laminar or turbulent.

Likewise, possible aortic regurgitation or a membranous ventricular (subaortic) septal defect should be ruled out.

Quantitative Analysis

In this image, the diameter of the aortic *annulus* should be measured in systole, as well as the ascending aorta level with the sigmoids and the sinotubular junction.

The diameter of the aortic *annulus* can vary in different breeds of dogs (in Boxers it is smaller than in other breeds of the same

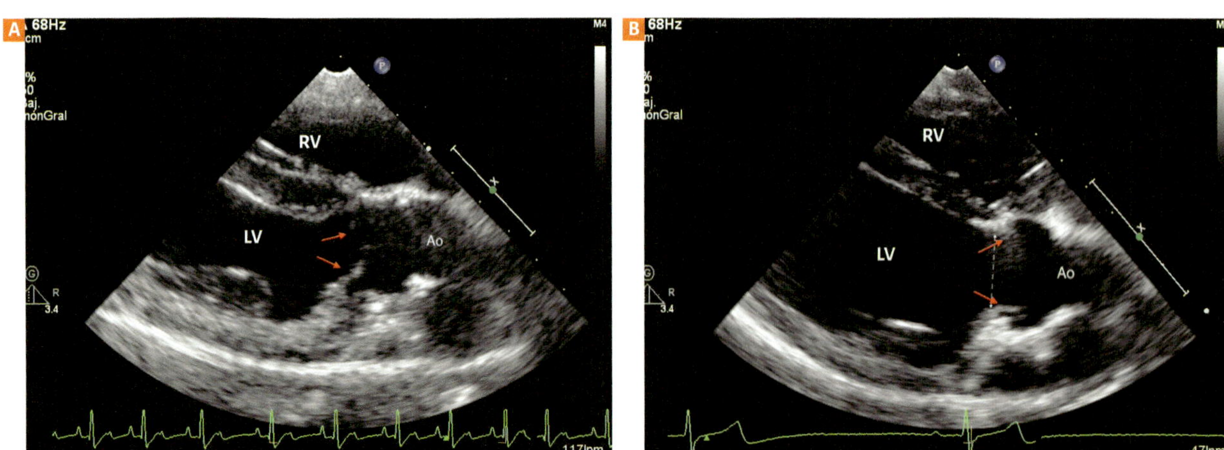

Figure 17. 2D echocardiogram in a normal dog, right-sided long axis parasternal view, showing the left ventricle (LV), the outflow tract and the ascending aorta (Ao). **A**. Two of the aortic sigmoids can be seen in the shape of a curve, closed during diastole. **B**. The aortic sigmoids are open during systole (arrows). In B measurement of the aortic *annulus*. RV: right ventricle.

weight) and is used to measure cardiac output using Doppler assessment of aortic flow (see the "Subxiphoid or Subcostal View" section).

Right-sided Short Axis Parasternal Views

Starting from a position on the long axis of the heart and turning the transducer 90° anticlockwise, transverse views of the heart are obtained, from the apex to the cardiac base, passing through the LV papillary muscles and the *chordae tendineae*, the mitral valve and the great vessels.

The views or images with diagnostic value that are explained below should be obtained.

Transventricular View

Obtained by placing the transducer with the marking directed cranially, over the 4th–5th intercostal space, almost perpendicular to the thorax (60°) and oriented caudally so that the transducer cable is directed slightly cranially (Figure 19 A).

Qualitative Analysis

- The LV appears with a circular shape in this image and the papillary muscles (anterior and posterior) are prominent in the ventricular cavity.
- The right ventricle, smaller than the left, is seen in the upper part of the image, with a crescent shape, within which one or more circular papillary muscles are seen.
- The very thin free wall of the right ventricle can be seen closest to the transducer.

Transmitral View

Obtained by orientating the transducer more parallel to the thorax than in the previous position and dorsally towards the back, so that the lead is positioned towards the sternum (Figure 19 B).

Qualitative Analysis

In this view, the following should be evaluated.

- The right ventricle is in the same position as in the transventricular view at the top of the image.
- The mitral valve appears in the left ventricular cavity, in the middle of the papillary muscles. It has an oval shape ("fish mouth") when it is open and appears as two parallel lines when the valve is closed. The septal (anterior) leaflet is the most dorsal and the parietal (posterior) leaflet is closest to the LV free wall.

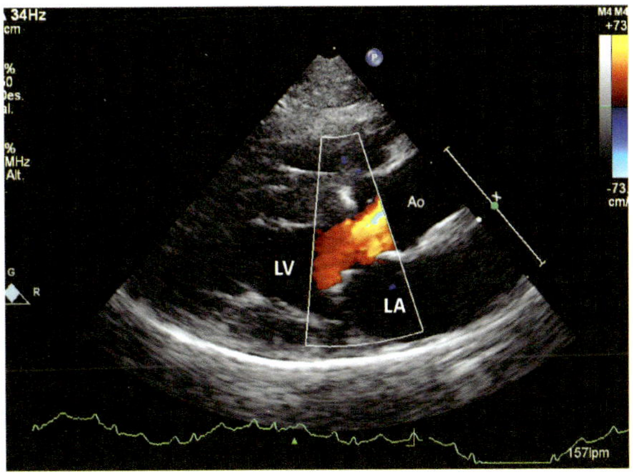

Figure 18. Colour Doppler echocardiogram in a normal cat, right-sided long axis parasternal view, showing the left ventricle (LV), the outflow tract and the ascending aorta (Ao). Laminar flow in red can be seen which goes from the LV towards the Ao. LA: left atrium.

Cardiac Base View, with the Aorta and Left Atrium

Obtained by positioning the transducer further towards the back (from the previous position), so that the lead is positioned ventrally and towards the xiphoid process (Figure 19 C). The transducer mark is still located cranially.

Qualitative Analysis

In this view, the following should be evaluated.

- The aorta appears as a circular structure located at the centre of the image.
- When closed the aortic sigmoids form an image similar to the Mercedes Benz logo (Figure 19 C). The sigmoid on the left is the non-coronary, the ventral one is the left coronary, and the one on the right is the right coronary.
- Dorsal to the aorta are the right atrium and ventricle with the tricuspid valve between them.
- To the left of the aorta is the left atrium with the appendage adjacent to the pulmonary artery.
- To the right of the aorta, the pulmonary valve and part of the main pulmonary artery can be seen.

Quantitative Analysis

In this view, the dimensions of the left atrium (LA) and aorta (Ao) are measured to obtain the LA/Ao ratio (<1.6 in dogs, <1.3 in cats).

Enlargement of the left atrium is a negative prognostic factor in patients with heart failure secondary to cardiomyopathies and mitral valve disorders (Figure 20).

Cardiac Base View with Aorta and Pulmonary Artery

Obtained by placing the transducer in a more cranial intercostal space (3rd intercostal space) and closer to the sternum than in the previous position and orientating it parallel and dorsal to the thorax of the animal, so that the transducer cable is positioned above the sternum (figure 19 D).

Qualitative Analysis

The following should be evaluated.

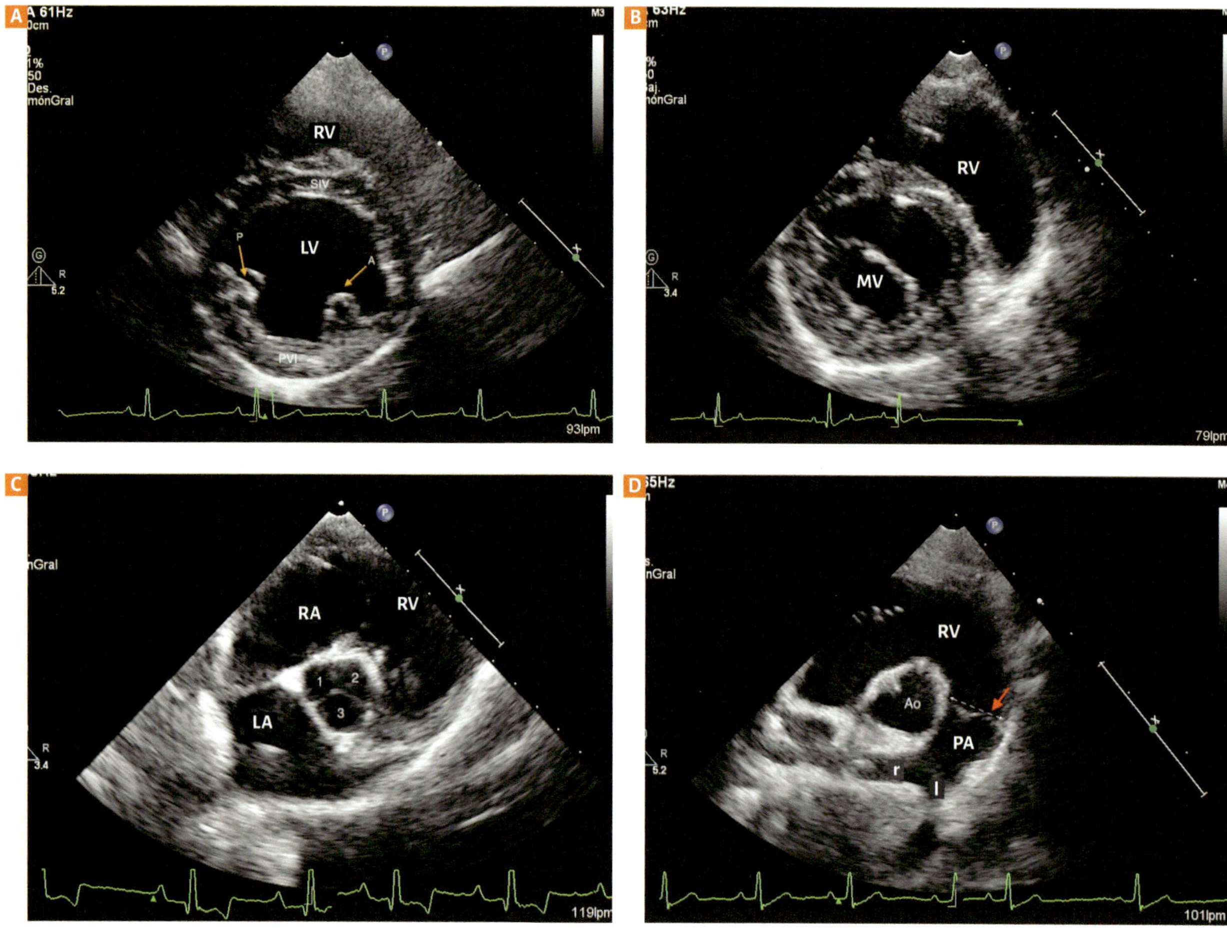

Figure 19. Bidimensional mode echocardiogram, right-sided short axis parasternal view at different levels. **A**. Transventricular where the left ventricle (LV) can be seen with the anterior (A) and posterior (P) papillary muscles towards the lumen (arrows) and the right ventricle (RV) in the upper part of the image in the shape of a half moon. **B**. Transmitral where the mitral valve (MV) can be seen with an oval shape in the centre of the LV. **C**. Transaortic cardiac base and left atrium (LA), where the aorta can be seen in the centre of the image with closed sigmoids ("Mercedes" logo) (1: non-coronary sigmoid, 2: right coronary sigmoid, 3: left coronary sigmoid), surrounded by the left atrium (LA), right atrium (RA), right ventricle (RV) and pulmonary infundibulum. **D**. Cardiac base with the aorta (Ao) and pulmonary artery (PA) and the sigmoids with a curved shape (red arrow). The Ao is visualised in the centre of the image of the RV in the upper part of the image and the pulmonary artery (PA) with bifurcation (r: right PA, l: left PA). Measurement of the PA *annulus* can also be seen.

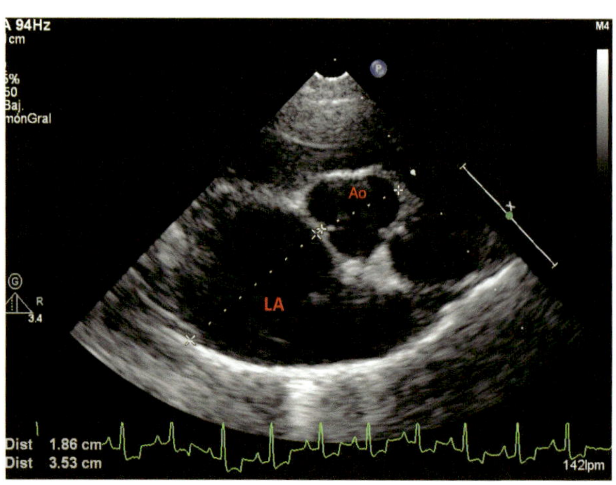

Figure 20. Bidimensional mode echocardiogram in a dog with chronic mitral disease and left atrial dilatation, right-sided short axis parasternal view at the transaortic cardiac base level, showing measurements for the aorta and left atrium for calculation of the LA/Ao ratio.

- In the centre of the image is the ascending aorta, dorsally the right ventricle and to the right of the image its outflow tract and the main pulmonary artery, on its long axis.
- In this view, two of the three pulmonary sigmoids are visualised as thin, curved lines when closed.
- The pulmonary artery bifurcates into two branches; the right one located ventrally to the aorta and the left ventrally into the pulmonary field. In cases of thromboembolism, the thrombus can be seen at the bifurcation, as is the case in cases of heartworm disease when parasite load is high.

Regarding the 2D image of this projection, **colour Doppler** mode is selected (Figure 21) to qualitatively evaluate the characteristics of pulmonary flow at the subvalvular, valvular and supravalvular levels, determining whether it is laminar or turbulent. Likewise, possible pulmonary insufficiency should be ruled out. Mild pulmonary insufficiency with a velocity less than 2 m/s is very common in normal dogs and cats.

To do this, the 2D mode sector is closed and colour Doppler is selected over the right ventricular outflow tract and the main pulmonary artery, adjusting the colour scale (pulse repetition frequency) to the pulmonary artery velocity (1 m/s) (Figure 22).

When turbulent flow is observed in the right ventricular outflow tract and/or main pulmonary artery, its velocity should be measured using spectral Doppler, first using pulsed Doppler and, if *aliasing* occurs, continuous Doppler. The ultrasound beam should be positioned as parallel as possible to the direction of blood flow (long axis of the pulmonary artery).

To determine the flow in the pulmonary artery, the pulsed Doppler sample volume is placed behind the pulmonary valve, within the main pulmonary artery. Normal pulmonary flow is laminar with slow acceleration and deceleration, as is appropriate for a low-pressure artery (Figure 21).

Quantitative Analysis

In this view the following should be measured.

- The diameter of the pulmonary valve *annulus* in systole (open sigmoid). This is used to calculate the pulmonary cardiac output (Qp) together with pulmonary flow, obtained by spectral Doppler, using the following formula to calculate the Velocity Time Integral (VTI):

$$\mathbf{Qp = VTI \times \pi(D/2)^2 \times HR}$$

($\pi = 3.1416$)

- The ratio between the diameter of the pulmonary artery *annulus* and the diameter of the aortic *annulus* in normal dogs (PA/Ao) should be in the range of 0.80–1.15. This is used to determine the type of congenital pulmonary stenosis (normal or hypoplastic *annulus*).
- Maximum pulmonary flow velocity and Doppler pressure gradient, VTI and systolic times (ejection time and pre-ejection period).

M-mode Echocardiographic Images

From the 2D-mode cross sections indicated above, the M-mode function is selected, and the cursor is placed on the structures to be examined, obtaining the standardised sections in which direct measurements of the cardiac structures (walls, chambers and great vessels) are performed (Tables 1, 2 and 3).

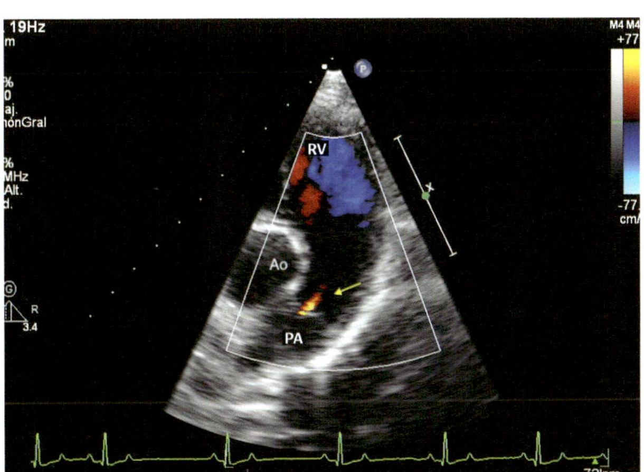

Figure 21. Colour Doppler echocardiogram in a normal dog, right-sided short axis parasternal view at the level of the cardiac base, aorta (Ao) and pulmonary artery (PA) showing a mild pulmonary insufficiency without clinical significance (arrow). RV: right ventricle.

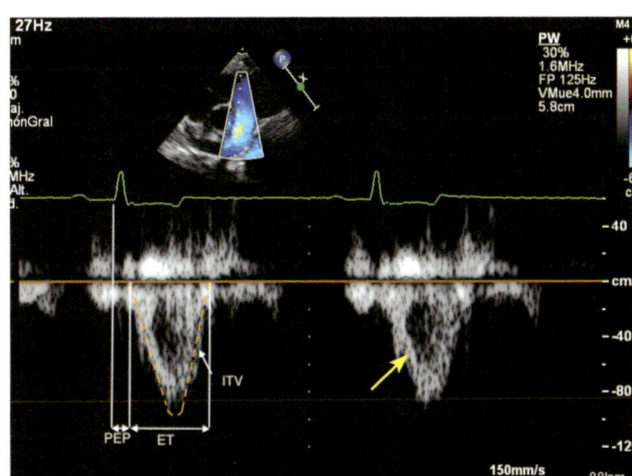

Figure 22. Spectral Doppler echocardiogram in a normal dog, right-sided short axis parasternal view at the level of the heart base, aorta and pulmonary artery showing pulmonary flow (arrow). Two measurement areas of the velocity time integral (VTI) are seen, using the spectral Doppler trace as well as systolic times, ejection time (ET) and pre-ejection period (PEP).

Table 1. Measurement of left ventricular (LV), interventricular septum and posterior wall size in dogs in relation to body weight (Cornell et al. 2004).

Body weight (kg)	LVd (cm)	LVs (cm)	PWd (cm)	IVSd (cm)
3	2.1 (1.8–2.6)	1.3 (1.0–1.8)	0.5 (0.4–0.8)	0.5 (0.4–0.8)
4	2.3 (1.9–2.8)	1.5 (1.1–1.9)	0.6 (0.4–0.8)	0.6 (0.4–0.8)
6	2.6 (2.2–3.1)	1.7 (1.2–2.2)	0.6 (0.4–0.9)	0.6 (0.4–0.9)
9	2.9 (2.4–3.4)	1.9 (1.4–2.5)	0.7 (0.5–1.0)	0.7 (0.5–1.0)
11	3.1 (2.6–3.7)	2.0 (1.5–2.7)	0.7 (0.5–1.0)	0.7 (0.5–1.1)
15	3.4 (2.8–4.1)	2.2 (1.7–3.0)	0.8 (0.5–1.1)	0.8 (0.6–1.1)
20	3.7 (3.1–4.5)	2.4 (1.8–3.2)	0.8 (0.6–1.2)	0.8 (0.6–1.2)
25	3.9 (3.3–4.8)	2.6 (2.0–3.5)	0.9 (0.6–1.3)	0.9 (0.6–1.3)
30	4.2 (3.5–5.0)	2.8 (2.1–3.7)	0.9 (0.6–1.3)	0.9 (0.7–1.3)
35	4.4 (3.6–5.3)	2.9 (2.2–3.9)	1.0 (0.7–1.4)	1.0 (0.7–1.4)
40	4.5 (3.8–5.5)	3.0 (2.3–4.0)	1.0 (0.7–1.4)	1.0 (0.7–1.4)
50	4.8 (4.0–5.8)	3.3 (2.4–4.3)	1.1 (0.7–1.5)	1.1 (0.7–1.5)
60	5.1 (4.2–6.2)	3.5 (2.6–4.6)	1.1 (0.7–1.6)	1.1 (0.8–1.6)
70	5.3 (4.4–6.5)	3.6 (2.7–4.8)	1.1 (0.8–1.6)	1.1 (0.8–1.6)

LVd, LVs: LV size in diastole (d) and systole (s), PWd: posterior wall diastole, IVSd: interventricular diastole.

Table 2. Reference ranges for spectral Doppler parameters and measurements and function indices for the left ventricle in normal adult dogs.

Parameter		Range or correct measurements
Mitral E (m/s)*		0.5–1.0
Mitral A (m/s)		0.3–0.6
E:A		1.63
Ao (m/s)		<1.7 left apical
		<2.2 subcostal
PEP/ET		0.24–0.38
PA (m/s)		<1.6 m/s
TD S'**	Lateral	5.8 ± 2.3
	Septal	4.1 ± 0.5
TD E'**	Lateral	7.4 ± 1.8
	Septal	5.5 ± 1.1
TD A'**	Lateral	3.3 ± 1.2
	Septal	3.9 ± 1.2
SF (%)		25–50
E-IVS (mm) M-mode		<7
EF (%) 2D mode		50–65
SVI (ml/m²)		≤30
LA/AO 2D mode		<1.6
SI		≥1.7

PEP: pre-ejection period. ET: ejection time. Ao: aorta. PA: pulmonary artery. SF: shortening fraction. E: point of maximum opening of the mitral valve. EF: ejection fraction. SVI: systolic volume index. SI: sphericity index. TD: tissue Doppler * Luis Fuentes et al. 2010; ** Hori et al. 2007.

Transventricular Level

Obtained by placing the M-mode cursor perpendicular to the ventricular septum between the two papillary muscles (Figure 2).

Qualitative Analysis

The free wall of the right ventricle and its chamber (smaller in relation to that of the LV), the interventricular septum, the left ventricular chamber (where the mitral valve chords can be observed) and the free wall of the LV. The septum and LV wall approach in systole and separate in diastole. The pericardium is visualised as a hyperechogenic line adjacent to the ventricular wall.

Quantitative Analysis

In this projection the following are measured.

- Systolic and diastolic septal and parietal thicknesses.
- The diameter of the diastolic right ventricular chamber and the dimensions of the LV chamber in both systole (s) and diastole (d). From these direct measurements the LV shortening fraction (SF) is obtained using the following formula:

SF (%) = LVd - LVs/LVd

- Standard measurements should be taken between the upper borders of each cardiac structure following the recommendations of the American Society of Echocardiography (Sahn & DeMaria, 1978). Due to the large variability in heart rate between dogs (sinus arrhythmia) performing at least three measurements in consecutive cardiac cycles is recommended.

Transmitral Level

Obtained by placing the M-mode cursor perpendicular to the ventricular septum in the centre of the LV over the mitral valve (Figure 23).

Qualitative Analysis

In this image the trace of the mitral valve should principally be evaluated. When it is open during diastole the leaflets are

Table 3. Echocardiographic measurements in adult cats (weight 3.2–7.2 kg) without signs of cardiopathy.

Parameter		Range or correct measurements
M-mode measurements*		
HR (bpm)		145–267
IVSd (mm)		≤5
LVd		11.5–17.8
PWd		≤5
IVSs		4.4–10.1
LVs		2.6–10.9
PWs		5.6–9.5
SF (%)		30–50
LA/Ao		<1.3
Spectral Doppler measurements*		
Ao (m/s)		0.8–1.9
PA (m/s)		0.5–1.6
Mitral E (m/s)		0.5–1.1
Mitral A (m/s)		0.3–0.9
E:A		1.1–2.9
TD S'** (cm/s)	Lateral	7.1 ± 2.34
	Septal	7.0 ± 1.8
TD E'** (cm/s)	Lateral	8.39 ± 2.58
	Septal	6.42 ± 1.83
TD A'** (cm/s)	Lateral	6.20 ± 2.43
	Septal	6.57 ± 2.4

HR: heart rate, IVSd, IVSs: interventricular septum diastolic (d) and systolic (s), LVd, LVs: left ventricle diastolic (d) and systolic (s), SF: shortening fraction, Ao: Aortic flow, PA: Pulmonary artery flow, TD: Tissue Doppler * Luis Fuentes V et al. 2010, ** Koffas et al. 2006.

thin, with the anterior leaflet appearing in an M shape and the posterior leaflet in a W shape. During systole the two leaflets appear as two parallel lines.

Quantitative Analysis

In this view the distance between the point of maximum opening of the mitral valve (E) and the interventricular septum (IVS) (Figure 23) (E – IVS <7 mm in dogs and almost non-existent in cats) is measured. This distance appears to be greater in patients with volume overload affecting the left-sided chambers or dilated cardiomyopathy.

Transaortic Level

Obtained by placing the M-mode cursor over the centre of the aorta and the left atrial appendage (Figure 24).

Qualitative Analysis

In this image the trace from the aortic valve and the set of

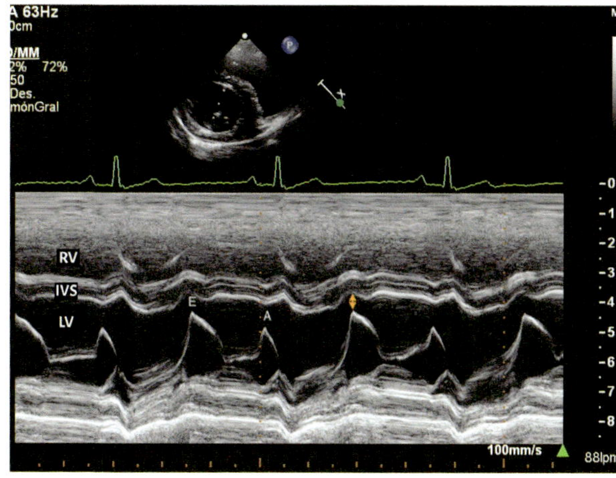

Figure 23. M-mode echocardiogram, transmitral level obtained using a right-sided parasternal view, where the image of the anterior leaflet can be seen with an 'M' shape and the posterior with a "W" shape. The measurement is shown from the point of maximum excursion of the mitral valve (E) to the interventricular septum. LV: left ventricle, RV: right ventricle, IVS: interventricular septum.

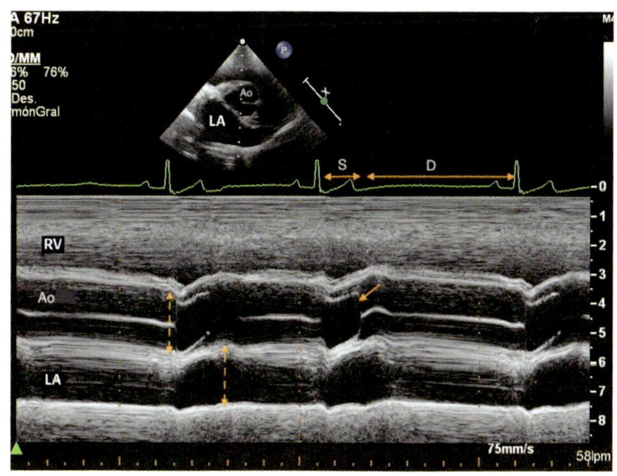

Figure 24. M-mode echocardiogram, transaortic level, where measurement of the size of the ascending aorta (Ao) is shown at the end of diastole and the size of the left atrium (LA) in systole. The open aortic valve appears to be box or rhombus shaped during systole (S) and closed during diastole (D). RV: right ventricle.

three spaces will be evaluated: right ventricle, aorta and left atrium. During systole the aortic valve appears as a box or rhombus shape and during diastole as a hyperechogenic line in the centre of the aorta.

Quantitative Analysis

In this view the size of the aorta at the end of diastole and that of the left atrium at the end of systole can be measured. In dogs these measurements are made in 2D echo because in M-mode the cursor passes through the appendage and not through the body of the left atrium.

Subxiphoid or Subcostal View

This view is primarily used to **measure aortic flow velocity in dogs**, especially those with suspected LV outflow tract stenosis. The animal should be in right or left lateral recumbency, depending on whether the operator is right or left-handed. A low frequency transducer (2–2.5 MHz) is selected to allow examination of the LV outflow tract and the ascending aorta. The transducer is positioned on the abdomen in a retroxiphoid position orientating it cranially and ventrally with the mark directed towards the spinal column (Figure 25). In this way a good alignment between the Doppler ultrasound beam and the aortic flow can be obtained and therefore the highest speed (V_{max} = 1.7–2.25 m/s).

In addition to velocity **ejection and pre-ejection times**, parameters used to evaluate ventricular functionality and the velocity time integral (VTI) can be measured (Figure 26). VTI is used to determine cardiac output (Qs) together with the diameter of the aortic *annulus* according to the formula given above for pulmonary cardiac output (Qp).

In large breed dogs with a deep chest the grey Doppler spectrum of blood flow may appear poorly defined, making measurements difficult. It can be improved by selecting the colour function in 2D mode and using the colour Doppler spectrum (Figure 26).

Animal Position: Left Lateral Recumbency

Diagnostic images are obtained by placing the transducer in two main positions, caudal or apical and cranial.

Caudal or Apical Left Parasternal View

These views are used for the evaluation of atrioventricular flows in both dogs and cats and also for aortic flow in cats.

Images in three cross-sectional planes are obtained:

Four Chamber Image

Obtained by placing the transducer over the 5th–6th left intercostal spaces near the cardiac apex (sternum) with the mark directed dorsally and caudally and orienting it towards the back and cardiac base (Figure 27).

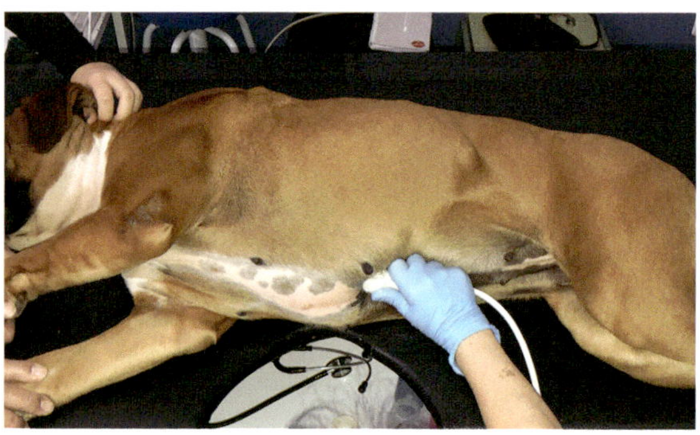

Figure 25. Positioning of the transducer in the dog to obtain aortic flow using a subcostal approach.

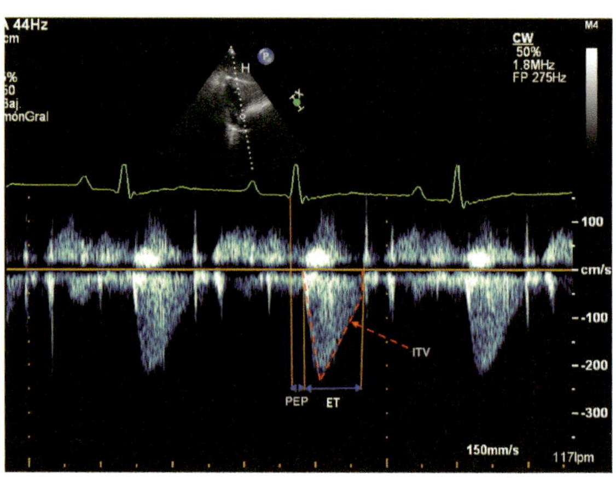

Figure 26. Continuous Doppler echocardiogram of aortic flow (arrows) in a normal dog, obtained using subcostal access. The places for measurement of the velocity time integral using the spectral Doppler trace can be seen along with systolic times, ejection time (ET) and pre-ejection period (PEP).

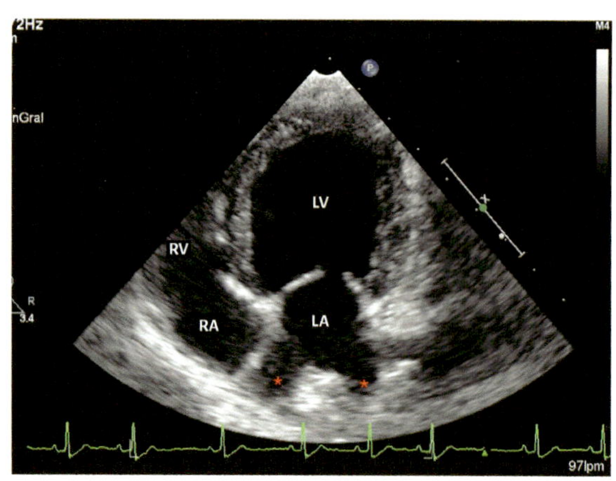

Figure 27. 2D echocardiogram in a normal dog obtained using a left-sided apical four chamber parasternal view. The group of cardiac chambers can be seen, right-sided ones are smaller in size than those on the left-side and the pulmonary veins in the lower part of the image (asterisks). LA: left atrium, LV: left ventricle, RA: right atrium, RV: right ventricle.

Qualitative Analysis

In this image the following should be evaluated.

- The set of four cardiac chambers with the right-sided chambers to the left of the image and smaller in size than the left-sided ones. Both atrioventricular valves are visualised, separating the atria from the ventricles.
- On the 2D image and selecting the colour Doppler function both left and right atrioventricular flow should be evaluated (Figure 28) in order to detect possible valvular stenosis or insufficiency.
- Pulsed Doppler is placed on the atrioventricular colour Doppler image in order to obtain the spectrum of atrioventricular flow (Figure 8).

Quantitative Analysis

In this image mitral and tricuspid flows will be obtained and measured in addition to the use of tissue Doppler.

- Transmitral flow is obtained by placing the pulsed Doppler sample volume behind the valve cusps when they open towards the LV in diastole. The Doppler spectrum consists of two waves or peaks, the E peak at the beginning of diastole and the A at the end, after the P wave of the ECG when atrial contraction occurs (Figure 8). The velocity of the E peak is greater than that of the A peak in dogs and cats without heart disease. If the heart rate is high as is often the case in cats the two peaks appear close together and the individual rates cannot be determined (Figure 29). The separation of both mitral waves can be achieved by lowering the heart rate using vagal manoeuvres (pressure on the eyeballs or nasal plane in cats and carotid sinus in dogs).
- For mitral flow the E and A velocities are measured as well as the deceleration time of the E wave (Figure 8).
- Left ventricular tissue Doppler is obtained by selecting the specific function for it and placing the sample volume on the lateral and medial *annulus* of the mitral valve. In both cases three peaks are obtained, one systolic (S') and two diastolic (E' and A') (Figure 10).
- Evaluation of the flow velocities of the pulmonary veins. Obtained by placing the sample volume (larger than that used for transmitral flow) into one of the pulmonary veins at the bottom of the four-chamber image. It consists of three peaks, systolic, diastolic and the reverse immediately after the ECG's P wave and atrial contraction.

Mitral flow, tissue Doppler and pulmonary vein measurements are used to assess LV diastolic function.

- Transtricuspid flow is obtained by optimizing the apical four-chamber image so that the right-sided chambers are better visualised. The Doppler spectrum also consists of two peaks: E and A with a velocity slightly lower than the velocities for transmitral flow and highly variable with the phases of respiration. It is also common for a systolic wave to be visualised.
- Right ventricular tissue Doppler is obtained by selecting the specific function for it and placing the sample volume on the lateral *annulus* of the tricuspid valve. The spectrum is also seen in three peaks, one systolic (S') and two diastolic (E' and A') (Figure 30).
- Evaluation of the RV and right atrial area (A) in systole (s) and diastole (d). They can also be measured in the right cranial parasternal view. From these values the right ventricular fractional area change (RVAC) is determined using the following formula:

RVAC = RVdA - RVsA/RVdA

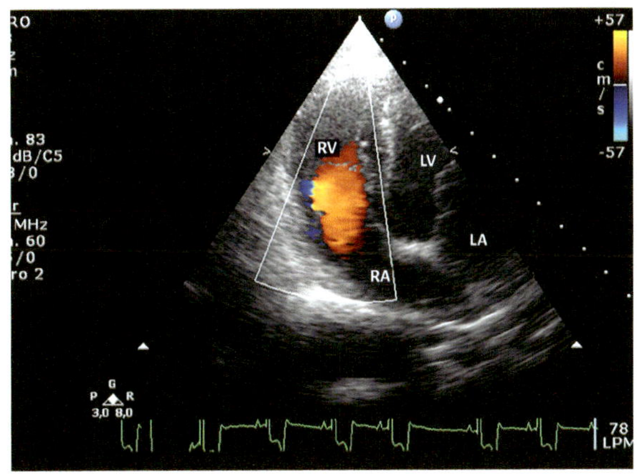

Figure 28. Colour Doppler echocardiogram of tricuspid flow in a normal dog obtained using a left apical parasternal view optimised for the visualization of the right-sided chambers. Flow with a red colour can be seen as it approaches the transducer (from the right atrium (RA) to the right ventricle (RV). On the right side of the image the colour scale can be seen with a numeration corresponding to the pulse repetition frequency which corresponds to the flow velocity to be measured. LA: left atrium, LV: left ventricle.

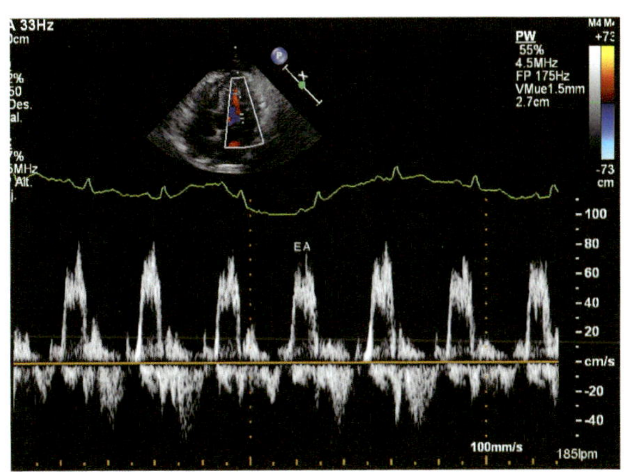

Figure 29. Pulsed Doppler echocardiogram showing transmitral flow in a normal cat obtained using a left apical parasternal view. Spectral Doppler shows the E and A peaks nearly merging due to the elevated heart rate.

– Evaluation of the excursion of the tricuspid *annulus* in systole known by the acronym TAPSE (tricuspid *annular* plane systolic excursion) (Figure 31). Measured using M-mode and placing the cursor on the tricuspid *annulus* and obtaining its systolic displacement in the form of variable depth waves. The reference values for TAPSE in relation to the aortic measurement (TAPSE/Ao) are 0.65–1.07.

Three-five Chamber Image

Obtained from the four-chamber projection by slightly rotating the mark cranially and directing the transducer towards the head of the animal so that the ultrasound beam is placed parallel to the long axis of the heart (Figure 32).

Qualitative Analysis

In this view the LV outflow tract and the anterior leaflet of the mitral valve are evaluated, especially in cats with hypertrophic cardiomyopathy. Likewise the LV, left atrium and right ventricle are observed.

Using colour Doppler the characteristics of the LV outflow tract can be evaluated determining whether flow is laminar or turbulent and detecting possible aortic regurgitation.

Quantitative Analysis

Aortic flow can be measured. Generally, the velocity is lower than that obtained through a subcostal approach (Figure 33).

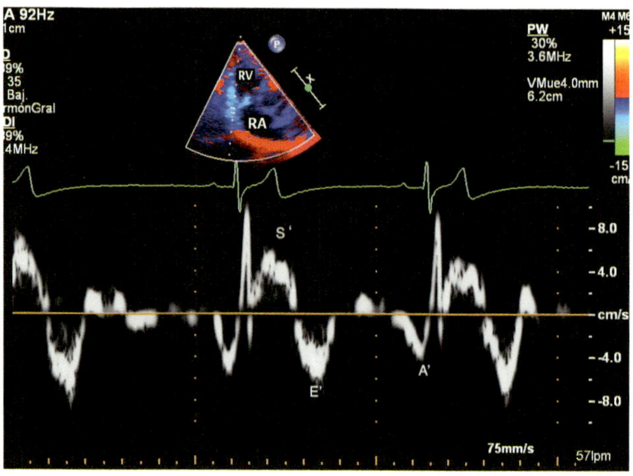

Figure 30. Tissue Doppler echocardiogram in a normal dog obtained using a left apical parasternal view, placing the sample volume over the tricuspid *annulus* showing one systolic (s') and two diastolic (E' and A') waves.

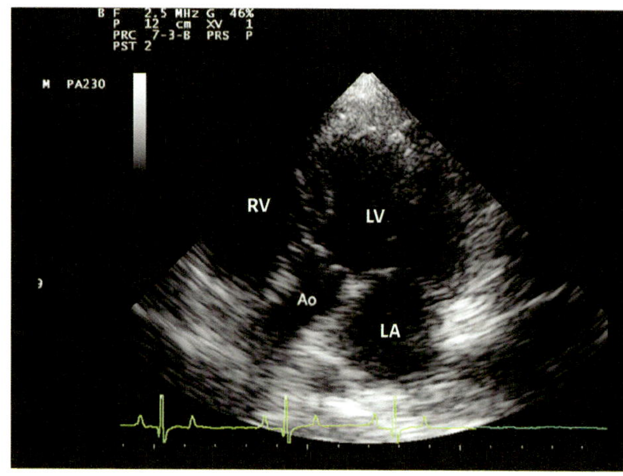

Figure 32. 2D echocardiogram in a normal dog obtained using a left-sided apical three-five chamber parasternal view. The left-sided chambers can be seen with the ascending aorta (Ao). LA: left atrium, LV: left ventricle, RV: right ventricle.

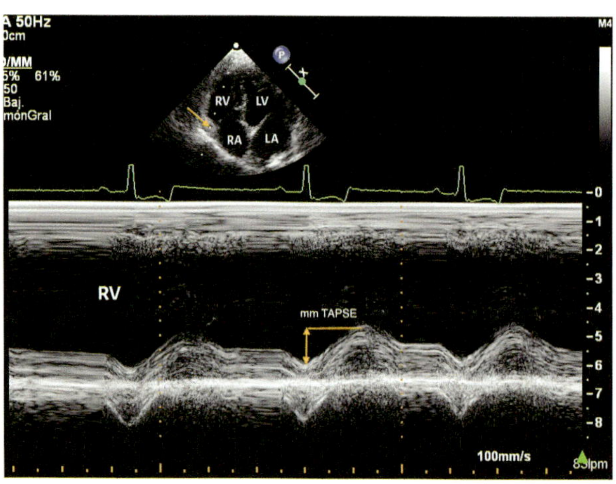

Figure 31. M-mode echocardiogram of the tricuspid annular plane systolic excursion (TAPSE) obtained using a right-sided apical four chamber parasternal view and placing the M-mode cursor over the tricuspid *annulus*. The method for measurement of the excursion (line of arrows) is also shown. LA: left atrium, LV: left ventricle, RA: right atrium, RV: right ventricle.

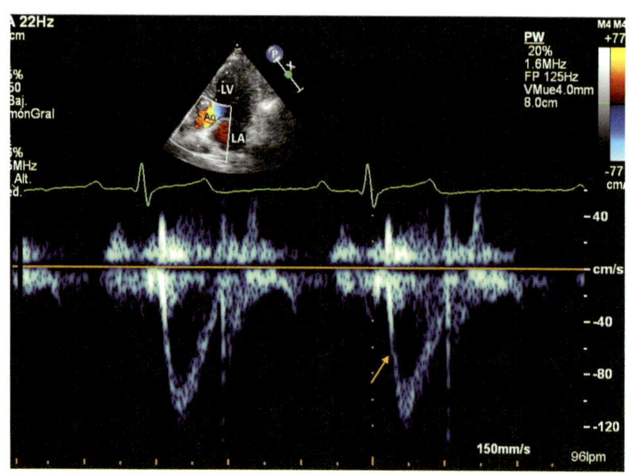

Figure 33. Pulsed Doppler echocardiogram in a normal dog obtained using a left-sided apical three-five chamber parasternal view, displaying aortic flow (arrow). LA: left atrium, LV: left ventricle, Ao: ascending aorta.

By enlarging the sample volume and placing it in the LV outflow tract between the mitral and aortic flow, the LV inflow and outflow are obtained simultaneously.

These are used to determine the myocardial function index which is useful to assess both LV systolic and diastolic function (Figure 34).

Two Chamber Image

Obtained from the apical position and with the ultrasound beam parallel to the long axis of the heart.

Qualitative Analysis

The LV and LA are seen separated by the mitral valve (Figure 35). This image allows visualization of the appendage, which is important in cats with cardiomyopathy and suspected thromboembolism.

Left-sided Cranial Parasternal Views

Obtained by placing the transducer in a more cranial position over the 3rd–4th intercostal spaces, between the sternum and the costochondral junctions and with the mark on the transducer directed cranially. Three long axis images and one short axis image are obtained.

Long Axis Views

Image of Entire Outflow Tract of the Left Ventricle

Obtained by placing the transducer with the mark directed cranially, the ultrasound beam along the long axis of the thorax and oriented slightly caudally towards the vertebral column (Figure 36).

Qualitative Analysis

This image allows visualization of the LV outflow tract and the ascending aorta with great precision, making it useful for characterisation of both valvular and subvalvular aortic stenoses. Using colour Doppler the characteristics of the flow in the outflow tract and ascending aorta can be determined.

Cranial Image of the Right Ventricle, Atrium and Appendage

Obtained with the transducer located cranially, close to the elbow of the animal and more perpendicular to the thorax than in the previous position (Figure 37).

Qualitative Analysis

This view is used to evaluate the right-sided chambers, tricuspid valve, entrance of the caudal vena cava to the right atrium and the right atrial appendage. The latter is important in dogs with neoplasms such as haemangiosarcoma.

Quantitative Analysis

Transtricuspid flow can be identified and measured using

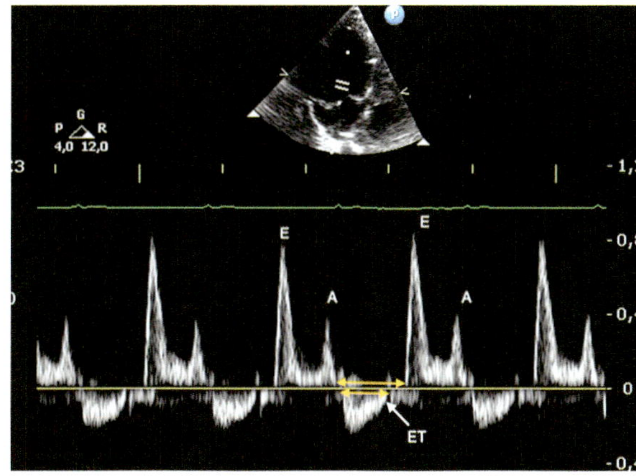

Figure 34. Pulsed Doppler Echocardiogram of mixed flow, transmitral and left ventricular outflow tract in a normal dog obtained using a left apical parasternal view. The location for measurement of ejection time (ET) and A-E duration can be seen for calculation of the myocardial performance index (MPI) using the formula: MPI = (A - E) - ET/ET.

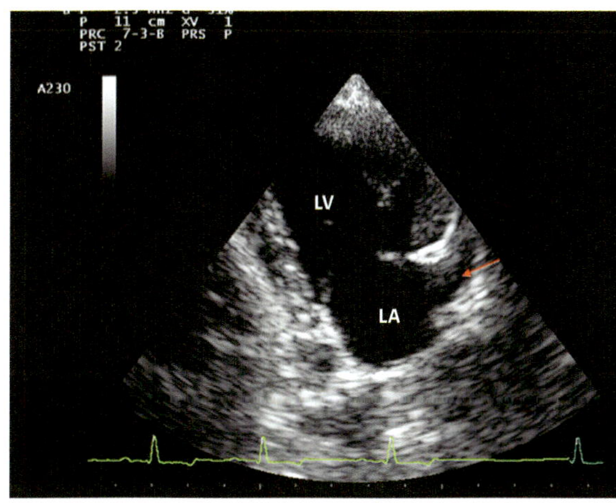

Figure 35. 2D echocardiogram, apical two chamber parasternal view, where the left ventricle (LV), left atrium (LA) and left appendage (arrow) can be seen.

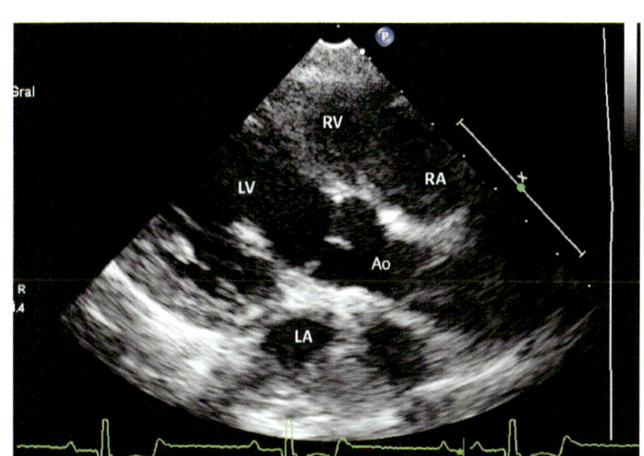

Figure 36. Long axis 2D echocardiogram obtained from a left-sided cranial parasternal view showing the left ventricular (LV) outflow tract and ascending aorta (Ao). RA: right atrium, RV: right ventricle.

spectral Doppler, as well as RV and RA area in systole and diastole to assess systolic and diastolic functions, respectively.

Cranial Image of the Right Ventricular Outflow Tract

Obtained by placing the transducer in a cranial position near the elbow of the animal, with the mark directed cranially and orienting the transducer towards the spine (Figure 38).

Qualitative Analysis

This image is used for visualization of the pulmonary artery and the descending aorta, which is important in patients with patent *ductus arteriosus* as it allows for characterisation and measurement of its size. Likewise, it complements the short-axis image obtained using the right-sided short axis parasternal view for the evaluation of the right ventricular outflow tract and pulmonary valve. Colour Doppler can be used to assess the flow through the pulmonary artery and descending aorta.

Quantitative Analysis

This image makes it possible to easily obtain information regarding pulmonary flow since the ultrasound beam and blood flow are parallel (Figure 39), as well as the velocity of a possible patent *ductus arteriosus*.

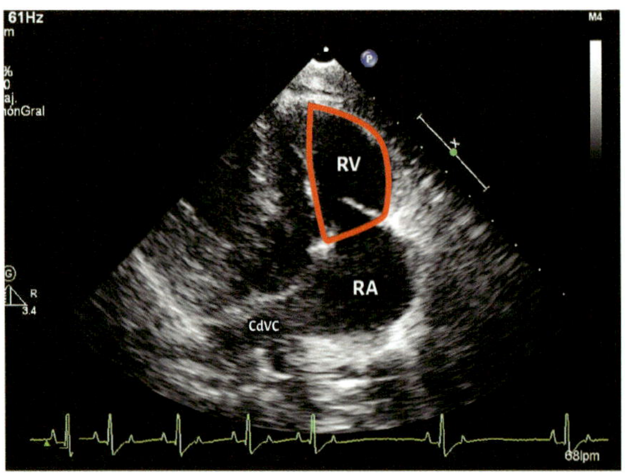

Figure 37. Long axis 2D echocardiogram obtained from a left-sided cranial parasternal view where the right-sided chambers and caudal vena cava (CdVC) entering the right atrium can be seen. Measurement of right ventricular area is shown round the endocardium from the *annulus* of the tricuspid valve. RA: right atrium, RV: right ventricle.

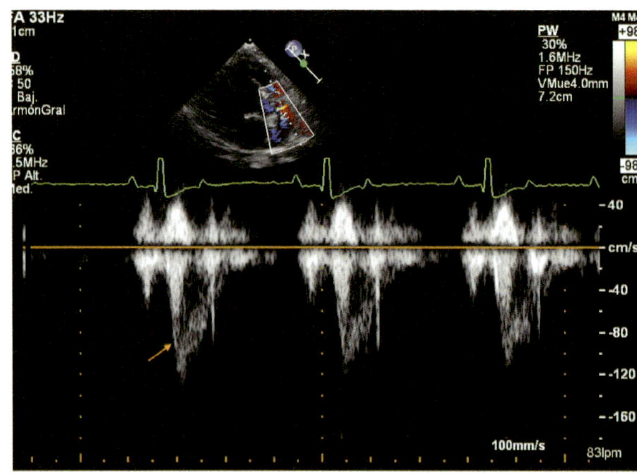

Figure 39. Long axis pulsed Doppler echocardiogram obtained from a left-sided cranial parasternal view showing pulmonary flow (arrow).

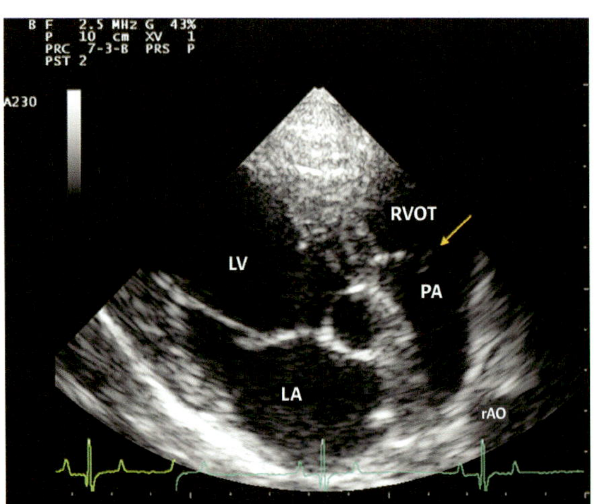

Figure 38. Long axis 2D echocardiogram obtained from a left-sided cranial parasternal view where the left-sided chambers, right ventricular outflow tract (RVOT) and pulmonary artery (PA) can be seen. RA: right atrium, RV: right ventricle.

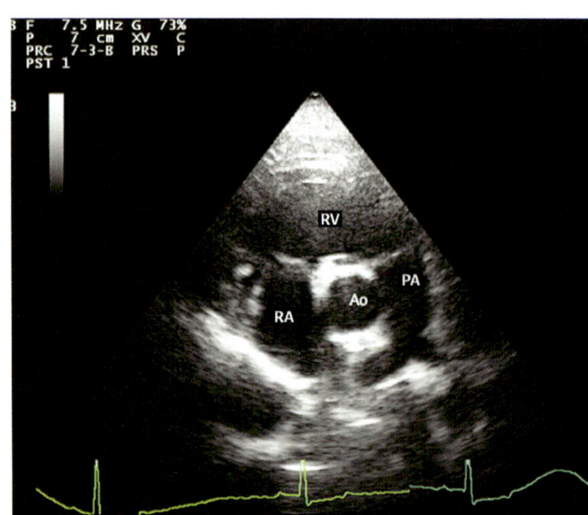

Figure 40. Short axis 2D echocardiogram obtained from a left-sided cranial parasternal view where the aorta can be seen surrounded by the right-sided chambers and the pulmonary artery with its bifurcation. RA: right atrium, RV: right ventricle.

Short Axis View

Obtained from the long axis images, rotating the transducer 90° in an anticlockwise direction with the mark facing dorsally (Figure 40).

Qualitative Analysis

This image makes it possible to assess the set of right-sided chambers and the pulmonary artery with its bifurcation.

Quantitative Analysis

Transtricuspid flow and pulmonary artery flow can be obtained from this image.

Main Parameters Indicative of Ventricular Functionality

Left ventricle:

- systolic function:
  - LV shortening fraction
  - LV ejection fraction
  - distance between the point of maximum opening of the mitral valve and the interventricular septum (E-IVS)
  - ventricular volumes
  - ventricular dimensions
  - myocardial performance index
- diastolic function:
  - left atrial dimension
  - isovolumic relaxation time
  - E/A ratio
  - E/E' ratio
  - duration of wave A
  - pulmonary veins: S/D ratio
  - pulmonary veins reverse R peak (speed and duration)
  - myocardial performance index.

Right ventricle:

- systolic function:
  - TAPSE
  - fractional change in RV area
  - S' tissue Doppler
- diastolic function:
  - RA size
  - tricuspid flow
  - tissue Doppler: diastolic velocities, tricuspid valve *annulus*.

Echocardiographic Report

The echocardiographic report is the means by which both the descriptive results of the echocardiographic examination and the clinical implications and diagnostic considerations are transmitted, in the context of the patient's clinical signs.

Ultrasound equipment often integrates the option to issue a report into its operating system, so that the measurements are automatically transferred to it along with some representative images of the heart disease.

A report should include:

- animal information: age, breed, sex, body condition;
- reason for echocardiographic examination in this patient;
- qualitative description of the cardiac structures from an anatomical point of view, highlighting the anomalies;
- quantitative data on the size of cardiac structures and great vessels, as well as ventricular systolic and diastolic function indices;
- haemodynamic Doppler data indicating the qualitative and quantitative characteristics of the transvalvular flows and possible pathological communications;
- summary and conclusions from a diagnostic and therapeutic viewpoint.

Bibliography

- Abbot, J.A., MacLean. (2003) Comparison of Doppler-derived peak aortic velocities obtained from subcostal and apical transducer sites in healthy dogs. *Vet Radiol & Ultrasound*, 44, pp. 695–698.
- Abraham, T.P., Dimaano, V.L., Liang, H-Y. (2007) Role of Tissue Doppler and Strain echocardiography in current clinical practice. *Circulation*, 116, pp. 2597–2609.
- Bonagura, J.D., Miller, M.W., Darke, P.G.G. (1998) Doppler echocardiography I. Pulsed-wave and continuous-wave examinations. *Vet Clinics North Am: Small Anim Pract*, 28, pp. 1325–1359.
- Bonagura, J.D., Miller, M.W. (1998) Doppler echocardiography II. Color Doppler imaging. *Vet Clinics North Am: Small Anim Pract*, 28, pp. 1361–1389.
- Boon, J.A. (2011) *Veterinary Echocardiography.* 2nd ed. Iowa: Wiley-Blackwell.
- Caivano, D., Dickson, D., Pariaut, R., et al. (2018) Tricuspid annular plane systolic excursion-to-aortic ratio provides a bodyweight-independent measure of right ventricular systolic function in dogs. *J Vet Cardiol*, 20, pp. 79–91.
- Chetboul, V., Sampedrano, C.C., et al. (2006) Quantitative Assessment of velocities of the *annulus* of the left atrioventricular valve and left ventricular free wall in healthy cats by use of two-dimensional color tissue Doppler imaging. *Am J Vet Res*, 67, pp. 250–258.
- Cornell, C.C., Kittleson, M.D., Della Torre, P., et al. (2004) Allometric scaling of M-mode cardiac measurements in normal adult dogs. *J Vet Intern Med*, 18, pp. 311–21.
- Fernandez del Palacio, Bayon, A., Agut, A. (1997) Dilated coronary sinus in a dog with persistent left cranial vena cava. *Vet Radiol & Ultrasound*, 38, pp. 376–379.
- Gomez, A., Fernandez-del Palacio, J., Latorre, R., et al. (2012) Plastinated heart slices aid echocardiographic interpretation in the dog. *Veterinary Radiology & Ultrasound*, 53, pp. 197–203.
- Haggstrom, J., Andersson, A.O., Falk, T., et al. (2016) Effect of Body Weight on Echocardiographic Measurements in 19.866 Pure-Bred Cats with or without Heart Disease. *J Vet Intern Med*, 30, pp. 1601–1611.
- Hansson, K., Haggstrom, J., Kvart, C., et al. (2002) Left atrial to aortic root indices using two-dimensional and M-mode echocardiography in Cavalier King Charles Spaniels with and without left atrial enlargement. *Vet Radiol & Ultrasound*, 43, pp. 568–575.
- Hoglund, K., Bussadori, C., Domenech, O., et al. (2007) Contrast echocardiography in Boxer dogs with and without aortic stenosis. *J Vet Cardiol*, 9, pp. 15–24.
- Hori, Y., Sato, Y., Hoshi, F., et al. (2007) Assessment of Longitudinal tissue Doppler Imaging of the left ventricular septum and free wall as an indicator of left ventricular systolic function in dogs. *Am J vet Res*, 68, pp. 1051–1057.
- Koffas, H., Dukes-McEvan, J., Corcoran, B.M., et al. (2006) Pulsed Tissue Doppler Imaging in normal cats and cats with hypertrophic cardiomyopathy. *J Vet Intern Med*, 20, pp. 65–77.
- Luis Fuentes, V. (2010) Echocardiography. In: Luis Fuentes, V., Johnson, L.R., Denis, S. (eds). *BSAVA Manual of Canine and Feline Cardiorespiratory Medicine.* 2nd ed, pp. 79–97.
- Rishniw, M., Erb, H.N. (2000) Evaluation of four 2-dimensional echocardiographic methods of assessing left atrial size in dogs. *J Vet Intern Med*, 14, pp. 429–35.
- Sahn, D.J., DeMaria, S., et al. (1978) Recommendations regarding quantitation in M-mode echocardiography: results of a survey of echocardiographic measurements. *Circulation*, 58, pp. 1072–1083.
- Schober, K., Savino, S., Yildiz, V. (2017) Reference intervals and allometric scaling of two dimensional echocardiographic measurements in 150 healthy cats. *J Vet Med Sci*, 10, 79, pp. 1764–1771.
- Thomas, W.P., Gaber, C.E., Jacobs, G.J., et al. (1993) Recommendations for standards in transthoracic two-dimensional echocardiography in the dog and cat. *J Vet Intern Med*, 7, pp. 247–252.

Test

Answers on Page 108

1. **Indicate which is correct regarding the echocardiographic examination:**
   a. Cats require low frequency sector transducers.
   b. Patients are preferably placed in lateral recumbency.
   c. The best images are obtained with animals in the supine position.
   d. Pleural effusion makes examination of the heart difficult.

2. **Indicate which is the correct answer:**
   a. Subcostal access is used to obtain maximum blood flow velocity in the pulmonary artery.
   b. High-frequency transducers (7.5–10 MHz) are best suited for Doppler echocardiographic examination in dogs over 20 kg.
   c. α-2 adrenergic agonists are the sedatives of choice in dogs and cats with heart disease for echocardiographic examination due to their minimal or null influence on the cardiovascular system.
   d. The acepromazine/buprenorphine or acepromazine/butorphanol combination is suitable for echocardiographic examination in dogs or cats.

3. **Indicate which is correct regarding echocardiographic projections (access):**
   a. Right parasternal and subcostal access is used.
   b. Using the right parasternal approach only short-axis sections of the heart are obtained.
   c. Subcostal access is used to obtain pulmonary flow velocities.
   d. Flow rates are obtained for the atrioventricular valves using the left parasternal access.

4. **Indicate which statement is false regarding M-mode echocardiography:**
   a. The heart is scanned using M-mode in each plane.
   b. It is used mainly for the measurement of cardiac structures.
   c. M-mode is derived from 2D mode images.
   d. M-mode is obtained from right-sided parasternal images of the short-axis.

5. **Indicate which statement is false regarding the left parasternal projection:**
   a. The transducer is placed in a cranial apical position.
   b. Using an apical position 4 and 5 chamber sections are obtained.
   c. Long and short axis sections are obtained using a cranial position.
   d. Aortic flow can be measured using a cranial position.

6. **Indicate which of the following statements is true:**
   a. 2D mode is the mode of choice to evaluate the size of the left atrium in dogs.
   b. M-mode allows accurate assessment of the relationship between the left atrium/aorta in dogs.
   c. The systolic size of the interventricular septum is measured at the end of the R wave on the electrocardiogram.
   d. The diastolic size of the interventricular septum is measured at the end of the T wave on the electrocardiogram.

Correct Answers:

1. b
2. d
3. d
4. a
5. d
6. a

NOTES

Therapeutic Principles and Treatment

Mª Josefa Fernández-del Palacio

Heart failure (HF) is a common reason for owners to take their pets to for a veterinary consult. The treatment of HF can be a challenge, both for cases managed as outpatients and those presented at emergency departments. This chapter focuses on the **definitions** related to the term "heart failure", the **causes** of HF, the **complex mechanisms** involved, types of treatment (including the drugs), and a summary of **treatment** protocols according to the clinical stage.

Box 1. Definitions

- **Heart disease:** any functional or structural abnormality of the heart that may or may not cause HF.
- **Heart failure (HF) or cardiac insufficiency:** a pathophysiological state in which cardiac output is inadequate to meet the metabolic needs of the tissues and exercise capacity can become limited despite normal or increased ventricular filling pressures. In other words, the heart has to adapt to "fulfil" the main functions of the cardiovascular system and the maintenance of blood pressure adequate for an individual's activity. The term heart failure is synonymous with cardiac insufficiency.
- **Congestive heart failure (CHF):** an oedematous state due to the combination of excessive sodium and water retention and a failing heart.

HF is characterised by vascular, renal, neurological, and endocrine responses that affect the heart, blood vessels, kidney, lungs, and central nervous system. **The aim of these responses is to maintain blood volume, venous and arterial pressures, heart rate, cardiac output, and ventilation,** within a range of sufficient levels to maintain tissue needs at rest, exercise, and in stressful situations. However, with **HF the failure of these mechanisms** is responsible, in the long term, for most of the clinical signs that appear in patients with CHF.

Treatment of HF should be tailored to the individual patient, based on the cause of the HF, the neurohormonal and cardiac remodelling mechanisms involved, and the patient's clinical stage.

Causes of Heart Failure and Compensatory Mechanisms

It is essential to understand the causes and pathophysiological mechanisms that occur in HF in order to provide an accurate prognosis and select the most appropriate treatment.

Causes of HF

Anatomical/Morphological

The lesions responsible for HF include both **congenital and acquired anomalies** affecting cardiac structures:

- **pericardium**: idiopathic pericarditis, haemopericardium due to haemangiosarcoma, etc.
- **myocardium**: dilated cardiomyopathy (DCM), myocarditis, etc.
- **heart valves**: congenital valvular dysplasia, chronic degenerative mitral disease (CDMD), etc.
- **communications between cardiac chambers or great vessels**: ventricular septal (VSD) and atrial defects and patent *ductus arteriosus* (PDA)
- formation and conduction of the **electrical impulse:** arrhythmias
- **blood vessels**: systemic arterial hypertension, pulmonary hypertension, etc.

Aetiological

Lesions can be **primary or secondary**:

- degenerative: chronic mitral and tricuspid valve disease (valvular endocardiosis)
- congenital malformations: patent *ductus arteriosus* (PDA), ventricular septal defect (VSD), etc.
- metabolic/endocrine: hyperthyroidism in cats, hypothyroidism in dogs
- nutritional: taurine deficiency in cats
- neoplastic: lymphoma in cats
- infectious: infective endocarditis
- inflammatory and immune-mediated: myocarditis
- iatrogenic: doxorubicin
- neoplastic: chemodectoma.

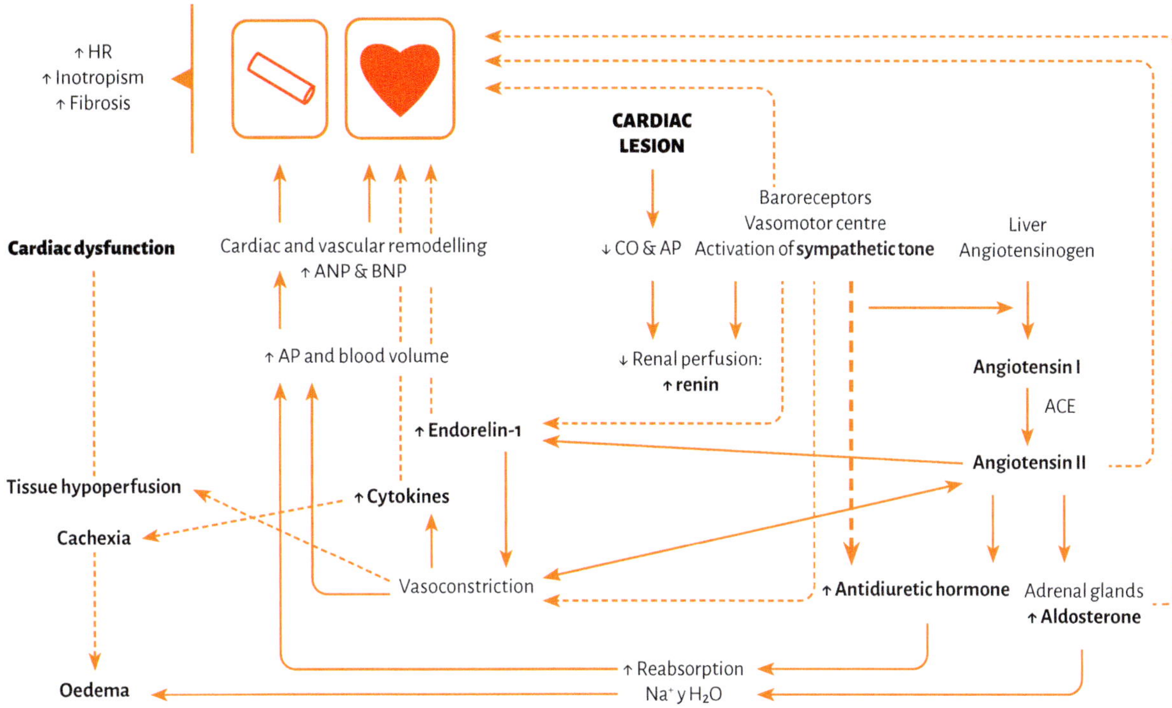

Figure 1. Diagram showing the compensatory mechanisms triggered in the course of heart failure and the clinical consequences (cardiac dysfunction, oedema, tissue hypoperfusion, cachexia). CO: cardiac output, AP: systemic arterial pressure, ACE: angiotensin converting enzyme, ANP: atrial natriuretic peptide, BNP: brain natriuretic peptide, HR: heart rate.

Pathophysiological

- **Myocardial dysfunction** and decreased systolic stroke volume: occur in primary and secondary DCM due to taurine deficiency (cats, Boxer, American Cocker Spaniel, Dalmatian and Golden Retriever), canine hypothyroidism, doxorubicin-induced cardiomyopathy, neoplasia (lymphoma), amyloidosis, and tachycardiomyopathy.
- **Valvular insufficiency** and volume overload: occurs in chronic disease of the atrioventricular valves, aortic insufficiency (endocarditis), congenital valvular dysplasia, dilatation of mitral and tricuspid annuli secondary to left-right intracardiac blood shunts (PDA and VSD). The consequence is chronic volume overload, elevated atrial and ventricular pressures, and CHF. In advanced stages, volume overload can also lead to myocardial dysfunction.
- **Diastolic function failure**: occurs in patients with hypertrophic and restrictive cardiomyopathies, and ventricular ischaemia. Diastolic dysfunction causes increased atrial, ventricular and venous system pressures, with consequent pulmonary oedema and/or ascites.
- **Increased afterload**: occurs in patients with pulmonary hypertension, systemic arterial hypertension, and obstructions of the ventricular outflow tracts (aortic and pulmonary stenosis). A chronic increase in afterload causes a reduction in systolic ejection, as well as an increase in myocardial oxygen consumption and a decrease in oxygen perfusion.
- **Decreased preload**: occurs in cases of severe pericardial effusion with tamponade, resulting in obstruction of venous return to the right-sided chambers, decrease in diastolic volume and, therefore, cardiac output.

Compensatory Mechanisms

The development of cardiac injury causes **haemodynamic changes related to decreased cardiac output and poor peripheral perfusion** (Figure 1). The decrease in arterial pressure is **counteracted by adaptations** by the neuroendocrine system, the kidneys and the heart muscle. These result in activation of the vasoconstrictor control systems and sodium and water retention, attenuation of vasodilator and natriuretic systems, activation of the foetal genes, and increased muscle hypertrophy, fibrosis and tissue inflammation mediators. In this scenario, **a "well compensated" patient generally maintains cardiac output and blood pressure within the normal range**. This is achieved by:

1. Vasoconstriction and Redistribution

- **Vasoconstriction and redistribution of blood flow**: mediated by the sympathetic nervous system (SNS), renin-angiotensin-aldosterone system (RAAS), vasopressin, and vascular endothelium.
- Early **activation of the SNS** (mediated by baroreceptors due to decreasing preload) helps maintain cardiac output, systemic blood pressure, tissue perfusion (by increasing venous return), and cardiac chronotropism and inotropism. However, increased myocardial work leads to high energy and oxgyen consumption, and over time this predisposes to myocardial damage and arrhythmias.
- Activation of the RAAS occurs when **cardiac output is reduced and the renal receptors detect it, releasing renin**. In the liver this contributes to the transformation of angiotensinogen into angiotensin I which is later transformed into angiotensin II by means of angiotensin converting enzyme (ACE). This, in turn, increases the synthesis of aldosterone (adrenal cortex) and antidiuretic hormone (arginine vasopressin). **Angiotensin II is a powerful vasoconstrictor** which also promotes remodelling of the vessels (hypertrophy, apoptosis, and cytokine activation) and myocardium (hypertrophy and fibrosis).
- Activation of these **neurohormonal systems** also promotes the release of endothelin-1 (E-1), a potent vasoconstrictor which participates in cell proliferation. Plasma E-1 is elevated in patients with HF, regardless of the aetiology, correlates with the severity of the disease, and plays an important role in the development of pulmonary hypertension.

2. Sodium and Water Retention

- **Sodium and water retention**: changes in renal flow, aldosterone, arginine-vasopressin, and inhibition of natriuretic hormones (ANP and BNP) occur.
- **Aldosterone causes sodium retention** in the distal renal tubules. Renal sympathetic stimulation causes **the release of antidiuretic hormone by the pituitary gland, which reduces the excretion of free water** (increasing preload) and contributes to worsening peripheral vasoconstriction and increasing endothelin production.
- **Natriuretic peptides** act as regulators of sodium and water homeostasis. They are increased in patients with HF due to distension of the cardiac chambers, and secondary to increased preload due to sodium and water retention. Their function is to neutralize the RAAS and SNS, inhibiting the release of vasopressin and avoiding sodium and water retention. In practice, **the increase in these peptides is used with diagnostic value for HF to differentiate between cardiac and respiratory involvement** and to monitor treatment.

3. Cardiac Structure and Remodelling

- **Changes in cardiac structure and function or cardiac remodelling**: a series of anatomical, geometric, histological, and molecular changes to the myocardium occur secondary to myocardial overload or damage. The heart responds to volume and/or pressure overload with **eccentric** (atrioventricular valve insufficiency, L-R blood shunts, chronic dilated cardiomyopathy, chronic bradycardia) or **concentric** (left or right ventricular outflow tract obstruction, systemic hypertension) **hypertrophy**, respectively.
- **Ventricular dilation** helps maintain the force of contraction and stroke volume, according to the mechanism in Frank Starling's law. However, the neurohormonal and E-1 systems **induce myocardial fibrosis in hypertrophic and dilated hearts**, causing stiffness (which makes ventricular filling difficult) and diastolic failure. This, in turn, predisposes the patient to high capillary pressures and oedema.

These **compensatory mechanisms** are very effective, so the **clinical signs of heart failure may be evident only with exercise**, that is, when pulmonary venous pressure increases, and skeletal muscle perfusion becomes limited. However, as heart disease progresses, a dependence on neurohormonal activity, myocardial hypertrophy, cardiac dilation, and heart rate is established, resulting in **maladaptation**, a key concept for the treatment of HF.

It is known that **HF progresses due to activation of neurohormonal systems** and also due to **proinflammatory cytokines**, which are related to morbidity and mortality in patients.

HF is a state of chronic immune activation. Adrenergic stimulation, together with tissue **hypoperfusion** (intestine and other tissues), are believed to be predisposing factors for the release of the main cytokines involved in HF (tumour necrosis factor (TNF), Interleukin 1 (IL-1) and interleukin 6 (IL-6)). These cytokines exacerbate haemodynamic changes, exert direct toxic effects on the heart, and contribute to tissue loss, weight loss, and cardiac cachexia.

From the above, it can be concluded that the clinical signs (Box 2) of congestive HF (CHF) are partially explained by:

- chronic **elevation of venous pressures**: pulmonary oedema, pleural effusion, jugular venous distention, hepatomegaly, and ascites;
- **inadequate tissue perfusion**: exercise intolerance, syncope and azotaemia; and
- **metabolic disorders**: weight loss, picky appetite, etc.

Diagnosing Cardiac Insufficiency

The diagnosis of HF fundamentally is clinically based and supported by paraclinical findings. The initial steps are to take

Box 2. Clinical Signs According to Types of HF

Left-sided HF

- **The clinical signs are mainly related to pulmonary oedema: e.g. tachypnoea, dyspnoea, orthopnoea, exercise intolerance, pulmonary crackles, cough, and cyanosis.**

Right-sided HF

- **Clinical signs are related to systemic venous congestion: e.g. enlarged liver and spleen, peritoneal effusion (ascites), cutaneous vein distention, and subcutaneous oedema in large breed dogs (lower thorax and abdomen).**

Biventricular HF

- **In most cases, it is the consequence of heart disease that occurs with left-sided heart failure (DCM and CDMD in advanced stages) which is complicated by pulmonary hypertension and atrial fibrillation. The result is the presence of signs of respiratory dysfunction (pulmonary oedema, pleural effusion) and ascites.**

Cardiogenic shock

- **This occurs when the signs of systolic dysfunction and signs of elevated venous pressure combine, resulting in severe hypotension and hypoperfusion.**

Other clinical signs

- **There are other signs at an individual level depending on the cause of HF, such as abnormalities on auscultation (murmur, gallop, arrhythmia, attenuation of heart sounds), cardiac cachexia (picky appetite, loss of muscle mass in large breed dogs with dilated cardiomyopathy), arterial thromboembolism in cats with any type of cardiomyopathy, and febrile signs and lameness in dogs or cats with infective endocarditis.**
- **Also, varying degrees of exercise intolerance, paleness, syncope, prerenal azotaemia, and arrhythmias may be present in all forms of HF.**

an **adequate clinical history** (anamnesis regarding the history and reason for consultation) and perform a **complete physical examination**, paying special attention to the cardiovascular and respiratory systems (similar clinical signs). Based on evaluation of the signalment, clinical signs, and physical exam (presence of respiratory distress, ascites, cough, auscultation of a murmur, arrhythmia or gallop rhythm, etc.), the clinician can guide the diagnosis and select the most appropriate **complementary tests**.

- **Thoracic radiographs**: radiographs allow evaluation of the lungs (to evaluate the presence of pulmonary oedema) and the cardiac silhouette (varying degrees of cardiomegaly). In addition, diseases other than HF can be diagnosed, which can explain the clinical signs (respiratory diseases).
- **Surface electrocardiogram (ECG)**: used to diagnose heart rhythm problems and cardiac repercussions from extracardiac conditions.
- **Echocardiography**: this technique makes it possible to assess the anatomical and/or functional causes that cause HF (cardiomyopathies, valvular heart disease, blood shunting, neoplasms, etc.). Currently it is the technique par excellence for the non-invasive diagnosis and assessment of the severity of most heart diseases in dogs and cats.
- **Laboratory tests**: in symptomatic patients, especially, it is necessary to perform a complete blood count and biochemistry to check kidney, liver and thyroid function, rule out anaemia, and look for indications of other diseases which can affect the heart. Additionally, troponin TnIc and natriuretic peptide nT-proBNP can help diagnose heart failure and be used to monitor treatment (especially the latter).

Functional Classification of Heart Failure

The treatment of HF patients should be undertaken as indicated by their clinical stage, regardless of the cause. For this, **functional classifications have been developed based on the patient's clinical signs** (Box 3).

Therapeutic Principles

The goals of treatment of patients with HF include:

- improve clinical status, functional capacity and quality of life
- prevent the need for hospitalization
- reduce mortality.

An appropriate treatment for HF is selected based on the aetiology, clinical stage, and current clinical signs; alongside considering the different types of patients such asymptomatic, with lung oedema or cardiogenic shock, chronic, with arrhythmias or complications (renal disease). Likewise, periodic reassessment of the patient is essential to assess the response to treatment and adjust doses or add/replace drugs.

Box 3. Functional Classifications of Patients with Heart Failure

New York Heart Association (NYHA): for human patients.

- Class I: asymptomatic patients in exercise and at rest.
- Class II: clinical signs only with exercise or intense activity.
- Class III: clinical signs with moderate activity.
- Class IV: obvious clinical signs both during exercise and at rest.

Animal Cardiac Health Council (ISACHC): developed for veterinary patients.

- Class I: no signs of heart failure (Class I NYHA).
  - Class IA: no signs of cardiomegaly.
  - Class IB: signs of cardiomegaly.
- Class II: the animal presents intolerance to significant and moderate exercise.
- Class III: obvious signs of heart failure at rest (NYHA Class IV).

American College of Cardiology and American Heart Association accepted by the European Society of Veterinary Cardiology and the study group of the American College of Veterinary Internal Medicine: have developed a classification system based on the progressive nature of HF that can be adapted to animals.

- **Class A**: dogs without structural cardiac changes, but with a risk of developing them, as occurs with certain breeds (Cavalier King Charles Spaniel and CDMD, Dobermann and Boxer and DCM) and elderly dogs (CDMD).
- **Class B**: dogs with structural heart disease but have not yet developed clinical signs of HF (small breed dogs with mitral regurgitation murmurs, Boxers with an elevated number of CPVS on Holter monitoring).
  - **Class B1**: no cardiomegaly on thoracic radiology or echocardiography.
  - **Class B2**: with cardiomegaly on thoracic radiology or echocardiography.
- **Class C**: patients with structural heart disease and previous or current clinical signs of HF (including those who are asymptomatic due to treatment) who require hospitalisation or outpatient treatment.
- **Class D**: patients with advanced structural heart disease, clinical signs of HF that are refractory to conventional therapy and require special intervention.

Where possible, treatment is diffentiated into corrective therapies (such as surgery or implanting a pacemaker) or medical (where lesions cannot be corrected or cured).

Specific corrective therapy is recommended in **heart diseases which can be corrected/minimised by surgery** (closure of the PDA), catheterization (balloon valvuloplasty in congenital pulmonary stenosis, closure of the PDA) or implantation of pacemakers (complete atrioventricular blocks, sinus syndrome patient, etc.) and pericardiocentesis/pericardiectomy (pericardial tamponade), amongst others. These procedures are covered in the corresponding chapters of this book.

Medical therapy is administered to patients with **HF secondary to lesions that cannot be corrected or cured**. This type of treatment involves drugs with a demonstrated and recognised prognostic benefit at recommended doses (evidence-based medicine) (Table 1), and avoiding drugs that may be harmful (NSAIDs, corticosteroids).

Neurohormonal Antagonists

Angiotensin Converting Enzyme Inhibitors (ACEI)

ACEI interfere with RAAS by inhibiting the enzyme responsible for converting angiotensin I (Ag I) into Ag II. These are true neurohormonal inhibitors as they also attenuate the sympathetic activity, inhibit the degradation of vasodilator quinines, the production of aldosterone, antidiuretic hormone and the activation of many pathways mediated by Ag II involved in the cardiac remodelling process. They are indirect vasodilators as blocking of Ag prevents the vasoconstriction mediated by it. Multicentre studies have shown safety and efficacy in dogs with CDMD and DCM secondary to HF.

The **different ACEI have similar haemodynamic effects**, but differ in the duration of effect and pharmacokinetic properties. Commercial preparations of benazepril, enalapril, imidapril and ramipril are available for use in veterinary medicine. The most important studies in veterinary patients have been conducted with benazepril and enalapril, through multicentre clinical trials, in which both drugs have demonstrated **good tolerance and similar efficacy and safety**, offering improvement of clinical signs of HF.

In dogs with CDMD there is **no clear evidence that administration of ACEI in asymptomatic patients prolongs the asymptomatic period**. There is a consensus that they should not be used in patients without cardiomegaly. However, many veterinarians recommend their use when there is significant cardiomegaly, pulmonary venous congestion, pulmonary hypertension or systemic high blood pressure, and of course in symptomatic patients. In dogs with DCM starting treatment when the disease is diagnosed is recommended, even in cases where the animal is asymptomatic. In cats with cardiomyopathies their use is recommended when there is recurrent pulmonary oedema or pleural effusion.

ACEI should not be used in unstable or dehydrated hospitalised patients. Even in stable patients, slight azotaemia may be observed after administration, as Ag II blockage may decrease glomerular infusion and filtration. Therefore, **renal function should be evaluated before administration and 5–7 days later**.

Aldosterone Inhibitors

The most commonly used is **spironolactone**, an aldosterone receptor blocker (also other corticosteroid hormones) which prevents its effects on the autonomous nervous system and acts directly on the cardiovascular system (vascular and myocardial fibrosis and baroreceptor dysfunction, among others). It also has diuretic effects as seen below.

Digoxin

Digoxin plays an important role in inhibiting HF-activated neurohormonal systems, because by sensitizing baroreceptors (over the course of HF they are progressively desensitised) it counteracts harmful friendly activation and produces indirect vasodilation. In addition, it has inotropic and antiarrhythmic effects.

Other Drugs

Inhibitors of inflammatory cytokines (etanercept, which inhibits tumour necrosis factor α), vasopeptidase inhibitors (omapatrilat, which inhibits ACE, and neutral endopeptidases that degrade endogenous vasodilator factors and natriuretic peptides), endothelin antagonists or receptors (bosentan, which antagonizes the effects of cardiac and vascular remodelling induced by endothelin) as well as endogenous (nesiritide) and synthetic (DNP or dendroaspis natriuretic peptide) natriuretic peptides, are also under investigation but without clinical application in animals.

Diuretics

Diuretics remain the cornerstone of treatment for CHF. These drugs **decrease preload** and are associated with improvements in symptoms and reduced hospitalizations (although there are no controlled studies on their effectiveness against mortality). The goal of diuretics is to **maintain adequate blood volume at the lowest possible dose**, which should be adjusted on an individual basis. Response to treatment is assessed using respiratory rate and pattern, hydration status, body weight, exercise tolerance, renal function, serum electrolyte concentrations and blood pressure.

General guidelines regarding the use of diuretics to optimize their use and avoid side effects include:

- the goal of diuretic treatment is to reduce fluid retention and relieve the symptoms of heart failure;
- in chronic therapy, diuretics should not be used in isolation but in **combination with ACEI and aldosterone receptor inhibitors**;
- the **minimum effective dose** should be used, adjusting the dosage according to the patient's needs;
- frequent **monitoring of the animal's weight** acts as a guide when evaluating the dose of diuretics;
- periodic evaluation of renal functionality and electrolytes;
- in patients with generalised oedema (pulmonary and ascites) initiation of diuretic administration intravenously (IV) or subcutaneously (SC) is recommended, as intestinal venous congestion makes oral absorption (PO) difficult;
- diuretics should be combined with **moderate salt restriction** in the diet.

Resistance to diuretics is frequently associated with clinical progression of HF, and must be identified and managed. This physiological resistance to diuretics has been called the "**brake phenomenon**", which occurs to prevent excessive losses of salt and fluids. Resistance to diuretics in an oedematous patient can be defined as the clinical state in which the "braking phenomenon" occurs before the goals of diuretic therapy have been achieved.

There are **three classes of diuretics**, depending on their mechanism of action and their ability to promote sodium and water excretion.

Loop Diuretics

These inhibit the cotransportation of $Na^+/K^+/2Cl^-$ in the ascending part of the loop of Henle, increasing the loss in urine of chlorine, sodium, potassium, magnesium, hydrogen ions and water. They can be used in a wide spectrum of doses and routes of administration, which allows treatment to be adjusted to the patient's clinical stage.

The most commonly used diuretics in dogs and cats are **furosemide and torsemide**. These drugs have different catabolic mechanisms, since furosemide is eliminated mainly through the kidney, while torsemide is eliminated through the liver.

Table 1. Main drugs and doses used in dogs and cats with heart failure.

Medication	Dose	Observations
Acepromazine	· Dogs: 0.01–0.03 mg/kg IM-IV · Cats: 0.02–0.03 mg/kg IM-IV	· Can be administered alone or in combination with opiates (butorphanol) · Especially useful in dogs with mitral regurgitation due to CDMD
Amiodarone	· Dogs: 10 mg/kg/24 h 7 days; reduce to 5 mg/kg/24 h PO · Cats: total 50 mg/24 h	Useful in atrial tachycardia, AF and ventricular arrythmias
Amlodipine	· Dogs: 0.05–0.1 mg/kg/12–24 h PO · Cats: total 0.625 mg/12–24 h PO	Monitor arterial pressure periodically
Atenolol	· Dogs: 0.2–1 mg/kg/12–24 h PO · Cats: total 6.25–12.5 mg/12–24 h PO	· Useful in atrial tachycardia, ventricular arrythmias · In cats with HOCM · Do not administer if there is congestive HF
Benazepril	Dogs and cats: 0.25–0.5 mg/kg/12–24 h PO	Do not administer in dehydrated patients. Monitor renal function
Butorphanol	· Dogs: acute HF 0.25 mg/kg IM-IV · Cats: 0.1–0.2 mg/kg IM, IV	Can be administered alone or in combination with acepromazine
Digoxin	· Small breed dogs: 0.0055 mg/kg/12 h PO · Large breed dogs: 0.22 mg/m2/12 h PO (maximum in the Dobermann: 0.25 mg/12 h) · Cats: 0.008 mg/kg/24–48 h PO	· Evaluate renal function and monitor digoxin levels 7–10 days after starting treatment and 8–10 hours after the last dose · Therapeutic doses: 0.8–1.5 ng/ml · Useful in AF and sinus tachycardia/supraventricular extrasystoles in patients with congestive HF. Do not use in cats with HCM or dogs with ventricular hypertrophy secondary to aortic or pulmonary stenosis
Diltiazem	· Dogs: 0.5–2.0 mg/kg/8–12 h PO · Cats: total 7.5 mg/8–12 h PO or 30–60 mg/24h PO, delayed release formula	Useful in atrial tachycardia and control of ventricular frequency in dogs with AF in combination with digoxin
Dobutamine	Dogs: starting at 2.5 µg/kg/min, increasing every 15–30 minutes until adequate systemic arterial blood pressure is achieved	Toxic effects occur at high doses (tachycardia, arrythmias, nausea, etc.)
Enalapril	· Dogs: 0.5 mg/kg/12–24 h PO · Cats: 0.25–0.5 mg/kg/12–24 h PO	Same observations as for benazepril
Esmolol	· Dogs: 50–100 g/kg bolus; repeat until a maximum of 50 µg/kg – CI: 50–200 µg/kg/min · Cats: 50–100 g/kg bolus; repeat up to a maximum of 500 µg/kg – CI: 50–200 µg/kg/min	· Do not use in cases of congestive HF · Ventricular tachycardia, AF, atrial tachycardia
Spironolactone	· Dogs: 1–2 mg/kg/24 h PO · Cats: 2 mg/kg/12–24 h PO	Administer in patients with HF stages C and D
Furosemide	· HF with pulmonary oedema – Dogs: 2–4 mg/kg IV; repeat in 30 min–1 h · CI: 0.5–1 mg/kg/h after initial bolus – Cats: 1–2 mg/kg IV · Chronic HF – Dogs: 2–4 mg/kg/8–12h PO (stages C and D) – Cats: 1–2 mg/kg/12–24h PO	· In patients with pulmonary oedema monitor RR to evaluate diuretic efficacy · Monitor renal function and electrolytes · Administer together with ACEI and spironolactone in long-term treatment
Hydralazine	· Dogs: 0.5–1 mg/kg/12 h PO · Cats: total 2.5 mg/12–24 h PO	Monitor arterial pressure regularly
Hydrochlorothiazide	Dogs: 2–4 mg/kg/12–24 h PO	Use in stages C and D
Lidocaine	· Dogs: 2 mg/kg IV in bolus; can be repeated up to 8 mg/kg · Cats: 0.25–1 mg/kg IV in bolus	· Ventricular tachycardia, AF occurring during anaesthesia or vagotonia · Use with care in cats
Mexiletine	Dogs: 4–8 mg/kg/8 h PO	Ventricular arrythmias together with β-blocker medications.
Morphine	Dogs: 0.1–1 mg/kg SC, IM	Useful as a sedative in dogs with CDMD
Nitroglycerin	· Small dogs and cats: a 5 mg nitroglycerin patch · Large dogs: a 10mg nitroglycerin patch	Effects last 24 h, after tolerance to the drug occurs
Sodium nitroprusside	Dogs: 0.5–5 µg/kg/min CI IV (maximum dose 10 µg/kg/min)	Monitor systemic arterial pressure

Medication	Dose	Observations
Pimobendan	· Dogs – Acute HF: 0.15 mg/kg IV – Chronic HF: 0.25–0.3 mg/kg/12 h PO · Cats: total 0.625–1.25/12 h PO	· Dogs: HF, stages B2, C and D · Cats: congestive HF · Do no administer in cats with HOCM and dogs with pulmonary or aortic stenosis
Ramipril	· Dogs: 0.125 mg/12 h PO · Cats: total 0.5 mg/24 h PO	Similar observations to those mentioned for benazepril
Sildenafil	Dogs and cats: 1–2 mg/kg/8h PO	Monitor systemic arterial pressure
Sotalol	· Dogs: 1–2 mg/kg/12 h PO · Cats: total 10–15 mg /12 h PO	AF and ventricular arrythmias
Torsemide	· Dogs: 0.2–0.3 mg/kg/12–24 h PO · Cats: 0.1–0.2 mg/kg/12–24 h PO	Monitor renal function and electrolytes Administer together with ACEI and spironolactone

PO: per os, IM: intramuscular, SC: subcutaneous, IV: intravenous, CI: continuous infusion, HOCM: hypertrophic obstructive cardiomyopathy, AF: atrial fibrillation, RR: respiratory rate, CDMD: chronic degenerative mitral disease, HF: heart failure, HCM: hypertrophic cardiomyopathy.

Furosemide

The **fastest-acting diuretic** used in the treatment of patients with CHF. When administered IV, it exerts an initial venous dilation effect which reduces pulmonary congestion before the start of diuresis, due to the release of prostaglandins (vasodilators).

In patients with acute pulmonary oedema, **high doses (2–4 mg/kg) are used parenterally**, and when the animal is stabilised the dosage is gradually decreased until the minimum effective dose is maintained. When furosemide is administered by IV and SC routes, the **maximum effect of diuresis occurs within 30 min**, returning to baseline levels two hours after IV administration and four hours after SC administration. If administered orally, the peak of diuresis occurs between 30 minutes and two hours later, returning to basal levels at six hours after administration. In continuous infusion, the maximum diuresis peak occurs at four hours.

There is controversy about the efficacy of furosemide doses in acute therapy and the form of administration, i.e. boluses or in continuous infusion. In human medicine, a double-blind DOSE (Diuretic Optimization Strategies Evaluation) trial revealed:

- greater symptom relief in the group of patients with high doses of furosemide (with improvement in volume reduction and weight reduction at 72 h);
- the efficacy of continuous infusion was similar to that of intermittent bolus therapy.

In chronic therapy, oral administration of furosemide is recommended at minimum effective doses to avoid adverse effects, with periodic review. In human medicine, furosemide dose is considered an independent marker of long-term mortality.

The **adverse effects** of furosemide include:

- **Drug resistance**: believed to be due to activation of neurohormonal systems (especially RAAS), hypertrophy of segments of the nephron, and increased renal absorption of solutes in other parts of the nephron.
- **Loss of electrolytes**: sodium, potassium, magnesium and chlorine. This can be avoided by combining it with potassium-sparing diuretics, such as spironolactone.
- **Hypotension and azotaemia**: these are usually due to volume depletion. In these cases, a dose reduction is recommended. However, in the event of volume overload, hypotension and azotaemia are due to a worsening of HF and, in this case, diuretic therapy should be maintained, and IV inotropic support added. The persistence of volume overload not only contributes to the persistence of symptoms, but also limits the efficacy and compromises the safety of other drugs used in the treatment of HF.

Torsemide

This loop diuretic is up to **ten times more potent than furosemide**, has a longer duration of diuretic effect, and induces less potassium loss.

The peak of maximum diuresis is estimated at 2–4 hours and persists for 12 hours. Studies in dogs with CDMD have shown good tolerance and efficacy when administered orally every 12 or 24 hours. In animal models this diuretic has been shown to have an inhibitory effect on aldosterone, reducing fibrotic remodelling of myocytes and improving the effects of the SNS.

Thiazide Diuretics

Thiazide diuretics block sodium and chloride cotransport, inhibiting reabsorption of chlorine, sodium, and water in the distal convoluted tubule.

Thiazides are less active than loop diuretics and are used when the response to furosemide is inadequate or in cases of resistance. The most widely used is hydrochlorothiazide.

Potassium-sparing Diuretics

Spironolactone is the most representative. It is a weak, potassium-sparing diuretic which acts on the collecting duct. It is rarely used in isolation and is usually administered together with furosemide in the chronic treatment of HF, especially when there is right-sided congestive heart failure. Orally, its diuretic effect begins between 48–72 h after administration.

Vasodilators

The goal of vasodilator therapy for patients with HF is to reduce oedema formation and improve minute volume. **Vasodilators are classified as arterial, venous, and mixed.** Arterial vasodilators are especially useful in animals with mitral regurgitation, aortic regurgitation, VSD, and PDA. Venodilators are used primarily to reduce the formation of pulmonary oedema. In all cases, **blood pressure should be monitored periodically**.

Nitroglycerin

Nitroglycerin is an organic nitrate that produces venous and arterial dilation through the nitric oxide pathway (endothelial relaxing factor), reducing preload.

For inpatient treatment of acute pulmonary oedema, nitroglycerin should be used together with intravenous furosemide and can cause tolerance when given repeatedly. Transdermal patches and aerosols are available for sublingual use.

Sodium Nitroprusside

Sodium nitroprusside is a potent mixed vasodilator with a similar mechanism of action to nitroglycerin, but does not lead to tolerance. Its main indication in HF is emergency intravenous treatment of dogs with acute pulmonary oedema secondary to severe or fulminant heart failure. It is used in a continuous infusion (due to its very short half-life) when HF is not controlled with oxygen, furosemide, and nitroglycerin or when the oedema is so fulminant that haemoptysis develops.

Amlodipine

Amlodipine is a dihydropyridine, a calcium channel blocker (L-type channels) in vascular smooth muscle. It induces arterial vasodilation and is the treatment of choice in systemic arterial hypertension together with an ACEI.

Likewise, in combination with standard treatment, it is shown to reduce the severity of mitral regurgitation in dogs with moderate to severe CDMD. It does not exhibit the effects of diltiazem on the heart muscle or sinus node. However, blood pressure must be controlled to avoid possible hypotension.

Hydralazine

Administered orally, hydralazine produces a powerful arteriolar dilation by direct action on vascular smooth muscle (via nitric oxide). Its effect begins at the time of administration and reaches maximum levels after 3 hours.

It should not be used if it is not possible to monitor blood pressure regularly. Chronic use is discouraged, as it can induce significant activation of the RAAS.

Sildenafil

Sildenafil is a phosphodiesterase V inhibitor that causes dilation of the pulmonary arteries by preventing the degradation of cGMP and, therefore, reduces resistance to blood flow. This drug is used for the treatment of precapillary pulmonary hypertension (heartworm disease, Eisenmenger physiology – left-right sided blood shunts that cause hypertension resulting in right-left shunts), although it is also considered useful in dogs with post-capillary PH secondary to CDMD and congenital heart disease.

The author has used sildenafil to treat PH in dogs with Eisenmenger syndrome and also postcapillary PH in cats, with good results.

Positive Inotropes

These are drugs that **increase myocardial contractility** by acting through various mechanisms regarding the interaction between calcium and contractile proteins. They are indicated in patients with systolic dysfunction, **mainly in dogs and cats with DCM**.

Digoxin

Exerts its effect through its ability to inhibit the (Na^+/K^+) ATPase pump, increasing intracellular calcium concentration which, in turn, interacts with the sarcoplasmic reticulum, releasing more calcium to interact with contractile proteins and increase cardiac contractility.

Its inotropic effect is weak. However, it has other benefits for patients with HF related to neurohormonal inhibition and ventricular rate control in dogs with supraventricular tachyarrhythmias.

Adrenergic Agonists

The most commonly used adrenergic agonists are dopamine and dobutamine. These increase myocardial contractility by stimulating cardiac β1-adrenergic receptors, which results in an increase in cAMP and favours the entry of calcium and its deposition in the sarcoplasmic reticulum, which increases the availability of calcium for interaction with contractile proteins.

They are indicated for short-term inpatient inotropic support and are not used in chronic treatments because the β-receptors are progressively desensitised. Dobutamine is used in continuous infusion (due to its short half-life) for the treatment of acute cardiogenic shock secondary to systolic failure (DCM). Dopamine has similar actions but produces more tachycardia and vasoconstriction. However, it improves renal perfusion and urine production, so it may be useful in patients with prerenal azotaemia and acute cardiogenic shock.

Pimobendan

Pimobendan is a drug (benzimidazole pyridazinone) considered as an "inodilator" due to its actions **as a potent positive inotrope and arterial and venous vasodilator**. As an inotrope, pimobendan works by increasing the sensitivity of calcium to contractile proteins (troponin C). The peripheral, coronary and pulmonary vasodilator effect is mediated by the inhibition of phosphodiesterase III and to a lesser extent by phosphodiesterase V.

Clinical studies have shown that pimobendan improves clinical signs and survival in symptomatic dogs with DCM and CDMD when added to standard treatments. More recent studies have also shown that when administered in stage B2 in dogs with CDMD and in stage B1 in Dobermanns with occult DCM (relative to placebo) it prolongs the asymptomatic period and survival.

β-blockers

The action of β-blockers is due to the blockage of β-adrenergic receptors. In addition to their antiarrhythmic properties, β-blockers are used mainly in dogs with myocardial hypertrophy secondary to aortic or pulmonary stenosis and in cats with hypertrophic obstructive cardiomyopathy (HOCM), since **they decrease myocardial oxygen demand and arrhythmias secondary to hypertrophy**.

The most widely used for this purpose is atenolol (selective β-blocker). It should not be used in patients with congestive HF due to its negative inotropic properties. Clinical studies have not shown increased survival in dogs with subaortic stenosis and in cats with HOCM, which have been treated with atenolol.

Antiarrhythmics

These are not used specifically for the treatment of HF, but they are used in cases of primary arrhythmias or those secondary to structural heart diseases such as atrial fibrillation (AF) or ventricular arrhythmias.

The management of arrhythmias is based on the precise diagnosis and the search for the primary causative aetiology. Specific treatment of the cause of the arrhythmia leads to resolution in many cases. The decision to use antiarrhythmic treatment is based on the presentation of associated clinical symptoms, haemodynamic instability or risk of aggravation.

Management of Bradyarrhythmia

The aetiology of bradyarrhythmia includes **pathologies of the sinus node or conduction system, and increased vagal tone**. Atropine response tests determine whether the arrhythmia is vagal in origin or not.

Sympathomimetics, such as terbutaline, can be used orally for outpatient treatment of bradyarrhythmia of vagal origin. Symptomatic non-vagal bradyarrhythmia requires implantation of a permanent pacemaker.

Management of Tachyarrhythmias

To select the appropriate antiarrhythmic medication it is **important to determine the origin of the arrhythmia, and whether it is ventricular or supraventricular**. The Vaughan Williams classification considers different classes of antiarrhythmic drugs (I to IV) depending on their mechanism of action.

Class I Antiarrhythmics

These work by blocking myocardial sodium channels and slowing the rate of transmission in Purkinje cells. Procainamide (Class Ia), lidocaine and mexiletine (class Ib) and flecainide (class Ic) belong to this group.

Lidocaine is the antiarrhythmic of choice during hospitalisation, for the treatment of rapid and morphologically dangerous ventricular arrhythmias. Given via the IV route of administration (initially in bolus form and later by continuous infusion) it has a rapid onset of action, is effective, and has a good safety margin.

The efficacy of lidocaine has also been shown to reverse atrial fibrillation secondary to vagotonia and anaesthetics. Mexiletine is the oral alternative to lidocaine with a similar mechanism. It has been shown to be effective in treating arrhythmias in Boxer dogs in combination with atenolol.

Class II Antiarrhythmics (β-blockers)

These act by competitive binding with β-adrenergic receptors, preventing the entry of calcium into cells, reducing late potentials that can cause premature complexes, and producing sinus node and atrioventricular (AV) conduction velocity depression.

Some of the most widely used in veterinary medicine are **propranolol** (non-selective β-blocker), atenolol, and esmolol (selective β-blockers. Esmolol is administered IV). Atenolol has been the most widely used to treat supraventricular arrhythmias (decreased AV conduction in AF). The main limitation of β-blockers is their negative inotropic effect.

Class III Antiarrhythmics

The most commonly used are **amiodarone and sotalol**. Their antiarrhythmic action is due to a delay in the repolarization of cardiac cells, which prolongs the refractory period and reduces the possibility of microentries and hence making it difficult for ventricular arrhythmias to develop.

Sotalol also has non-selective β-blocker properties, which is why it is widely used in the treatment of ventricular tachyarrhythmias in Dobermans and Boxers with arrhythmogenic cardiomyopathy. Both drugs are also used in the treatment of supraventricular arrhythmias (focal atrial tachycardia). Amiodarone is a complex drug, which can cause liver toxicity and thyroid dysfunction, both effects seen by the author in dogs undergoing chronic treatment of complex arrhythmias that did not respond to other drugs.

Class IV Antiarrhythmics

As represented by **calcium channel blockers**.

The most widely used is **diltiazem**. This drug selectively suppresses the flow of calcium through the membrane, reducing contractility, and slowing down sinoatrial depolarization and atrioventricular conduction. It also has vasodilator effects.

In dogs with AF, the combination of diltiazem and digoxin has been shown to control ventricular rate better than either alone. In cats with hypertrophic cardiomyopathy, it is used when there is moderate-severe ventricular hypertrophy, without left ventricular outflow tract obstruction, as it improves ventricular relaxation and reduces heart rate.

Digoxin

Although digoxin is not included in the aforementioned classification, digitalis is used in dogs for its vagotonic properties which cause a decrease in ventricular frequency in dogs with AF secondary to DCM (in combination with diltiazem) and in dogs with CDMD that also present AF and/or supraventricular extrasystoles.

It is administered orally, calculating the dose based on weight (small dogs and cats) or body surface area (large dogs). It should not be used in patients with subaortic stenosis or obstructive HCM.

Since several factors can affect serum levels of digoxin (electrolytes, thyroid and renal function – mainly renal elimination –, drug interactions, etc.) these should be monitored periodically to avoid toxicity. Serum concentrations are evaluated 7–10 days after starting treatment and 8–10 hours after the last administration, therapeutic levels are between 1 and 2 ng/ml. Intoxication can manifest itself with:

- gastrointestinal symptoms (vomiting, diarrhoea)
- neurological symptoms (depression, anorexia)
- cardiac symptoms (bradyarrhythmia or tachyarrhythmias).

Sedatives

These may be necessary in dogs and cats with HF and respiratory distress in order to **reduce anxiety and myocardial oxygen demand, facilitating handling** and reducing the risk for the patient. Agents with minimal impact on the cardiovascular system should be used, avoiding severe hypotension or decreased contractility.

Morphine (sulphate)

Morpine can be useful in dogs with CDMD and pulmonary oedema due to its properties as a splanchnic vasodilator and to decrease sympathetic tone.

Acepromazine

In addition to producing adequate sedation, it can also be useful in dogs with CDMD since, by producing peripheral vasodilation, it lowers systemic arterial pressure and secondarily, reduces the volume of mitral regurgitation and the pressure in pulmonary veins.

Butorphanol

Butorphanol is an opiate with little impact on the cardiovascular system that can be administered alone or in combination with acepromazine.

Management of Patients with HF

Physical Handling

In patients with heart failure, restriction of physical exercise is recommended. Excess exercise can lead to fatigue, exhaustion, and even collapse, causing cardiac work overload which can lead to decompensation of compensated chronic HF. However, mild but regular exercise can be beneficial in ambulatory patients.

Dietary Management

The development of HF causes a reduced appetite, resulting in cachexia in many animals, largely due to pro-inflammatory cytokines. **Weight loss during HF is considered a poor prognostic sign**.

Inadequate nutrition produces multiple adverse consequences, such as the deterioration of the immune system and tissue repair capacity, which may contribute to the appearance of hypalbuminaemia. Therefore, the first objective of dietary management is to ensure the animal does not stop eating and not to implement any change in feeding if this triggers rejection. Warming and the application of flavourings (such as garlic powder) can improve the palatability of prescription diets for patients with HF.

Dietary recommendations include the following.

Salt Restriction

In symptomatic patients and in those on diuretic treatment, a moderate restriction can be attempted if the diet is accepted. Commercial diets are more appropriate than homemade ones. However, it should not be introduced in the early stages of HF (B), as they can accelerate and/or exacerbate neurohormonal activation.

ω-3 Fatty Acid Supplementation

ω-3 supplementation is recommended in all phases of HF, as **it helps reduce the production of cytokines responsible for decreased appetite** and prevent the development of cardiac cachexia.

Supplementation with Taurine and L-carnitine

The benefits have been proven in deficient animals. Taurine supplementation is recommended in cats with dilated cardiomyopathy until it is established whether plasma levels of this amino acid are low.

In American Cocker Spaniel and Boxer dogs, supplementation with both amino acids improves myocardial function in cases of dilated cardiomyopathy. The recommended doses for supplementation with taurine and L-carnitine are 250–500 mg/12 h and 1–2 g/8–12 h, respectively.

Others

The effects of several micronutrients and vitamins, such as coenzyme Q10, vitamin E and magnesium, are under investigation and some have already shown their possible benefits in patients with HF.

Treatment Protocols According to Clinical Stage

Table 2 shows treatment for dogs with CDMD and DCM according to clinical stages, according to evidence-based medicine.

The medical treatment of cats with cardiomyopathies (dilated, hypertrophic, restrictive, arrhythmogenic right ventricular) is based on the **type of cardiomyopathy, severity (symptomatic, asymptomatic), and complications** (arterial thromboembolism).

- **Dilated cardiomyopathy (DCM)**: in cats with congestive failure, the administration of an ACEI, pimobendan, furosemide and topical nitroglycerin is recommended (if there is pulmonary oedema). Thoracentesis if there is pleural effusion. Taurine if it is found to be deficient.
- **Restrictive cardiomyopathy**: similar to cats with DCM.
- **Hypertrophic cardiomyopathy**:
  - **asymptomatic cats**: there is no consensus on which drugs to use for diastolic dysfunction (β-blockers or diltiazem). If there is tachycardia (>200 beats/min) and HOCM, atenolol is more effective than diltiazem. However, to date, no drug has been proven to increase survival in asymptomatic cats;
  - **symptomatic cats**: furosemide, ACEI at low doses and pimobendan are recommended. The latter should not be used if there is a dynamic obstruction. Thoracentesis, if pleural effusion is present. When congestive failure has been controlled, drugs that improve diastolic dysfunction (atenolol or diltiazem) can be administered.
- **Thromboembolism**: analgesics (butorphanol, fentanil), anticoagulants (heparin in inpatients, clopidogrel or aspirin in outpatients) and additional supportive treatment are recommended. In cats with significant left atrial dilation, the administration of preventive oral anticoagulants is recommended on an outpatient basis.

Table 2. Recommended treatment in dogs with chronic degenerative mitral disease (CDMD) and dilated cardiomyopathy (DCM) according to clinical stage.

Stage		Treatment
Stage A (No structural cardiopathy, patients at risk of HF)		Periodic monitoring of old dogs and predisposed breeds (CKCS, Dobermann, Boxer) No medical treatment
Stage B (Structural cardiopathy, asymptomatic patients)	**Stage B1** (Without cardiomegaly)	CDMD · No medication DCM (occult) · ACEI · Pimobendan · β-blockers Taurine in animals from breeds predisposed to deficiency (Spaniels, Golden Retriever, Terranova...)
	Stage B2 (With cardiomegaly)	CDMD · Pimobendan · ACEI? DCM · ACEI · Pimobendan in the Dobermann · β-blockers?
Stage C (Structural cardiopathy, patients which have or are currently symptomatic)	**Stage C1** (Hospital treatment)	CDMD · Furosemide IV · Pimobendan IV · O_2 · Nitroglycerin/nitroprusside? · Sedation? DCM · Furosemide IV · Pimobendan IV/dobutamine CI · Nitroprusside? · O_2 · Sedation? Centesis if there is effusion
	Stage C2 (Ambulatory treatment)	CDMD · ACEI · Pimobendan · Furosemide or torsemide · Spironolactone · Digoxin? DCM · ACEI · Pimobendan · Furosemide or torsemide · Spironolactone · β-blockers? · Digoxin/diltiazem? Ensure adequate nutrition. Moderate salt restriction
Stage D (Structural cardiopathy, refractory patients)		CDMD · ACEI · Pimobendan · Furosemide PO/SC or torsemide · Spironolactone · Digoxin? · Sildenafil? · Amlodipine? DCM · ACEI · Pimobendan · Furosemide SC or torsemide · Spironolactone · β-blockers? · Digoxin/diltiazem?
		Hospitalise if necessary Increase dose of ACEI and furosemide with respect to stage C Repeated centesis if effusion is produced Salt restriction if there is significant effusion

- **Cats with arrhythmogenic right ventricular cardiomyopathy**: if there is congestive failure, treatment with ACE inhibitors, furosemide and pimobendan is recommended. Specific antiarrhythmic treatment according to ventricular and/or supraventricular arrhythmias (sotalol, digoxin etc.).

For more comprehensive information on the treatment of specific heart diseases in dogs and cats the corresponding chapters in this book should be consulted.

Bibliography

- Atkins, C., Bonagura, J., Ettinger, S., et al. (2009) Guidelines for the diagnosis and treatment of canine chronic valvular heart disease. *Journal of Veterinary Internal Medicine*, 23, pp. 1142–1150.
- Boswood, A., Häggström J, Gordon SG et al. (2016) Effect of Pimobendan in Dogs with Preclinical Myxomatous Mitral Valve Disease and Cardiomegaly: The EPIC Study-A Randomized Clinical Trial. *J Vet Intern Med*, 30, pp. 1765–1779.
- Chow, S.L., Maisel, A.S., Anand, I. et al. (2017) Role of Biomarkers for the Prevention, Assessment, and Management of Heart Failure. A Scientific Statement from the American Heart Association. *Circulation*, 135:e1054–e1091.
- Cote, E., MacDonald, K.A., Meurs, K.M., et al. (2011) *Feline Cardiology*. Willey-Blackwell, Iowa, pp. 101–192.
- Fuentes, V.L., Corcoran, B., French, A., et al. (2002) A double-blind, randomized, placebo-controlled studyof pim obendan in dogs with dilated cardiomyopathy. *J Vet Intern Med*, 16, pp. 255–61.
- Häggström, J., Boswood, A., O'Grady, M. et al. (2008) Effect of pimobendan or benazepril hydrochloride on survival times in dogs with congestive heart failure caused by naturally occurring myxomatous mitral valve disease: the QUEST study. *J Vet Intern Med*, 22, pp. 1124–35.
- Harada K, Ukai Y, Kanakubo K et al. (2015) Comparison of the diuretic effect of furosemide by different methods of administration in healthy dogs. *J Vet Emerg Crit Care*, 25, pp. 364–71.
- Keene, B.W., Bonagura, J.D. (2014) Drugs for heart failure in dogs. In: Bonagura, J.D., Twedt, D. (eds.). *Kirk's Current Veterinary Therapy XV*. 15th Ed. St Luis (MO): Elsevier, pp. 762–772.
- Kittleson, M.D., Keene, B., Pion, P.D. et al. (1997) Results of the multicenter spaniel trial (MUST): taurine- and carnitine-responsive dilated cardiomyopathy in American cocker spaniels with decreased plasma taurine concentration. *J Vet Intern Med*, 11, pp. 204–211.
- Peddle, G.D, Singletary, G.E., Reynolds, C.A. et al. (2012) Effect of torsemide and furosemide on clinical, laboratory, radiographic and quality of life variables in dogs with heart failure secondary to mitral valve disease. *J Vet Cardiol*, 14, pp. 253–9.
- Ponikowski, P., Voors, A.A., Anker, S.D. et al. (2016) ESC Guidelines for the diagnosis and treatment of acute and chronic heart failure. *European Journal of Heart Failure*, 18, pp. 891–975.
- Strickland, K.N. (2016) Pathophysiology and therapy of heart failure. In: Smith, F.W.K., Tilley, L.P., Oyama MA, et al. (eds). *Manual of canine and feline cardiology*. 5th ed. St Luis (MO): Elsevier, pp. 287–312.

Test

Answers on page 126

1. Indicate which of the following is incorrect regarding cardiac insufficiency:

a. Neurohormonal mechanisms are responsible for the drop in cardiac output.
b. Neurohormonal mechanisms are responsible for the retention of sodium and water.
c. Neurohormonal mechanisms are responsible for the appearance of clinical signs in patients with cardiac insufficiency.
d. Angiotensin II is a powerful vasoconstrictor.

2. In cardiac failure, the sympathetic nervous system is activated due to:

a. An increase in blood pressure due to decreased renal perfusion.
b. A decrease in systemic blood pressure and stimulation of baroreceptors and the vasomotor centre.
c. The release of antidiuretic hormone.
d. The production of aldosterone.

3. Indicate which of the following is correct regarding the medications used to treat cardiac insufficiency:

a. Furosemide is a diuretic that decreases sodium and water reabsorption for more than 4 hours when administered intravenously as a bolus.
b. β-blockers increase blood pressure and are therefore contraindicated in severe cardiac insufficiency.
c. Spironolactone is a diuretic that acts on the ascending part of the loop of Henle.
d. ACE inhibitors should not be administered in dehydrated patients.

4. Indicate which of the following statements is false:

a. Atenolol is a selective β-blocker that is used in cats with hypertrophic obstructive cardiomyopathy.
b. Nitroglycerin is a vasodilator which is administered topically.
c. Dobutamine is an especially useful drug in dogs with dilated cardiomyopathy due to its negative inotropic properties.
d. Sodium nitroprusside is a vasodilator administered by continuous infusion, due to its short half-life in blood.

5. Indicate which is the correct answer:

a. An asymptomatic dog with chronic degenerative mitral disease and cardiomegaly should be treated with diuretics.
b. Furosemide should be administered in the congestive phase of cardiac insufficiency.
c. Spironolactone is administered as a first-line diuretic in dogs with right-sided heart failure and ascites.
d. The combination of hydrochlorothiazide and spironolactone has proven to be the ideal treatment for the treatment of pleural effusion in cats with dilated cardiomyopathy.

6. When is lidocaine used as an antiarrhythmic? Indicate which is the correct answer:

a. Ventricular tachycardia and atrial fibrillation secondary to vagotonia.
b. Focal atrial tachycardia.
c. Only ventricular tachycardia.
d. Symptomatic bradyarrhythmia.

7. Indicate the correct answer regarding positive inotrope medications:

a. Pimobendan works by increasing the release of calcium from the sarcoplasmic reticulum.
b. Digoxin is a negative inotropic drug that works by stimulating the Na^+/K^+ ATPase pump.
c. Dobutamine works by increasing myocardial contractility by stimulating β1-adrenergic receptors.
d. Pimobendan only has a positive inotropic effect when administered orally.

Notes

Correct Answers:

1. a
2. b
3. d
4. c
5. b
6. a
7. c

Notes

Pathophysiology, Diagnosis, and Management of Heart Failure

Andrew Francis

Heart Failure Basics

Heart failure is a clinical syndrome caused by the inability of the heart to function effectively within normal diastolic filling pressures. The primary function of the heart is to pump blood to meet the metabolic needs of the peripheral tissues. When it is unable to meet these metabolic needs, except with elevated diastolic filling pressures, then heart failure is present. The elevated diastolic filling pressures (increased preload) required to maintain the metabolic needs of the peripheral tissues in the failing heart are the root cause of the clinical signs seen in patients with heart failure, and directly lead to congestion/oedema, or poor peripheral perfusion.

Left heart failure is commonly the end result of severe left heart disease. Once left-sided heart disease is severe enough to require elevated left-sided filling pressures to maintain normal cardiac function, then left-sided heart failure is present. In Figure 1, elevated left ventricular end diastolic pressures (LVEDP) result in elevated left atrial pressures. **When the LVEDP exceeds 25 mmHg, pulmonary oedema develops**.

Right heart failure is commonly the end result of severe right heart disease. Elevated central venous pressures (CVP) are indicative of elevated right ventricular end-diastolic filling pressures (RVEDP) and consequently the presence of right-sided heart failure. **When RVEDP exceeds 10–15 mmHg ascites and/or pleural effusion develop**.

Common Types of Heart Failure in Dogs and Cats

In the majority of clinical cases, dogs and cats present with **backward failure, which is congestive heart failure (CHF)**. The physiological explanation is that the body's homeostatic mechanisms act to maintain the metabolic needs of the peripheral tissues by prioritising maintenance of normal

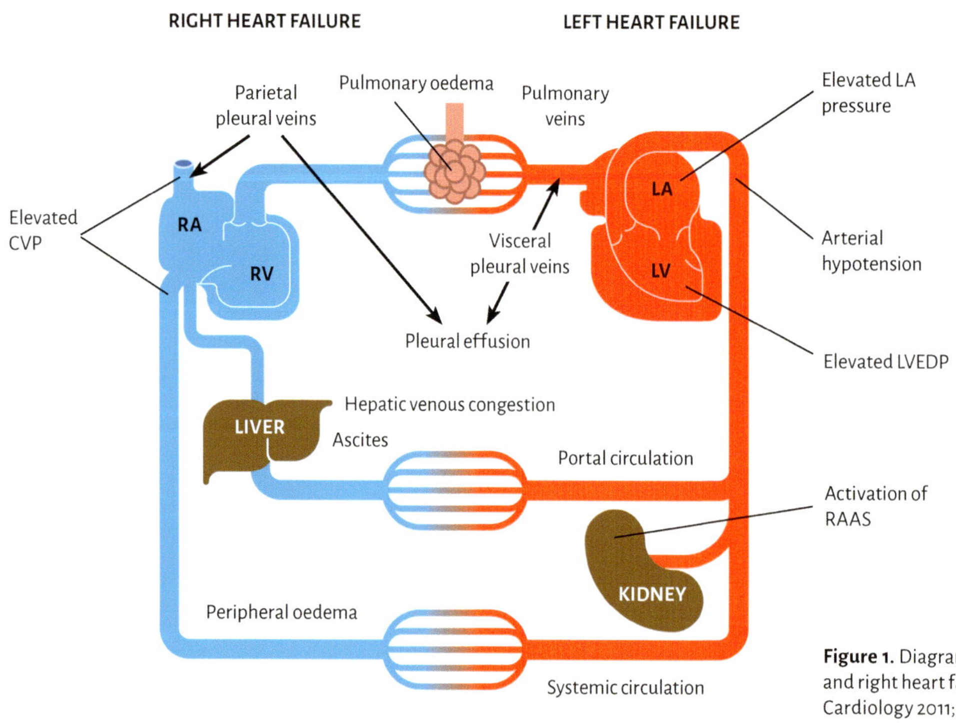

Figure 1. Diagram illustrating pathophysiology of left and right heart failure. (Adapted from Côté et al. Feline Cardiology 2011; Wiley Blackwell).

systolic blood pressure at the expense of normal capillary pressure. This is because **adequate cerebral perfusion is paramount to short-term survival**, whereas maintenance of LVEDP is less important for immediate survival.

Maintaining Blood Pressure

Decreases in cardiac output and blood pressure are detected by baroreceptors (pressure receptors) **and mechanoreceptors** (stretch receptors) located in the carotid sinus, aortic arch, and atrial walls (Figure 2). The firing rate of these receptors decreases, which results in a reduced number of inhibitory afferent impulses transmitted to the central nervous system (CNS) and vasomotor centres. Withdrawal of these inhibitory signals increases activity of the sympathetic nervous system and suppresses activity of the parasympathetic nervous system, resulting in increased delivery of cardiac noradrenaline (norepinephrine).

Elevated sympathetic nervous system activity results in tachycardia, increased cardiac contractility, vasoconstriction and activation of the renin-angiotensin-aldosterone axis.

Clinical Significance

- The predominant clinical signs result from congestive (backwards) failure; the hallmark of which is the **presence of effusion or oedema**.
- As a rule, patients with chronic heart failure exhibit signs of congestion and oedema before signs of low cardiac output.
- Signs of low cardiac output are generally only seen together with signs of oedema.
- All animals with heart failure have elevated sympathetic tone. Therefore, for a patient with suspected heart failure and a heart rate <160 for cats or <120 for dogs, other differential diagnoses should be considered.

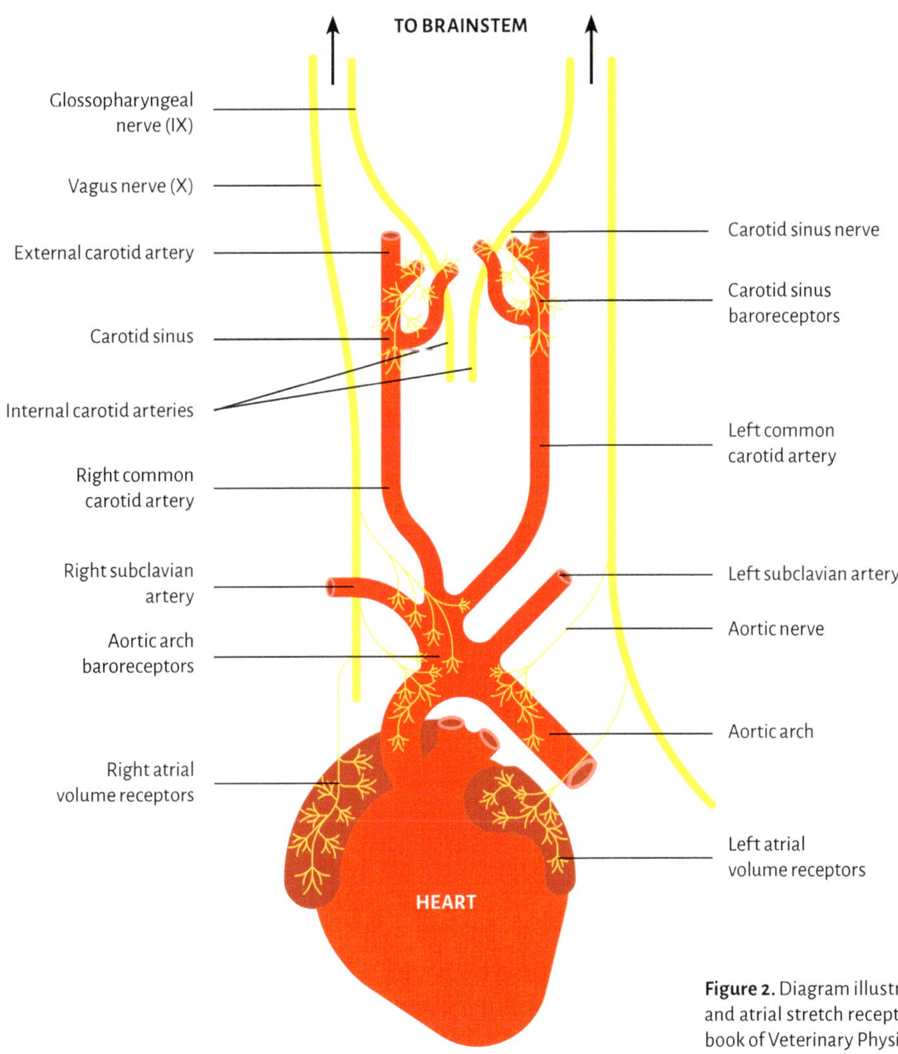

Figure 2. Diagram illustrating location of arterial baroreceptors and atrial stretch receptors. (Adapted from Cunningham. Textbook of Veterinary Physiology. 2007; Saunders Elsevier).

Causes of Heart Failure

Congestive heart failure is by far the most common type of heart failure seen in veterinary patients, therefore all references to heart failure from here onwards refer to congestive heart failure (CHF) unless specifically stated.

CHF is the end result of severe cardiac disease. However, it is important to remember many dogs and cats with heart disease never develop heart failure and often die of unrelated causes.

There are many diseases that can lead to CHF in dogs and cats, and one way to categorise them is to consider the part of the cardiac cycle that each disease primarily affects. This is known as **functional categorisation** (Figure 3).

Primary Myocardial Failure

Diseases that primarily result in systolic myocardial failure include **dilated cardiomyopathy (DCM) and arrhythmogenic right ventricular cardiomyopathy**. The hallmark of this group of diseases is a decrease in systolic function which may lead to pump failure over time, and subsequent increases in diastolic filling pressure.

DCM is the second most common acquired cardiac disease in dogs after myxomatous mitral valve disease (MMVD).

In cats diseases of primary myocardial failure are uncommon, especially since the introduction of taurine supplementation in commercial cat foods. When DCM is identified in cats it is often thought to constitute end-stage dilation in cats

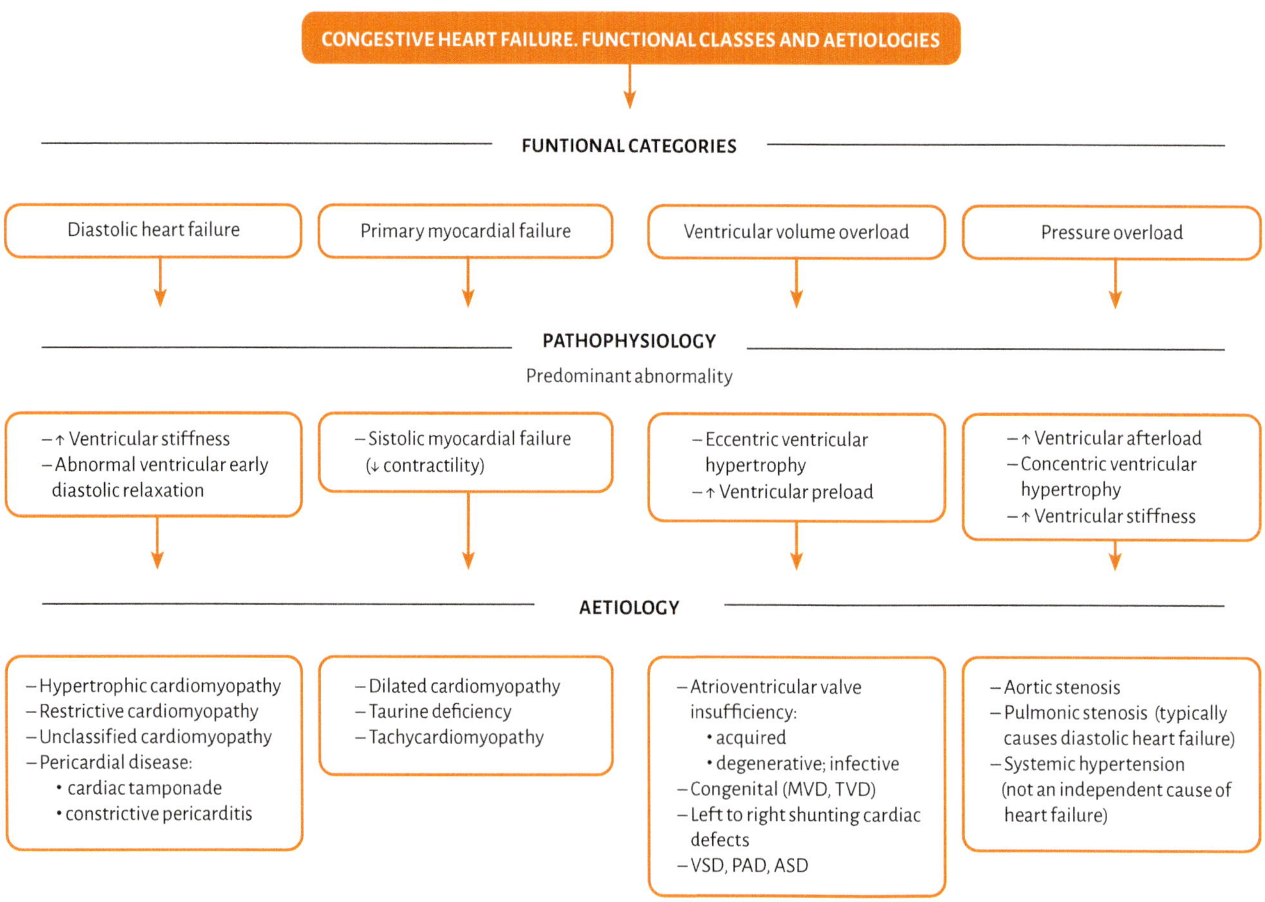

Figure 3. Algorithm illustrating functional categories and aetiologies of congestive heart failure. (Adapted from Côté et al. Feline Cardiology. 2011; Wiley Blackwell). MVD: mitral valve disease; TVD: tricuspid valve dysplasia; VSD: ventricular septal defect; PDA: patent *ductus arteriosus*; ASD: atrial septal defect

with severe hypertrophic cardiomyopathy (HCM) and CHF, rather than a primary myocardial failure

Ventricular Volume Overload

Any condition where the heart has to pump a stroke volume adequate to meet the metabolic needs of the peripheral tissues, whilst at the same time deal with increased blood volume resulting from regurgitation or shunting, may lead to elevated diastolic filling pressure and development of CHF. Typical diseases include, **myxomatous mitral valve disease** (the most common acquired heart disease in dogs), other valvular insufficiencies, and left to right shunting congenital heart defects such as patent *ductus arteriosus*.

Pressure Overload

Diseases that primarily result in pressure overload of the heart are less common. Essentially, any condition that increases the resistance through which the stroke volume is pumped (afterload) results in pressure overload. The heart must maintain stroke volume in order to meet the metabolic needs of the peripheral tissues, so when resistance to blood flow is higher than the systolic pressure generated by the left ventricle it must increase to compensate. Any condition that increases ventricular afterload will result in pressure overload over time. Examples include aortic stenosis, pulmonic stenosis and systemic hypertension.

Diastolic Heart Failure

As the functional classification indicates, **any disease that primarily impairs diastolic filling and leads to elevated diastolic filling pressure can result in diastolic heart failure**. It is important to remember that systolic function initially remains normal. However, with end-stage disease concurrent systolic function can develop. Essentially the ventricles are able to contract normally, but cannot accept the normal diastolic inflow of blood within normal pressures. This is often because the heart muscle is stiff or cannot relax properly. Elevated diastolic filling pressures lead to a backward transmission of elevated venous pressure to the capillary bed and ultimately leakage of fluid through the capillary wall causing oedema or effusion. Hypertrophic cardiomyopathy (HCM), unclassified cardiomyopathy (UCM), and restrictive cardiomyopathy (RCM) are all diseases which cause diastolic dysfunction that may lead to CHF.

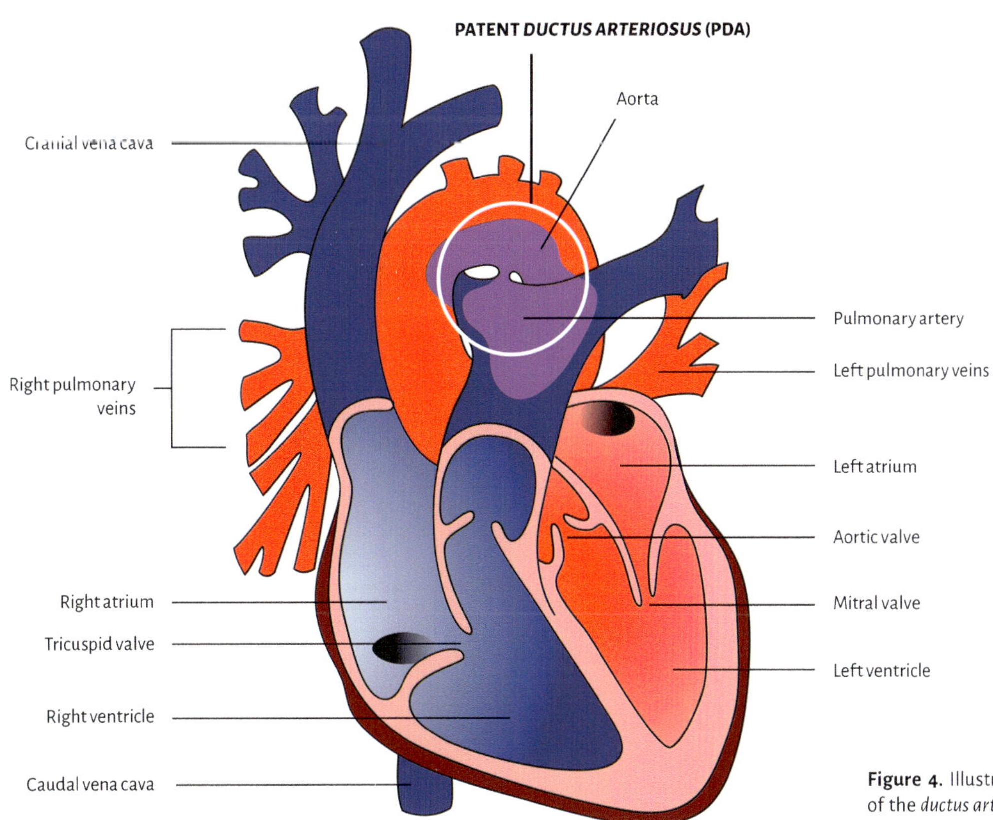

Figure 4. Illustration showing the position of the *ductus arteriosus* connecting the aorta (Ao) to the pulmonary artery (PA).

The Development of Heart Failure

Many cardiac diseases can result in heart failure, despite different primary functional abnormalities. This is because **the body tries to maintain the heart's ability to meet the metabolic needs of the peripheral tissues, through a progressive set of compensatory mechanisms**.

In early disease, the activation of compensatory mechanisms represents an attempt to maintain normal cardiac performance, but heightened neurohormonal activity quickly leads to **maladaptive changes which hasten the progression of disease and heart failure** (Figure 5).

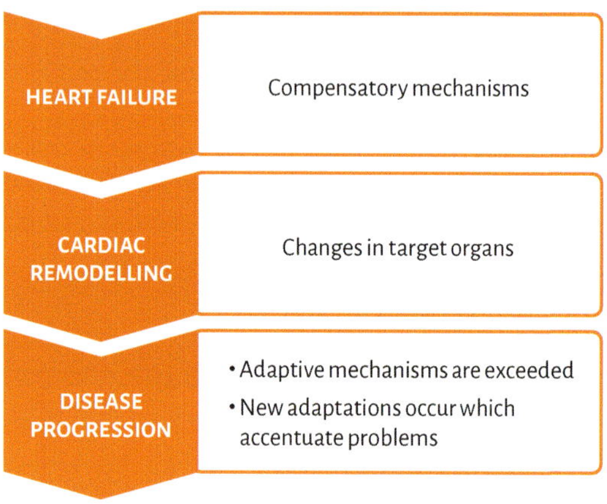

Figure 5. Flow chart illustrating the progressive nature of heart failure. (Diagram designed and created by Andrew Francis, Yellowfin Capital Ltd.).

As disease progresses, these mechanisms contribute to the development of clinical signs of heart failure, such as **respiratory distress, cough, and activity intolerance**; as well as abnormal physical examination findings, such as **tachycardia, heart murmur, pulmonary crackles, and ascites**.

These compensatory mechanisms are reviewed broadly in the order in which they occur once a cardiac insult occurs.

Acute Compensatory Mechanisms

Alterations in Autonomic Tone

Soon after a cardiac insult occurs, cardiac output and consequently arterial blood pressure are reduced. In order to maintain all-important cerebral blood flow, as well as coronary and renal blood supply, **the priority of the cardiovascular system is to maintain adequate arterial blood pressure**. The drop in blood pressure decreases the firing rate of the high-pressure baroreceptors. Withdrawal of these inhibitory signals increases activity of the sympathetic nervous system and suppresses activity of the parasympathetic nervous system, resulting in increased delivery of cardiac noradrenaline (norepinephrine).

The increased concentrations of cardiac noradrenaline act on:

- **cardiac β-receptors** to immediately increase cardiac output:
  - increased heart rate (positive chronotropy)
  - augmented cardiac contractility (positive inotropy)
  - early diastolic relaxation (positive lusitropy)
- **α-adrenergic receptors** to maintain arterial blood pressure:
  - arterial bed vasoconstriction increases total peripheral resistance
  - veno-constriction increases volume of venous return to the heart
- noradrenaline also directly activates the **renin-angiotensin-aldosterone system (RAAS)**.

These effects initially support dwindling cardiac performance, but this immediate response is not able to compensate for more than a few days, and more chronic compensatory mechanisms are necessary for the animal to survive. Worse still, these initially positive effects are countermanded by the detrimental effects of chronic activation of the sympathetic nervous system.

Chronic stimulation:

- Depletes cardiac noradrenaline stores, and then induces down regulation and uncoupling of myocyte β-adrenergic receptors. This blunts the beneficial positive inotropic and lusitropic (relaxation) effects of β-adrenergic stimulation.
- Causes myocardial cell loss through apoptosis and/or necrosis.

Chronic Compensatory Mechanisms

Activation of the Renin-angiotensin-aldosterone System

Noradrenaline directly activates the renin-angiotensin aldosterone system but the main driver of RAAS up regulation is reduced delivery of sodium to the macula densa as a result of decreased renal blood flow. RAAS up-regulation begins as soon as the initial cardiac insult occurs, but it takes time for circulating blood volume to increase. However, by the time the beneficial effects of sympathetic activation have begun to wane after about three days, significant RAAS up-regulation has occurred.

Reduced delivery of sodium to the macula densa stimulates renin release from the juxtaglomerular apparatus. Renin cleaves angiotensinogen in the liver to angiotensin I, which is further cleaved by angiotensin converting enzyme (ACE) in the lungs or other tissues to form the active hormone angiotensin II (ATII). **ACE also inactivates vasodilators such as bradykinin**.

ATII binds to the angiotensin II type 1 receptor (AT_1R) to exert powerful effects including, vasoconstriction, increased aldosterone synthesis from the adrenal gland, stimulation of thirst, vasopressin (ADH) release from the pituitary, induction of endothelin I synthesis, and increased sympathetic tone.

Overall, systemic vascular resistance is increased **because RAAS activation promotes an imbalance in favour of increased concentrations of vasoconstrictors** (ATII, vasopressin, endothelin-I, noradrenaline). Conversely **the concentrations of vasodilatory agents decrease**, including nitric oxide, natriuretic peptides, and prostaglandins. The net effect of RAAS activation is maintenance of systemic organ perfusion by increased systemic vascular resistance and increased blood volume through sodium and water retention, which occur within several days of activation.

Increased circulating blood volume helps maintain cardiac function in the short-term but, unfortunately, Angiotensin II is also the effector molecule for many of the maladaptive processes which promote heart failure, including vasoconstriction, renal sodium and water retention, elaboration of

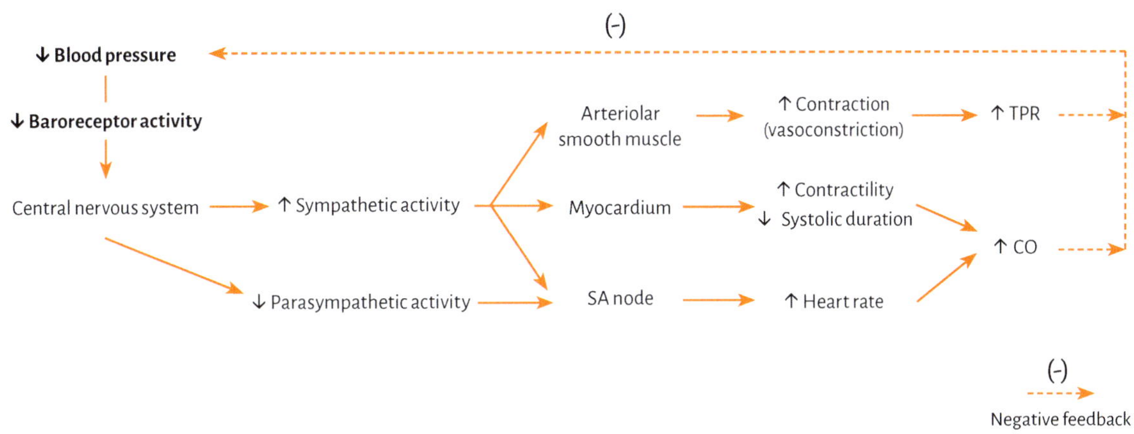

Figure 6. Arterial baroreceptor reflex response to a decrease in blood pressure resulting from a cardiac insult. (Adapted from Cunningham's Textbook of Veterinary Physiology. 2013; Elsevier Saunders).

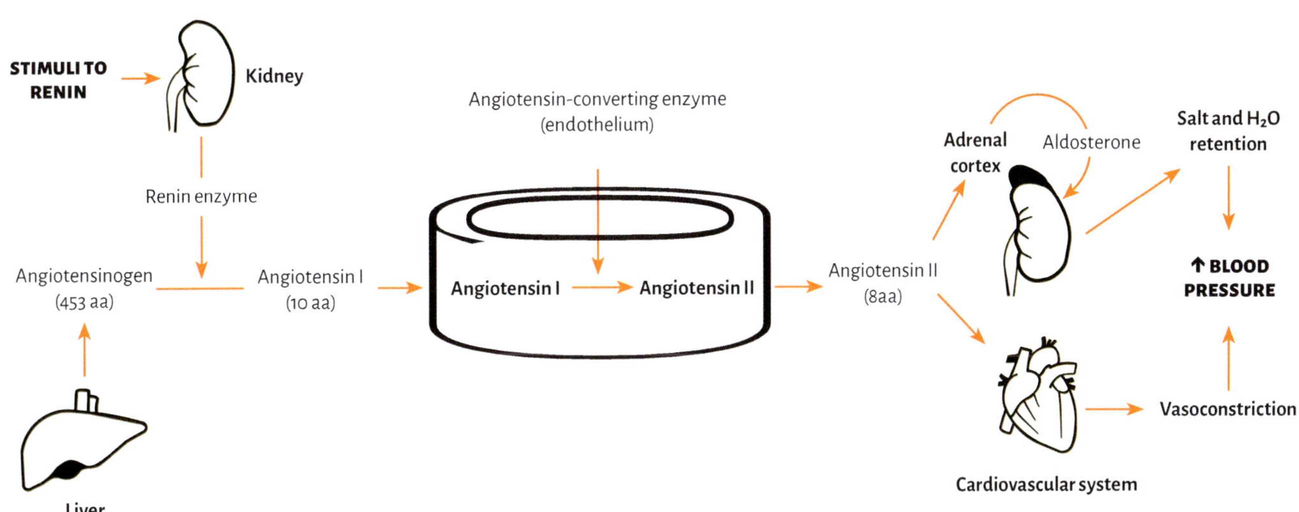

Figure 7. The renin-angiotensin-aldosterone system and the major effects of up-regulation. (Adapted from Ganong's Review of Medical Physiology 24th edition. 2012; McGraw Hill).

aldosterone, myocardial hypertrophy, increased thirst and water intake, apoptosis, and potentiation of the sympathetic nervous system.

Activation of Other Neuro-hormonal Pathways

Natriuretic Peptides

The heart products two natriuretic peptides, atrial natriuretic peptide (ANP) and B-type natriuretic peptide (BNP). The peptides are primarily produced and stored in the atrial muscle and **released in response to increased wall stretch**. Both natriuretic peptides elicit vasodilatation, natriuresis, and diuresis; and thus serve as counterbalances to the renin-angiotensin- aldosterone system and sympathetic nervous system. **Circulating levels of both ANP and BNP are increased in dogs and cats with heart disease**, roughly in proportion to disease severity. However, in advanced cases of disease, the counterbalancing effect of the natriuretic peptides is overwhelmed.

Arginine Vasopressin (ADH)

Arginine vasopressin is produced by the pituitary gland and increases resorption of free water in the collecting duct of the nephron. Unlike in other parts of the nephron sodium is not reabsorbed in tandem with the water. Consequently **excess vasopressin leads to dilution of total body sodium and chloride levels, leading to hypo-osmolarity**.

Plasma levels of vasopressin tend to mirror circulating levels of noradrenaline. Excess vasopressin leads to expansion of the extracellular fluid volume and **contributes to signs of congestion**. In patients with advanced disease, hyponatraemia and hypochloraemia are often detected on routine blood chemistry, and excessive vasopressin levels are the likely cause. This finding generally represents **a poor prognostic sign**.

Endothelin-1

Endothelin-1 is a potent vasoconstrictor and is elevated in patients with heart failure. It is primarily produced by vascular endothelial tissues in response to:

- angiotensin II;
- shear stress as a result of increased blood flow or resistance to blood flow;
- other vasoactive cytokines.

Together with angiotensin II, **endothelin-1 contributes to increased afterload and increased myocardial workload.**

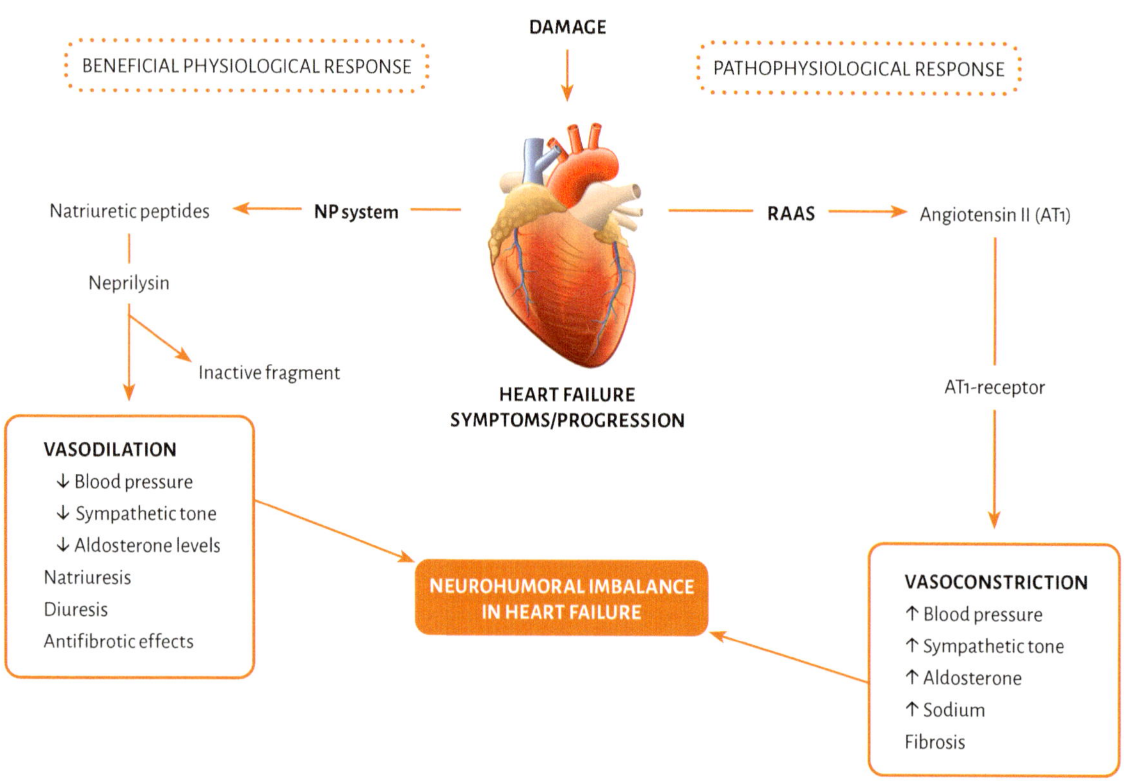

Figure 8. Heart failure is a state of neurohormonal imbalance. (Adapted from Langenickel TH, Dole WP. Angiotensin receptor-neprilysin inhibition with LCZ696: a novel approach for the treatment of heart failure. Drug Discovery Today: Therapeutic Strategies. 2012; 9:e131-e139).

Endothelin-1 is also thought to be directly toxic to myocardial cells and interfere with normal calcium ion cycling. Endothelin receptor blocking drugs have been licensed in human medicine to help moderate some of these negative effects.

Cardiac Remodelling and Hypertrophy

As a result of the initial cardiac insult, there are rapid changes in autonomic tone on cardiac function and systemic vascular resistance, and slower effects of up-regulation of RAAS to increase circulating blood volume. It is this **increase in circulating blood volume that helps drive cardiac remodelling**.

Remodelling of the myocardium, in the form of alterations in cardiac mass and geometry, represents one of the primary responses of the heart to sustained, increased workload.

There are two classic forms of ventricular remodelling, with the predominant type of remodelling depending on the type of increased workload. In other words, **the pattern of cardiac and cellular remodelling that occurs in response to haemodynamic overloading depends on the nature of the inciting stimulus**.

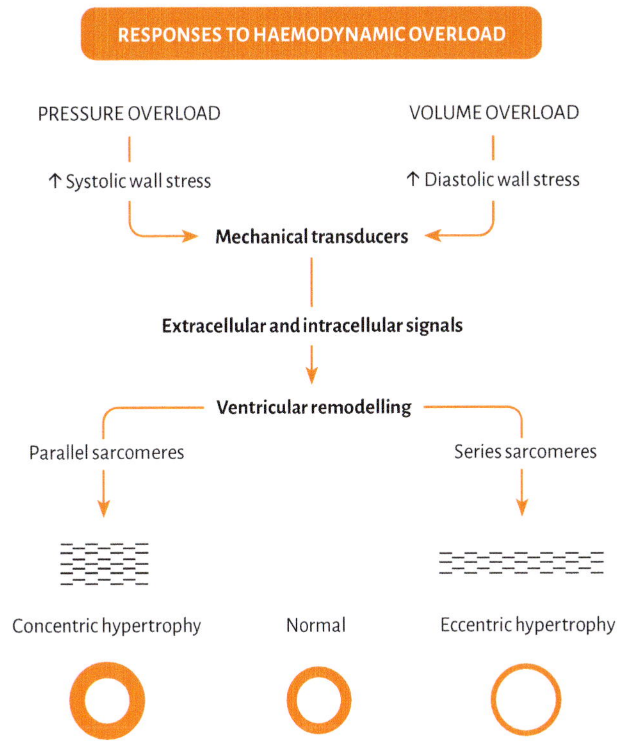

Figure 9. Patterns of cardiac and cellular remodelling. (Adapted from Braunwald's Heart Disease. 2012; Saunders).

Concentric Hypertrophy

A sustained increase in afterload requiring increased left ventricular systolic pressures (pressure overload) to maintain adequate stroke volume, results in predominantly **concentric hypertrophy**. Increased afterload triggers replication of sarcomeres in parallel, resulting in an increase in the relative thickness of the ventricular walls.

Eccentric Hypertrophy

Eccentric hypertrophy develops in response to volume overload. Common examples of volume overload conditions are **mitral regurgitation and patent *ductus arteriosus***. The sarcomeres replicate in series, leading to elongation of the myocytes, dilatation of the ventricular chamber, and a small increase in myocardial wall thickness. Thus, in some ways, eccentric hypertrophy is less adaptive than concentric hypertrophy in that dramatic increases in ventricular chamber diameter tend to increase ventricular wall stress beyond the point where the mild increases in wall thickness can compensate. Interestingly, although eccentric hypertrophy is less adaptive, dogs with myxomatous mitral valve disease remain stable for long periods of time. This is partly because a large proportion of the blood present in the left ventricle at the end of diastole can escape into the low-pressure left atrium rather than being pumped into the high-pressure aorta.

Unfortunately, every initially beneficial compensatory mechanism ultimately becomes maladaptive. In both forms of hypertrophy, myocardial remodelling is limited by eventual loss of viable myocytes through necrosis or apoptosis, abnormalities in calcium ion cycling, and dysfunction of myocardial energy production.

Myocyte Necrosis and Apoptosis

The heart has limited ability to regenerate myocytes lost to necrosis or apoptosis. In general, loss **of large numbers of myocytes is irreversible** and exacerbates the stress on the remaining viable cells.

Myocyte necrosis is triggered primarily by ischaemia (as in the case of excessive concentric hypertrophy) **or toxins** (such as doxorubicin), and is accompanied by an inflammatory response. Lost cells are replaced by fibrosis, which further impairs systolic and diastolic function.

Apoptosis, which is commonly referred to as programmed cell death, is non-inflammatory and triggered by:

- high catecholamine levels
- mitochondrial damage
- mechanical stress.

Abnormal Calcium Ion Cycling

Optimal calcium cycling within the cardiomyocyte is crucial for adequate contraction, and also appropriate relaxation. Depression of sarcomeric contractility seen in heart failure is largely due to abnormalities in intracellular handling of calcium ions.

The primary calcium store in every cardiomyocyte is within the sarcoplasmic reticulum. Lesser amounts of calcium are released from the mitochondria and during depolarisation flow in through specific calcium channels in the sarcolemmal membrane.

During cell depolarisation, calcium is released from the sarcoplasmic reticulum and binds to the troponin-C apparatus on the actinmyosin filaments, triggering contraction of the sarcomere.

Immediately following contraction the calcium is actively transported back in to the sarcoplasmic reticulum. Sarcomeric relaxation during diastole cannot occur without active calcium uptake. As a result, somewhat counterintuitively, cardiac relaxation during early diastole is an energy intensive process, requiring significant ATP hydrolysis.

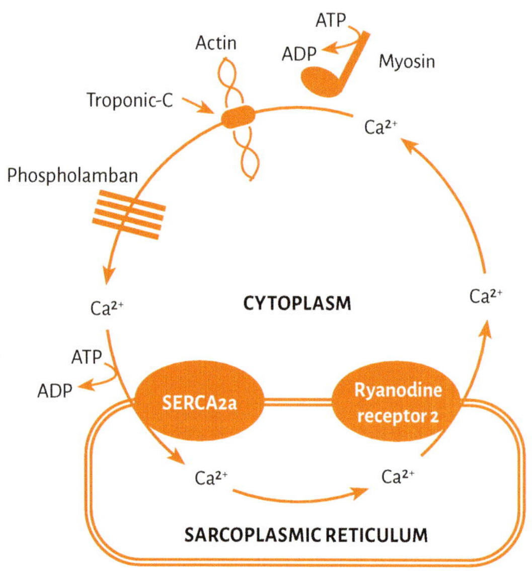

Figure 10. Calcium cycling in the myocardial cell. (Adapted from BSAVA Manual of Canine and Feline Cardiopulmonary Medicine 2nd Edition. 2010; BSAVA).

In heart failure, sarcoplasmic reticular calcium release is prolonged, resulting in systolic dysfunction, but active re-uptake is also inhibited causing concurrent diastolic dysfunction.

To make matters worse, the **sympathetically mediated tachycardia seen in animals with heart failure exacerbates the abnormalities in calcium cycling**. In healthy heart tissue, increases in heart rate have a positive force-frequency relationship. As heart rate increases, systolic and diastolic function are augmented. Due to abnormal calcium cycling in diseased heart tissue, cardiac contractility worsens as heart rate increases. This negative force-frequency relationship mitigates much of the positive effect that heart rate normally has on cardiac output.

Myocardial Energy Production Abnormalities

The normal heart is able to utilise a variety of substrates for energy production, including free fatty acids, glucose, and lactate. Cellular energy balance within cardiomyocytes is tightly regulated and extremely efficient. It is rare, except in the most severe cases of heart failure or acute ischaemia, that the heart is unable to maintain adequate perfusion, oxygen and substrate delivery.

Adenosine triphosphate (ATP), as in all cells is the key molecular store of energy in the cardiomyocyte. ATP hydrolysis fuels contraction and relaxation of the sarcomere, operation of ion pumps and exchangers, especially those involved in calcium cycling, action potential propagation, maintenance of the resting cell membrane, and phosphorylation of various enzymes and proteins.

In dogs with myocardial failure, cytochromes and enzymes critical to mitochondrial oxidative phosphorylation are variably absent. Cardiomyocyte energy stores in the form of creatine phosphate and ATP are also depleted in advanced disease, and a deficiency of ATP production may well contribute to the development and progression of heart failure.

To try and compensate there is a shift in substrate metabolism within the heart. In the healthy heart metabolism of free fatty acids meets a large proportion of energy demands. In diseased hearts, a greater proportion of energy needs are met by metabolism of glucose and lactate. Although less energy dense, glucose and lactate metabolism requires less oxygen consumption per unit of ATP produced. **This helps to reduce myocardial oxygen demand at a time of severe cardiac stress**.

Global Cardiac Function

The detailed physiological changes and metabolic derangements reviewed above constitute a current model of how heart disease can develop into heart failure in some animals and the mechanisms that underpin the progressive nature of heart failure.

Global cardiac function is affected by the complex interplay of the positive and negative effects of these mechanisms. It is this overall pump function that clinicians are attempting to assess during clinical examination of patients with heart failure.

The three primary clinical determinants of global cardiac performance are:

- **preload**: the volume of blood or hydrostatic pressure within the ventricles at the end of diastole;
- **afterload**: the force that opposes ejection of blood into the peripheral arterial system, of which arterial blood pressure is the primary factor;
- **contractility**: the intrinsic ability of the myocardium to generate force to eject blood. Contractility is not dependent on the degree of heart loading.

Clinical examination of the cardiac patient allows indirect evaluation of each of these three determinants. However, true contractility is difficult to quantify accurately because all the available measurement techniques are affected by preload and afterload, and true contractility is independent of heart loading.

- **Preload**
  - assessment of jugular venous distension
  - evaluations of effusions, oedema or ascites
  - degree of cardiac eccentric hypertrophy using radiography or echocardiography.
- **Afterload**
  - measurement of systemic blood pressure
  - indirect measurement of pulmonary artery pressures on echocardiography.
- **Contractility**
  - overall visual assessment of systolic function
  - indices of systolic performance such as fractional shortening.

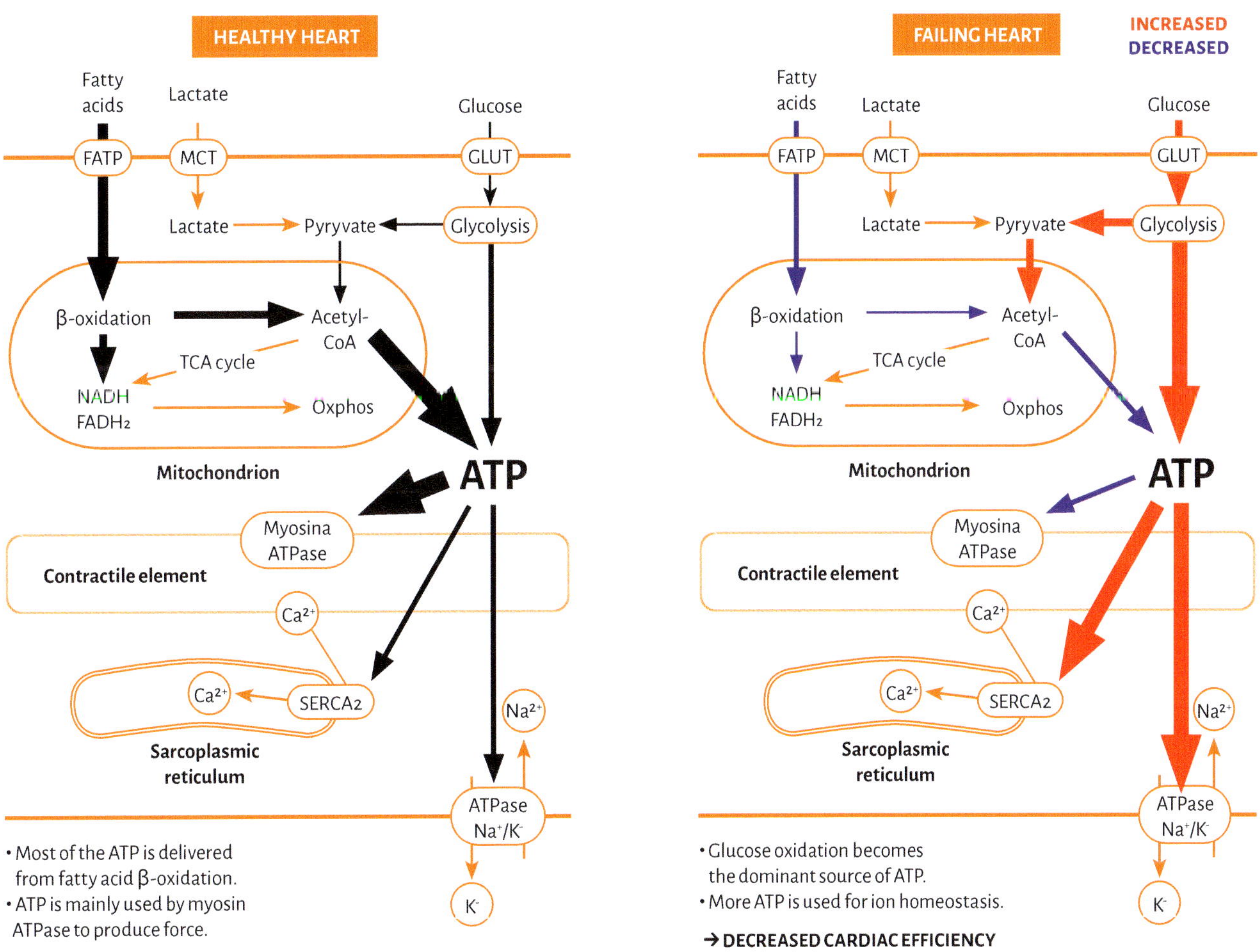

Figure 11. ATP usage in the healthy heart and the failing heart. (Adapted from Toumainen T, Pasi T. The role of cardiac energy metabolism in cardiac hypertrophy and failure. Experimental Cell Research 2017;360:12-18).

In patients with heart failure, the complex compensatory mechanisms drive increased preload through fluid volume retention and increased afterload due to peripheral arteriolar vasoconstriction, which **increases total peripheral resistance**. In patients with myocardial disease where systolic function is primarily affected (e.g. DCM), then decreased contractility is a cardinal sign of early disease. In most other cardiac diseases that result in failure, decreased contractility develops with disease progression as a result of the maladaptive compensatory mechanisms.

Cardiac Performance and Preload

When the heart is healthy, and cardiac function is normal small increases in ventricular volume elicit considerable improvement in cardiac function, indicating **significant cardiac reserve is available during periods of exercise**. The curve illustrating this relationship is known as the Frank-Starling Curve (Figure 12).

In the diseased heart the acute and chronic compensatory mechanisms ultimately reduce the heart's response to adrenergic drive, decrease the number of viable myocytes, increase afterload and cardiac work, reduce energy production and alter the normal extracellular matrix. In effect, the heart operates in an environment of increased afterload and decreased contractility.

See Figure 12 for the impaired relationship between preload and cardiac performance in the diseased heart.

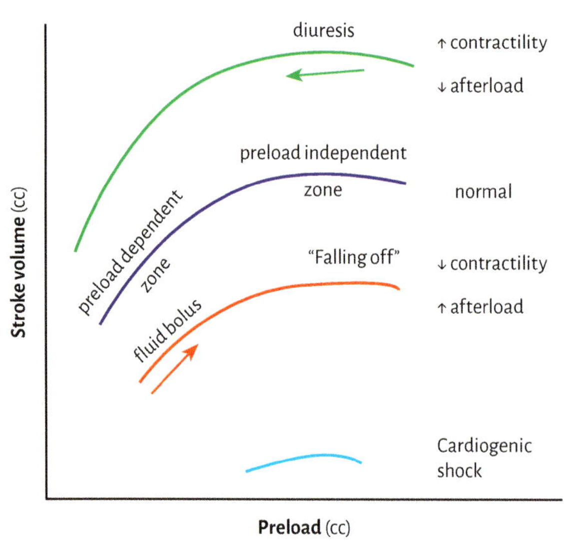

Figure 12. The relationship between preload and stroke volume, and how changes in contractility and afterload affect this relationships. This is known as the Frank-Starling Curve. (Adapted from https://rk.md/2017/frank-starling-curves).

In diseased hearts cardiac output is decreased for any given level of preload (red dashed lines in Figure 12 A), and the incremental gains in cardiac output for any increase in loading (preload) are less than in a healthy patient (blue dashed arrows in Figure 13 A).

Activation of the renin-angiotensin-aldosterone axis results in sodium and water retention, which maximises ventricular volume, and therefore increases preload. This acts to augment cardiac performance (cardiac output).

However, increased preload comes at a cost in the form of increased ventricular and venous pressure. In the short-term the heart is able to accommodate this increased preload because eccentric hypertrophy increases ventricular compliance. Increased ventricular compliance allows the ventricle to accept a greater volume of blood in diastole without a significant increase in ventricular end-diastolic pressures. **Longer term, once venous pressure rises above approximately 25 mmHg, transudation of fluid occurs across the capillary membrane and congestive failure (effusion and/or oedema) develops** (Figure 13 B).

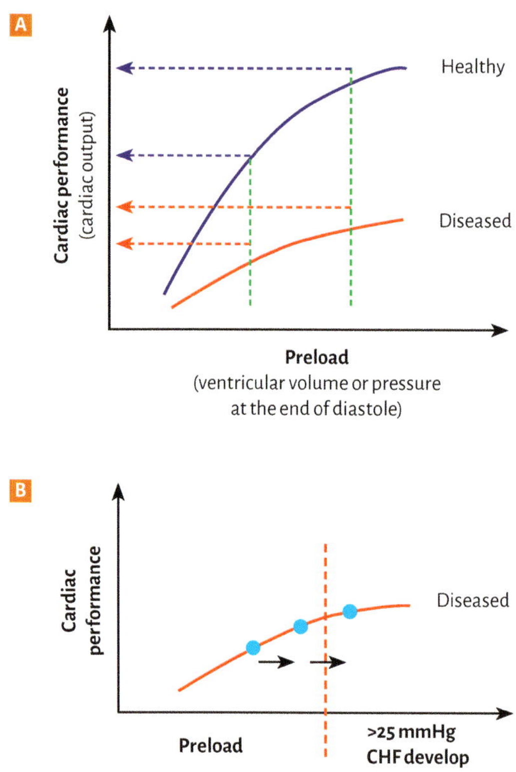

Figure 13. A. Graph illustrating the effect of significant cardiac disease on cardiac function. **B**. Graph showing the preload threshold for development of congestive heart failure.

The Effects of Diastolic Dysfunction

Some forms of heart disease are primarily due to diastolic dysfunction, as opposed to systolic myocardial failure. The most commonly encountered diastolic heart disease in veterinary medicine is **feline hypertrophic cardiomyopathy (HCM)**.

The primary functional abnormality in hypertrophic cardiomyopathy is **concentric hypertrophy of the left ventricle**. This hypertrophy, if severe enough, often results in progressive diastolic dysfunction, in the face of normal or near normal systolic function.

Diastolic dysfunction in HCM usually results from a primary impairment in ventricular relaxation. With significant hypertrophy left ventricular compliance becomes impaired, which results in increased filling pressures. Even though primary diastolic dysfunction is the primary abnormality in HCM, rather than primary systolic dysfunction, or primary volume overload, **left-sided congestive heart failure remains the end result**. Consequently, treatment options for cats with congestive heart failure secondary to HCM are very similar to treatment options for dogs with DCM or MMVD.

In healthy patients, increases in ventricular volume are achieved with little change in ventricular pressure because of normal early ventricular relaxation and high ventricular compliance during mid- and late diastole.

In patients with impaired ventricular relaxation, early filling is achieved at the expense of higher ventricular pressures. In patients with poor ventricular compliance, mid- and late-diastolic filling is hindered and only achieved at the expense of higher ventricular pressures.

Diastolic Dysfunction and Congestive Heart Failure

When diastolic filling is reduced, cardiac output falls. Subsequent reduction of cardiac output triggers activation of the same neurohormonal and adrenergic responses that are seen in cases of systolic dysfunction, and fluid and sodium retention leads to CHF.

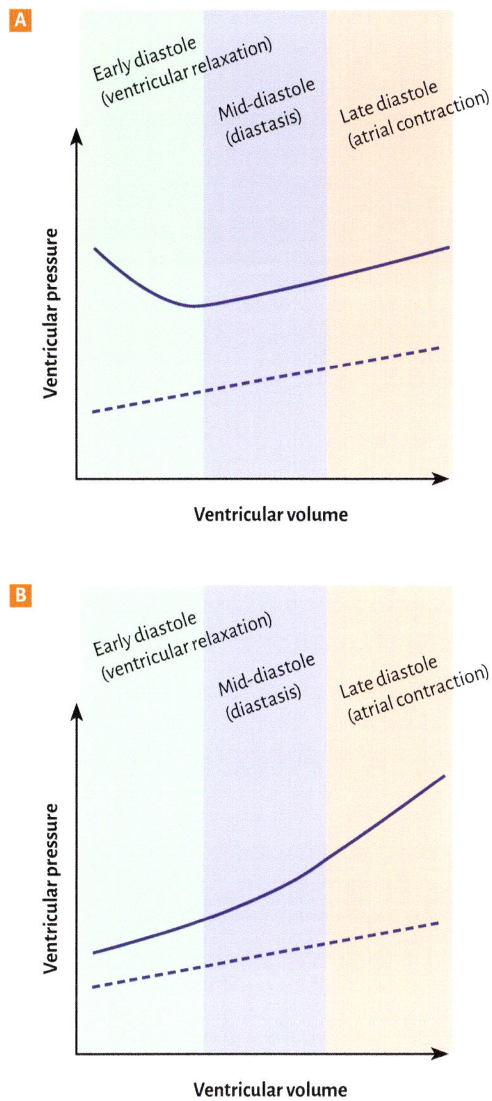

Figure 14. Diagram illustrating the relationship between pressure and volume within the ventricle in patients with impaired ventricular relaxation (**A**), and patients with poor ventricular compliance (**B**). (Adapted from BSAVA Manual of Canine and Feline Cardiopulmonary Medicine 2nd Edition. 2010; BSAVA).

Clinical Examination

Clinical Presentation of Heart Failure

When assessing a patient with suspected cardiac disease, a thorough history should be obtained, including the onset and nature of clinical signs, rate of progression, risk factors, previous medical examinations, and treatment.

Importantly, **the owner should be questioned specifically regarding the patient's exercise tolerance, respiratory effort and rate**.

Respiratory Abnormalities

Many pets do not exercise to any significant degree. Consequently, **owners do not notice dyspnoea until it is evident at rest**.

When dogs or cats present with **severe dyspnoea due to pulmonary oedema or pleural effusion, they generally have a marked inspiratory effort** and may have an expiratory effort to their breathing pattern. Other dogs may be primarily hyperpnoeic, with rapid, deep respirations.

Coughing is a commonly noted in dogs with heart failure. It is much less common in cats. Unfortunately, many small dogs prone to developing heart failure secondary to mitral regurgitation due to myxomatous mitral valve degeneration also have concomitant respiratory disease. Consequently, it is **difficult to determine if the cough is due to respiratory or cardiac disease**.

Almost all dyspnoeic patients with left-sided congestive heart failure are also tachypnoeic. **Tachypnoea usually precedes clinical evidence of dyspnoea**. Tachypnoea is a subtler clinical sign, however, so owners commonly miss this sign.

Ascites

Right heart failure commonly produces ascites in dogs. Ascites secondary to heart failure is less common in cats. Right heart failure as a result of tricuspid valve dysplasia is the most common cardiac reason for ascites in cats.

Ascites secondary to right heart failure generally accumulates slowly over weeks to months, although owners commonly think of it as an acute event because they do not notice the increase in abdominal size until it is severe. Chronic pericardial tamponade can result in subacute (days) accumulation of peritoneal fluid. Large accumulations place pressure on the diaphragm, which impedes breathing. Consequently, dogs with severe ascites may be dyspnoeic or tachypnoeic.

Syncope

Syncope (fainting) is defined as an episodic and transient loss of consciousness and postural tone. It most commonly occurs because of a brief cessation of blood flow to the brain as a result of either a bradyarrhythmia or short period of asystole, or a burst of non-sustained and severe tachycardia. However, syncope, episodic collapse, and episodic weakness can occur secondary to many non-cardiac abnormalities as well. **Distinguishing between seizures and episodic collapse or syncope can be difficult**, especially if the owner cannot provide a detailed and accurate history of at least one witnessed event.

Weakness

Generalised weakness can occur secondary to cardiac disease. Dogs and cats with advanced heart failure can be weak. This is due to poor perfusion resulting in decreased oxygen delivery to skeletal muscles or to generalised muscle wasting or both. Dogs with severe tachycardia (a heart rate usually greater than 300 beats/min) or severe bradycardia (a heart rate usually less than 30 beats/min) have a severely decreased cardiac output and therefore poor tissue perfusion and weakness. The decrease in cardiac output occurs with tachycardia because of inadequate ventricular filling time and with the bradycardia because of the slow heart rate.

Exercise Intolerance

Exercise intolerance is an occasional complaint by an owner of an animal with cardiac disease. It is not a more common complaint, because many animals do not exercise vigorously. **It is more common in dogs with subaortic stenosis** than in other cardiac disease. Owners of dogs with pulmonic stenosis often describe an increase in activity following successful balloon valvuloplasty. Consequently, it appears these dog owners often may not recognize exercise intolerance or decreased activity resulting from cardiac disease. Exercise intolerance as a result of cardiac disease can also be an early indication of heart failure.

Cyanosis

Cyanosis is commonly both a historical finding and a physical sign. It is a blue to blue-grey discoloration of the mucous membranes, and/or nail beds.

Cyanosis can be central or peripheral:

- **Central cyanosis** affects the mucous membranes of the oral cavity and tongue, and usually **results from an increased quantity of reduced** (deoxygenated) **haemoglobin due to poor pulmonary circulation or impaired ventilation**. Rarely, it is due to abnormal haemoglobin pigments in the blood (e.g. congenital methaemoglobinaemia). Treatment with supplemental oxygen usually rapidly corrects central cyanosis.
- **Peripheral cyanosis** is due to the stasis of blood in capillary beds resulting in increased extraction of oxygen in the capillary beds. This is most commonly **due to low cardiac output with peripheral vasoconstriction**. The decrease in cardiac output must be severe for peripheral cyanosis to become evident. It can also be caused by arterial thromboembolism localised to individual limbs. Peripheral cyanosis is much less responsive to supplemental oxygen therapy.

In cardiovascular medicine, cyanosis is most common in patients with arterial hypoxaemia as a result of right-to-left shunts such as tetralogy of Fallot. Patients with right-to-left shunts with hypoxaemia usually also have polycythaemia. The increased red cell mass results in a greater quantity of reduced haemoglobin and so contributes to the cyanosis.

Cardiac Physical Examination

The physical examination should be performed systematically and include:

- observation of respiratory rate, pattern and effort
- determination of hydration status
- evaluation of mucous membranes
- inspection of the jugular veins
- auscultation of the heart and lungs
- palpation of the systemic arterial pulses
- detection of pleural or abdominal effusions through percussion, palpation and/or auscultation.

Clinical Signs of Congestive (backward) Heart Failure

Clinical signs of congestive heart failure in patients with CHF can be subtle; mild tachypnoea, slight abdominal effort, decreased appetite. In some cases, the clinical signs are overt; severe respiratory distress, haemoptysis, shock.

Signs of disease chronicity include weight loss, muscle wasting or severe cachexia.

Whereas most dogs with heart failure have either an obvious heart murmur or a diastolic gallop, many **cats with significant disease have intermittent murmurs or soft gallop sounds** which are difficult to detect, particularly in an animal in respiratory distress.

CHF can manifest as predominantly left- or right-sided failure, or occasionally as biventricular failure. Pulmonary oedema, pleural effusion, abdominal effusion (ascites), and even occasionally pericardial effusion (especially cats) can occur, depending on the underlying cardiovascular disease, and which ventricle is primarily affected.

Left-sided Congestive Heart Failure

In dogs, acquired mitral valve disease, mitral regurgitation, and volume overload affect the left ventricle (LV), left atrium (LA), pulmonary veins, and capillaries; thus, heart failure is manifested as left-sided heart failure in the form of pulmonary oedema. **In both dogs and cats, pulmonary oedema is exclusively a sign of left-sided heart failure**.

Right-sided Congestive Heart Failure

In dogs, right heart failure manifests as pleural effusion and/or ascites. In the cat, pleural effusion can occur as a result of either left- or right-sided heart failure, and in most cases is actually due to left-sided heart disease. The explanation for this discrepancy between species is because a portion of the visceral pleural surface actually empties into the pulmonary veins, and this anatomic arrangement appears to be more prominent in cats than in humans or dogs.

Ascites as a sign of right heart failure in the cat is relatively uncommon, and **most cats with ascites suffer from non-cardiac diseases**.

Peripheral oedema that affects the limbs or subcutaneous tissues is uncommon, and is seen only in the most severe cases of right-sided CHF in small companion animals.

Congestive versus Low Output Heart Failure

The majority of cases of heart failure in companion animals predominantly involve CHF rather than low output failure. There is a sound physiological reason for this. The body's homeostatic mechanisms act to maintain the metabolic needs of the peripheral tissues by prioritising maintenance of normal systolic blood pressure at the expense of normal capillary pressure. This is because adequate cerebral perfusion is paramount to short-term survival, whereas maintenance of LVEDP is less important for immediate survival.

In cases of severe myocardial dysfunction, global cardiac performance may be insufficient to provide adequate cardiac output, and patients present with signs of low output heart failure. This can manifest as **depressed mentation, skeletal muscle weakness, oliguria or anuria, hypothermia, and cardiac shock**.

Acute versus Chronic Heart Failure

Acute heart failure occurs with a rapid deterioration in cardiac function. Sometimes these patients have no history of any prior problems, while in other situations they may already be receiving medical therapy for congestive heart failure. In acute cases that are already on medical therapy for congestive heart failure acute deterioration is a possibility, but chronic deterioration over a number of days that goes unnoticed by the owner can culminate in a sudden deterioration which appears to be acute. **Educating owners to monitor resting respiratory rate at home can help them to identify subtle deterioration early**, and avoid precipitous end-stage decompensation.

With acute deterioration there may be little time for sodium and water retention, and sympathetic compensatory mechanisms can be overwhelmed. Consequently, low cardiac output signs may predominate. **Patients with acute heart failure are also at risk of developing cardiogenic** shock secondary to markedly decreased blood flow. Cardiogenic shock in patients with chronic heart failure is much less common, though overzealous furosemide administration can precipitate a drop in blood pressure in animals that stop eating and drinking, and become markedly dehydrated.

Therapy in animals with acute heart failure must be focused on trying to optimize haemodynamic function. Trying to neutralise neurohormonal activation in this setting may be counterproductive, as the compensatory mechanisms help to support arterial pressures. These cases require rapid aggressive management if they are to survive.

Diagnosis of Heart Failure

In many cases, diagnosis of congestive heart failure is relatively straight forward, especially for experienced clinicians. The clinical history and physical examination are a key part of diagnosis, and there is often a high clinical index of suspicion that congestive heart failure is present, before any diagnostic tests are undertaken.

Once a diagnosis of congestive heart failure has been made, further diagnostic tests can be used to identify the underlying cardiac disease process that resulted in heart failure.

In the acute setting a definitive diagnosis of the underlying cardiac disease is not required for appropriate medical management, and further diagnostics should not be performed until the patient is stable. Once the patient has been medically stabilised, then a definitive diagnosis helps guide long-term management and allows the clinician to provide the owner with a more accurate prognosis for their pet.

Diagnostic Modalities

Thoracic Radiography

One primary reason for obtaining thoracic radiographs is to **detect evidence of heart failure**.

Radiographic evidence of heart failure is dependent on **the identification of pulmonary oedema or pleural effusion**. There are other possible causes of oedema or effusion, so there should also be evidence of cardiomegaly, particularly severe left atrial enlargement when pulmonary oedema is present. **Pulmonary vessels should also be evaluated for evidence of venous distension**, though obvious distension is not present in all cases.

If the patient is severely compromised, then **one dorso-ventral thoracic radiograph** is often the only view required to make a diagnosis of congestive heart failure. However, if the patient will not tolerate restraint for radiography then the attending clinician can perform a slap-stick probe test, or administer a furosemide treatment trial.

The clinician should also bear in mind that **patients with mild or early congestive heart failure may not have had time to develop alveolar oedema when radiographed**. Therefore, the classic peri-hilar alveolar lung pattern consistent with pulmonary oedema may not be visible in every case. Some patients with congestive heart failure may only have a diffuse interstitial lung pattern on radiography, consistent with oedema in the interstitial space.

Echocardiography

Echocardiography is the diagnostic test of choice for detailed evaluation of structural cardiac disease and evidence of specific chamber enlargements. Congestive heart failure can be diagnosed with echocardiography but advanced spectral Doppler echocardiography is required.

In the acute setting echocardiography can be used to quickly rule in or rule out cardiac disease as a cause of the presenting clinical signs. Most heart diseases compromise left ventricular function, **resulting in left atrial enlargement, and left-sided congestive heart failure**. Therefore, a slap-stick probe test is quite a sensitive screening test. One right parasternal short axis (RPSA) 2D view will provide an estimation of left atrial size.

Animals with clinical signs consistent with congestive heart failure and evidence of pulmonary oedema on thoracic radiography, **have significant left atrial enlargement** in most cases. In rare cases, when acute heart failure develops and there is insufficient

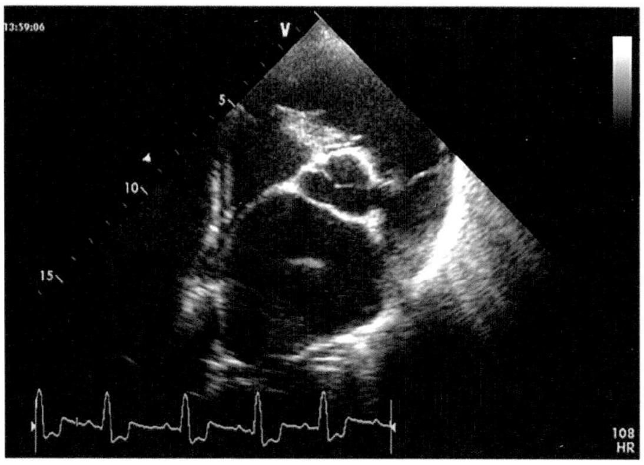

Figure 15. Right parasternal short axis 2D echo view in a dog; severe left atrial enlargement.

time for fluid volume retention, then left atrial size may be normal or not enlarged enough to be considered clinically significant. **Caution should also be observed in patients that have already received furosemide treatment, as this can decrease left atrial size significantly in some cases, particularly in cats.**

A detailed echocardiographic examination is often not possible in animals with significant congestive heart failure at the time of presentation. Acute management of congestive heart failure is not dependent on detailed echocardiographic evaluation in most cases, and complete echocardiography can often be delayed by a day or two in these cases.

Electrocardiography

A hallmark of heart failure is sympathetic up-regulation. Consequently, patients with heart failure should have **elevated heart rates**. Healthy animals that are very stressed in the consult room can also have elevated heart rates. However, conversely, **a dog with a heart rate less than 120 beats per minute, or a cat with a heart rate less than 160–180 beats per minute is unlikely to have congestive heart failure**.

Electrocardiography is not required to make a diagnosis of heart failure, but tachyarrhythmias are commonly found in patients with heart failure, and high heart rates can contribute to clinical signs of congestion. An ECG diagnosis of a specific tachyarrhythmia is important to ensure appropriate antiarrhythmic therapy is chosen.

Blood Pressure Measurement

Evaluation of blood pressure is important in animals that present with clinical signs of forward failure in order to identify those patients with cardiogenic shock.

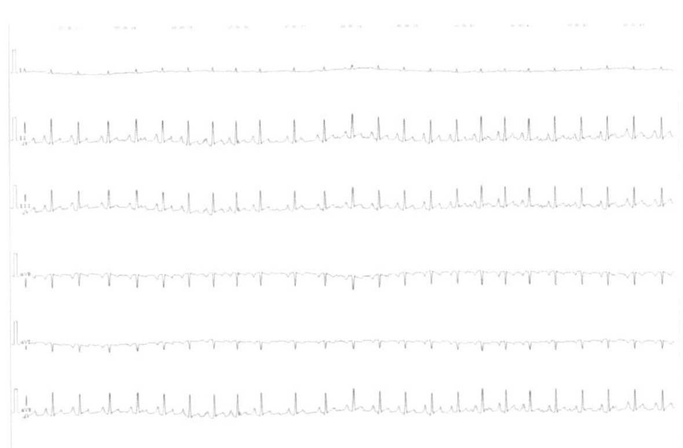

Figure 16. Six lead ECG from a dog with respiratory sinus arrhythmia.

Cardiogenic shock occurs when low cardiac output due to forward failure is no longer adequately compensated for by elevations in total peripheral resistance. The result is markedly decreased blood flow and low systemic blood pressure.

Low blood pressure is uncommon in patients with heart failure. The body's homeostatic mechanisms act to maintain the metabolic needs of the peripheral tissues by prioritising maintenance of normal systolic blood pressure at the expense of normal capillary pressure. This is because adequate cerebral perfusion is paramount to short-term survival, whereas maintenance of LVEDP is less important for immediate survival. This prioritisation of pressure over flow persists in chronic heart failure. **In most patients with chronic severe heart failure, systemic arterial blood pressure is normal** or only mildly decreased, whereas cardiac output is decreased.

Treatment Options in Heart Failure

Where possible, specific therapies should be selected based on the evidence of randomised controlled clinical trials carried out in the relevant patient group.

Animals with gradual onset CHF may not require hospitalisation for management, and stabilisation may be possible with oral medications. However, patients with acute-onset, severe CHF can be very unstable and usually require hospitalisation for careful clinical monitoring. Wherever possible, IV formulations of appropriate medications should be used in these patients.

Treatment Goals in Acute Heart Failure

Rapid improvement in oxygenation and haemodynamic function is crucially important in patients with acute-onset left-sided congestive heart failure. A suggested step-wise approach to management of these patients is outlined below:

- provision of oxygen supplementation if required;
- identification and drainage of any significant volume pleural effusions;
- treatment of pulmonary oedema with diuresis and venodilation if required;
- augmentation of cardiac output using positive inotropes;
- augmentation of cardiac output with judicious arteriodilation if required, though most patients can be stabilised without use of arteriodilators.

In patients with congestive heart failure there is **an impaired relationship between preload and cardiac performance**. Increases in preload can effectively augment cardiac function in the earlier stages of haemodynamically significant structural cardiac disease. However, with disease progression the compensatory mechanisms become progressively maladaptive, and incremental increases in preload have very little impact on cardiac function. Ultimately, patients with CHF operate on the far right side of the Frank-Starling curve and resolution of signs is accomplished via preload reduction (i.e. diuretics and venous vasodilators), and use of positive inotropes or afterload reducers.

Treatment of heart failure with **preload reducers, diuretics or venous vasodilators shifts a patient leftward** along the Frank-Starling curve, helping to reduce signs of congestion.

Removal of abnormal fluid accumulation (pulmonary oedema, pleural effusion, ascites) **is a priority**, and the aim is to get the patient dry without causing unacceptable azotaemia or polyuria/polydipsia which compromises quality of life. The general approach is to titrate a loop diuretic to effect, using the lowest dose that is effective.

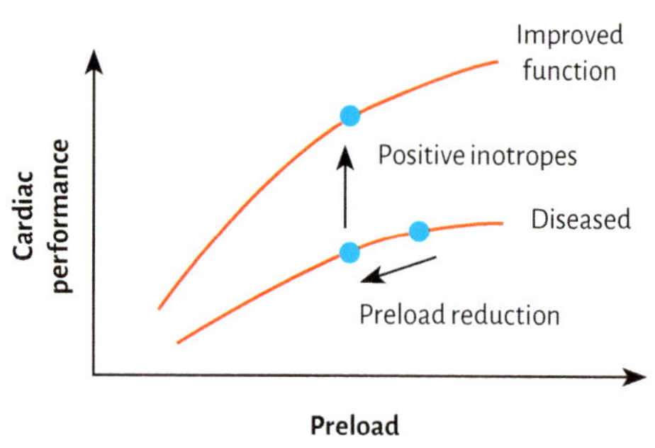

Figure 17. Improvement in cardiac performance resulting from treatment.

Treatment of heart failure with afterload reducers, arterial vasodilators, or positive inotropes, dobutamine, pimobendan, shifts the Frank-Starling curve upwards with a steeper slope, helping to restore the normal relationship between preload and cardiac performance.

Treatment goals in chronic heart failure

Once the patient is adequately haemodynamically stable, **the minimum effective dose of loop-diuretic dose should be administered orally** for the long-term.

Pimobendan has been shown to prolong survival time in patients with left-sided congestive heart failure secondary to myxomatous mitral valve disease (MMVD) and dilated cardiomyopathy (DCM). Consequently, treatment with pimobendan should be started or continued long-term if the patient is already being treated.

Neurohormonal blockade medications are designed to blunt the effects of the maladaptive chronic compensatory mechanisms up-regulated in patients with heart failure. While a number of these medications make sense from a pathophysiological perspective, large prospective randomised controlled trials (RCTs) proving efficacy are not available for all indications. See Table 1 for summary of the available evidence.

Table 1. Neurohormonal blockade medications; recommendations for when to use agents.

	ACE Inhibitors	Spironolactone	β-blockers
Preclinical DCM	Equivocal evidence	Equivocal evidence	Detrimental
DCM with CHF	Recommended	Recommended	Contraindicated
Preclinical MMVD	Equivocal evidence	Positive pilot study	Equivocal evidence
MMVD with CHF	Recommended*	Recommended	Contraindicated

*There is some evidence that addition of ramipril to patients receiving furosemide and pimobendan does not change outcome, though the data has yet to be published in a peer-reviewed journal.

Treatment goals in refractory congestive heart failure

This category includes animals already receiving standard treatment for heart failure, but their heart failure signs persist despite upwards titration of furosemide doses. By this stage there may be surprisingly few signs of diuresis (or polydipsia) as the animal becomes increasingly refractory.

Signs consistent with right heart failure are common.

Sequential nephron blockade is often necessary, as the combination of multiple diuretics achieves greater diuresis than high doses of a single diuretic. The addition of other diuretics (without withdrawing the furosemide) often restore diuresis, but cardiac cachexia becomes a common problem as the disease progresses.

Diet

By this stage, appetite is often poor and essential ω-3 fatty acid supplementation can be tried in an attempt to counteract cardiac cachexia. However, few clinical trials have been carried out to investigate the effect of diet on management of CHF in dogs.

- **Low-salt diets should not be used before the onset of CHF**, as low sodium intake can activate the renin-angiotensin aldosterone system.
- Salt loading should be avoided, but modest salt restriction is probably better than aggressive salt restriction.

Other dietary additives include the nutraceuticals (co-enzyme Q10, L-carnitine, taurine). There may be benefit in selected cases (taurine deficiency in cats and American Cocker Spaniels; canine familial L-carnitine deficiency) but in most cases the effect of supplementation appears minimal.

There is much more justification for **ω-3 fatty acid supplementation**, which may have an effect in cachexic dogs in particular. There may also be some antiarrhythmic benefits.

Exercise

There are no studies examining the effect of exercise in canine heart failure.

Advice for dogs with CHF is generally to **restrict exercise until signs of CHF resolve**. There is less agreement on appropriate advice for animals with a history of previous CHF.

In chronic heart failure in humans, regular moderate exercise training improves exercise tolerance. Heart failure results in skeletal muscle changes similar to deconditioning, and exercise can reverse this. Both for these reasons and for optimal quality of life, it seems reasonable to **recommend continuation of exercise for dogs with stable heart disease**.

Regular exercise is more likely to be beneficial than intermittent exercise. Conversely, sudden sprinting or extremes of exercise should be avoided in dogs with exertional syncope, or those at high risk of sudden death due to arrhythmias.

Bibliography

- Côté, E., MacDonald, K.A., Montgomery, K. et al. (2011) *Feline Cardiology*. Wiley Blackwell.
- Cunningham, J.G., Bradley, G.K. (2007) *Cunningham Textbook of Veterinary Physiology*, 4th edition. Saunders Elsevier.
- Barrett, K.E., Barman, S.M, Boitano, S. et al. (2012) *Ganong's Review of Medical Physiology*, 24th edition. McGraw-Hill Medical.
- Bonow, R.O., Mann, Zipes et al. (2012) *Braunwald's Heart Disease*. Elsevier Saunders.
- Luis Fuentes, V., Jonhson, L.R., Dennis, S. (2010) *BSAVA Manual of Canine and Feline Cardiopulmonary Medicine*, 2nd Edition. BSAVA.
- Kittleson, M.D., Kienle, R.D. (1998) *Small Animal Cardiovascular Medicine*. Mosby.

Test

Answers on Page 148

1. Heart failure is a clinical syndrome caused by the inability of the heart to function effectively within which normal parameter?
  a. Blood pressure.
  b. Heart rate.
  c. Diastolic filling pressures.
  d. Respiratory rate.

2. What is the most common type of heart failure in dogs and cats?
  a. Backward failure.
  b. Pressure overload.
  c. Forward failure.
  d. Volume overload.

3. Which disease is a common cause of ventricular volume overload?
  a. Myxomatous mitral valve disease.
  b. Hypertrophic cardiomyopathy.
  c. Aortic stenosis.
  d. Pulmonic stenosis.

4. Which disease is a common cause of diastolic heart failure?
  a. Myxomatous mitral valve disease.
  b. Hypertrophic cardiomyopathy.
  c. Aortic stenosis.
  d. Pulmonic stenosis.

5. In patients with heart failure there are alterations in autonomic tone. Which heart rhythm is associated with this change in autonomic tone?
  a. Tachycardia.
  b. Bradycardia.
  c. Sinus arrhythmia.
  d. Asystole.

6. Pulmonary oedema develops when left ventricular end diastolic pressure exceeds which value?
  a. 10 mmHg.
  b. 15 mmHg.
  c. 20 mmHg.
  d. 25 mmHg.

7. Which feedback mechanism acts to rapidly maintain blood pressure in the face of a cardiac insult?
  a. Myocardial apoptosis.
  b. The renin angiotensin aldosterone system.
  c. Myocardial remodelling.
  d. Baroreceptors – autonomic nervous system.

8. Dilated cardiomyopathy (DCM) is an example of what functional category of heart failure?
  a. Diastolic heart failure.
  b. Ventricular volume overload.
  c. Pressure overload.
  d. Primary myocardial failure.

9. When increased concentrations of cardiac noradrenaline act on cardiac β-receptors which effect below is seen?
  a. Heart rate is decreased.
  b. Early diastolic relaxation is impaired.
  c. Cardiac contractility declines.
  d. Early diastolic relaxation is augmented.

10. When angiotensin II binds to the angiotensin II type 1 receptor (AT1R), which powerful effect shown below occurs?
  a. Aldosterone is released from the adrenal gland.
  b. ADH release from the pituitary is prevented.
  c. Vasodilation.
  d. Decreased sympathetic tone and increased parasympathetic tone.

11. Which option best describes the underlying pathophysiology of acute heart failure?
  a. Acute heart failure occurs in most animals with significant underlying cardiac disease.
  b. Acute heart failure is more common in dogs with DCM than in dogs with myxomatous mitral valve disease.
  c. Diseases causing left ventricular pressure overload result in decreased afterload, and a rapid deterioration in cardiac function.
  d. With a rapid deterioration in cardiac function, there is little time for sodium and water retention, and low cardiac output signs may predominate.

12. Which medication listed below is recommended in the acute management of congestive heart failure of both dogs and cats?
  a. Furosemide.
  b. Spironolactone.
  c. Digoxin.
  d. Benazepril.

13. Which medication listed below is an aldosterone antagonist?
  a. Torasemide.
  b. Pimobendan.
  c. Spironolactone.
  d. Diltiazem.

14. Which of the following is correct?

a. Right to left shunting congenital cardiac defects cause peripheral cyanosis but never central cyanosis.
b. Feline aortic thromboembolism causes central cyanosis and never peripheral cyanosis.
c. Central cyanosis is always caused by primary lung disease whereas peripheral cyanosis is not.
d. Central cyanosis is blue discolouration of the mucous membranes of the head and neck.

Correct Answers:

1. c
2. a
3. a
4. b
5. a
6. d
7. d
8. d
9. d
10. a
11. d
12. a
13. c
14. d

Notes

Acquired Valvular Disease

Andrew Francis

This chapter covers acquired valvular disease of the atrioventricular (AV) valves and valvular endocarditis.

Myxomatous Mitral Valve Disease

Myxomatous mitral valve disease (MMVD) of the atrioventricular (AV) valves is characterised by the accumulation of glycosaminoglycans (myxomatous proliferation), and **fibrosis of the valve leaflets and chordae tendinae**.

Historically, **many names** have been used to describe this condition including:
- endocardiosis
- chronic degenerative valvular disease
- chronic valvular disease
- chronic valvular heart disease
- chronic valvular fibrosis
- acquired mitral or tricuspid regurgitation or insufficiency.

Valvular degeneration and involvement of the chordae tendinae **affects the function of the entire mitral valve structure.** This leads to insufficient coaptation of the mitral valve during systole and consequently, **valvular regurgitation**. In some patients the degree of valvular regurgitation is relatively mild and remains **haemodynamically insignificant**. In other animals, the volume of valvular regurgitation leads to progressive elevations in left ventricular end-diastolic volume over time which can **eventually result in congestive heart failure (CHF)**.

The mitral valve is by far the most commonly affected valve. In some animals the tricuspid valve is also affected, but isolated tricuspid myxomatous degeneration is less common.

Myxomatous degeneration of the pulmonic and particularly the aortic valves does occur, but infrequently. This is rarely of clinical importance unless aortic regurgitation is severe.

Causes

Despite huge research efforts **the underlying cause of myxomatous degeneration remains unknown**. The current scientific belief is that the primary defect lies within the connective tissue (ground substance) within the valve.

Affected individuals are born normal but, because of this inherent weakness of the valve, degenerative changes develop unusually early in life. There is no scientific evidence of any association between the disease and vaccination or haematological spread of bacteria from the oral cavity.

Pathology

Mitral valve competence requires complex interplay between the structures comprising the mitral apparatus.

The **structures that constitute the mitral valve apparatus include**:
- mitral *annulus*
- mitral valve leaflets
- *chordae tendineae*
- papillary muscles
- left atrial and left ventricular myocardium.

Histologically, the mitral valve comprises four main layers.
1. **Atrialis layer**: a thin layer on the inflow side of the mitral leaflet lined by endothelial cells overlying elastin fibres.
2. **Spongiosa layer**: extends from the *annulus* to the free edge of the leaflet and comprises glycosaminoglycans, proteoglycans, and loose, fine collagen fibres.
3. **Fibrosa layer**: comprises a dense, circumferentially orientated layer of collagen fibres that continues with the *annulus* proximally, and the central core of *chordae tendineae* distally.
4. **Ventricularis layer**: a thin layer facing the left ventricular chamber, similar to the atrialis that contains elastic and collagen fibres covered by endothelium.

Myxomatous valvular remodelling is associated with characteristic histopathologic features, including:
- expansion of the extracellular matrix of the spongiosa with glycosaminoglycans and proteoglycans;
- valvular interstitial cell alteration from fibroblast to myofibroblast phenotype to maintain mechanical valve function and tone; and
- attenuation or loss of the collagen-laden fibrosa layer, resulting in scattered fibrosa layer remnants throughout the valve spongiosa.

These **structural changes lead to malformation of the mitral apparatus, biomechanical dysfunction, and mitral incompetence**.

Mitral regurgitation is the most common manifestation of mxyomatous valve disease and in advanced stages, associated volume overload promotes progressive valvular regurgitation, left atrial and left ventricular remodelling, atrial tears, chordal rupture, and congestive heart failure.

Epidemiology and Inheritance

Myxomatous mitral valve degeneration is **prevalent in the canine**, and most adult dogs develop some degree of mitral valve disease as they age, highlighting the apparent vulnerability of canine heart valves to injury.

Despite the ubiquity of myxomatous mitral valve degeneration, the prevalence of clinically identified disease is **highly variable among different breeds**. The disease is encountered in all breeds, but is most common in **small to medium-sized breeds**, such as:

- Papillon
- Poodle
- Chihuahua
- Dachshund
- Cavalier King Charles Spaniel.

The condition is uncommon in young individuals, but **prevalence increases with age**. Indeed, the prevalence in some affected breeds may be >90% in dogs over 10 years of age, with cardiac mortality exceeding all other causes of death in many affected breeds.

The prevalence of MMVD in cats is unknown but seems to be extremely low and rarely of clinical importance.

The exact **genetic basis for MMVD is unknown**. Because of the variable prevalence of the disease in different breeds, a genetic basis has long been suspected. However, it was not until fairly recently that MMVD was shown to be inherited in Cavalier King Charles Spaniels (CKCS) and Dachshunds (Figure 1).

The mode of inheritance is not simple, and the age of disease onset is inherited as a polygenetic trait, meaning more than one gene is involved in the disease process. **Males have an earlier onset**, and the disease progresses more rapidly than in females.

The major role played by genetic factors suggests that other factors, such as level of exercise, obesity, and quality of diet play only a small role in the pathogenesis of the disease.

Pathophysiology

The likelihood of disease progression in an affected dog involves two pathophysiological events:

- the **degree of valve degeneration** and the rate of progression
- the progressive **haemodynamic significance** of mitral regurgitation.

The severity of mitral regurgitation and its haemodynamic significance is dependent on the degree of valve degeneration. However, mild MMVD can be present without any evidence of mitral regurgitation.

There are other causes of mitral regurgitation other than MMVD. Two salient examples are **mitral valve dysplasia** and mitral regurgitation due to annular dilation in dogs with **dilated cardiomyopathy**.

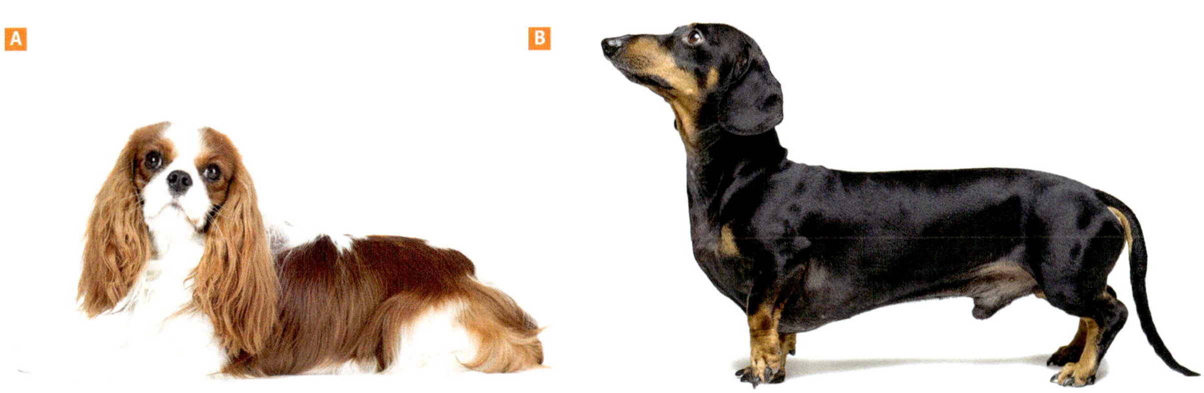

Figure 1. Breeds in which myxomatous mitral valve disease has been shown to be inherited. **A**. Cavalier King Charles Spaniel; **B**. Dachshund.

Progression of Valve Degeneration in Dogs with MMVD

Abnormal valve motion with **prolapse of the leaflets** increases the shear stresses on the leaflets, both directly (abnormal leaflet apposition) and indirectly (increased regurgitant flow).

Regurgitation and valve stress lead to endothelial damage and subsequent **activation of valvular interstitial cells (fibroblasts)** in the valve. The activation of valvular interstitial cells leads to **subendothelial deposition of glycosaminoglycans**, particularly within the spongiosa layer, and fibrosis, resulting in further **distortion of valve morphology** and regurgitation.

The abnormal stress on the valve caused by prolapse and the altered ultrastructure of the leaflets predispose to **rupture of *chordae tendineae***, which leads to increased regurgitation.

The end-stage valve is characterised by **thickened, fibrotic and contracted leaflets** (Figure 2), usually with evidence of ruptured low-order *chordae tendineae*.

Progression of Valvular Degeneration into Congestive Heart Failure

With progression, the valvular lesions cause **insufficient coaptation of the leaflets**, leading to **regurgitation into the left atrium**. The severity and progression of mitral regurgitation is dependent on the severity and progression of the valvular lesions. Initially compensatory mechanisms allow accommodation of the mitral regurgitation. For example, to compensate for increased preload eccentric hypertrophy increases left ventricular compliance.

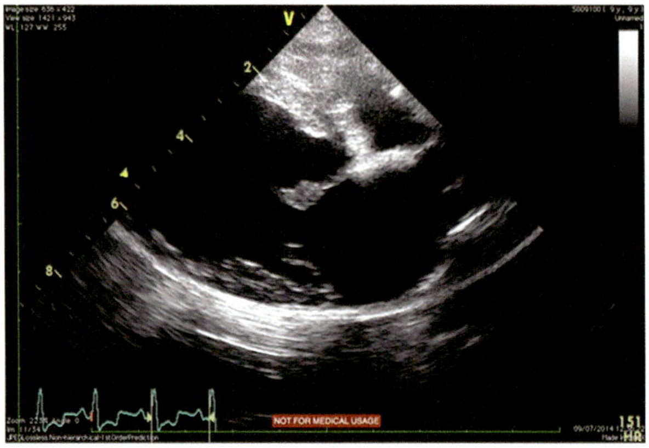

Figure 2. Thickened, fibrotic and contracted leaflets visible during echocardiography (right).

Sympathetic up-regulation to maintain forward stroke volume results in tachycardia, increased inotropy, and improved lusitropy. Neuro-hormonal modulation results in fluid retention, which further increases preload in an attempt to maintain forward stroke volume.

Increased pulmonary lymphatic drainage allows the left ventricular end diastolic pressures to increase to 25 mmHg before pulmonary oedema forms. Ventricular dilatation further increases the regurgitation by causing secondary valvular regurgitation.

With progression, compensation of the regurgitation is no longer possible, leading to reduced cardiac output and increased venous pressures with subsequent pulmonary oedema (left-sided CHF) or ascites (right-sided CHF).

Pulmonary hypertension may develop as a consequence of left-sided heart failure,

Prognosis

Although cardiac mortality exceeds other causes of death in many breeds with a high prevalence of MMVD, **most dogs with disease actually do not develop congestive heart failure**.

In one study including 558 dogs affected by MMVD at different stages of CHF, more than 70% of asymptomatic dogs were alive at the end of the follow-up period of 6.6 years. In another recent study, 82% of asymptomatic dogs remained asymptomatic at 12 months from inclusion in the study.

Classification

The diagnosis of mitral regurgitation caused by MMVD is usually straightforward, given the easily recognised characteristic murmur and the echocardiographic changes. However, it is clear many patients with mitral valve disease remain compensated in the long-term and never develop clinical signs consistent with left-sided congestive heart failure. Consequently, a classification system that links severity of clinical signs to appropriate treatments at each stage of the disease process is very useful.

The **classification system** outlined in Table 1 was formulated by the American College of Veterinary Internal Medicine (ACVIM) and published in the Journal of Veterinary Internal Medicine (JVIM) in 2009.

Table 1. Classification system for chronic valvular heart disease (myxomatous mitral valve disease).

ACC/AHA score ACVIM modified		Stages of heart disease and failure	Examples
Stage A		Identifies patients at high risk for developing heart disease but that currently have no identifiable structural disorder of the heart	Healthy CKCS and Dobermanns
Stage B	Stage B1	Asymptomatic patients with structural heart disease and no evidence of cardiac remodelling in response to the cardiac insult	A murmur but normal heart size
	Stage B2	Asymptomatic patients that have a haemodynamically significant cardiac defect as evidenced by radiographic or echographic finding of heart enlargement	A murmur with evidence of cardiomegaly
Stage C		Patients with past or current clinical signs of heart failure associated with structural heart disease. Patients in stage C can also be subclassified according to the requirement for hospitalization or outpatient management of clinical signs	A murmur with cardiomegaly and current or previous CHF
Stage D		Patients with end-stage disease with clinical signs of heart failure that are refractory to standard therapy. Patients in stage D can also be subclassified according to whether hospital-based or outpatient therapy is necessary	A murmur with cardiomegaly and refractory CHF

Clinical Signs

Heart Murmur

The most important clinical manifestation of MMVD is the **characteristic left apical systolic heart murmur**. It often takes years to progress from the development of a soft heart murmur in a dog without clinical signs, to severe heart failure in advanced MMVD. However, some **large dogs appear to be less tolerant of the disease**, and in these dogs the disease has a more rapid progression.

In MMVD the murmur grade correlates well with the severity of disease. A dog with a characteristic grade II/VI murmur is likely to have mild disease, whereas a grade IV/VI murmur is likely to indicate more severe disease. In fact, the murmur grade is useful to assess whether an asymptomatic patient with a characteristic left apical murmur has a dilated heart or not.

A retrospective study published in the Journal of Small Animal Practice by Ljungvall et al. looked at whether murmur intensity in small-breed dogs with myxomatous mitral valve disease reflected clinical and echocardiographic disease severity. The author combined the data from this study with the classification system documented above to create the diagnostic flow chart shown below (Figure 3).

Clinicians can therefore use murmur grade to inform their index of suspicion as to whether to recommend further diagnostic tests for an individual patient, and what the most appropriate diagnostic tests might be (Table 2).

Table 2. Diagnostic test selection is somewhat dependent on murmur grade. In patients with low-grade murmurs cardiomegaly is less likely; consequently, thoracic radiography is likely to be unremarkable and therefore less useful.

Soft murmur (grade 1–2/6)	Echocardiography
Moderate murmur (grade 3/6)	Echocardiography
Loud murmur (grade 4/6)	Echocardiography or radiography
Thrilling murmur (grade 5–6/6)	Echocardiography or radiography

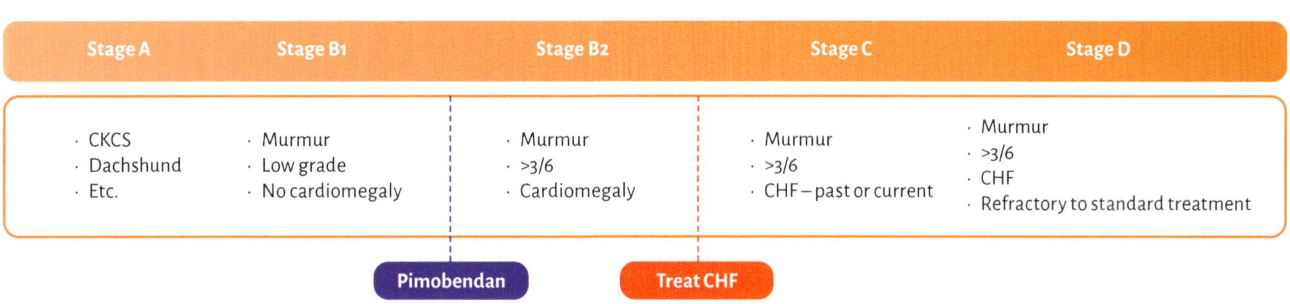

Figure 3. Flow chart using the ACVIM classification system and data from the study by Ljungvall et al. JSAP 2014 to map out the diferent stages of myxomatous mitral valve disease.

Coughing

Coughing can occur in the absence of congestive heart failure. Cardiomegaly as a result of moderate to severe valvular regurgitation may cause compression of the mainstem bronchi, triggering a cough. Recognition of this situation is complicated by the fact that MMVD and bronchial collapse or chronic bronchitis frequently coexist. (Figure 4).

Coughing is reportedly a common clinical sign in dogs with congestive heart failure. The cough is often reported to be **worse in the morning or evening**. While dogs with congestive heart failure are reported to cough, the author's experience is that many dogs with congestive heart failure do not. There are **no cough receptors within the alveoli so pulmonary oedema itself is unlikely to be the inciting cause of cough**. Mainstem bronchus compression due to severe cardiomegaly and/or bronchomalacia are the most likely triggers of cough in dogs with CHF.

General

CHF is most commonly left-sided, and **typical clinical signs** include:

- cough
- tachypnoea
- respiratory distress
- orthopnoea
- lethargy
- anorexia
- reduced exercise tolerance
- syncope
- weight loss with very advanced disease (cardiac cachexia).

Ascites is sometimes present if there is concurrent right-sided congestive heart failure. This may occur because of triscuspid myxomatous valvular degeneration, but can also occur as a result of pulmonary hypertension secondary to left-sided CHF.

Syncope

Syncope can occur in dogs with MMVD, but the **triggers are poorly understood**. Syncope may be vasovagal or associated with supraventricular tachyarrhythmias, and is often triggered by exercise or excitement, as well as by coughing (tussive syncope).

In patients with MMVD that are syncopal, pulmonary hypertension is a common finding. Humans with significant pulmonary hypertension often report exercise intolerance and syncopal episodes, although the mechanism remains unclear.

Sudden Death

Sudden death may occur as a consequence of an acute development of a complication, but it is uncommon in the absence of preceding clinical signs of CHF. This reflects the low incidence of malignant ventricular arrhythmias (Figure 5) in dogs with MMVD.

Diagnosis

The diagnosis of mitral regurgitation due to MMVD is straightforward, because both the characteristic murmur and the echocardiographic changes are easily recognised.

The effect on the circulation of mild mitral regurgitation is minimal, and clinical signs usually develop relatively late in

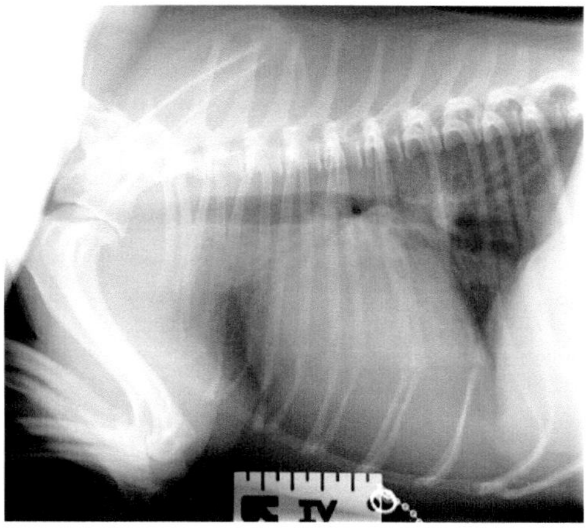

Figure 4. Severe cardiomegaly and mainstem bronchus collapse in a dog with MMVD.

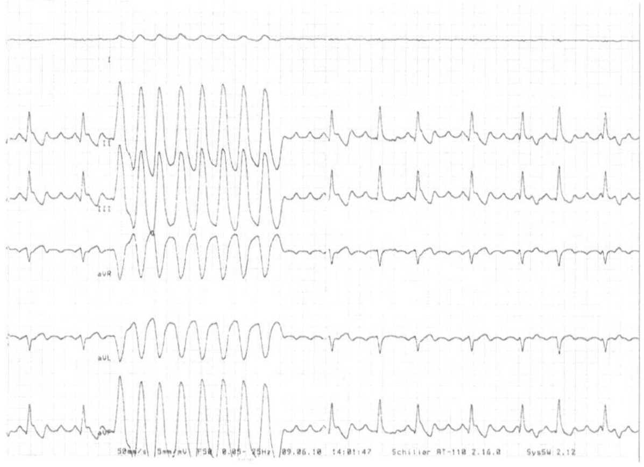

Figure 5. Six lead ECG from a patient with paroxysmal ventricular tachycardia and underlying atrial flutter.

the course of the disease. Consequently, in some cases it is difficult to determine whether mitral regurgitation is the true underlying cause for the reported clinical signs. This can be particularly difficult in patients with concurrent respiratory disease or systemic disease causing lethargy and a low-grade mitral murmur.

The clinical investigation should be tailored to the individual patient and aim to explain the cause of the presenting clinical signs and owner's problem list.

Physical Examination

Dogs without Clinical Signs of Disease

- A **systolic click**: high pitched, sharp sound between S1 and S2 heart sounds. Easily mistaken for a gallop rhythm. Indicative of early-stage disease.
- An **apical systolic heart murmur**.
- **Mild regurgitation**: grade I–II/VI soft, early, late or holosystolic murmur.
- **Moderate to severe regurgitation**: grade IV–VI/VI loud holosystolic or pansystolic murmur.

If sinus arrhythmia is present the mitral regurgitation is often less severe. Sinus arrhythmia is rare in dogs with congestive heart failure.

Isolated atrial premature complexes are common in some small dogs and the presence of a few such complexes on the electrocardiogram (ECG) does not necessarily indicate severe disease. (Figure 6).

Dogs with Congestive Heart Failure

- A **loud heart murmur** (grade IV–VI/VI).
- The first heart sound is loud (unless there is significant systolic dysfunction from concurrent myocardial disease), and the second heart sound is decreased in intensity (may often be difficult to hear).
- **Tachycardia** and loss of respiratory sinus arrhythmia.
- An arrhythmia, most commonly frequent **supraventricular premature complexes**.
- **Atrial fibrillation** (Figure 7) or frequent ventricular premature complexes indicate severe disease and a poor prognosis.
- Weak femoral pulses and **pulse deficits**.
- **Prolonged capillary refill time** and pale mucous membranes indicate forward failure.
- **Tachypnoea**, respiratory distress, and orthopnoea.
- **Respiratory crackles and wheezes** due to pulmonary oedema. However, they are absent in many dogs with severe congestive heart failure.
- **Pink froth** in the nostrils and oropharynx with acute, severe pulmonary oedema (fulminant CHF).
- Concurrent right-sided CHF, then ascites and jugular venous distension may be noted.

Echocardiography

Echocardiography is the method of choice to diagnose MMVD and estimate the severity of mitral regurgitation. However, the technique cannot accurately diagnose the presence of CHF unless the operator is experienced in advanced spectral Doppler interrogation.

The assessment of valvular insufficiency uses all echocardiographic modalities to assess the significance and severity of the leak.

Two-dimensional and M-mode echocardiography are used to define valve morphology and structure, including the type

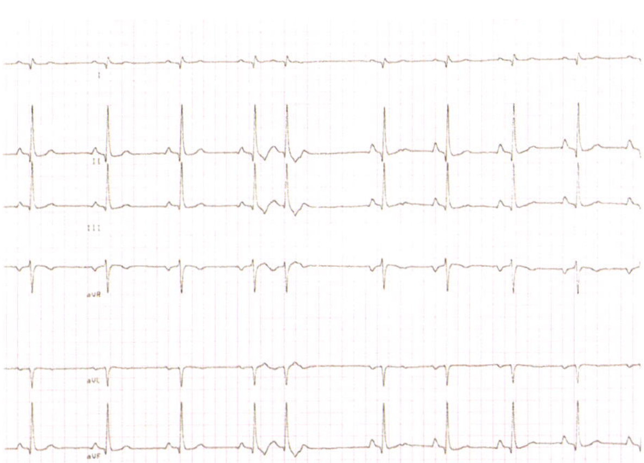

Figure 6. Six lead ECG from a patient with an isolated supraventricular premature complex.

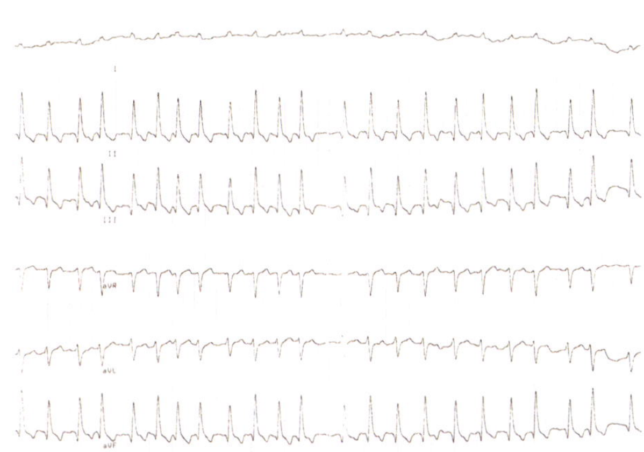

Figure 7. Six lead ECG from a patient with atrial fibrillation.

of lesion and the presence of valvular prolapse or ruptured *chordae tendineae*. Measurement of chamber size and function help define both the chronicity and the extent of remodelling.

Colour-flow Doppler rapidly identifies the presence of regurgitation. Attention to the jet area with respect to the receiving chamber, the width of the jet at its orifice, and the area of flow convergence adds accuracy in assessing the severity of regurgitant volume. However, colour-flow Doppler is notoriously variable when the technical factors are not set properly.

Spectral Doppler helps measure regurgitant volume and fraction and is used to measure regurgitant orifice area. **Pulsed-wave Doppler** and continuous-wave Doppler assess haemodynamic severity by evaluating spectral trace density, velocity of flows, and flow profiles.

Two-dimensional and M-mode Evaluation

The typical characteristics of myxomatous degeneration include **left ventricular and atrial dilation**, wall and septal **hypertrophy**, increased thickness, nodularity and prolapse of one or both **mitral valve leaflets**, elevated systolic function parameters, and hyper-dynamic wall and septal motion. (See Figure 2). Thickened, fibrotic and contracted leaflet, left ventricular volume overload and left atrial dilation, consistent with a diagnosis of myxomatous mitral valve disease, visible during echocardiography).

Less common features include pericardial effusion, lack of hypertrophy, decreases in systolic function, and ruptured *chordae tendineae*.

The lesions are generally smooth and small creating a **club-shaped appearance to the leaflet** tips during early stages of the disease but may become large and irregular as the disease progresses. Generally, but not always, larger lesions are associated with more severe insufficiency.

Large breed dogs with acquired mitral valve insufficiency seem to have fewer observable changes of the valve leaflets despite significant regurgitation and prolapse that may be observed without any abnormal thickness or irregularity of the leaflets.

Right parasternal four-chamber views of the heart are excellent for imaging the mitral valve. The left ventricular inflow outflow view is also good, but the valves may appear to be thicker than they truly are if the imaging plane is not perfect. Transverse images of the valve are useful for identifying large lesions but can be misleading when looking for small ones.

Ruptured *Chordae Tendineae*

Degenerative mitral valve disease is the most common cause of ruptured *chordae tendineae* in the dog. Vegetative growths on the mitral valve, including mitral valve endocardiosis, rarely result in ruptured *chordae tendineae*.

CT rupture is classically described as a devastating complication of canine MVD responsible for acute left heart failure, which commonly results in pulmonary oedema and death despite aggressive medical therapy.

However, the prognosis may not be as bad as initially thought. In one study, long-term follow-up was available for 57 treated dogs (angiotensin-converting enzyme inhibitors and diuretics) with *chordae tendineae* rupture and 58% of these (33/57) survived for one year after initial *chordae tendineae* rupture diagnosis (median survival time, 425 days).

The echocardiographic examination for mitral flail in dogs with rupture of the first or second order CT is very similar, although the pathologic consequences and therefore the clinical signs and survival may be different.

The majority of dogs with echocardiographic evidence of ruptured *chordae tendineae* have **severe mitral insufficiency**. Most instances of ruptured chordae **affect the septal leaflet** of the mitral valve, and rupture of chordae to the parietal (posterior) leaflet is much less common. Rupture of a *chordae tendineae* resulting in a flail leaflet is diagnosed when the leaflet points back into the left atrial chamber during systole.

These findings are visible on both **parasternal and apical images**. Minor chordal rupture may be seen in only one echocardiographic plane, while major chordal rupture tends to be seen in several imaging planes.

The colour-flow jet of mitral regurgitation caused by chordal rupture is usually eccentric. When Doppler confirms the presence of severe mitral insufficiency without the concurrent left ventricular and atrial dilation that is usually present in a chronic process, a ruptured chordae should be looked for.

Papillary muscle rupture can occur but is usually the result of trauma.

Mitral Valve Prolapse

In dogs, prolapse of the mitral valve (MVP) is usually secondary to myxomatous degeneration of the leaflets, chronic stretch of the *chordae tendineae*, and reflux into the atrium during systole.

Mitral valve prolapse may be seen without any evidence of insufficiency and seems to be genetically influenced in Cavalier King Charles Spaniels (CKCS) and Dachshunds. These dogs tend to show prolapse as early as three-years of age without any clinical signs or murmurs and have a high incidence of mitral valvular insufficiency later in life.

MVP in dogs is associated with a greater incidence of degenerative valvular disease. Dogs also have more significant insufficiency and higher classes of heart failure with mitral valve prolapse than without.

In patients with mitral valve prolapse, one or both leaflets buckle back toward the left atrium during systole. To identify the mitral valve *annulus* a line should be drawn joining the attachment points of both mitral leaflets on right parasternal four-chamber views. (Figure 8).

Normally, the body of the mitral valve leaflets does not extend beyond the line into the left atrium. Buckling of either leaflet into the atrium beyond this line indicates mild mitral valve prolapse.

Left Ventricular Size

Volume overload of the left atrium and ventricle is seen with haemodynamically significant chronic mitral valvular insufficiency. Significant insufficiencies without concurrent chamber enlargement are suggestive of an acute process and ruptured chordae.

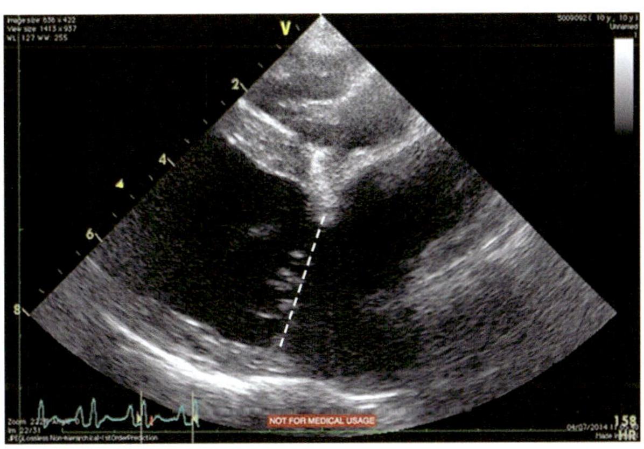

Figure 8. White dashed line indicates position of the mitral valve *annulus*. No part of the mitral valve is seen on the atrial side of this line. No mitral valve prolapse.

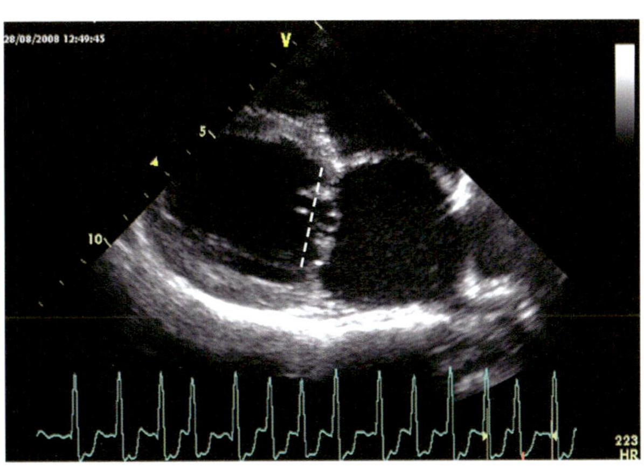

Figure 9. White dashed line indicates position of the mitral valve *annulus*. Parts of both mitral valve leaflets can be seen on the atrial side of this line. Mitral valve prolapse.

Gross left atrial (LA) dilation (significantly larger than (LVIDd) the diameter of the left ventricle in diastole) indicates MMVD is likely. Conversely, if LVIDd is much bigger than left atrial size, then dilated cardiomyopathy should be suspected.

Left Atrial Size

The left atrial to aortic root ratio is used to evaluate atrial size.

Many methods for evaluating left atrial size echocardiographically, and indexing measurements to body weight or to aortic diameter have been described. The most commonly adopted method in Europe is the left atrium to aorta ratio measured on 2D short axis views of the heart base.

All measurements are made from **inside edge to inside edge**.

- The **aortic diameter** should be measured by drawing a line from the middle of the right coronary cusp to the commissures between the left and non-coronary cusp.
- The **left atrial diameter** is a line extending from the aortic measurement out to the lateral wall of the left atrium. The measurement should try to avoid the pulmonary vein.

The left atrial measurement is divided by the aortic diameter measurement to obtain a ratio. **An LA:Ao ratio of <1.59:1 is the cut-off for normal atrial size in dogs**.

It is still quite common for left atrial size to be measured in long-axis views, particularly in the USA. While this is not wrong, it is important to be aware that the cut-offs for normal atrial size are different, and the short-axis cut-off value of 1.6:1 cannot be used.

Atrial Rupture

Severe left atrial enlargement and concurrent high left atrial pressures in dogs with mitral valvular disease can, on rare occasions, result in rupture of the left atrial wall. The tear may occur within the atrial septum creating an atrial septal defect. The tear may occur in the lateral wall of the atrium or auricular appendage resulting in **fluid accumulation within the pericardial sac**, evident on echocardiography.

Pericardial effusion occurs secondary to congestive heart failure, but the **presence of a thrombus within the pericardial space confirms the diagnosis of atrial rupture**. This is because pericardial effusions secondary to neoplasia, pericarditis, or heart failure do not tend to form clots.

Thrombi within the pericardial space develop linear layers of hyperechoic material that **conforms to the shape of the heart**. Tumours within the pericardial sac are generally more rounded and not laminar in appearance.

Left Ventricular Function

Fractional shortening (FS), as a measure of myocardial function in dogs with chronic degenerative mitral valve insufficiency, should be **elevated** because of the presence of increased preload, decreased afterload, and generally increased contractile properties. Using fractional shortening to separate dogs with abnormal myocardial function from those with normal myocardial function can be problematic, because **fractional shortening is dependent upon preload, afterload, and contractility**.

FS is greater than normal in dogs with MMVD and no systolic dysfunction. This is because preload is increased but end-systolic diameter remains within reference range. Hearts with normal myocardial contractility will shorten to normal systolic dimensions regardless of how dilated the heart becomes. FS in dogs with MMVD and systolic dysfunction is often within reference range. Consequently, the following cut-offs should be used to divide dogs with chronic mitral valve insufficiency into various categories of impaired contractility:

- no myocardial dysfunction: FS >45%
- mild to moderate myocardial dysfunction: FS 33–45%
- severe myocardial failure: FS below reference range.

Systolic diameters or end systolic volume index are better indicators of systolic dysfunction in MMVD dogs.

Colour-flow Doppler Evaluation

Colour-flow Doppler readily identifies regurgitant flows (Figure 10). This modality should be used and attention paid to the jet area with respect to the receiving chamber, the area of flow convergence, jet width at its origin, vena contracta, and its use can significantly improve the evaluation of severity of the regurgitation.

Jet Size

Measuring the size of the colour-flow jet within the left atrium can semi-quantitatively assess the pathological regurgitation. In humans, the proportion of the left atrium filled by the regurgitation flow classifies severity of insufficiency as follows:

- less than 20% of LA filled = mild insufficiency
- 20–40% of LA filled = moderate insufficiency
- more than 50% of LA filled = severe insufficiency.

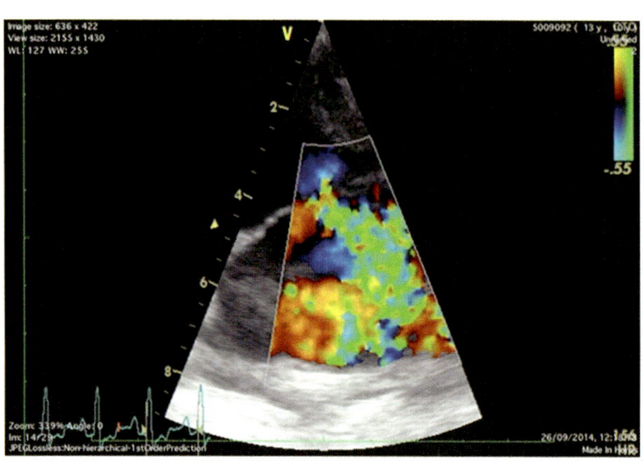

Figure 10. Colour Doppler interrogation documenting severe mitral regurgitation.

This method uses the largest regurgitant jet found in any plane. Studies that average the jet size over several imaging planes do not show any significant improvement in predicting severity.

Assessment of mitral insufficiency based upon colour jet area is the poorest of colour-flow assessment methods, because of the inherent inaccuracies of quantification of colour flow Doppler. When the regurgitant jet is centrally directed and there is a normal sinus rhythm, then the assessment of severity using color-flow Doppler is usually reliable.

Other methods that attempt to overcome some of the limitations of colour-Doppler evaluation of MR have been investigated. The ratio of MR jet area to LA area can be useful:

- <30% = mild MR
- 30–70% = moderate MR
- >70% = severe MR.

Vena Contracta

Measuring the proximal regurgitant **jet height** as it enters the left atrium through the mitral valve has also been studied in an effort to eliminate the other limitations of colour-flow evaluation. The smallest regurgitant colour-flow jet, the vena contracta, at the mitral regurgitant orifice is identified by carefully angling the sound beam in various directions.

Long-axis parasternal images, or imaging planes that identify the vena contracta perpendicular to the sound plane are recommended as it minimises error arising from poor lateral resolution.

Views that orient the vena contracta parallel to the sound beams should not be used.

Tips for measuring the vena contract accurately include:

- keeping the colour sector small to provide the best lateral and temporal resolution;
- identification of the proximal flow convergence, vena contracta, and jet expansion into the left ventricular chamber. The vena contracta should then be zoomed in to minimise measurement error;
- the smallest regurgitant jet width should be measured through the valve.

Vena contracta based estimates of mitral regurgitation in humans are the following:

– <3 mm = mild regurgitation
– >6 mm = severe regurgitation
– there is much overlap in between.

Applying the area equation to the vena contracta width provides another measure of EROA. This measurement defines the orifice at its smallest if done correctly. Assuming the vena contracts is a circular configuration, the area of the vena contracta is calculated using the following equation:

Vena contracta area = π x (vena contracta width/2)²

Identification of Proximal Flow Convergence

The colour flow jet is composed of three distinct segments.

- The **proximal flow convergence zone** is the area of flow acceleration into the orifice.
- The **vena contracta** is the narrowest and highest velocity region of the jet, at or just downstream from the orifice.
- The **mitral regurgitant jet** itself projects into the left atrium.

In patients with mild mitral regurgitation the proximal flow convergence zone is very small and essentially not present. As **the mitral regurgitation increase in severity the proximal flow convergence becomes progressively more visible as it gets bigger** (Figure 11).

Identification and subjective evaluation of the size of the proximal flow convergence zone is therefore a useful additional way of assessing severity of mitral regurgitation. This principle is also useful to assess the severity of insufficiency in other cardiac valves.

Spectral Doppler Evaluation

To further quantify mitral regurgitation there are complex calculations to define regurgitant volume and fraction from spectral Doppler traces. Their complexity tends to limit their clinical use.

Evaluation of transmitral flow velocity is a simple measure of MR severity. **A flow velocity greater than 1.2 m/sec is predictive of poor survival time.**

Regurgitant Jet Appearance

The velocity of a mitral regurgitant jet does not provide any information regarding severity of the insufficiency, but the flow profiles and density of the signal yield some useful information. Regurgitant jet flow profiles provide some indication

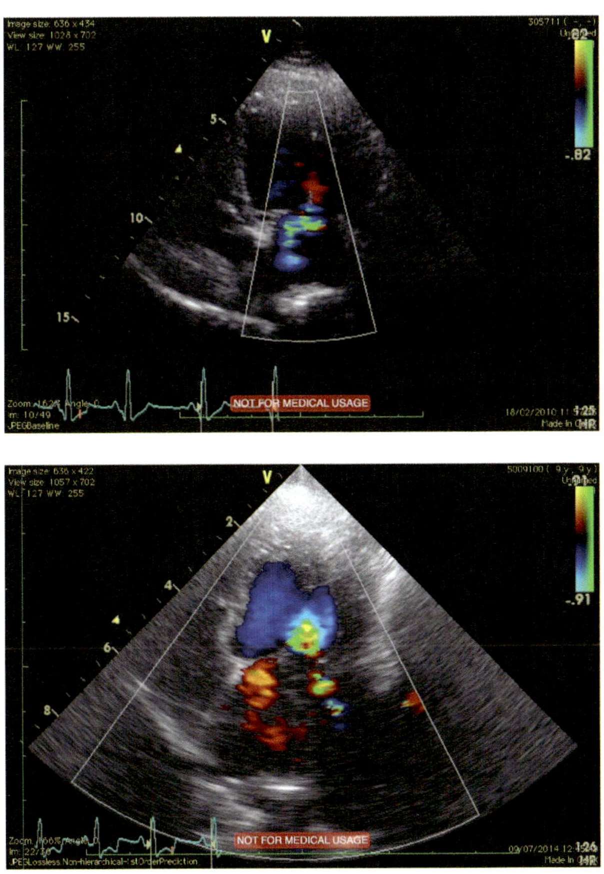

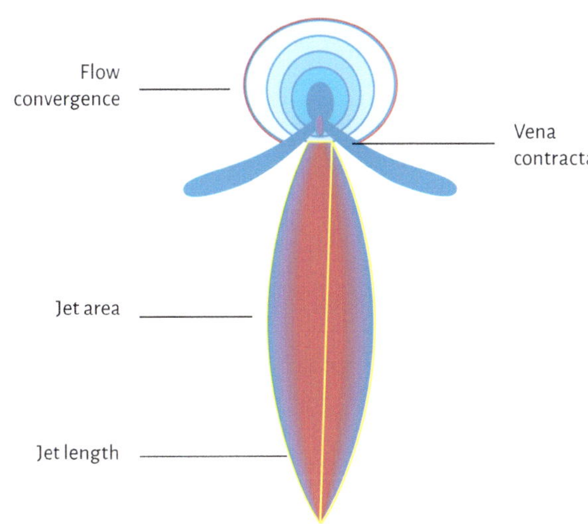

Figure 11. Identification and assessment of proximal flow convergence in patients with myxomatous mitral valve disease.

regarding the haemodynamic significance of the insufficient volume and left atrial pressures. Mitral regurgitant jet appearance is usually symmetrical (Figure 12).

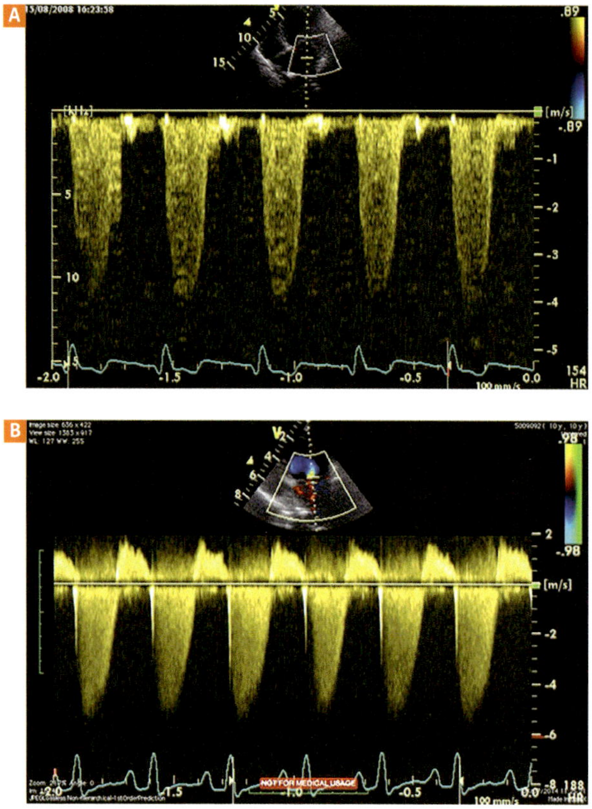

Figure 12. Continuous wave Doppler (CWD) jets showing symmetrical envelopes (**A**) and cut-off on the deceleration side of the flow profile (**B**). Also note the differences in density of the flow profiles in the two images.

A cut-off flow profile, a v-wave, on the deceleration side of the flow profile suggests a rapid increase in left atrial pressures secondary to the regurgitant volume. The result of this rapidly elevated atrial pressure is a decrease in regurgitant flow in mid to late systole. The flow profile is no longer symmetrical as seen in patients without high atrial pressures and compliant atrial chambers. This type of flow profile is often seen in **acute severe mitral insufficiency**.

The strength or density of the regurgitant flow profile represents the number of red blood cells within the regurgitant jet. A CWD flow profile that is as dense as forward diastolic flow through the mitral valve represents a significant regurgitant volume. Flow profiles that are barely discernable or do not show complete envelopes suggest the regurgitant volume is small.

Overall Assessment of Mitral Regurgitation

The overall assessment of mitral regurgitation **should never rely on a single method** of assessment. Multiple parameters to assess severity of MR should be used to account for inaccuracies inherent in any individual method, and to ensure an accurate assessment of severity of mitral regurgitation (Table 3).

Electrocardiography

Electrocardiography does not allow a definitive diagnosis of MMVD, mitral regurgitation, or CHF. Abnormal duration or amplitude of the PQRS complexes are common findings in severe disease and such findings usually indicate secondary changes in cardiac size. Unfortunately, electrocardiography is an insensitive method to detect such abnormalities; echocardiography and radiography are preferred.

Table 3. Summary table of methods of determining severity of mitral regurgitation. Adapted from the BSAVA Manual of Canine and Feline Cardiorespiratory Medicine – 2nd Edition.

Technique	Feature	Normal	Mild myxomatous mitral valve disease	Moderate myxomatous mitral valve disease	Severe myxomatous mitral valve disease
2D	Valve prolapse	None	Just extending beyond annular line	Partial prolapse beyond annular line	Large segments prolapsing with fixed distortion
	Flaid leaflets	None	None	None	+/-
	LA size	Normal	Normal	Normal/mildly dilated	Dilated
Colour Doppler	Jet position	None or trace	Single central	Multiple or eccentric	Filing chamber
	Jet area	None or trace	Narrow or short	Less than half LA area	More than half LA area
	Vena contracta width	N/A	N/A	<2 mm	>2 mm
	Proximal flow convergence	N/A	None	None	Present
Spectral Doppler	Mitral E wave velocity	<1.2 m/s	<1.2 m/s	<1.2 m/s	>1.2 m/s

ECG is the most useful diagnostic test to detect and characterise arrhythmias. The presence of a tachyarrhythmia, such as atrial fibrillation or ventricular premature depolarisations, usually indicates severe disease, presence of a complication (acute chordal rupture or myocardial infarction) or other concurrent cardiac disease.

Supraventricular premature complexes (SVPCs) (Figure 13) **are the most common arrhythmia** in patients with myxomatous mitral valve disease. However, they are frequently identified in the earlier stages of the disease and are **rarely of clinical consequence**.

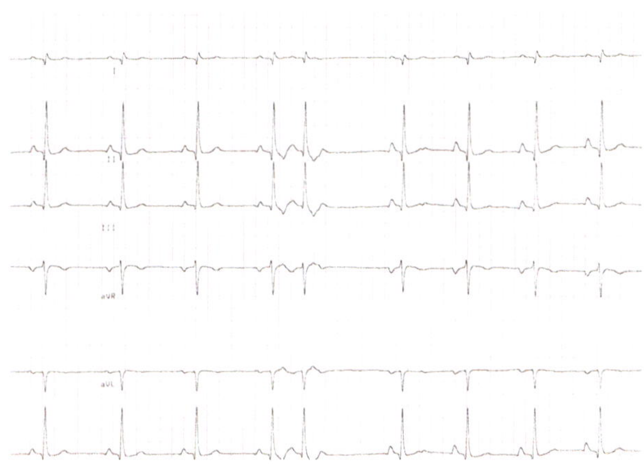

Figure 13. 6 lead ECG showing a supraventricular premature complex (SVPC).

Thoracic Radiography

Radiography cannot be used to diagnose MMVD or mitral regurgitation, but it is the **method of choice to detect left-sided congestive heart failure**. It also identifies cardiomegaly in patients with more advanced disease and is important for **excluding concurrent primary respiratory disease**.

Radiographic findings include left-sided cardiomegaly and left atrial dilatation in dogs with moderate or severe mitral regurgitation (Figure 14). **A vertebral heart size (VHS) of >10.5 is suggestive of cardiac enlargement**, but there is breed variation as outlined in Table 4.

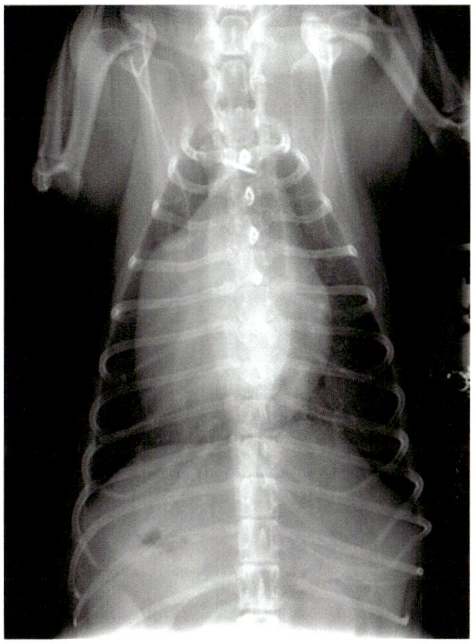

Figure 14. Dorsovental thoracic radiograph of a dog with MMVD and severe cardiomegaly.

Table 4. Breed variation in the normal vertebral heart size (VHS) in dogs. Adapted from the BSAVA Manual of Canine and Feline Thoracic Imaging.

Breed	VHS	Range
Boxer	11.6	+/-0.8
CKCS	10.6	+/-0.5
Dobermann	10.0	+/-0.6
GSD	9.7	+/-0.7
Labrador	10.8	+/-0.6
Whippet	11.0	+/-0.5
Yorkshire Terrier	9.7	+/-0.5

It is also known that the **phase of respiration and the cardiac cycle affects the VHS** by up to 0.97 and 1.11 vertebral units respectively. Interobserver variability in the assessment of vertebral heart size has been calculated at 1.05 plus or minus 0.32 vertebral units.

Recognition of left atrial dilatation is very important.

Left-sided CHF is characterised by perihilar to caudodorsal pulmonary infiltrates (interstitial, mixed or alveolar pattern) and pulmonary venous distension.

Compression of the left mainstem bronchus is seen by widening of the left bronchial angle at the body of the left atrium on dorsoventral (DV)/ventrodorsal (VD) views and splitting apart of the bronchi on the lateral view.

Blood Pressure

Blood pressure should be measured to identify dogs with systemic hypertension. Mitral regurgitation is greatly worsened by increased afterload. Hypotension with low output signs may occur with arrhythmias, secondary systolic dysfunction, excessive vasodilator therapy or overzealous diuresis. Primary cardiac disease does not cause systemic hypertension. **In most dogs with congestive heart failure secondary to MMVD systemic blood pressure is either normal or low normal**.

Laboratory Evaluation

Biochemistry should be performed to:

- detect concurrent disease
- identify secondary consequences of mitral valve disease, such as prerenal azotaemia
- detect and monitor electrolyte imbalances
- guide therapeutic decisions.

Complete blood count is less useful but often run as part of a routine profile and can identify concurrent anaemia. Complete blood count and biochemistry panels are usually unremarkable in mild cases.

Biomarkers

Troponins

The troponin complex is a group of proteins (I, T and C) which regulate the interaction between actin and myosin and have distinct myocardial isoforms.

Troponins are intracellular proteins and thus increased concentrations of these proteins are **only found in the circulation when a significant number of myocardial cells are compromised or die simultaneously**. In veterinary patients troponins I and T have been evaluated in a number of different circumstances, and circulating concentrations are elevated in association with many cardiac diseases in both cats and dogs.

The problem with troponin concentrations lies in their **lack of specificity**. They increase in response to numerous cardiac diseases, yet their **concentration does not correlate predictably with the severity of the cardiac disease** or failure in dogs. Consequently, if it is already known that the patient has heart disease, **the test simply confirms that the patient has heart disease**; it does not give any further information.

Their greatest clinical value is in cases where a **diagnosis of infarction or myocarditis is suspected**, both of which are rare diagnoses in small animals. In such cases dramatic elevations of troponin can be seen; in contrast to the relatively modest elevations seen in most animals with cardiomyopathy or valvular heart disease.

As well as a diagnostic value, it is suggested troponin concentrations have prognostic value. It is possible patients with more rapidly progressive disease tend to have higher concentrations of these proteins.

Natriuretic Peptides

Natriuretic peptides are hormones manufactured in **and released from the ventricular and atrial myocardium**. Their manufacture is increased in **response to myocardial stretch** and increased end-diastolic wall stress.

The heart releases two peptides:

- atrial natriuretic peptide (ANP)
- B-type natriuretic peptide (BNP).

Both these peptides are manufactured as larger pro-peptides and the active peptide is cleaved from the C-terminal end of the molecule (Figure 15). This means equimolar quantities of the N-terminal pro-peptide are manufactured and released into the circulation. Concentrations of either the active peptides or their N-terminal pro-peptides can be measured in the circulation.

NT-proBNP is a more stable marker of disease and recent attention focuses on the measurement of this polypeptide in both dogs and cats.

Sensitivity and specificity have been shown to be in the region of 80–85% for NT-proBNP for the discrimination of dogs with heart disease from dogs with respiratory disease.

Summarising published values:

- patients with NT-proBNP concentrations below about 450 pmol/l are unlikely to have clinically significant cardiac disease;
- patients with overt signs of heart failure are likely to have concentrations above 800 pmol/l;
- most severely affected patients have values well over 1000 pmol/l.

Unlike in human medicine, natriuretic peptide concentrations are currently not helpful for prognostication. Knowledge of these proteins is not yet at the stage of being able to treat patients on the basis of NT-proBNP concentrations. However, a recent study in dogs with mitral valve disease suggests dogs with a NT-proBNP concentration greater than about 750 pmol/l are much more likely to succumb to heart disease in the near future than dogs with lower concentrations.

These tests are unlikely to provide unequivocal yes/no answers in many patients. They need to be interpreted in conjunction with other clinical and diagnostic information and the clinician consider whether or not the result increases or decreases the likelihood of the presence of the abnormality in question.

There are also a number of confounding factors that affect the interpretation of these tests. NT-proBNP concentrations have been shown to be significantly increased in dogs with azotaemia and no cardiac disease, although the magnitude

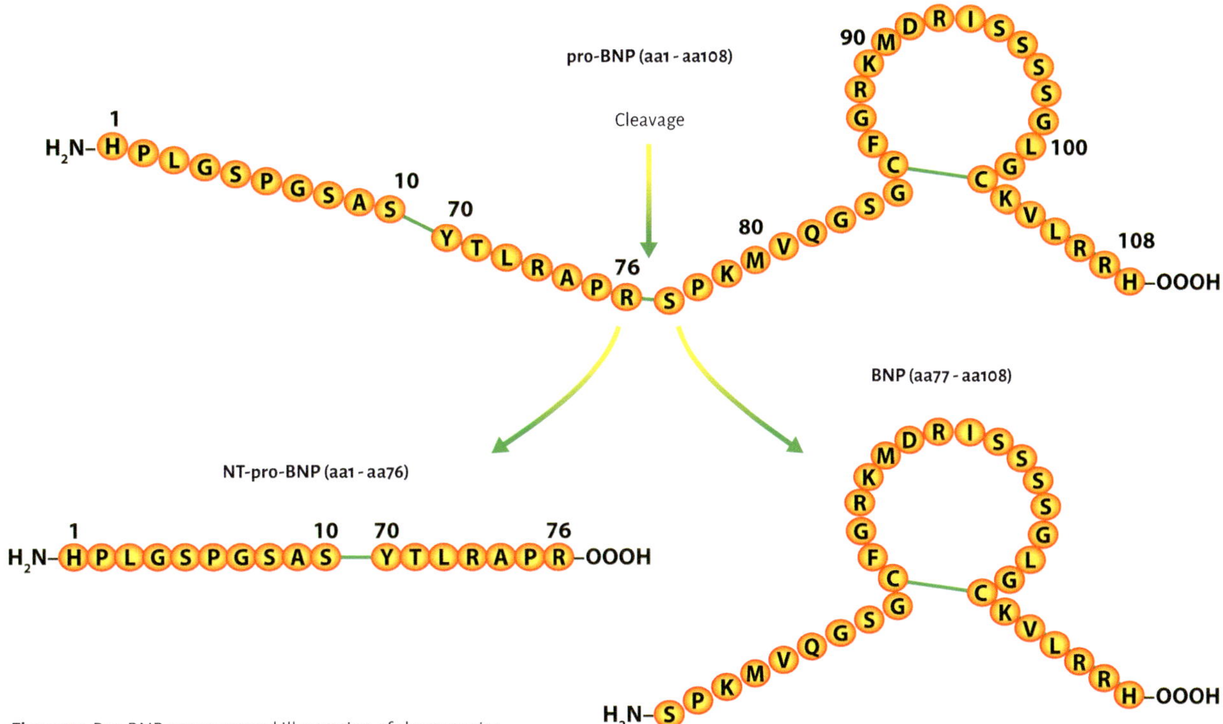

Figure 15. Pro-BNP structure and illustration of cleavage site.

of increase is typically not as great as with heart failure. Knowledge of a patient's serum creatinine concentration is therefore likely to be important for accurate interpretation of concentrations of NT-proBNP.

There is also some concern that there may be some **breed variation in NT-proBNP** reference ranges.

Differential Diagnoses

The differential diagnoses for mitral regurgitation include:

- mitral regurgitation secondary to a primary cardiomyopathy
- mitral dysplasia
- mitral regurgitation secondary to congenital heart disease, resulting in left ventricle dilatation (e.g. patent *ductus arteriosus*)
- infective endocarditis of the mitral valve
- systemic hypertension.

Treatment

The ideal therapy for MMVD is to **halt the progression of the valvular degeneration or improve valvular function** (e.g. by surgical repair or valve replacement). However, no therapy is currently known to inhibit or prevent the valvular degeneration, and surgery is not technically or economically practical in most veterinary patients.

A group of surgeons and cardiologists in Japan performed mitral annuloplasty under cardiopulmonary bypass in more than 48 small breed dogs. They have reported good initial outcomes in dogs with MMVD. Surgeons at The Royal Veterinary College, University of London have also recently started operating on cases. This is therefore now a viable treatment option for those clients with adequate resources.

In most dogs however medical management remains the mainstay treatment option, and is palliative. The aim is to ameliorate the clinical signs and improve survival.

Treatment of Asymptomatic Myxomatous Mitral Valve Disease (Stage B)

Most animals with myxomatous mitral valve disease are asymptomatic. In early heart disease, haemodynamic function may be relatively unaffected and there may be little or no neurohormonal activation. Therapy at this stage is only worthwhile if it slows or reverses the underlying disease progression, or if the onset of CHF is delayed or prevented.

In 2016 the EPIC study, a prospective randomised placebo-controlled trial (RCT), was published in the Journal of Veterinary Internal Medicine. Treatment with pimobendan was compared with placebo in patients with stage B2 MMVD. Inclusion criteria were as follows:

- dogs >6 years of age
- body weight within the range 4.1–15 kg
- a typical mitral murmur (≥ grade 3/6)
- characteristic valvular lesions on echocardiography
- regurgitation noted on colour Doppler interrogation of the mitral valve
- left atrial dilation; left atrium to aorta ratio >1.6:1
- left ventricular dilation; normalised LVIDd ≥1.7
- radiographic vertebral heart size >10.5.

All patients were classed as having stage B2 myxomatous mitral valve disease, and 360 dogs between the ages of 7 and 11 years of varying breeds were included; 180 patients in the pimobendan group and 180 patients in the placebo group. The primary endpoint of the study was onset of left-sided congestive heart failure or cardiac death (stage C MMVD). The secondary endpoint was all cause mortality.

The onset of stage C MMVD was delayed by approximately 15 months (median) in the pimobendan group compared to the placebo group. This time extension was not offset by a reduction in overall survival time. Treatment was safe and well-tolerated (See Figure 3. Intervention points for medical management of patients with myxomatous mitral valve disease).

Monitoring at Home

The main goal of monitoring is to detect early signs of heart failure. Owner education is particularly important, as the owner is best placed to identify the earliest signs. **A normal dog's respiratory rate should be less than 30–40 breaths/min when at rest**. A respiratory rate exceeding 50 breaths/min at rest is clear evidence that respiratory function is abnormal, and to contact the veterinarian.

Treatment: Mild to Moderate Congestive Heart Failure (CHF) (Stage C)

Animals with mild to moderate CHF usually show clinical signs, but **do not require hospitalisation** for management. It is logical to attempt to counteract the neurohormonal mechanisms leading to sodium and water retention. Most clinical trials in canine heart failure are carried out with this stage of heart disease and selection of therapy should be evidence-based.

Treatment Goals

Patients with CHF operate on the far right side of the Frank-Starling curve and resolution of signs is accomplished via **preload reduction** (i.e. diuretics and venous vasodilators), and use of **positive inotropes or afterload reducers** (Figure 16).

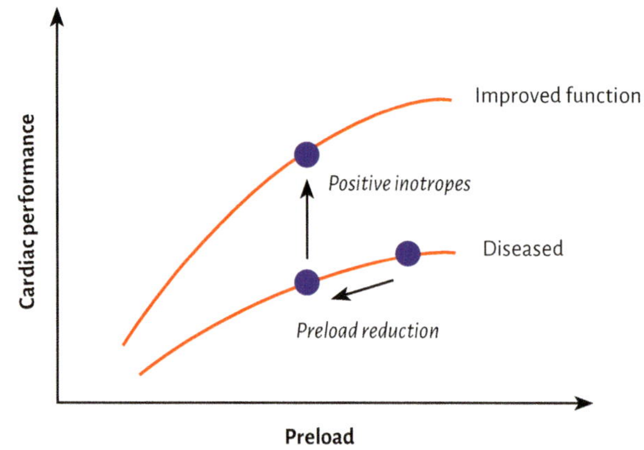

Figure 16. Treatment goals in patients with left-sided congestive heart failure; preload reduction and augmentation of cardiac performance. Image adapted from the BSAVA Manual of Canine and Feline Cardiorespiratory Medicine – 2nd Edition.

Treatment of heart failure with preload reducers, diuretics or venous vasodilators shifts a patient leftward along the Frank-Starling curve, helping to reduce signs of congestion. **A priority is removal of abnormal fluid accumulation** (pulmonary oedema, pleural effusion, ascites), and the aim is to reduce and eliminate fluid accumulation without causing unacceptable azotaemia or polyuria/polydipsia which compromises quality of life.

The general approach is to titrate a loop diuretic to effect, using the lowest effective dose. Furosemide and torasemide are the most commonly used loop diuretics.

Treatment of heart failure with afterload reducers, arterial vasodilators, or positive inotropes, shifts the Frank-Starling curve upwards with a steeper slope, helping to restore the normal relationship between preload and cardiac performance.

Treatment with pimobendan is recommended in patients with acute-onset left-sided congestive heart failure, if not already administered prior to the onset of CHF.

Neurohormonal blockade may be associated with prolonged survival, and drugs with beneficial haemodynamic effects may also improve outcome, these include:

- ACE inhibitors
- spironolactone.

Monitoring

The goals of monitoring include using thoracic radiographs to assess resolution of CHF, **checking respiratory rate at home**, and checking for adverse effects of medications by monitoring biochemistry (electrolytes and urea/creatinine).

Life-threatening Congestive Heart Failure (Stage C)

Many cases present acutely, sometimes without any history of prior problems or sometimes already receiving medical therapy for CHF. With acute deterioration there may be little time for sodium and water retention, and **low cardiac output signs may predominate**. This can manifest as depressed mentation, skeletal muscle weakness, oliguria or anuria, hypothermia and cardiac shock.

In the worst of circumstances, both congestive and low output failure may be simultaneously present.

Patients with **low output failure operate** on the bottom portion of the Frank-Starling curve (Figure 17) and resolution of signs is accomplished by **increasing contractility** (i.e. positive inotropes). **Judicious arterial vasodilation** may help to improve cardiac output, if it does not compromise arterial blood pressure.

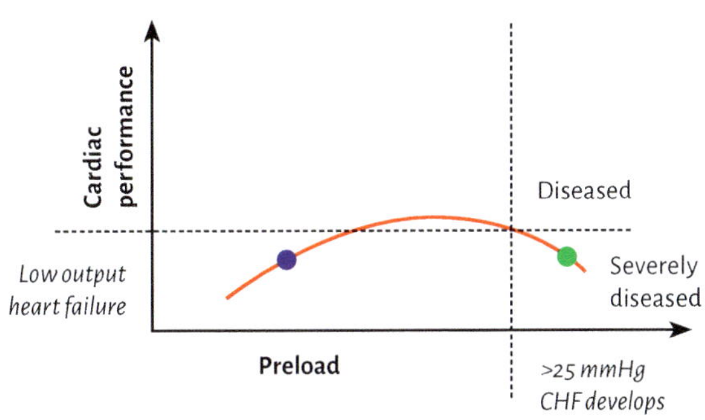

Figure 17. Blue circle - low output heart failure; green circle – combined low output failure and CHF in instances of severely depressed myocardial function. Image adapted from the BSAVA Manual of Canine and Feline Cardiorespiratory Medicine – 2nd Edition.

In rare instances, patients with low output failure actually benefit from volume (preload) expansion to shift their operating point rightward and higher on the Frank-Starling curve. Conversely, overly aggressive diuretic use in a patient with depressed myocardial function could precipitate or worsen low output failure.

Therapy must be focused on **optimising haemodynamic function**. Trying to neutralise neurohormonal activation in this setting is counterproductive, as the compensatory mechanisms help to support arterial pressures. These cases require rapid aggressive management if they are to survive.

Management Goals

- Rapid improvement in oxygenation and haemodynamic function.
- Oxygen supplementation.
- Drainage of pleural effusions.
- Treatment of pulmonary oedema with diuresis and sometimes venodilation.
- Augmentation of cardiac output using positive inotropes.
- Augmentation of cardiac output with judicious arteriodilation.

Monitoring

Monitoring must not compromise patient safety, but the minimum requirement is to monitor **respiratory rate/effort** to chart resolution of pulmonary oedema and, ideally, **blood pressure** if low output signs are present.

Electrolytes and renal function should also be monitored, as the adverse effects of medications include azotaemia and hypokalaemia (loop diuretics).

Monitor heart rate and rhythm (particularly ventricular arrhythmias) closely when using catecholamines.

Refractory Congestive Heart Failure (Stage D)

This category includes animals already receiving standard treatment for heart failure, but with heart failure signs which persist despite upwards titration of furosemide doses to greater than 6 mg/kg PO q 12 hours. By this stage there may be surprisingly few signs of diuresis (or polydipsia) as the animal becomes increasingly refractory.

Clinical signs consistent with concurrent right-sided congestive heart failure are common.

Addition of other diuretics (without withdrawing the furosemide) often restors diuresis, but as the disease progresses cardiac cachexia is a common problem. Sequential nephron blockade is usually necessary, as the combination of **multiple diuretics** achieves greater diuresis than high doses of a single diuretic.

Appetite may be poor by this stage and **essential ω-3 fatty acid supplementation** can be tried in an attempt to counteract cardiac cachexia.

Monitoring and Follow Up

Client education is vital for successful management of the dog at home:

- the common clinical signs of CHF
- what to do if signs of CHF develop
- how to monitor resting respiratory rates
- administration of parenteral furosemide when required.

Preclinical dogs with slight to moderate regurgitation are rechecked every 6–12 months and those with moderate to severe regurgitation rechecked every 3 months.

Table 5. Treatment options for different stages of myxomatous mitral valve disease (MMVD). Adapted from the BSAVA Manual of Canine and Feline Cardiorespiratory Medicine – 2nd Edition.

MMVD disease stage	Standard treatment	Optional use	Diet/exercise
Stage A	No treatment	None	Normal diet and exercise (decrease calorie intake if obese)
Stage B1	No treatment	None	Normal diet and exercise (decrease calorie intake if obese)
Stage B2	Pimobendan	No other drugs have been shown to be effective at this stage. Some clinicians use ACE inhibitors, β-blockers and spironolactone	· Normal diet and exercise (decrease calorie intake if obese) · Consider ω-3 fatty acid supplementation
Stage C	· Pimobendan · Furosemide or torasemide · ACE inhibitor · Spironolactone	· Spironolactone · Digoxin/diltiazem if atrial fibrillation	· Avoid excessive salt consumption · Restrict exercise until CHF resolved, then avoid extreme exertion
Stage D	· Furosemide (increase dose until no further effect or 6 mg/kg PO q 12 hours · Pimobendan · ACE inhibitor · Spironolactone	· Thiazide diuretics · Parenteral furosemide · Abdominocentesis if refractory ascites · Amlodipine or hydralazine · Sildenafil if severe pulmonary hypertension · Digoxin if atrial fibrillation	· Avoid excessive salt consumption · Avoid undue exertion
Severe/life-threatening CHF	· Intravenous furosemide · Supplemental oxygen · Pimobendan	· Glyceryl trinitrate · Sedation (e.g. butorphanol) if distressed · Thoracocentesis if large pleural effusions · Dobutamine if hypotensive · Intravenous sodium	· Encourage eating · Cage rest

In dogs with CHF, a follow up examination should be scheduled for 1–2 weeks after discharge to check for resolution of clinical signs, level of dehydration, electrolytes, renal function, and radiographic evidence of CHF. If the dog is stable, follow up examinations are scheduled every 3–6 months thereafter.

Infective Endocarditis

Infective endocarditis (IE) is caused by invasion of the valvular endothelium by microbes, resulting in proliferative or erosive lesions and consequently valvular insufficiency. Vegetative lesions may result in embolism or metastatic infection involving multiple body organs, producing a large variety of clinical signs. The **mitral and aortic valves** are almost exclusively infected in small animals. Endocarditis has a low incidence, in the order of 0.04–0.13% of all dogs referred to one veterinary medical teaching hospital. The incidence in cats is considerably lower.

Aetiology

Transient or persistent bacteraemia is a prerequisite for the development of IE.

Common routes of infection include:

– discospondylitis
– prostatitis
– pneumonia
– urinary tract infections
– pyoderma
– periodontal disease
– long term indwelling central venous catheters.

The condition has been associated with **subaortic stenosis and high-velocity shunting diseases** such as patent *ductus arteriosus* and ventricular septal defects. However, IE has not been found to have any association with myxomatous mitral valve disease (MMVD) in dogs.

The risk of IE seems to be very small following conditions or procedures that cause bacteraemia such as dental scaling or GI endoscopy, unless another predisposing factor coexists.

The most common bacteria isolated from diseased patients are:

– *Staphylococcus spp.* (*aureus*, *intermedius*, coagulase positive and coagulase negative)
– *Streptococcus spp.* (*canis*, *bovis*, and *betahaemolytic*)
– *Escherichia coli*.

Less commonly isolated bacteria include:

– *Pseudomonas spp.*, *Erysipelothrix rhusiopathiae*, *Enterobacter spp.*, *Pasteurella spp.*, *Corynebacterium spp.*, *Proteus spp.*

The majority of cases (60–70%) are culture negative, presumably because many dogs are already receiving antibiotic therapy prior to blood culture.

In addition, *Bartonella spp.*, which are intracellular bacteria, have recently emerged as an important cause of endocarditis in dogs. *Bartonella spp.* were reported to be the causative agent of endocarditis in 28% (5 out of 18) of dogs with IE in a recent North American study, representing 45% (5 out of 11) of dogs with negative blood cultures.

Pathophysiology

The development and progression of infectious endocarditis involves **four key stages**.

Stage 1. Non-bacterial Thrombotic Endocarditis (NBTE)

Endothelial damage and a hypercoagulable state predispose to the development of platelet-fibrin deposition on damaged valve tissue.

Damage to endothelial surfaces can occur secondary to inflammation (e.g. vasculitis) or mechanical damage (e.g. from high-velocity flow secondary to subaortic stenosis). The resulting cellular deposits are referred to as **non-bacterial thrombotic endocarditis** (NBTE).

Stage 2. Infectious Endocarditis (IE)

During bacteraemia, microorganisms adhere to these sites via exposed fibronectin, converting NBTE to infectious endocarditis.

The coagulum of fibrinogen, fibrin, platelet proteins and fibronectin forms and avidly binds **bacteria, protecting them from host defence and antibiotics**. Bacterial pathogenicity is also an important factor in both adherence to endothelial surfaces and subsequent valve damage.

Stage 3. Valve Tissue Destruction

The **destruction of valvular tissue** can be caused by the action of bacteria or the cellular response of the immune system.

Immune complexes form, which primarily consist of immunoglobulins, complement factors and bacterial antigens. These are deposited in the basement membrane and cause further complement activation and tissue destruction.

In addition, **immune-mediated glomerulonephritis, polyarthritis, and skin diseases are common sequelae** of immune complex deposition.

Stage 4. Embolisation

Septic or aseptic emboli frequently lodge in the kidneys, spleen, heart, brain, systemic arteries and other organs.

These emboli do not always cause clinical signs, but evidence of systemic embolisation is common at postmortem examination in dogs with infectious endocarditis.

Effects of Infectious Endocarditis on Heart Function

The haemodynamic effects depend on the severity and rate of development of structural changes to valve morphology. Severe mitral or aortic insufficiency leads to **elevated left ventricular end diastolic pressure, left atrial pressure and pulmonary capillary pressure, with subsequent left-sided congestive heart failure (CHF)**. With severe acute valvular disruption, pulmonary oedema may develop early in the clinical course. With less disruptive lesions, progressive left ventricular remodelling may develop before the onset of CHF.

Clinical Signs

Infectious endocarditis can easily be overlooked as the history and clinical signs are nonspecific and predisposing factors are not always present.

Medium to large breeds and middle-aged to older male dogs are more commonly affected with IE.

The most common clinical signs include:

- lameness
- lethargy
- anorexia
- respiratory abnormalities
- weakness and collapse
- neurological signs
- haematuria.

Diagnostic Approach

Infectious endocarditis often presents with **nonspecific clinical signs associated with septic embolisation of organs**. Making a definitive diagnosis of IE is therefore challenging, and a set of criteria for diagnosis of IE has been developed in human medicine called the Modified Duke Criteria (Table 6).

Table 6. Modified Duke criteria for diagnosis of infectious endocarditis in humans. Table adapted from the BSAVA Manual of Canine and Feline Cardiorespiratory Medicine – 2nd Edition.

Major criteria of IE	· Positive echocardiographic findings (vegetative, erosive lesion or abscess) · Newly developed moderate to severe aortic insufficiency in the absence of congenital disease, aortic disease, or severe systemic hypertension · Positive blood culture for typical microorganism (≥2 positive blood cultures)
Minor criteria of IE	· Fever · Medium to large dog (>15 kg) · Subaortic stenosis · Thromboembolic disease · Immune-mediated disease · Immunocompromised (such as chronic systemic corticosteroid therapy) · Polyarthritis/glomerulonephritis · Single positive blood culture or atypical organism
Definitive diagnosis of IE	· Histopathology of valve · 2 major criteria · 1 major and 2 minor criteria
Possible diagnosis of IE	· 1 major and 1 minor criterion
No diagnosis of IE	· Other cardiac disease diagnosed · Resolution of regurgitation or valvular abnormality within 4 days of treatment. · No pathological evidence of IE on post-mortem examination

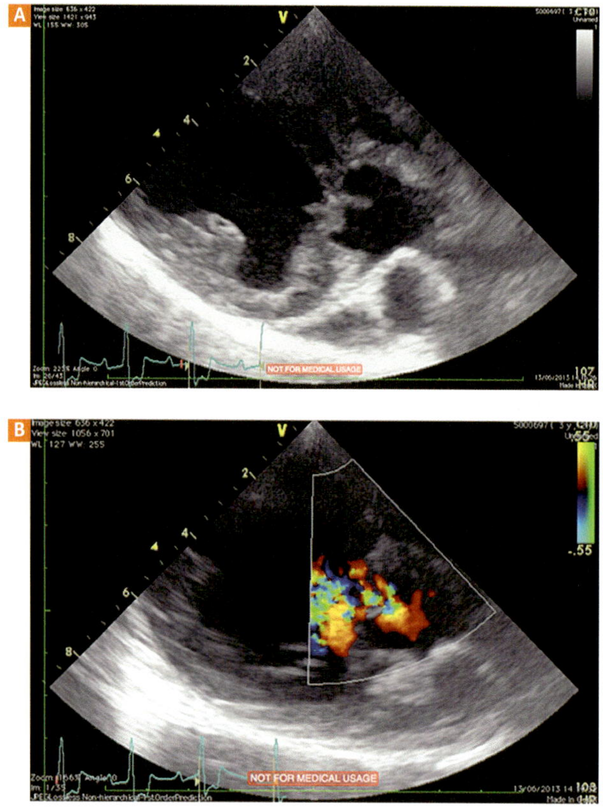

Figure 18. Vegetative lesions (**A**) on the aortic valve of a patient with infectious endocarditis. Significant valvular regurgitation (**B**) is often noted on colour Doppler interrogation of the affected valve.

Physical Examination

- Murmur present in most (89–96%) dogs.
- Left apical holosystolic murmur occurs with mitral regurgitation.
- Left basilar diastolic murmur with bounding femoral arterial pulses is highly suggestive of aortic valve involvement.
- Arrhythmia in 40–70% of dogs, including ventricular arrhythmias, supraventricular tachycardia, atrioventricular block and atrial fibrillation.
- Respiratory distress, cough, or crackles on lung auscultation present in animals with CHF.
- Fever is present in 70% of dogs, with joint effusion and lameness also common.

Echocardiography

Valvular vegetations may be detected using two-dimensional echocardiography (Figure 18), but small or less advanced lesions are difficult to distinguish from myxomatous disease. Mitral vegetations do not normally result in valve prolapse.

Echocardiographic identification of a **hyperechoic oscillating vegetative lesion on the valve** is the principal method of diagnosing endocarditis.

Left atrial enlargement may be present with chronic endocarditis of the mitral valve, but **left atrial size is normal in acute disease**.

Thoracic Radiography

Thoracic radiographs help exclude the presence of coexisting thoracic disease, assess global cardiac size, and evaluate for CHF (reported in approximately 50% of dogs with IE).

Blood Culture

Positive blood cultures help to confirm the disease.

Contrary to previous opinion, it is more likely that **the bacteraemia associated with IE is a continuous rather than intermittent event**.

For Bartonella species serum may be submitted for measurement of antibody titres to *Bartonella spp.* A titre ~1:1024 is strongly suggestive of bartonellosis. There is strong cross reactivity between species. Culture is not recommended because *Bartonella spp.* are rarely cultured from dogs despite long-term incubation in an enriched medium. Because of these methodological problems, PCR-based detection of *Bartonella spp.* DNA from blood is also recommended.

Differential Diagnoses

- Mitral regurgitation from MMVD or mitral dysplasia.
- Aortic insufficiency secondary to aortic valve degeneration or a large VSD.
- Aortic insufficiency and stenosis due to congenital aortic stenosis.
- Lameness from immune-mediated polyarthritis.
- Septic arthritis, tick-borne diseases or degenerative arthritis.
- Fever from other systemic diseases such as sepsis, pneumonia, neoplasia.

Treatment

The main goals of therapy are:

- eradication of the infective microorganism
- treatment of all secondary complications.

Long-term bactericidal antibiotic treatment is generally necessary. The ideal duration of therapy is unknown, but at least 4–6 weeks is recommended and therapy may be required for 3–4 months.

Selection of the appropriate antibiotic is based on **culture and sensitivity testing** (minimum inhibitory concentration of the antibiotic), whenever possible. While the culture results are pending, or if the microbial cause is not known, **empirical treatment with broad-spectrum** antibiotics is recommended.

Initially, intravenous antibiotics are administered for 1–2 weeks, followed by oral antibiotics.

If congestive heart failure is present, then standard CHF treatment is required.

Prognosis

Prognosis depends on the infective agent, the aggressiveness and severity of valve colonisation, the immunological status of the animal and how promptly therapy has been initiated.

The prognosis is poor to guarded, with an overall median survival of 54 days in one study.

The prognosis tends to be worse for aortic endocarditis with a median survival time of 3 days versus 476 days for mitral IE in another study that included mostly bartonellosis.

Bibliography

- Côté, E., MacDonald, K.A., Montgomery, K. et al. (2011) *Feline Cardiology*. Wiley Blackwell.
- Cunningham, J.G., Bradley, G.K. (2007) *Cunningham Textbook of Veterinary Physiology*, 4th edition. Saunders Elsevier.
- Barrett, K.E., Barman, S.M, Boitano, S. et al. (2012) *Ganong's Review of Medical Physiology*, 24th edition. McGraw-Hill Medical.
- Bonow, R.O., Mann, Zipes et al. (2012) *Braunwald's Heart Disease*. Elsevier Saunders.
- Luis Fuentes, V., Jonhson, L.R., Dennis, S. (2010) *BSAVA Manual of Canine and Feline Cardiopulmonary Medicine*, 2nd Edition. BSAVA.
- Kittleson, M.D., Kienle, R.D. (1998) *Small Animal Cardiovascular Medicine*. Mosby.

Test

Answers on Page 172

1. Which heart disease is the most common acquired heart disease in the dog?
a. Dilated cardiomyopathy (DCM).
b. Subaortic stenosis.
c. Myxomatous mitral valve disease (MMVD).
d. Patent *ductus arteriosus*.

2. In dogs with mitral valve disease, which option best describes the characteristic murmur?
a. A holosystolic or pansystolic murmur with a point of maximal intensity (PMI) over the left apex.
b. A continuous murmur with a PMI over the left heart base, and often radiation apically.
c. A systolic murmur with a PMI over the right apex.
d. A crescendo-decrescendo heart murmur with a PMI over the left heart base.

3. Which medication has been shown to delay the progression of disease in asymptomatic dogs with myxomatous mitral valve disease?
a. No medication.
b. Pimobendan.
c. Benazepril.
d. Spironolactone.

4. Infective endocarditis involves almost exclusively which two of the heart valves in small animals?
a. Tricuspid and mitral valves.
b. Aortic and mitral valves.
c. Aortic and pulmonic valves.
d. Pulmonic and tricuspid valves.

5. Which antibiotic class should not be used in animals with infective endocarditis and secondary congestive heart failure?
a. Aminoglycosides.
b. Fluoroquinolones.
c. Tetracyclines.
d. Penicillins.

6. Which option indicates the correct structure of the mitral valve from atrium to ventricle?
a. Atrialis, fibrosa, spongiosa, ventricularis.
b. Spongiosa, fibrosa, atrialis, ventricularis.
c. Atrialis, spongiosa, fibrosa, ventricularis.
d. Atrialis, ventricularis, spongiosa, fibrosa.

7. In dogs with mitral valve disease, which cell type is a key player in valve degeneration?
a. Valvular interstitial cells.
b. Neutrophils.
c. Platelets.
d. Endothelial cells.

8. What changes in audibility of the heart sounds are characteristic of severe MMVD?
a. Loud S1, quiet or sometime inaudible S2.
b. Quiet S1, loud S2.
c. S1 equal to S2.
d. Presence of an S3 gallop.

9. Which feature below must be demonstrated on echocardiography to make a diagnosis of *chordae tendineae* rupture?
a. There is mitral valve prolapse.
b. The leaflet tip points back into the left atrium.
c. Mitral regurgitation suddenly worsens.
d. Acute heart failure develops without time for significant volume retention.

10. Proximal isovelocity surface area measurements should be performed on which echocardiographic view?
a. Left parasternal four chamber.
b. Right parasternal long axis.
c. Right parasternal short axis at the level of the papillary muscle.
d. Right parasternal short axis at the level of the left atrium.

Notes

Correct Answers:

1. c
2. a
3. b
4. b
5. a
6. c
7. a
8. a
9. b
10. a

Notes

Syncope

Mª Josefa Fernández-del Palacio

Definitions

- **Syncope is a symptom characterised by a sudden, transitory and complete loss of consciousness**, associated with an inability to maintain postural tone and spontaneous recovery. The loss of real consciousness is a cognitive state in which the individual lacks self-awareness and awareness of the situation, with the inability to respond to stimuli.
- **Collapse** describes a loss of postural tone without loss of consciousness.
- **Presyncope or "near syncope"** describes a state similar to prodromal syncope, such as dizziness or difficulty standing, but is not followed by complete loss of consciousness. In some animals, presyncope can progress to syncope or stop without evolving.

Syncope is manifested by sudden-onset ataxia and disorientation, followed by a loss of musculoskeletal tone and consciousness. These signs may appear suddenly or be preceded by profound disorientation, vocalization, and signs of significant distress. By definition, **one of the characteristics of syncope is that it rarely lasts more than 30 seconds**, with recovery of an almost normal mental state in a few seconds, although in some cases it can end in death.

Syncope must be differentiated from other causes of temporary loss of consciousness, real or apparent, for example seizures, hypoglycaemia, anaemia, metabolic abnormalities, drugs, neurological abnormalities, intoxications or cataplexy. **The syncope mechanism is presumably due to cerebral hypoperfusion**, while non-syncope loss of consciousness is attributable to other mechanisms. For example, epilepsy is caused by uncontrolled cortical neuronal discharge.

There is no specific data on the prevalence of episodes of syncope in small animals, although it is known to be a frequent cause for consultation in dogs and is rare in cats.

Creating a differential diagnosis list of the causes of temporary loss of consciousness is essential in both general and referral practice. An appropriate initial approach may be enough to guide the clinician as to the correct steps to take and if necessary advise referral to an internal medicine, neurology, or cardiology specialist.

Causes and Pathophysiology of Syncope

Once it is established the patient presented with syncope, the next step is **evaluation of the cause**. In physiological terms, **blood pressure (BP) depends on cardiac output (CO) and vascular resistance**, so any cause that reduces CO or causes excessive arterial vasodilation can reduce BP and cerebral perfusion, causing loss of consciousness. In addition, BP is regulated by pressure receptors and the autonomic tone of the cardiovascular system, controlled in part by the **baroreceptor reflex**. Inadequate activation of this reflex causes bradycardia and vasodilation, especially during activity, resulting in hypotension and possibly syncope.

The consensus, regarding the aetiology of syncope is that most of the episodes are due to one of the following mechanisms.

- **Reflex or neuro-mediated mechanism**: due to bradycardia, vasodilation, or both.
- **Cardiogenic**: due to arrhythmias and/or structural heart disease.
- **Orthostatic hypotension**: due to primary autonomic dysfunction, secondary to an underlying pathology or triggered by hypotensive drugs or hypovolaemia.

In some patients more than one of these mechanisms contributes to the syncopal episode and so establishing causality is difficult.

Reflex or Neurally Mediated Syncope

This is characterised by inappropriate activation of cardiovascular reflexes (baroreceptor reflex) which normally control circulation, by triggering stimuli that can cause bradycardia, vasodilation, or both. **Pressure receptors** are located in the carotid artery, aorta, and also in the ventricular myocardium (C fibres).

There are three notable forms of reflex syncope.

Vasovagal Syncope

Preceded by **prodromal signs of autonomous activation** (paleness, nausea). In predisposed dogs, triggers such as fear, beginning of exercise, or excitement increase sympathetic activity, causing less ventricular filling, increased myocardial contraction, and stimulation of ventricular mechanoreceptors (innervated by afferent vagal fibres), sending signals to spinal and cerebral centres which cause an **intense vasovagal reflex** response from the vasomotor centre in the brain (Bezold Jarish reflex) producing bradycardia and syncope in predisposed dogs.

In practice the author has documented several cases of hunting dogs that are anxious when they head out to the countryside and suffer syncopal episodes within minutes of starting activity.

Likewise, syncope episodes with a bimodal pattern have been documented in Boxer dogs, that is, more frequent between 6 and 24 months and then at 7–10 years.

Situational Syncope

In this case, **the triggers are physical situations**, such as coughing (cough syncope, common in dogs), urination, or defaecation which cause vagotonia, sympathetic inhibition, vasodilation, and hypotension.

In the author's experience, **cough syncope** is common in brachycephalic breeds of dogs and dogs with chronic tracheobronchial conditions such as tracheal collapse. Several mechanisms appear to contribute to **triggering the baroreceptor reflex** during coughing episodes including: increased intrathoracic pressure, decreased venous return and cardiac output, vagus nerve stimulation, reflex bradycardia, and decreased intracranial pressure of cerebral blood flow.

Micturition syncope is due to vagal activation of the bladder and pelvic nerve mechanoreceptors (afferent pathway). Defaecation can activate parietal tension of receptors in the intestine and cause syncope.

Prolonged **neurocardiogenic bradycardia** during sleep (2–6 h) has been considered the cause of syncope episodes in dogs with advanced mitral disease associated with pulmonary hypertension. These dogs wake up and howl (vegetative response to hypoxia) and then collapse. Bradycardia is noted by the owners and has also been seen during Holter monitoring.

Carotid Sinus Hypersensitivity Syncope

In some susceptible dogs, **compression of the carotid sinus** has been associated with syncope. The author has been able to demonstrate this in some Boxer dogs.

Reflex or neuro-mediated syncope is difficult to demonstrate in dogs and has been suggested in patients with and without structural heart disease. However, the inability to measure BP and perform the tilt table test on an outpatient basis prevents an accurate diagnosis. Evaluation of heart rate and rhythm using a 24-hour Holter monitor or an event monitor can help exclude malignant tachyarrhythmias as the cause of syncope.

In cats, the reflex mechanism as a cause of syncope is poorly documented.

The initial evaluation should include a risk assessment to guide treatment and prevent morbidity and mortality, in both the short and long term, since a patient with arrhythmogenic heart disease is not at the same risk as one with reflex syncope.

Syncope of Cardiac Origin

The main causes of cardiac syncope are **arrhythmias and structural cardiopathies**.

Arrhythmias

Bradyarrhythmias such as sick sinus syndrome, atrioventricular blocks, and atrial standstill are the **main causes of syncope in dogs**. Episodes of loss of consciousness occur when the escape rhythm is very low or unstable, or during exercise.

The **most common tachyarrhythmias** as a cause of syncope in dogs include ventricular tachycardias, especially in the Boxer, English Bulldog, and Dobermann, secondary to **arrhythmogenic cardiomyopathies**. Other cases have been associated with genetic channelopathies such as long QT syndrome.

In some Boxer dogs with arrhythmogenic right ventricular cardiomyopathy and syncope, the concurrence of ventricular tachyarrhythmias with episodes of bradyarrhythmias and asystole, presumably of a reflex or vagal type, has been revealed by 24-hour Holter monitoring.

Structural Cardiopathies

The main structural conditions which cause loss of consciousness are generally associated with **obstructive lesions of the ventricular outflow tracts**, such as pulmonary stenosis or aortic or subaortic stenosis, cardiac tamponade (idiopathic or due to neoplasia), diseases of the mitral and tricuspid valves (congenital insufficiency or stenosis), and cardiomyopathies. In the latter, low cardiac output can be associated with tachyarrhythmias as the cause of syncope. At least a third of dogs with moderate/severe pulmonary hypertension have syncope associated with exercise or excitement.

In cats, the most common cause of transient loss of consciousness is structural heart disease, often coexisting with significant tachyarrhythmias or bradyarrhythmias: hypertrophic cardiomyopathy and ventricular arrhythmias, cardiac dirofilariasis, atrial septal defects, arrhythmogenic right ventricular cardiomyopathy, arrhythmogenic right ventricular cardiomyopathy, cardiac lymphoma, and hyperthyroidism associated with third degree atrioventricular (AV) block.

In some publications concerning cats with syncope, the cause has not been established. In the author's experience, complete AV block with absence of stable ventricular escape rhythm has been the most common cause of syncope in elderly cats (in some cases, it has been associated with cardiomyopathy).

Orthostatic Hypotension Syncope

Refers to the loss of consciousness as a consequence of **an abnormal decrease in systolic BP (due to standing)**, related to the following mechanisms:

- primary autonomic system failure
- secondary autonomic failure: diabetes, uraemia, spinal cord damage
- medications: diuretics, vasodilators
- volume depletion: bleeding, diarrhoea, vomiting.

It is difficult to demonstrate this mechanism in animals as they are quadrupeds. However, episodes of syncope have been documented in dogs due to insufficient blood volume, venous return deficits and hypotension.

Related conditions include severe dehydration due to gastrointestinal losses, hypoadrenocorticism, and drugs which cause bradycardia, cardiac depression, vasodilation, or hypotension (such as acepromazine, diltiazem, β-blockers, and amlodipine). The author has documented dogs referred for syncope in which the diagnosis on presentation was acute haemolytic anaemia (similar to that described in cases of splenic rupture).

In small animals, hypoglycaemia as a cause of collapse is generally due to the presence of an insulinoma (tumour that secretes excess insulin), as the brain needs a constant supply of energy since it does not store or synthesize it.

Signs of collapse-syncope in Labrador Retriever dogs when performing intense exercise have been associated with a genetic predisposition due to DNM1 mutation. However, such a mechanism has not been demonstrated in the Pembroke Welsh Corgi, Boykin Spaniel, and Chesapeake Bay Retriever which suffer with similar clinical signs.

Clinical Evaluation and Diagnosis

Evaluation of these patients includes:

- **history** from the owner;
- complete **physical examination**, paying special attention to the cardiovascular system;
- **complementary tests** according to findings on physical examination: initially complete blood count and biochemistry, ECG and, later, possible 24-hour Holter monitoring, echocardiography, etc.

Table 1. Diagnostic criteria for the initial examination of the patient with syncope.

Type of syncope	Most significant clinical findings
Vasovagal syncope	· Normal physical examination and ECG · Emotional/stress triggers and not a breed predisposed to arrhythmogenic cardiopathy
Situational syncope	· Normal physical examination and ECG · Triggers such as coughing episodes, urination or defaecation and not a breed predisposed to arrhythmogenic cardiopathy
Syncope due to carotid sinus hypersensitivity	· Normal physical examination and ECG · Syncope associated with carotid sinus pressure and not a breed predisposed to arrhythmogenic cardiopathy
Syncope due to orthostatic hypotension	· When symptoms which occur with hypotension become evident, such as loss of blood volume or due to vasodilator drugs
Syncope due to structural cardiopathy	· Detection of murmur due to significant pulmonary, aortic or subaortic stenosis · Signs of left-sided heart failure in small breed and old dogs. In endemic areas suspicion of dirofilariasis
Syncope due to bradyarrhythmia or sinus node dysfunction	· When persistent sinus node bradycardia is documented <60 bpm during the daytime or the presence of episodes of sinoatrial block or sinus pauses >6–8 s
Syncope secondary to AV block	· Presence of episodes of complete AV block or second-degree high grade Mobitz type II
Syncope secondary to tachyarrhythmia	· When rapid sustained VT or SVT are documented · When frequent PVC are documented on ECG in consults of breeds predisposed to arrhythmogenic cardiopathy (Boxer and Dobermann)

History

The history should encompass **the symptoms before, during and after syncopal episodes**, their duration, and whether or not they are associated with coughing, exercise, rest or urination. Any **medications** the patient is taking should be noted.

It is helpful for the owner to **video episodes** of the dog or cat showing symptoms, since the owner's interpretation often does not coincide with that of the veterinarian.

The **description of a typical syncope** is as follows: it can be precipitated by exercise, excitement or coughing, but also when the animal is at rest. This is followed by a transient loss of consciousness, followed by a collapse or fall, usually in a lateral recumbent position. The patient appears flaccid or, quite the opposite, with stiff limbs, presence of opisthotonos, head turned back, and even urination and defaecation.

In dogs with **symptomatic bradyarrhythmias** (high-grade or complete second-degree AV block), the author has seen **syncope in resting** dogs and cats. Patients start looking disorientated and fall sideways, turn their heads back, some vocalize and, after a few seconds of limb movements, regain consciousness and normal behaviour.

Likewise, dogs with severe bradyarrhythmias may show significant tonic-clonic movements which must be differentiated from seizures due to cerebral hypoxia. In these cases, recovery to a normal state is generally slower. Cerebral hypoxia is considered to be responsible for the seizure threshold being passed.

In cats the clinical signs of syncope are highly variable:
- intermittent weakness and lethargy
- clinical signs with preserved consciousness: stumbling, ataxia, confused behaviour
- syncope
- cardiogenic convulsions
- sudden death.

Signalment

The following should be taken into account.
- **Dobermann and Boxer** dogs: in these breeds, it is most likely that syncope is due to rapid ventricular tachycardia, although it has been described in some cases due to vasodilation. Since both can occur in the same animal, diagnosis requires **24-hour Holter monitoring** to determine the cause, since the drugs administered for arrhythmias can increase the frequency of syncope.
- Miniature Schnauzers, West Highland White Terriers and American Cocker Spaniels: these breeds of dogs are highly predisposed to **sick sinus syndrome** due to a bradycardia-tachycardia heart rhythm which can cause syncope.
- Small breeds of dogs with advanced chronic degenerative mitral disease and those with severe pulmonary hypertension: may present with **neurally mediated syncope**, both during exercise and at rest.
- **Apparently healthy dogs**, even young ones, without signs of cardiovascular disease: can present syncope associated with excitement or intense exercise due to a reflex mechanism.

Appearance

When the episodes occur should be taken into consideration, such as:
- following activities such as coughing, urination, and defaecation: situational syncope;
- at the end of exercise: reflex syncope;
- associated with exercise: syncope of cardiac origin (ventricular tachycardia);
- at rest: symptomatic bradyarrhythmias such as complete AV block.

Symptoms

The main differential diagnosis includes **differentiating syncope from seizure activity/epilepsy**. Literature data indicates that in many cases of seizures, in some patients treated for months for epilepsy where no improvement is seen have turned out to be reflex syncope. The main cause of confusion is due to the fact that, although most syncope episodes present with flaccidity of the limbs, they can also present stiffness in extension and, as indicated above, tonic-clonic movements.

In epilepsy, seizures appear from the onset of the condition, are generalised and present broad movements that affect the entire limb, while in syncope patients initially present muscle hypotonia and only after several seconds of cerebral hypoperfusion can muscle movements of less amplitude than in epileptic seizures appear, that usually affect the most distal part of the upper extremities.

Hypersalivation or facial movements are rarely associated with syncope, except in cats, in which some facial movements that simulate partial seizures are frequent. When, following an episode of this type, the animal seeks water or food, a seizure should be suspected. Significant tonic-clonic motor activity should lead to suspicions of a seizure.

Physical Examination

A comprehensive physical examination is essential, and for the patient with syncope there should be particular emphasis on the **cardiovascular and neurological systems**. Certain findings, such as auscultation of a murmur, arrhythmia, or gallop, may suggest possible heart disease, although they are not necessarily related to the cause of syncope.

In patients with a normal physical examination and syncope associated with intense exercise, once an arrhythmia has been excluded, it may be useful to exercise them and evaluate the response together with a neurologist.

Cats with seizures and physical examination findings consistent with heart disease should be further evaluated using ECG and echocardiography, to identify or exclude heart disease as the cause.

Diagnostic Tests

Electrocardiogram (ECG)

When an arrhythmia is detected on physical exam, a surface ECG is indicated in order to classify the arrythmia's characteristics. However, in cases of suspected transient arrhythmias not detectable during a routine examination, as sometimes occurs in Boxer and Dobermann dogs, **24-hour Holter monitoring** (Figure 1) or event monitors are recommended.

In cases of bradycardia, sick sinus syndrome, or high grade 2nd and 3rd degree AV blocks, **the atropine test** is recommended. The author administers atropine 0.04 mg/kg SC and performs a new ECG at 30 minutes. In animals with normal sinus node function, the heart rate increases to 180 beats/minute. Dogs with high vagal tone may show significant sinus bradycardia, so a positive atropine test suggests these dogs may respond to treatment with anticholinergic drugs.

Echocardiography

Echocardiography in patients with a murmur helps identify underlying structural heart disease which may be the cause of syncope. Indeed, Doppler echocardiography makes it

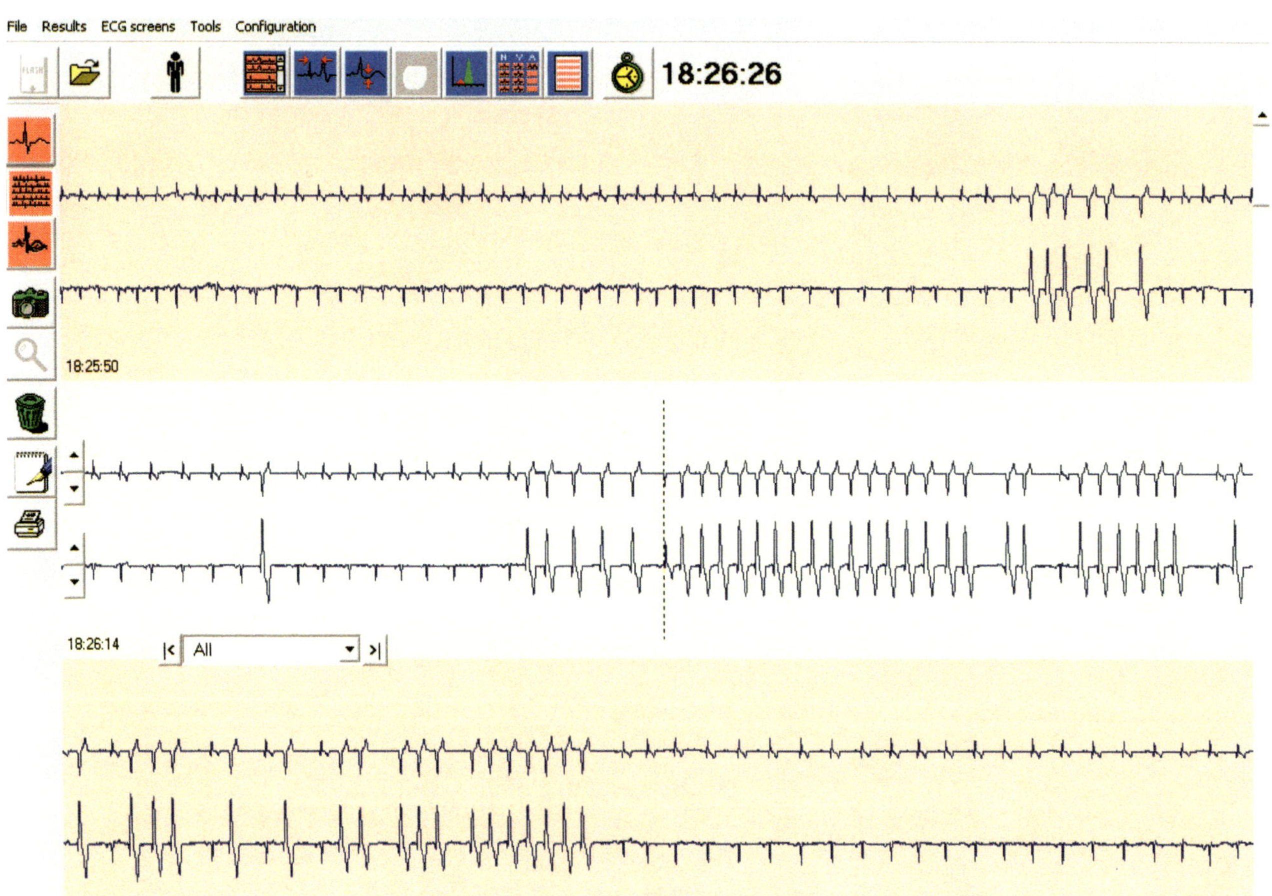

Figure 1. Image showing ECG traces from a dog with syncope where 24 h Holter monitoring was performed. Ventricular arrhythmias can be seen consistent with isolated and double ventricular complexes and episodes of ventricular tachycardia.

possible to document the severity of pulmonary hypertension or ventricular outflow tract obstructions, by assessing the Doppler pressure gradient.

Thoracic Radiographs

Radiography is an important tool for use in patients with congestive heart failure, pulmonary thromboembolism, or other pulmonary diseases such as angiostrongyliasis or pulmonary fibrosis.

Arterial Blood Pressure (AP)

Periodic evaluation of BP is recommended in patients presenting with syncope who receive vasodilator drugs, ACE inhibitors or antiarrhythmic drugs.

Laboratory Tests

In specific cases where the physical examination is not conclusive, performing a complete blood count and biochemistry with electrolytes, together with endocrine studies (hypothyroidism, hypoadrenocorticism) and tests to diagnose dirofilariasis in endemic areas are recommended. Measurement of serum cardiac troponin (TnIc) can help in the differentiation of syncope of cardiac origin and seizures.

Treatment

Treatment of these patients is aimed at controlling the cause of syncope once it has been identified.

Syncope of Cardiac Origin

In principle, syncope due to cardiac causes is usually the easiest to treat, despite being the most serious.

- **Symptomatic bradyarrhythmias** (sick sinus syndrome, atrial standstill (Figure 2), high grade 2nd degree and 3rd degree AV blocks). The treatment of choice is implantation of a permanent pacemaker. In dogs with sinus bradycardia and a positive response to atropine, anticholinergic drugs such as hyoscyamine (0.005 mg/kg/8 h) have been recommended.
- **Ventricular tachyarrhythmias**: sotalol or atenolol together with mexiletine are the **drugs that shown to be most effective**.
- **Supraventricular tachyarrhythmias**: radiofrequency therapy may be necessary for arrhythmias such as AV reentry tachycardia.

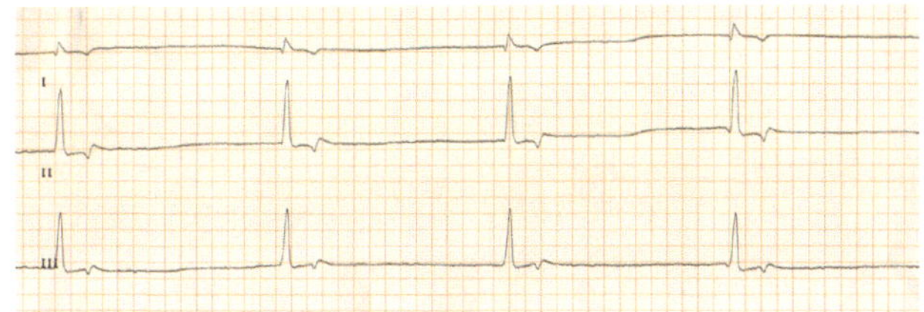

Figure 2. Surface ECG in a Springer Spaniel with episodes of syncope, showing atrial standstill. Note that P waves can be seen, and the ventricular frequency is 40 beats/minute (50 mm/s; 0.5 cm = 1 mV).

- **Structural heart disease**: therapy for congestive failure (pimobendan, ACEI, diuretics, spironolactone) or balloon valvuloplasty in pathologies that present with obstruction of the ventricular outflow tracts.
- **Pulmonary hypertension (PH)**: sildenafil (1 mg/kg/8 h) is the drug of choice in patients with moderate-severe PH with syncope, in addition to treating the cause of it.

Syncope of Reflex or Neurally Mediated Origin

The treatment of this type of syncope is complex and not well standardised in animals. In general, it does not require special therapeutic measures beyond informing the owner of the animal about the benign nature of the condition. Still, the following recommendations can be considered.

- **Vasovagal syncope**. It is desirable to reduce the stressors that trigger sympathetic activity, although this is not always achievable in animals. The use of β-blockers has been suggested, although there is no consensus that they work in dogs. In severe cases, the implantation of a pacemaker may be necessary since it can be difficult to differentiate bradycardias due to a reflex mechanism from those due to sinus dysfunction.
- **Situational syncope**. Actions to avoid the trigger factors are necessary. In patients with cough syncope, control of the tracheobronchial disease together with cough suppressants is the therapy of choice to avoid syncopal episodes.
- **Syncope due to carotid sinus hypersensitivity**. In the author's experience, dogs with this type of syncope improve when the collar is replaced by a harness, since the cause is pressure on the carotid sinus by the collar when pulling on walks.

Syncope Due to Orthostatic Hypotension

Treating the causes of hypotension is necessary and rehydration measures should be actioned.

Prognosis

Syncope due to structural heart disease has a reserved prognosis depending on the specific cause, so determining the risk factors is essential.

Thus, the conditions with highest risk are dilated cardiomyopathy, arrhythmogenic right ventricular cardiomyopathy and systolic dysfunction, hypertrophic cardiomyopathy, and pulmonary, and aortic stenosis. All these cardiopathies can present with loss of myocytes and substitution by fibrosis and fat, interstitial fibrosis and, sometimes, myocardial ischaemia.

In all these cases, sudden death can occur even when antiarrhythmic treatment is implemented, as occurs in young Dobermann, Boxer, and German Shepherd dogs with ventricular arrhythmias.

Also, reflex bradycardias in dogs with chronic degenerative mitral disease and pulmonary oedema can be fatal.

Although data in the literature suggest that syncope of reflex origin is benign in terms of survival and, in many cases, with a self-limiting course, there are also references to sudden death in dogs in extreme situations of stress or intense fear.

Bibliography

- Barnett, L., Martin, M.W.S., Todd, J. (2011) A retrospective study of 153 cases of undiagnosed collapse, syncope or exercise intolerance: the outcomes. *J Small Anim Pract*, 52, pp. 26–31.
- Cote, E., MacDonald, K.A., Meurs, K.M., et al. (2011) *Feline Cardiology*. Iowa: Willey-Blackwell, pp. 13–17.
- Kraus, M., Thomason, J.D., Calvert, C.A. (2008) Syncope. In: Bonagura, J.D., Twedt, D. (eds.). *Kirk's Current Veterinary Therapy XIV*. 14th Ed. Saunders, pp. 324–331.
- Moya-i-Mitjans, A., Rivas-Gandara, N., Sarrias-Merce, A. et al. (2012) Síncope. *Rev Esp Cardiol*, 65, pp. 755–765.
- Penning, V.A., Connolly, D.J., Gajanayake, I. et al. (2009) Seizure-Like Episodes in 3 Cats with Intermittent High-Grade Atrioventricular Dysfunction. *J Vet Intern Med*, 23, pp. 200–205.
- Rasmussen, C.E., Falk, T., Domanjko, A. et al. (2014) Holter Monitoring of Small Breed Dogs with Advanced Myxomatous Mitral Valve Disease with and without a History of Syncope. *J Vet Intern Med*, 28, pp. 363–370.
- Shen, W.K., Sheldon, R.S., Benditt, D.G. (2017) ACC/AHA/HRS guideline for the evaluation and management of patients with syncope: A report of the American College of Cardiology/American Heart Association Task Force on Clinical Practice Guidelines and the Heart Rhythm Society. *Heart Rhythm*, 14:e155–e217.
- Thomason, J.D., Kraus, M.S., Surdyk, K.K., et al. (2008) Bradycardia-associated syncope in 7 Boxers with ventricular tachycardia (2002–2005). *J Vet Intern Med*, 22, pp. 931–6.

Test

Answers on Page 182

1. Which of the following statements is false?

a. Syncope is a disease.
b. Syncope is a clinical sign.
c. During syncope, there is loss of consciousness.
d. During collapse, there is loss of muscle tone.

2. Which of the following is true regarding syncope:

a. It is due to a sudden drop in glucose in the brain.
b. It is due to a sudden interruption of blood flow to the brain.
c. It is due to a cortical neuronal problem.
d. It is due to a problem related to cataplexy.

3. Which of the following causes of syncope is rare in cats?

a. Symptomatic bradyarrhythmias.
b. Syncope due to carotid sinus hypersensitivity.
c. Ventricular tachycardia.
d. Hypertrophic cardiomyopathy.

4. Which of the following statements is false regarding situational syncope?

a. Coughing is a frequent cause of this type of syncope in small breed dogs.
b. The mechanism is related to the Hering nerve, which sends signals to the vasomotor centre in the brain.
c. Physical examination and ECG are normal.
d. Urination as a cause of situational syncope is due to vagal activation of the mechanoreceptors of the bladder and pelvic nerve.

5. What is the most likely cause of syncope in a Miniature Schnauzer?

a. Ventricular tachycardia.
b. Subaortic stenosis.
c. Sick sinus syndrome.
d. Situational syncope.

6. Regarding the treatment of syncope, which of the following is false?

a. Hyoscyamine can be used to treat sinus bradycardia that does not respond to the atropine test.
b. To treat carotid sinus pressure syncope, changing the collar for a harness is recommended.
c. The recommended treatment in dogs with syncope secondary to symptomatic bradyarrhythmias is permanent pacemaker implantation.
d. In Boxer dogs with ventricular arrhythmias that worsen upon initiation of treatment with β-blockers, 24-hour Holter monitoring should be performed to rule out vagal reflex bradyarrhythmias.

Correct Answers:

1. a
2. b
3. b
4. b
5. c
6. a

Notes

Pulmonary Hypertension and *Cor Pulmonale*

Mª Josefa Fernández-del Palacio

Pulmonary hypertension (PH) is a complex and progressive cardiopulmonary disorder. PH is characterised by high pulmonary vascular resistance, sustained vasoconstriction, progressive vascular remodelling, and irreversible right ventricular dysfunction. PH is a haemodynamic and pathophysiological abnormality, which involves and complicates multiple cardiovascular and respiratory diseases, with limited treatment options, and a **poor prognosis**.

PH is a relatively frequent diagnosis in canine practice, **but is only diagnosed sporadically in cats. The diagnosis can be made non-invasively** (cardiac catheterization is not necessary) thanks to specialist veterinarians and ultrasound.

The following chapter reviews:

- an overview of pulmonary circulation
- definitions
- clinical classification
- causative mechanisms
- clinical signs
- diagnosis
- treatment.

An Overview of the Pulmonary Circulation

The pulmonary circulation constitutes a low pressure, low resistance, and high compliance vascular system. The range of pressures in normal pulmonary arteries in dogs and cats are as follows:

- systolic: 15–25 mmHg
- diastolic: 5–10 mmHg
- mean: 10–15 mmHg.

The **low physiological pressure within the pulmonary arteries** and vessels of the pulmonary parenchyma, means minimal changes in intravascular pressure will change the haemodynamics within the pulmonary circulation.

In the pulmonary circulation, only the small muscular arteries and arterioles have vasoactive properties; these are the resistant vessels or precapillary vessels. **Pulmonary vasoconstriction is a normal response to alveolar hypoxia**, which allows adjustment of pulmonary perfusion to alveolar ventilation to ensure the ventilation/perfusion ratio is optimal. Also, the pulmonary circulation is unique in terms of its double function of gas exchange and pulmonary circulation haemodynamics. The latter is related to its function regarding the regulation of systemic blood pressure, via synthesis of Ag II and endothelin in numerous pulmonary endothelial cells.

Definitions of PH

PH is defined as a sustained increase (above reference values) in pulmonary arterial pressure.

In human medicine, a patient is considered to have PH when the mean **pulmonary arterial pressure (PAP)** is ≥25 mmHg or systolic PAP is ≥35 mmHg at rest, when evaluated using right ventricular catheterization. In dogs and cats, the PAP is evaluated clinically using Doppler echocardiography. The overall consensus indicates that PH exists when systolic arterial blood pressure is ≥30 mmHg at rest.

When PH is associated with pulmonary or thoracic diseases, it is called ***cor pulmonale***.

Classification of Pulmonary Hypertension

PH has conventionally been classified as **primary** (idiopathic) and **secondary** (to pulmonary, cardiac or systemic conditions), depending on the presence or absence of identified causes or risk factors. More recently, **pathophysiological, haemodynamic, and clinical mechanisms** have been used to classify patients with PH (Box 1).

The **main cause of PH in dogs is heart disease affecting the left side of the heart**, such as chronic degenerative mitral disease, dilated cardiomyopathy and, to a lesser extent, left ventricular outflow tract obstruction. The second most common cause of PH are primary pulmonary diseases (pulmonary fibrosis, tracheobronchial disease), followed by congenital defects (septal defects and patent *ductus arteriosus*) which cause blood shunting, thromboembolic diseases, and dirofilariasis (except in endemic areas) and to a lesser extent miscellaneous causes such as neoplasms and immune-mediated haemolytic anaemia.

Box 1. Classification of Pulmonary Hypertension According to its Pathophysiological, Haemodynamic and Clinical Mechanisms

HAEMODYNAMIC CLASSIFICATION. Two types are considered.

- **Precapillary PH.** Pulmonary capillary pressure or left ventricular pressure at the end of diastole is ≤15 mmHg (assessed by right ventricular catheterization). Causes include:
  - — primary PH
  - — PH due to lung conditions
  - — PH due to thromboembolic conditions.
- **Postcapillary PH.** Pulmonary capillary pressure or left ventricular pressure at the end of diastole is >15 mmHg (assessed by right ventricular catheterization).
  - — It mainly includes PH due to left-sided heart diseases.

CLINICAL CLASSIFICATION. Six categories are considered with their corresponding causes.

1. **Arterial PH:** idiopathic PH (little referenced in dogs and not at all in cats), congenital conditions with systemic-pulmonary shunts, vascular collagen diseases and Eisenmenger syndrome.
2. **PH associated with left sided heart diseases:** chronic degenerative mitral disease, valvular endocarditis, congenital mitral dysplasia, cardiomyopathies, aortic stenosis etc.
3. **PH associated with pulmonary diseases and/ or hypoxaemia:** chronic obstructive pulmonary conditions (collapse of the trachea/main bronchi, bronchomalacia), interstitial pulmonary conditions (interstitial pulmonary fibrosis, eosinophilic pneumonia, infectious pneumonia, alveolar proteinosis, diffuse pulmonary neoplasia), altitude sickness and reactive arterial pulmonary vasoconstriction (hypoxia due to pulmonary oedema).
4. **PH associated with thromboembolic diseases:** embolism, pulmonary thromboembolism, acute and chronic.
5. **PH associated with parasitic diseases:** *Dirofilaria* or *Angiostrongylus* infection.
6. **PH associated with multifactorial or unknown mechanisms** (miscellaneous): chronic haemolytic anaemia, lymphadenopathy, systemic conditions, neoplasms compressing pulmonary arteries etc.

Pathophysiology of Pulmonary Hypertension

General Pathophysiological Mechanisms

Regardless of the type of PH, the central pathophysiological mechanisms that cause the clinical development of PH are **changes in the pulmonary arteries and arterioles**, due to poor adaptation of their phenotype to the causative agent. The mechanism that initiates PH is **endothelial dysfunction**, which, in turn, causes **an imbalance between the production of vasoconstrictor and vasodilator agents**. This has an effect on smooth muscle cells, thrombotic mediators, and inflammatory cytokines (Figure 1). As a consequence, there is a migration and proliferation of muscle cells towards the small precapillary pulmonary arterioles, (which normally lack a smooth muscle layer) resulting **in the abnormal presence of myofibroblasts**.

This cell proliferation causes **narrowing of the vascular lumen** and an inability to dilate with the subsequent increase in pressure. In very advanced stages there are areas of disorganised neovascularization, called **plexiform lesions.** In addition to the proliferation of the medial layer of smooth muscle, there are alterations of the extracellular matrix. Vasoactive mediators converge in the calcium in the cytosol, which triggers smooth muscle contraction. Since the small vessels contribute to resistance, there is an increase in pressure transmitted to the large vessels, reducing compliance in the proximal arteries. The net effect is transmitted to the right ventricle and eventually leads to congestive heart failure.

Specific Pathophysiological Mechanisms

Arterial PH

Congenital heart defects that cause blood shunts from the systemic to the pulmonary circulation can cause PH.

The increase in blood flow to the lungs from the systemic to the pulmonary circulation through a septal defect or CAP generates an increase in pressure and circumferential distention of the pulmonary arterial walls. This causes stress on the intima with endothelial cells, which promotes **increased pulmonary vascular resistance** and remodelling (hypertrophy).

This is a panvasculopathy, meaning that **all layers of the vascular wall** are involved. As the lesions progress and the obstruction of the vascular lumen grows, in some animals the deviation becomes bidirectional, or is mostly from the pulmonary to the systemic circulation (Eisenmenger syndrome). The size of the defect and, therefore, of the shift in blood and individual predisposition dictate the development of PH.

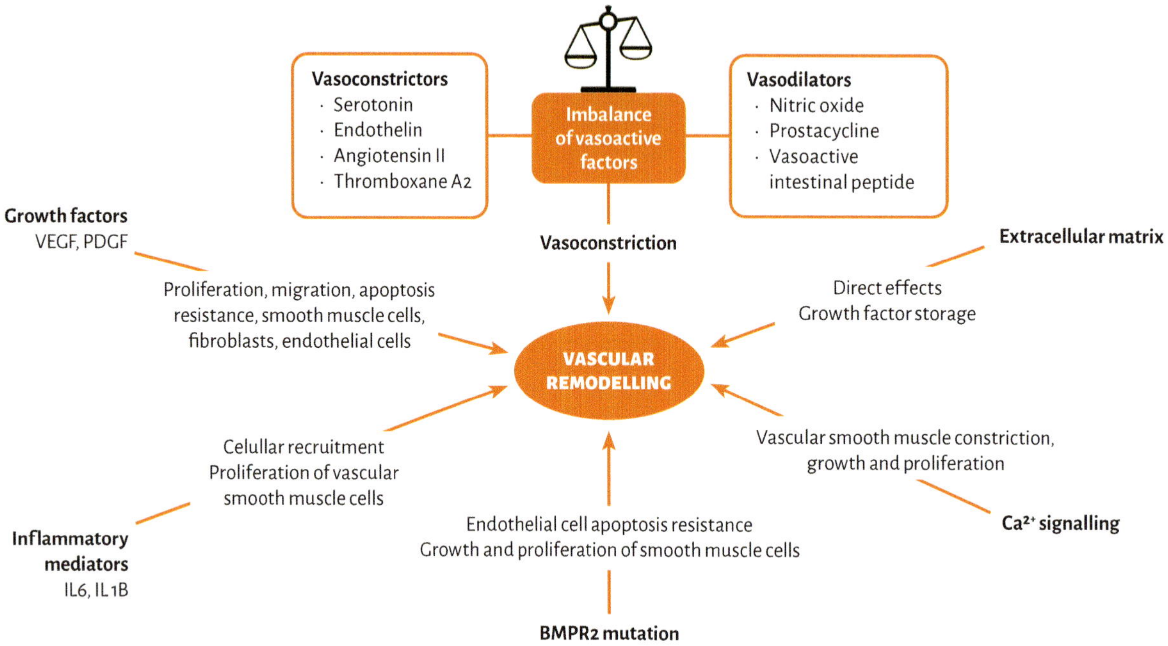

Figure 1. Pathophysiological mechanisms behind arterial pulmonary hypertension. (PDGF: platelet derived growth factor, FGF: foetal growth factor, VEGF: vascular endothelial growth factor, IL: interleukin, BMPR2: bone morphogenetic protein receptor type II).

PH Associated with Left-sided Heart Diseases

During the course of these heart diseases, there is a **progressive increase in pulmonary venous pressure which is transmitted to the venous capillaries**. This causes an increase in the vascular tone of the arteries and/or remodelling of these vessels, possibly due to reflex vasoconstriction of the pulmonary arteries, decreased oxygen levels, and desensitization to natriuretic peptides, which contribute to the extent of PH.

The structural changes translate into thickening of the alveolar capillary membrane, hypertrophy of the tunica media, fibrosis of the tunica intima and adventitia, and occlusion of the lumen of small vessels. All of these changes are adaptive, as they protect against pulmonary oedema due to chronic increases in ventricular filling pressures. As left chamber dysfunction progresses, the right ventricle begins to disengage with the pulmonary artery, leading to RV dysfunction and ultimately systemic venous congestion, kidney dysfunction, and ascites.

PH Associated with Pulmonary Diseases and/or Hypoxaemia

Severe conditions of the lung parenchyma or fibrosis cause destruction and reduction of the pulmonary vascular bed, stimulating hypoxic vasoconstriction, and increasing pulmonary vascular resistance.

PH associated with chronic lung conditions is related to hypoxia, persistent inflammation with marked expression of growth factors, vasoactive mediators and increased vascular stress. Furthermore, vasoconstriction is related to the enhanced activity of thromboxane and endothelin 1. The result is morphological changes in the pulmonary arteries such as muscle hypertrophy, proliferation of the tunica intima and fibrosis, and increased extracellular matrix deposition.

PH Associated with Thromboembolic Diseases

Obstructive pulmonary vascular diseases can be the **consequence of thromboembolism, pulmonary thrombosis, or dirofilariasis**.

Vascular obstruction mechanically affects the pulmonary vascular area, since organised thrombi replace the tunica intima of the proximal and distal arteries, adhering to the tunica media and causing varying degrees of stenosis or occlusion of the vascular lumen.

In dogs and cats, dirofilariasis causes proliferative lesions of the tunica intima of the pulmonary arteries, obstruction due to dead worms, and inflammation of the surrounding parenchyma which damages vascularization, causing sustained PH.

Impact of PH on the Heart

Increased pulmonary vascular resistance and pressure in the pulmonary artery impose a **pressure overload on the right ventricle, which results in hypertrophy**.

Normally, RV myocardial perfusion is maintained in both systole and diastole due to low intraventricular pressures. When PH is severe, RV perfusion depends on diastolic pressure and duration of diastole (heart rate), and any change in these factors can lead to reduced RV function and cardiac output (CO). The interventricular septum flattens and protrudes into the LV, interfering with its diastolic filling and raising diastolic pressure and lowering the CO. The interventricular septum contributes to both LV and RV function and is responsible for one-third of the RV work under normal conditions. All this contributes to increasing RV afterload and, in advanced stages, triggers right congestive heart failure.

Diagnosis

The diagnostic plan for PH is based on clinical suspicions arising from the symptoms and physical examination. With the data obtained, complementary diagnostic tests (thoracic radiographs, echocardiography, computed tomography – CT –) are selected to confirm the haemodynamic criteria are met and describe the aetiology and severity of the functional and haemodynamic involvement. It is important to also **establish if there is more than one cause of PH**.

Clinical signs are generally nonspecific to PH, since most patients begin with signs of the causative condition, and signs corresponding to RV dysfunction appear only in advanced stages. The most common signs manifest with exercise, such as **tachypnoea, dyspnoea, weakness, and syncope**. The presence of coughing is less common. In severe cases, the signs also appear at rest and, as the process progresses, patients may present with right congestive heart failure with ascites. In other cases, the appearance of PH can be modified and masked by the diseases that cause PH or other concurrent conditions.

General physical examination is characterised by **changes in cardiac auscultation** such as doubling of the second heart sound, a pansystolic murmur due to tricuspid regurgitation, a diastolic murmur due to pulmonary regurgitation, and **abnormalities in lung sounds** such as crackles in cases of pulmonary parenchyma or airway obstruction. In advanced stages with severe PH, elevated jugular venous pressure, hepatomegaly, and ascites may be observed.

Cardiac catheterization is the most accurate method for directly measuring pressures in the pulmonary artery, through the introduction of a catheter. However, given the invasive nature and the fact that many patients are in a critical condition, this method is not performed routinely and is only performed in specific complex cases or in an experimental setting.

Thoracic radiographs are abnormal in most patients with PH at the time of diagnosis (Figure 2). The main findings include an increased size of the silhouette of the main pulmonary artery (in contrast to the peripheral arteries) and of the right-sided chambers in advanced stages. Likewise, radiographs can help differentiate between arterial or venous PH depending on whether the artery/vein ratio is lower or higher. Infiltrates in the pulmonary parenchyma are common when there is an underlying disease.

In patients with PH due to dirofilariasis, lobar pulmonary arteries are enlarged in the centre, tortuous and thin in the peripheries, together with protrusion of the silhouette of the main pulmonary artery and, sometimes the RV. In general, widening of the lobar arteries without coexisting venous distention of the veins is highly suggestive of PH.

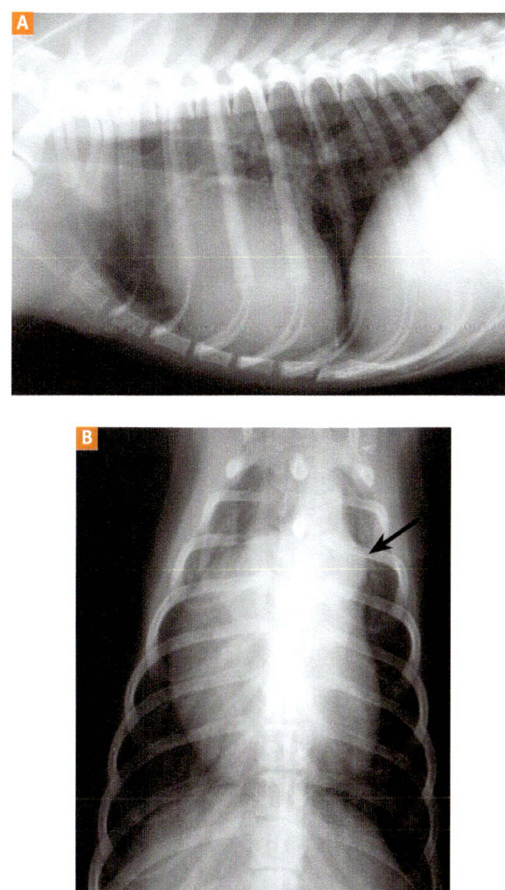

Figure 2. Lateral and ventrodorsal thoracic radiographs of a dog with severe pulmonary hypertension which show an increase in size of the silhouette of the right-sided cardiac chambers and the main pulmonary artery (arrow).

However, the severity of PH does not always correlate with radiographic abnormalities, so **apparently normal images do not exclude the presence of PH**.

Transthoracic echocardiography is the standard non-invasive imaging modality to visualize the effects of PH on the heart, estimate pulmonary artery pressure using continuous Doppler, and determine possible causes of PH (e.g. left-sided heart lesions or congenital defects).

The most characteristic findings determined using 2D, M, and colour and spectral Doppler modes are the following.

- Variable degrees of **RV hypertrophy** (concentric or eccentric) and dilatation of the right atrium (Figure 3) and main pulmonary artery (Figure 4).
- **Flat interventricular septum** and paradoxical septal movement (Figure 5). In cases of moderate-severe PH, a decrease in the size of the left-sided chambers is observed.
- **Hypertrophy of the RV free wall** and interventricular septum in patients with Eisenmenger syndrome.
- Presence of **septal defects or patent *ductus arteriosus*** in cases of precapillary PH, as well as bidirectional or systemic pulmonary shunts, using colour Doppler.
- Alterations to the left-sided chambers, myocardium or valves in cases of postcapillary PH.
- **Visualization of a possible thrombus or *Dirofilaria*** in the main pulmonary artery.
- **Evaluation of pulmonary arterial pressure using colour and spectral Doppler**. Colour Doppler helps to identify the presence of flow due to tricuspid (Figure 6) and pulmonary (Figure 7) regurgitation. In addition, by placing the cursor on the appropriate point, the speed of tricuspid (V) and pulmonary regurgitation can be accurately measured using spectral Doppler with subsequent transformation into a Doppler pressure gradient (DPG) using the modified Bernoulli formula DPG = $4V^2$. Pulmonary hypertension is considered to be present when the velocity of tricuspid regurgitation is >2.8 m/s (DPG = 31.6 mmHg) and the velocity of pulmonary regurgitation is >2.2 m/s (DPG = 19.36 mmHg) (Figure 6). The grade of severity is shown in Table 1.
- **The Doppler spectrum of pulmonary flow changes with the severity of PH**, showing rapid acceleration and abrupt deceleration with a dent (Figure 8). The ratio of acceleration time/ejection time (AT/ET) of pulmonary flow can be used to predict PH, especially when tricuspid regurgitation is not present or could not be measured.

Computed tomography (CT) is an increasingly affordable technique for veterinary patients and provides important information about vascular, cardiac, parenchymal, and mediastinal abnormalities, as well as important prognostic information. Specifically, this imaging technique visualises the pulmonary parenchyma in detail, facilitating the diagnosis of interstitial lung diseases and emphysema, e.g. pulmonary fibrosis in West Highland White Terriers.

Table 1. Grades of severity of pulmonary hypertension (PH) according to tricuspid regurgitation (TR) velocity and the corresponding Doppler pressure gradient (DPG).

Velocity	Mild PH	Moderate PH	Severe PH
Tricuspid regurgitation (m/s)	2.8–3.5	3.5–4.3	>4.3
TR systolic DPG (mmHg)	31.4–50	50–75	>75

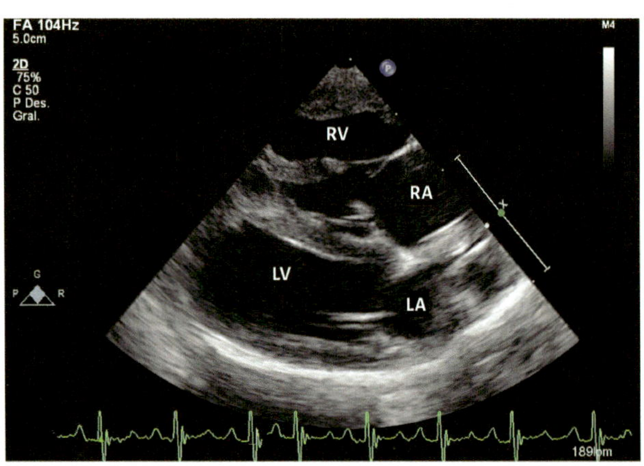

Figure 3. Two-dimensional echocardiogram, right parasternal approach, four chamber long axis, of a dog with PH. Dilation of the right-sided cardiac chambers, reduction in size of the left-sided ones and displacement of the interventricular septum towards the left ventricle (LV), due to the increased pressure in the right ventricle (RV). (RA: right atrium, LA: left atrium).

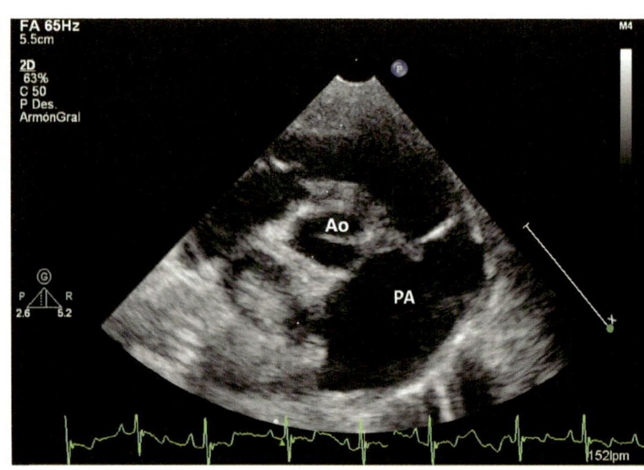

Figure 4. Two-dimensional echocardiogram, right parasternal approach, short axis at the level of the aorta (Ao) and pulmonary artery (PA) of a dog with PH, with significant dilation of the main pulmonary artery.

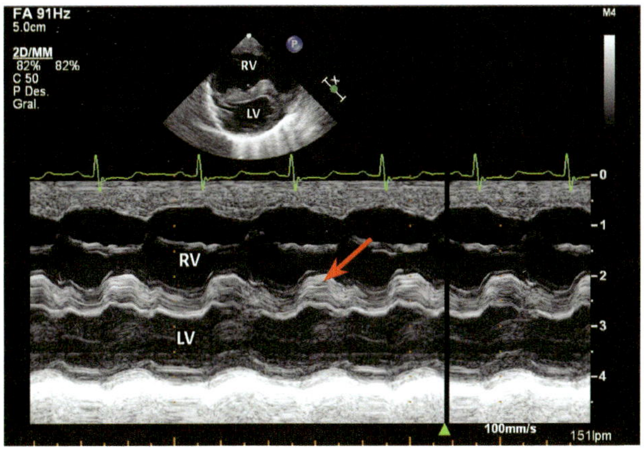

Figure 5. M-mode echocardiogram, right parasternal approach, short axis at a ventricular level, of a dog with PH. Significant dilation of the right ventricle can be seen as well as paradoxical septal movement in systole (arrow).

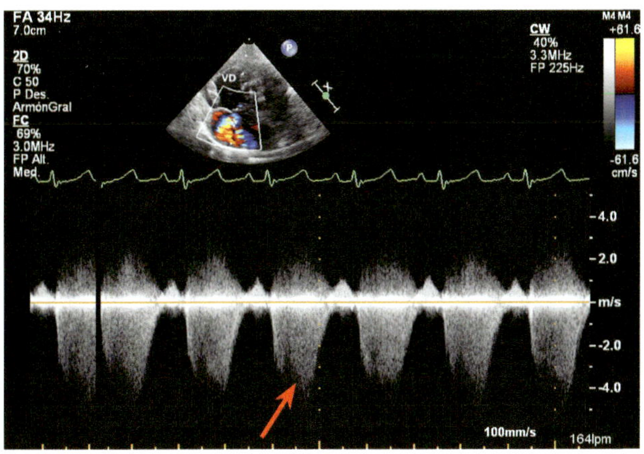

Figure 6. Continuous Doppler echocardiogram via a left apical approach, optimised to visualise the right-sided chambers. High speed (4 m/s) systolic tricuspid regurgitation (arrow) flow can be seen compatible with PH.

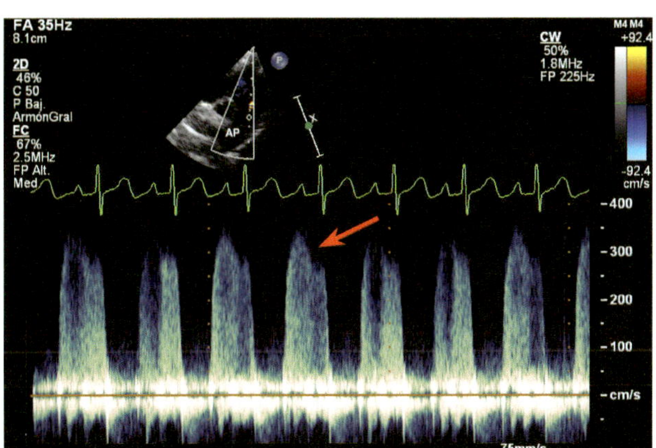

Figure 7. Continuous Doppler echocardiogram obtained using a right parasternal approach, short axis at the level of the aorta and pulmonary artery. High speed (3.5 m/s) diastolic pulmonary regurgitation (arrow) flow can be seen compatible with PH.

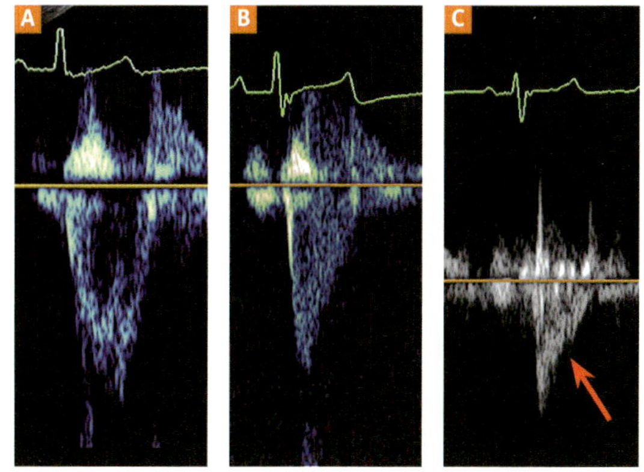

Figure 8. Doppler profiles of systolic flow in the pulmonary artery. **A**. Normal dog with type 1 spectrum, where the acceleration and deceleration curves are similar. **B**. Type II pulmonary spectrum consistent with a dog with moderate pulmonary hypertension (PH), where the peak of maximum velocity occurs at the start of systole, the acceleration is rapid, and the deceleration is slower. **C**. Doppler spectrum type III from a dog with severe PH where rapid acceleration and a dent (arrow) in the deceleration phase is seen, caused by the reverse flow from the pulmonary artery.

In most patients with PH the ECG is normal. When significant RV hypertrophy is present, signs of right-sided chamber enlargement may be seen such as tall P waves, right deviation of the electrical axis in the frontal plane and deep S waves on leads I, II, III and aVF (mainly in patients with Eisenmenger syndrome). However, it is neither a sensitive nor a specific technique for the detection of PH and, as with thoracic radiographs, **a normal ECG does not exclude the presence of PH**.

Laboratory tests are not used to diagnose PH, but they are useful to **identify diseases associated with PH and assess the patient's condition**. Tests should include complete blood count, biochemistry, thyroid function, coagulation tests, D-dimer (when thromboembolism is suspected), and

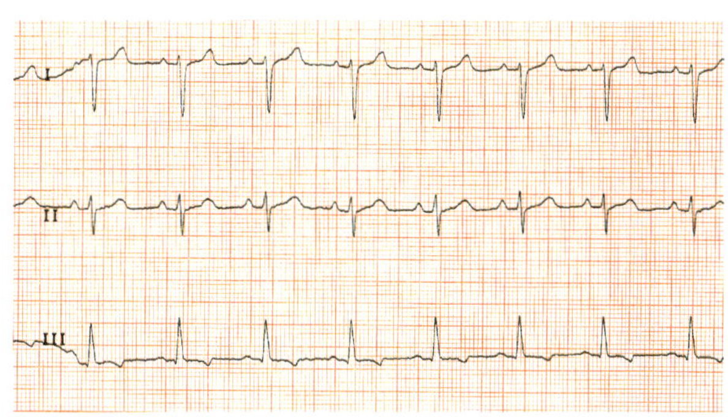

Figure 9. Surface electrocardiogram of a dog with PH associated with a reverse patent *ductus arteriosus* (Eisenmenger syndrome) with deep S waves on leads I and II and an electrical axis on the frontal place of +155°, compatible with right ventricular hypertrophy (50 mm/s, 0.5 cm = 1 mV).

specific tests for the diagnosis of dirofilariasis. Measurement of arterial blood gases provides information on the existence of hypoxia and acidosis which contribute to hypertension.

The biomarker NT-proBNP may be elevated in patients with PH, providing in an independent predictor of risk in these patients.

Treatment

Despite advances in new classes of drugs for the treatment of pathological pulmonary vasoreactivity, the majority of patients with PH are not cured and the prognosis is poor. For this reason, the goals of treatment are to improve the clinical signs and quality of life of patients, as well as treat the underlying cause if established.

The general principles of PH treatment include:

- **reduction of physical activity**: adapted to each patient so they are able to exercise without symptoms;
- **oxygen therapy** when there is chronic hypoxaemia or in acute crises, to achieve an O_2 saturation >90%;
- **vasodilator agents** specific to pulmonary arteries, aimed at controlling pulmonary arterial vasoconstriction and endothelial dysfunction. The main groups of drugs in human medicine include:
    - **prostacyclin analogues**: epoprostenol, treprostinil, iloprost, beraprost
    - **endothelin receptor antagonists**: bosentan, sitaxentan
    - **phosphodiesterase inhibitors** present in the pulmonary arteries. These are the most widely used in dogs and cats for the treatment of PH. There are two types:
        - **selective phosphodiesterase V inhibitors**, such as sildenafil and tadalafil. They exert their vasodilator action on the main pulmonary arteries, since degradation of cGMP results in relaxation of the smooth muscles of pulmonary vessels, with little action on the systemic circulation. Studies in dogs with PH secondary to pulmonary diseases, Eisenmenger syndrome, and left-sided congestive heart failure, have shown that sildenafil is well tolerated, contributes to reducing pulmonary pressure, improving quality of life and prolonging survival. The dose for dogs' ranges from 0.5 to 2 mg/kg/8–12 h. The author recommends 1 mg/kg/8 h PO;
        - **phosphodiesterase III inhibitors**, such as pimobendan, also known as an inodilators or calcium sensitizers, exert their vasodilator action on the small and large pulmonary arteries, enhancing adrenergic relaxation. Due to their dual vasodilator and inotropic action, they are especially indicated for the treatment of PH secondary to left-sided congestive heart failure.
- **calcium channel blockers** such as diltiazem may be an alternative due to their vasodilator properties, although the long-term benefit is unclear as they can cause significant systemic hypotension.

Treatment of the Underlying Cause of PH (if known)

Left-sided Congestive Heart Failure

Patients with left-sided congestive heart failure (cardiomyopathies and chronic mitral degenerative disease) should be adequately treated with ACE inhibitors, appropriate doses of diuretics (furosemide, torsemide), aldosterone inhibitors (spironolactone), digoxin, and inodilators (pimobendan).

Chronic Respiratory Conditions

Treatment of patients with PH secondary to chronic respiratory conditions depends on the aetiology and the clinical signs in the patient. In general, treatment includes cough suppressants, bronchodilators, specific antibiotic therapy, and corticosteroids. Theophylline may be beneficial both due to its bronchodilator properties and the increase in diaphragmatic contractility, which reduces respiratory muscle fatigue. In addition, it inhibits phosphodiesterase's, inducing pulmonary vascular relaxation.

Eisenmenger Syndrome

Treatment for PH associated with Eisenmenger syndrome includes exercise restriction, periodic phlebotomies if there are clinical signs, and severe polycythaemia (haematocrit >68%) and/or hydroxyurea.

Thromboembolism

The treatment of patients with PH secondary to thromboembolism includes the **administration of anticoagulants** and specific treatment of the cause.

Dirofilariasis

In dogs and cats with PH secondary to cardiac dirofilariasis, treatment is aimed at stabilizing the patient and adequately treating the parasite infestation. When the parasite load is high, removing parasites by catheterization may be necessary.

In conclusion, the current treatment of PH in small animals is based on the following points:

- oxygen therapy
- treatment of the cause of PH
- sildenafil administration.

Bibliography

- Borgarelli, M., Abbott. J., Braz-Ruivo, L. et al. (2015) Prevalence and prognostic importance of pulmonary hypertension in dogs with myxomatous mitral valve disease. *J Vet Intern Med*, 29, pp. 569–74.
- Galié, N., Humbert. M., Vachiery, J.L. et al. (2016) 2015 ESC/ERS Guidelines for the diagnosis and treatment of pulmonary hypertension. *Eur Heart J*, 37, pp. 67–119.
- Kellihan, H.B., Stepien, R.L. (2010) Pulmonary hypertension in dogs: diagnosis and therapy. *Vet Clin North Am: Small Anim*, 40, pp. 623–641.
- Kellihan, H.B., Waller, K.R., Pinkos, A. et al. (2015) Acute resolution of pulmonary alveolar infiltrates in 10 dogs with pulmonary hypertension treated with sildenafil citrate: 2005–2014. *J Vet Cardiol*, 17, pp. 182–91.
- Murphy, L.A., Russell, N., Bianco, D. et al. (2017) Retrospective evaluation of pimobendan and sildenafil therapy for severe pulmonary hypertension due to lung disease and hypoxia in 28 dogs (2007–2013). *Vet Med Sci*, 3: 99–106.
- Nakamura, K., Yamasaki, M., Ohta, H. et al. (2011) Effects of sildenafil citrate on five dogs with Eisenmenger's syndrome. *J Small Anim Pract*, 52, pp. 595–8.
- Reinero, C., Visser, L.C., Kellihan, et al. (2020) ACVIM consensus statement guidelines for the diagnosis, classification, treatment, and monitoring of pulmonary hypertension in dogs. *J Vet Intern Med*, 34, pp. 549–573.
- Schober, K.E., Baade, H. (2006) Doppler Echocardiographic prediction of pulmonary hypertension in West Higland White Terriers with chronic pulmonary disease. *J Vet Intern Med*, 20, pp. 912–920.
- Tidholm, A., Höglund, K., Häggström, J. et al. (2015) Diagnostic Value of Selected Echocardiographic Variables to Identify Pulmonary Hypertension in Dogs with Myxomatous Mitral Valve Disease. *J Vet Intern Med*, 29, pp. 1510–7.
- Toshner, M., Tajsic, T. et al. (2010) Pulmonary hypertension: advances in pathogenesis and treatment. *British Med Bull*, 94, pp. 21–32.

Test

Answers on Page 194

1. Which of the following statements is false regarding pulmonary hypertension (PH):
   a. PH is very common in cats.
   b. PH can cause syncope.
   c. Chronic degenerative mitral disease is a common cause of right-sided congestive heart failure due to pulmonary hypertension.
   d. PH can occur in all age groups.

2. Regarding types of PH, which of the following statements is false?
   a. Arterial PH can occur as a consequence of systemic-pulmonary blood shunts.
   b. Hypertension associated with chronic degenerative mitral disease is the least common in dogs.
   c. In patients with precapillary PH, the LV end diastolic pressure is ≤15 mmHg.
   d. Postcapillary PH may appear secondary to dilated cardiomyopathy.

3. Regarding the pathophysiology of PH, which of the following statements is correct?
   a. There is an increase in pulmonary venous resistance.
   b. Chronic hypoxaemia protects against PH.
   c. An increase in pulmonary vascular resistance and right-sided congestive heart failure can occur.
   d. Thromboembolic disease is only associated with PH if the thrombi occur in the pulmonary tree.

4. Regarding PH, which of the following statements is correct?
   a. The presence of exercise intolerance in patients with PH is rare.
   b. Chronic hypoxia can cause PH.
   c. Wide ventricular septal defects protect against PH.
   d. Subaortic stenosis is a common cause of PH in Boxer dogs.

5. Regarding the diagnosis of PH, which of the following statements is correct?
   a. The tricuspid regurgitation murmur is pathognomonic.
   b. The electrocardiogram helps detect PH in the early hours of development.
   c. Thoracic radiographs show varying degrees of pulmonary hypoperfusion in most cases.
   d. Echocardiography allows the severity of PH to be measured based on the tricuspid regurgitation velocity and the Doppler pressure gradient between right ventricle and right atrium.

6. Regarding the treatment of PH, which of the following statements is correct?
   a. Mannitol is the diuretic of choice in right-sided congestive heart failure.
   b. Sildenafil is used in the treatment of PH because it inhibits aldosterone production.
   c. Sildenafil causes pulmonary vasodilation because it is a phosphodiesterase V inhibitor.
   d. Pimobendan is contraindicated in dogs with PH secondary to chronic degenerative mitral disease.

7. Indicate which molecule is not related to vasodilation of the pulmonary arteries:
   a. Nitric oxide.
   b. Diltiazem.
   c. Endothelin.
   d. Prostacyclin.

Notes

Correct Answers:

1. a
2. b
3. c
4. b
5. d
6. c
7. c

Notes

Cardiac Biomarkers

Ashley B. Saunders

The diagnosis and management of heart disease requires a variety of tests. For each patient it is important to **decide which are the most relevant and productive tests to perform**. When assessing heart disease, **basic laboratory tests** include a minimum data base (complete blood count, biochemistry profile, electrolytes, urinalysis) to determine if a patient has concurrent systemic disease, and monitor medical therapy to prevent adverse effects and drug interactions.

Cardiac biomarkers are blood-based tests used to assess the cardiovascular system. Biomarkers potentially improve the diagnosis and management of heart disease in dogs and cats. In veterinary cardiology, **cardiac troponins and natriuretic peptides** have been studied the most.

Signs of heart disease are often nonspecific and overlap with other diseases. In particular, with acute breathing difficulty it can be difficult to **differentiate between cardiac and respiratory causes**. Also, in many patients with cardiomyopathy, an audible heart murmur is not present, and in other cases a heart murmur does not mean cardiac distress is responsible for the symptoms. Cardiac imaging can be expensive and echocardiography in particular requires training. In which case, a cardiac biomarker can serve as additional information in the evaluation of heart disease.

Researched and proposed use of biomarkers in veterinary cardiology

- **Distinguishing between cardiac and non-cardiac causes of dyspnoea (dog, cat).**
- **Screening test for congenital heart disease (dog).**
- **Screening test for asymptomatic heart disease (dog, cat).**
- **Predicting severity of disease (dog, cat).**
- **Predicting risk of congestive heart failure (dog, cat).**
- **Assessing response to treatment (dog, cat).**
- **Predicting outcome (dog, cat).**

Types of Cardiac Biomarkers

Troponin

What It Is

Cardiac troponins are released from cardiac myocytes into circulation in response to myocardial damage. The troponin complex is made up of three subunits (cTnI, cTnT, cTnC) of which **cTnI and cTnT are cardiac specific** and have been evaluated in small animals.

Assays

Standard and high sensitivity assays are available for humans and can be used to measure cTnI concentrations in dogs and cats. The **high sensitivity assays** allows detection of much lower concentrations of cTnI. For example, lower detection limits for high sensitivity assays are 0.006 ng/ml compared to 0.2 ng/ml for standard assays. High sensitivity assays are preferred.

Utility

In normal dogs the circulating levels of cTnI are undetectable or low. Therefore, elevated cTnI concentrations indicate recent or on-going damage to the myocardium.

Obstacles

Troponin concentrations correlated with age in some studies where older dogs can have concentrations that overlap with disease. **Elevations can indicate underlying disease or increased cardiac myocyte turnover in older pets**. Elevated concentrations can occur with decreased glomerular filtration rate based on a study in which dogs with azotaemia had increased values compared to healthy dogs and dogs with heart disease and heart failure. Elevated concentrations can occur in hyperthyroid cats and cats with systemic hypertension. Additionally, while a high value indicates myocardial damage, the test is not specific for a particular disease.

B-type Natriuretic Peptide

What It Is

B-type natriuretic peptide (BNP) is released by cardiac myocytes primarily in the ventricle in response to stretch.

It is cleaved into two parts including an inactive N-terminal portion (NT-proBNP) with a longer half-life which can be measured in plasma and serum.

Assays

Multiple commercial assays are available for dogs and cats. Assays are species specific. A second-generation assay is able to detect higher concentrations of NT-proBNP. A **SNAP© point-of-care proBNP test is available for cats** through IDEXX laboratories.

Utility

High NT-proBNP concentrations can be an indicator of heart disease and heart failure, and in some cases correlate with the severity of disease. Testing the general population leads to false positive results. The ideal use is to test based on index of suspicion in animals suspected of having heart disease (auscultation abnormality, respiratory signs, heart disease in a related animal) or based on screening recommendations in specific diseases or breed groups.

Obstacles

Elevated values are reported in animals with kidney disease, systemic hypertension (cat), hyperthyroidism (cat), and pulmonary hypertension (dog), and increase with age. Biologic variability and breed variation are reported. Additionally, while high values suggest the presence of heart disease or heart failure, **the test is not specific for a particular disease**.

Cardiac Biomarkers: A Canine Literature Review

Healthy Dogs

In healthy dogs studies using different assays analysing samples, the reported median (range) cTnI were similar at **0.02 ng/ml (<0.03–0.07) in 41 dogs**, 0.03 ng/ml (0.01–0.15) in 176 dogs, and 0.017 ng/ml (0.006–0.128) in 24 dogs.

Congenital Heart Disease

Plasma NT-proBNP (ELISA assay) and phonocardiography were used to assess healthy dogs and dogs with innocent murmurs and congenital heart disease in a study including 186 asymptomatic dogs (83% Cairn Terriers). The median NT-proBNP was similar for 90 healthy puppies without a murmur (300 pmol/l; range: 102–1340) and 45 puppies with an innocent murmur based on echocardiography (326 pmol/l; range: 102–1224).

Higher NT-proBNP values were found in 31 dogs with congenital heart disease (1102 pmol/l; range: 102–8970), although some dogs with congenital heart disease (small patent *ductus arteriosus*, severe pulmonic stenosis, ventricular septal defect) did not have elevated NT-proBNP. **Thus, NT-proBNP is not recommended as a screening test for congenital heart disease in dogs.**

Median plasma NT-proBNP was 895 pmol/l (490–7118) in 10 dogs with patent *ductus arteriosus* and a concentration >1224 pmol/l identified dogs that had radiographic vertebral heart size and echocardiographic left ventricular internal dimensions above reference values.

Median serum cTnI in 19 dogs with congenital heart disease including patent *ductus arteriosus*, pulmonic stenosis, subaortic stenosis, tricuspid valve dysplasia, and ventricular septal defect was 0.088 ng/ml (range: 0.035–1405) using a high sensitivity assay. Cardiac troponin I has been evaluated in dogs with severe pulmonic stenosis (23 dogs; median cTnI 0.2 ng/ml; range: 0.2–1.29; standard assay) and subaortic stenosis (30 dogs; median cTnI 0.08 ng/ml; range: 0.01–0.94; high sensitivity assay). **Values are more likely to be elevated in symptomatic dogs or in dogs with severe disease**. Increases in cTnI concentrations following balloon valvuloplasty for pulmonic stenosis were attributed to trauma to the heart from balloon inflation.

In a puppy with a murmur, normal NT-proBNP or cTnI does not rule out congenital heart disease. An echocardiogram is recommended when NT-proBNP is elevated, in the presence of clinical signs, or when a murmur does not have the characteristics that are typically identified as non-pathologic. Non-pathologic "innocent" murmurs are typically soft, systolic and located at the left base while a loud murmur or the presence of clinical signs would suggest the presence of heart disease.

Acquired Heart Disease

Degenerative Mitral Valve Disease

On physical exam the presence of a left sided systolic murmur is characteristic of myxomatous mitral valve disease (MMVD). Detecting disease is not the primary use for cardiac biomarkers in dogs with MMVD. Biomarkers have been evaluated as a tool to classify severity of disease, predict risk of congestive heart failure, determine prognosis, assess response to therapy, and differentiate cardiac from respiratory causes of dyspnoea.

Elevations of both biomarkers, NT-proBNP and cTnI, have been identified in dogs with MMVD and values are positively correlated with severity of disease. There is overlap between values in the early stages of disease that limit the utility of the tests. In a study investigating factors that could predict heart failure, NT-proBNP >1500 pmol/l and vertebral heart size >12 were identified as risk factors with the ability to predict congestive heart failure (Figure 1). Elevated NT-proBNP >738.5 pmol/l combined with other markers, including increased left ventricular internal dimension normalised to body weight, suggested a higher risk of heart failure within the subsequent 12 months. In a study of 202 dogs, a shorter survival time was associated with elevations in both serum cTnI (>0.025 ng/ml) and NTproBNP (>524 pmol/l).

A reduction in NT-proBNP with heart failure therapy has also been identified in dogs and can be associated with a better outcome. A prespecified treatment escalation algorithm has been described with the objective of treating heart failure based on NT-proBNP values >1500 pmol/l without elevated creatinine and while carefully monitoring kidney function. This requires future study to assess outcomes and develop guidelines which can be incorporated into clinical practice.

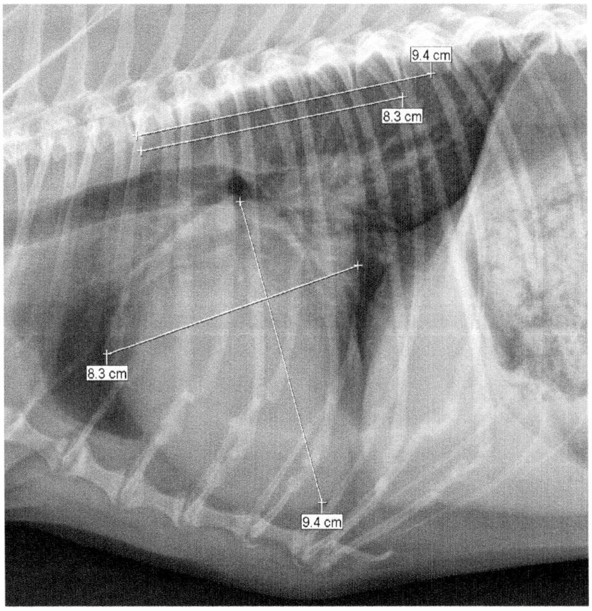

Figure 1. Right lateral thoracic radiograph in a 9-year old Cavalier King Charles Spaniel with a grade 5/6 systolic left apical murmur and a history of cough for three weeks. The cardiac silhouette is enlarged. Specifically, the heart is tall and there is evidence of left atrial enlargement. The pulmonary veins are not enlarged and the lungs are clear without evidence of pulmonary oedema. The vertebral heart size (VHS) is 12.5. Plasma NT-proBNP at this visit was elevated at 1825 pmol/l. A VHS >12 and NT-proBNP >1500 pmol/l suggest a high risk of congestive heart failure in dogs with degenerative mitral valve disease.

Dilated Cardiomyopathy

In studies evaluating the use of biomarkers to detect all forms of heart disease, small numbers of dogs with dilated cardiomyopathy of varying breeds are often included. Multiple studies have specifically evaluated cTnI and NT-proBNP as screening tests and predictors of clinical outcome in Dobermanns with dilated cardiomyopathy.

Elevations in NT-proBNP are found in all stages of dilated cardiomyopathy (ventricular arrhythmias, left ventricular dilation, both preclinical and heart failure). NT-proBNP does not replace echocardiography and Holter monitoring for identifying occult dilated cardiomyopathy but can serve as a screening test for Dobermanns where high values indicate a need for further testing with echocardiography and Holter monitoring. In two studies, similar NT-proBNP values were reported (>400 and >457 pmol/l) as an indicator of an increased likelihood of dilated cardiomyopathy.

Elevations in cTnI concentrations have also been reported in Dobermanns with dilated cardiomyopathy. Concentrations >0.113 ng/ml suggested the presence of dilated cardiomyopathy and concentrations >0.34 ng/ml were associated with a higher risk of sudden death. Similar to NT-proBNP, cTnI is not meant to replace evaluation with echocardiography or Holter monitoring.

In 2017, the European Society of Veterinary Cardiology published screening guidelines for dilated cardiomyopathy in Dobermanns including cardiac biomarkers. Dogs with a NT-proBNP >500 pmol/l or cTnI >0.22 ng/ml have a higher likelihood of occult dilated cardiomyopathy and further work up is recommended.

Arrhythmogenic Right Ventricular Cardiomyopathy (ARVC)

Both cTnI and BNP (not NT-proBNP) have been evaluated in small studies of Boxers with ARVC. While cTnI was elevated, there was overlap between Boxers with and without ARVC. **Based on the BNP assay results, it is not a reliable indicator of ARVC in Boxers.**

Pulmonary Hypertension

Precapillary pulmonary hypertension is caused by **diseases that affect the pulmonary arteries**. In a study of 12 dogs with precapillary pulmonary hypertension caused by pulmonary disease, pulmonary neoplasia, heartworm disease, and Eisenmenger's syndrome in congenital heart disease,

NT-proBNP but not cTnI was elevated compared to dogs with respiratory disease that did not have pulmonary hypertension. Median NT-proBNP in dogs with pulmonary hypertension was 2011 pmol/l (range: 274–7713). Additionally, NT-proBNP concentrations correlated with tricuspid regurgitation gradients derived from the echocardiogram.

In a separate study evaluating cTnI concentrations in pulmonary hypertension, dogs with precapillary pulmonary hypertension, and postcapillary pulmonary hypertension associated with pulmonary venous hypertension secondary to MMVD had elevations in cTnI concentrations compared to healthy controls and dogs with MMVD without pulmonary hypertension. Serum cTnI was not different between dogs with precapillary pulmonary hypertension (median 0.25 ng/ml; range: 0.10–1.9) and dogs with MMVD and pulmonary hypertension (median 0.21 ng/ml; range: 0.10–2.1).

In a study evaluating pimobendan therapy in dogs with pulmonary hypertension secondary to MMVD, NT-proBNP was shown to decrease in the short term after starting pimobendan as compared to placebo. Median NT-proBNP at baseline was 2143 pmol/l (range: 450–3981) and decreased to 1329 pmol/l (range: 123–2411).

These studies demonstrate elevations in biomarker values can occur in dogs with pulmonary hypertension caused by a range of underlying diseases.

Pericardial Disease and Cardiac Neoplasia

Troponin has been measured in three studies evaluating pericardial effusion and cardiac neoplasia in dogs. In two of the studies that used different assays to analyse peripheral blood samples in dogs with pericardial effusion, the reported median (range) cTnI was 0.19 ng/ml (0.04–6.89) in 15 dogs and 0.64 ng/ml (0.03–47.18) in 37 dogs. Elevations in peripheral blood and pericardial fluid were found in one study. In two studies evaluating cardiac haemangiosarcoma and pericardial effusion, concentrations of cTnI >2.45 ng/ml in one study and median concentration 2.77 ng/ml (range: 0.09–47.18) reported in a second study indicated haemangiosarcoma that involved the heart was more likely than idiopathic effusion or other types of cardiac neoplasia.

Because of the low numbers of histologically confirmed neoplasia, it is important to recognize that **elevations cannot differentiate between causes of pericardial effusion** but can identify dogs that would benefit from further evaluation with echocardiography.

Myocarditis, Infectious Disease and Arrhythmias

Myocarditis can result in a variety of conduction abnormalities and arrhythmias including atrioventricular block, atrial standstill, supraventricular, and ventricular arrhythmias. Elevations in cTnI have been reported with infectious diseases which can cause myocarditis including *Babesia canis*, *Bartonella* spp, *Ehrlichia canis*, *Leishmania infantum*, and *Trypanosoma cruzi* (Figure 2). Some of the dogs in these reports had histologic confirmation of myocardial inflammation, fibrosis, and necrosis and identification of parasitic organisms (i.e. *Trypanosoma cruzi* amastigotes). In one report, elevated cTnI was the only abnormal test in a dog suggesting it could be a better screening test for myocarditis than other routine cardiac diagnostics (electrocardiography, echocardiography). High cTnI concentrations (>1 ng/ml) were reported in dogs in these studies. In humans, high values that are much greater than the top end of the reference range can be associated with acute myocardial necrosis and a higher risk of death.

In a retrospective study of 14 dogs paced for bradyarrhythmias, cTnI was elevated at initial evaluation and decreased after pacing while staying above reference range in the majority of dogs suggesting possible continued myocardial damage despite artificial pacing. Four of the dogs with the highest initial cTnI concentrations developed progressive cardiac enlargement and dysfunction.

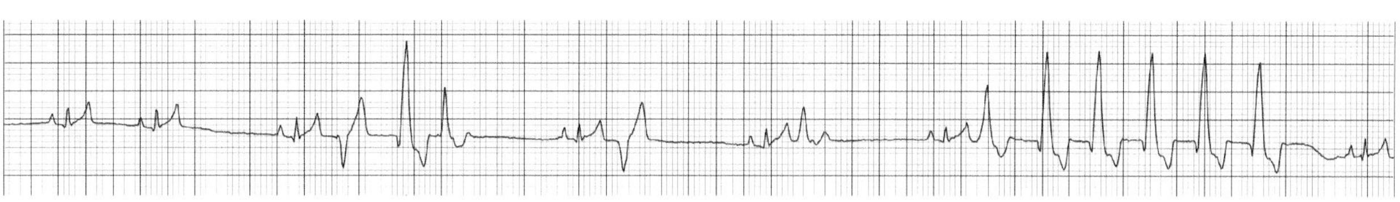

Figure 2. A lead II electrocardiogram from an 8-year old Mastiff with a history of acute panting and abnormal behaviour. On physical exam, an arrhythmia was detected. The ECG documents a sinus rhythm (three sinus beats) followed by three multiform ventricular premature beats, two bigeminal beats (sinus, ventricular premature beat) and a paroxysm of ventricular tachycardia. Cardiac troponin I was elevated at 2.12 ng/ml. Myocarditis was suspected in this case. Serum biochemistries were normal, and an immunofluorescent antibody titre for *Trypanosoma cruzi* was high (1:160) indicating Chagas disease.

In a study of 20 heartworm infected dogs, NT-proBNP and cTnI were elevated in dogs with more severe disease characterised by persistent clinical signs, often right sided heart failure, and caval syndrome. In dogs with caval syndrome, NT-proBNP was >2530 pmol/l, mean cTnI was 1.99 ng/ml, and C-reactive protein, a marker of inflammation, was also significantly increased. The authors pointed out that biomarker values could be affected by concurrent pulmonary hypertension and kidney dysfunction in this population of dogs.

In summary, biomarkers can be elevated in dogs with infectious or parasitic diseases, myocarditis, and arrhythmias but further evaluation is required to determine if they predict outcome.

Systemic Disease

Cardiac troponin I is elevated in many systemic diseases including dogs with systemic inflammatory response syndrome (SIRS), immune mediated haemolytic anaemia, gastric dilatation volvulus, pyometra, meningitis, and seizures.

In 38 critically ill dogs with systemic inflammation, cTnI concentrations were increased in non-survivors (median 1.74 ng/ml in non-survivors vs. 0.22 ng/ml in survivors). In 60 dogs with SIRS, elevated cTnI concentration based on the peak value during hospitalization was associated with poor outcome (median 0.63 ng/ml in non-survivors vs. 0.09 ng/ml in survivors). In dogs with gastric dilatation volvulus, increased cTnI concentration especially when combined with elevated serum alanine transferase activity was a predictor of poor outcome. In multiple studies, it was suggested that dogs with elevated values can benefit from more frequent monitoring.

Snake Bite

Elevations in cTnI concentration, as **an indicator of myocardial damage**, have been identified in dogs within 48 hours of presenting with a snake bite. A higher percentage of dogs with elevated cTnI concentration are identified when a high sensitivity assay is used (33% with a standard assay vs. up to 81% with a high sensitivity assay). Studies have evaluated dogs bitten by a variety of snakes and dogs envenomated by cobras in particular were more likely to have detectable and often higher cTnI elevation compared to other types of snakes suggesting variability in the cardiotoxicity of snake venom.

Dyspnoea: Distinguishing Between Cardiac and Non-cardiac Causes

Patients with dyspnoea can be difficult to assess, and a quick blood test that would identify the cause of dyspnoea would be clinically useful. In multiple studies, **cTnI** was elevated in dogs with respiratory signs but with **too much overlap between cardiac and respiratory causes to be recommended for this purpose**. Concentrations of cTnI were elevated in both groups of dogs and thus could not distinguish between groups (congestive heart failure group mean 0.42 ng/ml, 95% CI 0.12–0.72; respiratory disease group mean 0.29 ng/ml, 95% CI 0.18–0.97).

In a study using a first-generation NT-proBNP assay, serum and plasma samples were compared from 32 dogs with congestive heart failure from a variety of causes including MMVD and dilated cardiomyopathy, 28 with heart disease but without congestive heart failure, and 17 with respiratory disease. Plasma and serum samples were similar and NT-proBNP was higher in dogs with congestive heart failure and heart disease compared to dogs with respiratory disease and no heart disease. Use of a second-generation assay to measure plasma NT-proBNP provided measurements that exceed the first-generation upper limit of 3000 pmol/l. The second-generation assay was used to measure plasma samples in 39 healthy dogs, 74 with heart disease and 178 with respiratory distress from respiratory or cardiac disease. Median NT-proBNP was higher in dogs with congestive heart failure (5110 pmol/l) compared to respiratory disease (1287 pmol/l). The authors of this study described **a cut-off >2447 pmol/l to discriminate congestive heart failure from respiratory disease** as the cause of dyspnoea using this assay. A point-of-care test would provide more rapid results for this patient population.

Cardiac Biomarkers: A Review of the Feline Literature

Healthy Cats

In studies using different assays analyzing samples from healthy cats, the reported median (range) cTnI was similar at 0.03 ng/ml (0.03–0.16) in 21 cats, 0.03 ng/ml (0.03–0.16) in 33 cats, and 0.027 ng/ml (0.012–0.048) in 88 cats. **NT-proBNP <100 pmol/l suggests clinically significant heart disease is less likely**.

Acquired Heart Disease

Cardiomyopathy

Detecting feline heart disease can be challenging. **Murmurs are not present in all cats with heart disease and murmurs can occur in the absence of heart disease**. To complicated matters, echocardiography is the ideal test for assessing the heart but is not always routinely available and can be expensive. Multiple studies have been performed to evaluate the possibility of using biomarkers to aid in the detection of heart disease in cats.

Concentrations of cTnI were significantly elevated in 20 cats with hypertrophic cardiomyopathy (median 0.66 ng/ml; range, 0.05–10.93). In a recent study, cTnI >0.06 ng/ml indicated a higher likelihood of hypertrophic cardiomyopathy compared to normal cats. In 41 cats with hypertrophic cardiomyopathy, cTnI >0.7 ng/ml predicted a higher risk of cardiac death. The highest values were often reported in cats with arterial thromboembolism. Occult cardiomyopathy (hypertrophic, hypertrophic obstructive) was more likely when NT-proBNP was >46 pmol/l in a study of 113 cats and >100 pmol/l in a study of 102 cats. However, **biomarker values can overlap between healthy controls and cats with mild to moderate cardiac disease**. In addition, elevations in both biomarkers are possible when systolic anterior motion of the mitral valve is identified, both in the absence of left ventricular hypertrophy or left atrial enlargement and in cats with hypertrophic cardiomyopathy. Therefore, high values should be pursued further with additional diagnostic tests (echocardiography) to confirm and stage heart disease.

In cats hospitalised for congestive heart failure, a larger reduction in NT-proBNP from admission to discharge and resolution of CHF at recheck were associated with longer survival times.

Systemic Disease

Systemic Hypertension, Hyperthyroidism

Both cTnI and NT-proBNP have been shown to be elevated in cats with systemic hypertension and with hyperthyroidism. Biomarker concentrations decrease with appropriate treatment. Initial biomarker values are indistinguishable from cats with hypertrophic cardiomyopathy; thus blood pressure and thyroid status should be considered in cats evaluated for heart disease or based on biomarker elevations.

Dyspnoea – Distinguishing Between Cardiac and Non-cardiac Causes

Distinguishing between cardiac and non-cardiac causes of dyspnoea has been the subject of more than ten studies in cats. Both biomarkers are elevated in cats with congestive heart failure. Veterinarians had increased confidence levels and made a more accurate diagnosis when NT-proBNP results were provided during the evaluation of cats with respiratory signs. **NT-proBNP concentrations are elevated in plasma and pleural fluid samples in cats with cardiac disease**. Median plasma cTnI concentration was 1.59 ng/ml (range: 0.20 to 30.24 ng/ml) in 31 cats with congestive heart failure. **A cTnI >1.42 ng/ml was able to distinguish most cats with congestive heart failure** from non-cardiac causes of dyspnoea; and a cTnI <0.2 ng/ml suggested a high likelihood that respiratory signs were not related to heart disease.

Evaluation of point-of-care tests is of major interest in cats with respiratory signs. Cardiac troponin I values >0.24 ng/ml were found in 25 cats with congestive heart failure measured with the i-stat analyzer cage side test. The median cTnI concentration was 1.68 ng/ml (range: 0.24 to 50.00 ng/ml) compared to 0.16 ng/ml (range: 0.02 to 0.66 ng/ml) in the 14 cats with respiratory signs from non-cardiac causes. A point-of-care NT-proBNP test detected high plasma values in cats with a cardiac cause for pleural effusion but was not able to distinguish between cardiac and respiratory causes when testing pleural fluid samples.

A second-generation ELISA test (not point-of-care) could distinguish between cardiac and respiratory disease on pleural fluid samples and **values >240 pmol/l suggested cardiac disease as the cause of the pleural fluid**. Using this same assay, plasma concentrations >199 pmol/l suggested cardiac disease was more likely cause of respiratory signs. Combining point-of-care tests that included NT-proBNP, focused ultrasound of the heart to identify left atrial size and presence of pericardial effusion, and lung ultrasound to identify pleural effusion and B lines was useful for identifying congestive heart failure in cats with respiratory signs.

Bibliography

- Bijsmans, E.S., Jepson, R.E., Wheeler, C. et al. (2017) Plasma N-terminal probrain natriuretic peptide, vascular endothelial growth factor, and cardiac troponin I as novel biomarkers of hypertensive disease and target organ damage in cats. *J Vet Intern Med*, 31, pp. 650–60.
- Borgeat, K., Sherwood, K., Payne, J.R. et al. (2014) Plasma cardiac troponin I concentration and cardiac death in cats with hypertrophic cardiomyopathy. *J Vet Intern Med*, 28, pp. 1731–37.
- Borgeat, K., Connoly, D.J., Luis Fuentes, V. (2015) Cardiac biomarkers in cats. *J Vet Cardiol*, 17, pp. S74–S86.
- Boswood, A., Dukes-McEwan, J., Loureiro, J. et al. (2008) The diagnostic accuracy of different natriuretic peptides in the investigation of canine cardiac disease. *J Sm Anim Pract*, 49, pp. 26–32.
- Boswood, A. (2009) Biomarkers in cardiovascular disease: Beyond natriuretic peptides. *J Vet Intern Med*, 11:S23–S32.
- Carreton, E., Morchon, R., Simon, F. et al. (2014) Cardiopulmonary and inflammatory biomarkers in the assessment of the severity of canine dirofilariosis. *Vet Parasti*, 206, pp. 43–47.
- Chetboul, V., Serres, F., Tissier, R. et al. (2009) Association of plasma N-terminal pro-B-type natriuretic peptide concentration with mitral regurgitation severity and outcome in dogs with asymptomatic degenerative mitral valve disease. *J Vet Intern Med*, 23, pp. 984–94.
- Chun, R., Kellihan, H.B., Henik, R.A. et al. (2010) Comparison of plasma cardiac troponin I concentrations among dogs with cardiac hemangiosarcoma, noncardiac hemangiosarcoma, other neoplasms, and pericardial effusion of nonhemangiosarcoma origin. *J Am Vet Med Assoc*, 237, pp. 806–11.
- Dutton, E., Carmichael, N., Michal, U. et al. (2018) Serum cardiac troponin I concentrations in dogs with generalised seizures. *J Sm Anim Pract*, 59, pp. 167–173.
- Ferasin, L., Kilkenny, E., Ferasin, H. (2020) Evaluation of N-terminal prohormone of brain natriuretic peptide and cardiac troponin-I levels in cats with systolic anterior motion of the mitral valve in the absence of left ventricular hypertrophy. *J Vet Cardiol*, 30, pp. 23–31.
- Gomart, S., Allaway, D., Harrison, M. et al. (2020) Long-term biological variability and the generation of a new reference interval for plasma N-terminal pro-B-type natriuretic peptide in Labrador retrievers. *J Sm Anim Pract*, 61, pp. 368–73.
- Guglielmini, C., Civitella, C., Diana, A. et al. (2010) Serum cardiac troponin I concentration in dogs with precapillary and postcapillary pulmonary hypertension. *J Vet Intern Med*, 24, pp. 145–52.
- Hamacher, L., Dorfelt, R., Muller, M. et al. (2015) Serum cardiac troponin I concentrations in dogs with systemic inflammatory response syndrome. *J Vet Intern Med*, 29, pp. 164–70.
- Hariu, C.D., Saunders, A.B., Gordon, S.G. et al. (2013) Utility of N-terminal pro-brain natriuretic peptide for assessing hemodynamic significance of patent ductus arteriosus in dogs undergoing ductal repair. *J Vet Cardiol*, 15, pp. 197–204.
- Herndon, W.E., Kittleson, M.D., Sanderson, K. et al. (2002) Cardiac troponin I in feline hypertrophic cardiomyopathy. *J Vet Intern Med*, 16, pp. 558–64.
- Hertzsch, S. Roos, A., Wess, G. (2019)Evaluation of a sensitive cardiac troponin I assay as a screening test for the diagnosis of hypertrophic cardiomyopathy in cats. *J Vet Intern Med*, 33, pp. 1242–50.
- Hezzell, M.J., Boswood, A., Chang, Y.M. et al. (2012) The combined prognostic potential of serum high-sensitivity cardiac troponin I and N-terminal pro-B-type natriuretic peptide concentrations in dogs with degenerative mitral valve disease. *J Vet Intern Med*, 26, pp. 302–11.
- Hezzell, M.J., Rush, J.E., Humm, K. et al. (2016) Differentiation of Cardiac from noncardiac pleural effusions in cats using second-generation quantitative and point-of-care NT-proBNP measurements. *J Vet Intern Med*, 30, pp. 536–42.
- Hezzell MJ, Block CL, Laughlin DS, et al. (2018) Effect of prespecified therapy escalation on plasma NT-proBNP concentrations in dogs with stable congestive heart failure due to myxomatous mitral valve disease. *J Vet Intern Med*, 32, pp. 1509–16.
- Hori, Y., Iguchi, M., Heishima, Y. et al. (2018) Diagnostic utility of cardiac troponin I in cats with hypertrophic cardiomyopathy. *J Vet Intern Med*, 22, pp. 653–58.
- Joonbum, S., Payne, J.R., Matos, J.N. et al. (2020) Biomarker changes with systolic anterior motion of the mitral valve in cats with hypertrophic cardiomyopathy. *J Vet Intern Med*, 34, pp. 1718–27.
- Kellihan, H.B., Oyama, M.A., Reynolds, C.A. et al. (2009) Weekly variability of plasma and serum NT-proBNP measurements in normal dogs. *J Vet Cardiol* 2009;11(Suppl1):S93–S97.
- Kellihan HB, Mackie BA, Stepien RL. (2011) NT-proBNP, NT-proANP and cTnI concentrations in dogs with pre-capillary pulmonary hypertension. *J Vet Cardiol*, 13, pp. 171–82.
- Kluser, L., Holler, P.J., Simak, J. et al. (2016) Predictors of sudden cardiac death in Doberman Pinschers with dilated cardiomyopathy. *J Vet Intern Med*, 30:722–732.
- Kluser, L., Maier, E.T., Wess, G. (2019) Evaluation of a high-sensitivity cardiac troponin I assay compared to a first-generation cardiac troponin I assay in Doberman Pinschers with and without dilated cardiomyopathy. *J Vet Intern Med*, 33, pp. 54–63.
- Machen, M.C., Oyama, M.A., Gordon SG, et al. (2014) Multi-centered investigation of a point-of- care NT-proBNP ELISA assay to detect moderate to severe occult (pre-clinical) feline heart disease in cats referred for cardiac evaluation. *J Vet Cardiol*, 16, pp. 245–55.
- Marinus, S.N., van Engelen, H., Szatmari, V. (2017) N-terminal pro-B-type natriuretic peptide and phonocardiography in differentiating innocent cardiac murmurs from congenital cardiac anomalies in asymptomatic puppies. *J Vet Intern Med*, 31, pp. 661–67.
- Moonarmart, W., Boswood, A., Luis, F.V. et al. (2010) N-terminal pro B-type natriuretic peptide and left ventricular diameter independently predict mortality in dogs with mitral valve disease. *J Small Anim Pract*, 51, pp. 84–96.

■ Oyama, M.A., Sisson, D.D. (2004) Cardiac troponin-I concentration in dogs with cardiac disease. *J Vet Intern Med*, 18, pp. 831–39.
■ Oyama, M.A., Fox, P.R., Rush, J.E. et al. (2008) Clinical utility of serum N-terminal pro-B-type natriuretic peptide concentration for identifying cardiac disease in dogs and assessing disease severity. *J Am Vet Med Assoc*, 232, pp. 1496–1503.
■ Oyama, M.A. (2015) Using cardiac biomarkers in veterinary practice. *Clin Lab Med*, 35, pp. 555–66.
■ Pierce, K.V., Rush, J.E., Freeman, L.M. et al. (2017) Association between survival time and changes in NT-proBNP in cats treated for congestive heart failure. *J Vet Intern Med*, 31, pp. 678–84.
■ Reynolds, C.A., Brown, D.C., Rush, J.E. et al. (2012) Prediction of first onset of congestive heart failure in dogs with degenerative mitral valve disease: the PREDICT cohort study. *J Vet Cardiol*, 14, pp. 193–202.
■ Sangster, J.K., Panciera, D.L., Abbott, J.A. et al. (2014) Cardiac biomarkers in hyperthyroid cats. *J Vet Intern Med*, 28, pp. 465–72.
■ Saunders, A.B., Smith, B.P., Suchodolski, J.S. et al. (2009) Cardiac troponin I and C-reactive protein levels prior to and following balloon valvuloplasty in dogs with severe pulmonic stenosis. *J Vet Cardiol*, 11, pp. 9–16.
■ Serres, F., Pouchelon, J.L., Poujol, L. et al. (2009) Plasma N-terminal pro-B-type natriuretic peptide concentration helps to predict survival in dogs with symptomatic degenerative mitral valve disease regardless of and in combination with the initial clinical status at admission. *J Vet Cardiol*, 11, pp. 103–21.
■ Sharkey, L.C., Berzina, I., Ferasin, L. et al. (2009) Evaluation of serum cardiac troponin I concentration in dogs with renal failure. *J Am Vet Med Assoc*, 234, pp. 767–70.
■ Shaw, S.P., Rozanski, E.A., Rush, J.E. (2004) Cardiac troponin I and T in dogs with pericardial effusion. *J Vet Intern Med*, 18, pp. 322–24.
■ Singletary, G.S., Rush, J.E., Fox, P.R. et al. (2012) Effect of NT-pro-BNP assay on accuracy and confidence of general practitioners in diagnosing heart failure or respiratory disease in cats with respiratory signs. *J Vet Intern Med*, 26, pp. 542–46.
■ Sjöstrand, K., Wess, G., Ljungvall, I. et al. (2014) Breed differences in natriuretic peptides in healthy dogs. *J Vet Intern Med*, 28, pp. 451–57.
■ Trafny, D.J., Oyama, M.A., Wromser, C. et al. (2010) Cardiac troponin-I concentratinos in dogs with bradyarrhythmias before an after artificial pacing. *J Vet Cardiol*, 12, pp. 183–90.
■ Ward, J.L., Lisciandro, G.R., Ware, W.A. et al. (2018) Evaluation of point-of-care thoracic ultrasound and NT-proBNP for the diagnosis of congestive heart failure in cats with respiratory distress. *J Vet Intern Med*, 32, pp. 1530–40.
■ Wess, G., Daisenberger, P., Mahling, M. et al. (2011) Utility of measuring plasma N-terminal pro-brain natriuretic peptide in detecting hypertrophic cardiomyopathy and differentiating grades of severity in cats. *Vet Clin Path*, 40, pp. 237–44.
■ Wess, G., Butz, V., Mahling, M. et al. (2011) Evaluation of N-terminal pro-B-type natriuretic peptide as a diagnostic marker of various stages of cardiomyopathy in Doberman Pinschers. *Am J Vet Res*, 72, pp. 642–49.
■ Winter, R.L., Saunders, A.B., Gordon, S.G. et al. (2014) Analytical validation and clinical evaluation of a commercially available high-sensitivity immunoassay for the measurement of troponin I in humans for use in dogs. *J Vet Cardiol*, 16:81–89.
■ Winter, R.L., Saunders, A.B., Gordon, S.G. et al. (2017) Biologic variability of N-terminal pro-brain natriuretic peptide in healthy dogs and dogs with myxomatous mitral valve disease. *J Vet Cardiol*, 19, pp. 124–31.
■ Winter, R.L., Saunders, A.B., Gordon, S.G. et al. (2017) Biologic variability of cardiac troponin I in healthy dogs and dogs with different stages of myxomatous mitral valve disease using standard- and high-sensitivity immunoassays. *Vet Clin Path*, 46, pp. 299–307.

Test

Answers on page 206

1. Measuring NT-proBNP in a patient is not indicated for which of the following:
- a. Distinguish between respiratory and cardiac disease in a cat with respiratory signs.
- b. Determine if there is myocardial damage in a dog with gastric dilatation volvulus.
- c. Screen for cardiomyopathy in a cat with a heart murmur.
- d. Screen for cardiomyopathy in a 6-year-old Dobermann without a heart murmur.

2. In which case scenario would NT-proBNP be more likely to provide useful results?
- a. To screen the littermate of a cat recently diagnosed with hypertrophic cardiomyopathy and congestive heart failure.
- b. To screen a healthy, geriatric cat for heart disease.
- c. As part of a minimum data base before a dental cleaning in a healthy small breed dog.
- d. To screen a cat with a murmur and concurrent hyperthyroidism and chronic kidney disease.

3. Biomarker concentrations can be elevated with:
- a. Increasing age.
- b. Kidney disease.
- c. Hyperthyroidism.
- d. All of the above.

4. Elevated NT-proBNP in combination with which of the following increases the likelihood that a Dobermann has occult (asymptomatic) dilated cardiomyopathy?
- a. Abnormal Holter monitor results.
- b. Elevated heart rate.
- c. Elevated alanine transferase on a biochemistry panel.
- d. Elevated respiratory rate.

5. An elevated cTnI concentration of 2.2 ng/ml in a dog with third degree atrioventricular block and paroxysmal ventricular arrhythmias would suggest which of the following as the most likely cause:
- a. Dilated cardiomyopathy.
- b. Pulmonary hypertension.
- c. Myocarditis.
- d. Subaortic stenosis.

6. NT-proBNP is a marker of _____ in the heart and cTnI is a marker of _____.
- a. myocardial injury; chamber dilation or stretch.
- b. chamber dilation or stretch; oxidative stress.
- c. oxidative stress; myocardial injury.
- d. chamber dilation or stretch; myocardial injury.

Clinical Case 1

Signalment. Devon Rex, 10-year old, male neutered, 6.1 kg.

History. A new heart murmur was auscultated prior to dental cleaning. Anaesthesia was postponed to evaluate the murmur and determine if the cat has heart disease.

Physical exam. The cat was bright and alert with pink mucus membranes. The heart rate was 165 beats/min and respiratory rate was 32 breaths/min. A grade 3/6 systolic left sternal murmur was auscultated. The lung sounds were normal. Abdominal palpation did not reveal any pain or abnormalities. Femoral pulses were strong bilaterally.

Diagnostic tests performed
- Complete blood count: all parameters within normal limits.
- Serum biochemistry panel: all parameters within normal limits.
- Thyroid testing with serum T4: within the normal range.
- Systemic blood pressure: 145 mmHg (Doppler, taken on the front limb).
- NT-proBNP: 646 pmol/l (>100 pmol/l heart disease is likely).

Discussion. Diagnostic tests were offered to the owner including thoracic radiographs, and echocardiography. The owners approved blood work and blood pressure but were reluctant to spend the money initially on imaging. The elevated NT-proBNP value suggested an increased possibility of heart disease, and an echocardiogram was considered an ideal next step for evaluating the heart for cardiomyopathy. The owners approved further diagnostic testing with thoracic radiographs and echocardiogram. The radiographs showed overall increased heart size with normal size pulmonary vasculature. The echocardiogram documented left ventricular hypertrophy, reduced left ventricular free wall motion, and left atrial enlargement.

Conclusion. In this case, the elevated NT-proBNP result suggested an increased risk of heart disease in this cat with a heart murmur and encouraged the owners to pursue echocardiography and hypertrophic cardiomyopathy was diagnosed. Clinical management of heart disease could be initiated prior to elective anaesthesia for a dental cleaning.

Clinical Case 2

Signalment. Dobermann, 8-year old, female, 34 kg.

History. Presented for evaluation of a mammary mass which requires surgical removal.

Physical exam. No murmur or arrhythmia detected. There is a large, painful mass associated with a portion of the mammary chain.

Based on the breed predilection for dilated cardiomyopathy, screening tests were recommended.

Diagnostic tests performed

- NT-proBNP: 821 pmol/l.
- Holter summary: overall sinus rhythm with a heart rate ranging from 55 to 180 beats/min. There were 1300 ventricular ectopic beats consisting of singlets, couplets (**A**), trigeminy (**B**), and paroxysms of ventricular tachycardia (see figure below).
- Echocardiogram:
  - left ventricular internal dimension in diastole 46 mm (normal <47 mm)
  - left ventricular internal dimension in systole 36 mm (normal <38 mm)
  - fractional shortening 22%
  - ejection fraction based on Simpson's method of disks 47%
  - serum biochemistry panel: all parameters within normal limits
  - systemic blood pressure: 139 mmHg (Oscillometric, taken on the front limb).

Discussion. The elevated NT-proBNP value (>500 pmol/l) and identification of ventricular arrhythmias on the Holter study indicate the arrhythmic form of occult dilated cardiomyopathy in this breed. Based on results of these tests, the dog could be started on medical management with antiarrhythmics prior to anaesthesia for the mass removal and set up for recheck evaluations to monitor for progressive heart disease.

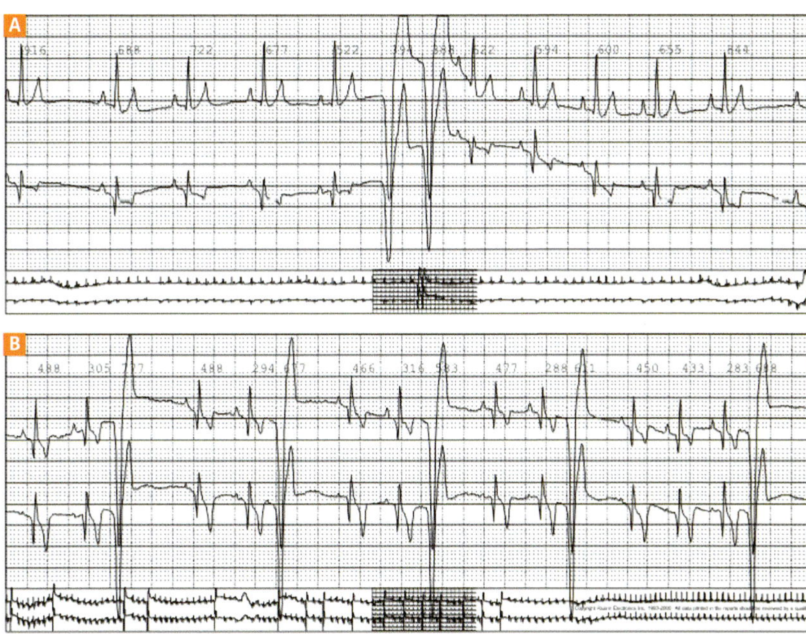

Correct Answers:

1. b
2. a
3. d
4. a
5. c
6. d

Notes

Congenital Cardiac Pathologies

Oriol Domenech

This chapter covers **congenital heart diseases of the dog and cat**, including vascular shunts and valve abnormalities. Each pathology is explained from an **anatomical and functional perspective**, along with any genetic predisposition, pathophysiology, diagnosis, and treatment. Both medical and surgical treatment of each condition are discussed (see chapter 18 for detailed information on surgical interventions).

Patent *Ductus Arteriosus* (PDA)

PDA is the failure of the *ductus arteriosus* (DA) to close after birth. This anomaly produces **pulmonary over-circulation** due to the diversion of blood from the high-pressure aorta to the low-pressure pulmonary artery. As a consequence of this pulmonary over-circulation, secondary **left cardiac volume overload develops**. Eventually, the pathology degenerates into left-sided congestive heart failure (CHF) which may be associated with pulmonary hypertension and less frequently into Eisenmenger syndrome.

Anatomical and Functional Considerations

Structurally, the DA originates from the left sixth aortic arch and allows **direct communication between the descending aorta and the pulmonary artery**.

In foetal development, since oxygenation of the blood occurs in the placenta and not in the lungs, the DA allows the diversion of blood from the pulmonary to the systemic circulation. Direct communication between the pulmonary and systemic circulation is due to the collapsed lungs, resulting in high pulmonary vascular resistance.

After delivery there is a decrease in pulmonary pressure when the lungs begin to ventilate. This produces an increase in oxygen saturation and, combined with reduced levels of prostaglandins, **induces functional closure of the duct** followed by anatomical obliteration during the successive weeks of life. **Failure of ductal closure is due to lack of normal ductal musculature**. The duct wall in normal dogs is made up predominantly (approximately 98%) of smooth muscle uniformly distributed along the wall, which is mainly circumferential and contractile. The remaining tissue consists of loose subadventitial elastic fibres interspersed with free collagen in the adventitia.

A line of dogs descended from Miniature Poodles with hereditary PDA anomalies in the wall of the DA, has provided an histopathological explanation for the failure of closure after birth. The two main histological features in these cases were **the smooth muscle of the hypoplastic, asymmetric duct**, and the presence of **non-contractile aortic-type elastic tissue** (segments of the wall of the DA that should be muscular had an elastic, non-contractile wall similar to the aorta instead). The muscular portion was always located close to the pulmonary artery and the thinner elastic portion (aorta-like tissue) was always adjacent to the aorta.

Histology of serial sections of foetuses predisposed to PDA identified **six degrees of abnormality**. These are characterised by an asymmetric reduction of smooth muscle and an increase in elastic aorta-like tissue which correlated with an increase in the concentration of the PDA gene in experimental breeds (Box 1).

The duct is widest at the end of the aorta and narrowest at the end of the pulmonary artery, where the smallest hole of the PDA is located, also called the ***ostium***.

The PDA's *ostium* provides resistance to blood flow and determines the pressure gradient between the aorta and the pulmonary artery, which can be measured non-invasively using **Doppler echocardiography**.

Genetics and Breed

An increase in the prevalence is observed in certain dog breeds, which indicates there are genetic factors involved in the pathogenesis of PDA. This is how a line of Poodle crossbreed dogs with hereditary PDA has been developed.

It is proven that heritability does not follow simple Mendelian genetics. It has been suggested that **heritability is most likely polygenic** (at least two genes contribute to development). Heritability in other breeds has not been studied in

Box 1. Degrees of *Ductus Arteriosus* Abnormalities that Determine Severity of PDA

- **Grade 1–2.** Lack of muscle to close the aortic end of the duct, but the presence of enough muscle to close the pulmonary artery end means PDA does not develop. This causes a ductal aneurysm, a blind diverticulum (non-patent type). This mild defect is an occult form that can only be diagnosed by autopsy and angiography.
- **Grade 3–5.** The lesions produce small, medium, and large ducts respectively, depending on the amount of muscle that remains at the end of the pulmonary artery. The ductal musculature is absent at the aortic end of the duct and mostly present at the pulmonary end, with some muscle remaining along the duct. This distribution produces a partial closure: the less muscle there is at the pulmonary end, the greater the size of the opening and the larger the PDA. This distribution of the remaining muscle gives rise to the characteristic cone-like or tunnel-like shape of the left to right sided PDA.
- **Grade 6.** The most serious type, but the least frequent. The DA remains as it was in foetal life (large communication) due to ductal constriction failure. This type of PDA results in a large left-to-right communication, which can lead to perinatal death, as well as the development of pulmonary hypertension early in life (Eisenmenger syndrome, see the pathophysiology section below) creating a right-to-left sided or two-way communication.

depth, but several breeds are likely to be strongly predisposed to PDA.

In the author's experience, PDA is the **third most common congenital heart disease**. There is a breed and sex predisposition (**it affects more females than males** in a 2:1 or 3:1 ratio). The breeds in which it occurs most frequently are:

- German Shepherd
- American Cocker Spaniel
- Border Collie
- Pomeranian
- Shetland Sheep Dog
- Maltese
- English Springer Spaniel
- Keeshond
- Yorkshire Terrier
- Rottweiler.

Pathophysiology

After birth, as a consequence of high systemic pressures compared to pulmonary pressures, **blood is shunted through the DA from left to right during systole and diastole**. Blood flowing from the aorta to the low-pressure pulmonary circulation through the PDA passes through the lungs and returns to the left-side of the heart. To accommodate the increased return of blood, the left ventricle increases in size. The result is an increase in end-diastolic volume of the left ventricle, termed **volume overload**. The increase in the end-diastolic volume of the left ventricle causes an increase in the parietal stress to the end-diastolic left ventricle, which causes **eccentric hypertrophy** as a compensatory mechanism.

The amount of blood diverted depends on the smallest diameter of the PDA and the relative resistances in the pulmonary and systemic circulation. If it is small, it may not produce serious haemodynamic consequences, since compensatory mechanisms may adapt to a slight volume overload. However, in the long run, **even a small PDA can cause CHF**. Larger-calibre PDAs often exceed the left ventricle's ability to compensate by eccentric hypertrophy and result in increased telediastolic pressure in the left ventricle, left atrial enlargement, which often leads to CHF.

Less frequently, a **bidirectional or complete reversal of the direction of communication** (right to left) is found. In these cases, the lumen of the PDA remains wide open after birth, with the aortic and pulmonary parts of equal size, offering no resistance to blood flow. Blood flows between the aorta and the pulmonary artery without resistance and the aortic pressure is transmitted to the pulmonary circulation, balancing both aortic and pulmonary pressures.

These patients do not develop left-sided heart failure after birth because it is likely that pulmonary vascular resistance does not decrease to normal levels but remains partially elevated to prevent mass diversion. Increased pressure in the pulmonary artery along with increased pulmonary blood flow causes pathological responses in the pulmonary arteries over time. Histopathological changes observed in these cases include mean hypertrophy and thickening of the intima of the small and medium pulmonary arteries. This causes a decrease in dimensions of the lumen, producing pulmonary hypertension (physiology of **Eisenmenger syndrome**).

The exact mechanism of this process is unknown, but injury to the endothelial cells which triggers growth factors is likely to be involved. These lesions are considered irreversible. Blood flow from the aorta to the pulmonary artery through the PDA begins to decrease due to increased pulmonary vascular resistance.

Therefore, the rate of blood flow decreases. When the pulmonary vascular resistance is greater than the systemic vascular resistance, the blood shunts from right to left (i.e., from the pulmonary artery to the aorta). **This phenomenon is called reversed PDA**.

A large amount of deoxygenated blood is diverted from the pulmonary artery to the descending aorta, causing **differential cyanosis**. This is because the communication occurs distally to the brachiocephalic trunk and left subclavian artery, which irrigate the head, neck and thoracic limbs.

Exercise results in a decrease in systemic vascular resistance, causing an increase in right-left shunting which worsens **cyanosis**. This mechanism, along with increased demand for oxygen for the muscles explains why some of these patients suffer from **hind end weakness during exercise**. Renal oxygenation decreases leading to increased production of erythropoietin secondary to activation of oxygen receptors. **Compensatory polycythaemia** occurs and can become harmful if haematocrit exceeds 70–75% because it increases the viscosity of the blood and resistance to blood flow. This compromises systemic blood flow and decreases oxygen release in tissues.

In the pulmonary circulation, systemic hypoxaemia causes vasoconstriction. Pulmonary vasoconstriction, combined with increased viscosity, worsens the pulmonary hypertension.

Although it is a rare situation, a dog with a moderate to severe left-right communication may develop pulmonary hypertension and, with age, a gradual reversal may occur. This type of pulmonary hypertension may be due to chronic pulmonary venous congestion, but the exact mechanism is not fully understood.

Diagnosis

Clinical Presentation

Although some affected puppies and kittens may appear smaller, thinner, or tachypnoeic, most are described as asymptomatic and develop normally at the time the condition is discovered. **Clinical signs are rarely recognised in the first few weeks of life** and most dogs are not diagnosed until their first veterinary examination, at 6–8 weeks of age. In some dogs the condition is not detected in the first months of life and may occur with CHF and a history of coughing, dyspnoea, and tachypnoea.

The main feature of a PDA is a **continuous murmur over the third intercostal space**. The PMI is in the left axillary area, which means auscultation should be performed carefully (sometimes stretching the forelimb forward) to properly explore the cranial region, otherwise, it is easy to miss the murmur. This usually happens if the veterinarian only auscultates the base and left cardiac apex. In some cases, the intensity of the murmur differs during the cardiac cycle, with an increase in the intensity in systole and decrease in diastole, but the murmur is actually continuous as it can be completely auscultated at any point of the cycle.

The murmur can be of any intensity but is often loud (grade 4–6/6) and radiates cranially (towards the sternum) and into the right cranial thorax. A palpable thrill may be felt in the cranial thorax, especially in patients with a large PDA. When the PDA is small, the murmur may be localised, and the thrill is not palpable. Neonates or older dogs with a large left-to-right PDA and balanced diastolic pressures (elevated pulmonary artery pressure or low systemic pressure) only have a systolic murmur rather than a continuous one. Dogs with large shunts may have mitral regurgitation secondary to dilation of the mitral *annulus*, with a systolic murmur over the left apex.

The pulse from the femoral artery is often stronger and is described as a hammer pulse. This is because pulse pressure is the difference between systolic pressure and diastolic pressure. With PDA, the increased left ventricular ejection volume causes an increase in systolic pressure and the rapid outflow of blood from the aorta into the pulmonary artery (and to the lower pressure pulmonary circulation) through the PDA causes a decrease in diastolic pressure. As a consequence, the pulse pressure is higher and can be seen clinically as a hyperkinetic or hammer pulse.

Murmurs in dogs with pulmonary hypertension and bidirectional shunts or right-to-left PDA are difficult to detect on physical examination, because they usually have a mild systolic murmur or no murmur at all. There may be a split-second heart sound, but it is not always detectable.

Radiography

Radiographic abnormalities reflect the degree of cardiac volume overload, CHF, and pulmonary overcirculation. These **changes depend on the size of the PDA**, the presence of concomitant cardiac abnormalities, and the presence or absence of pulmonary hypertension. In mild cases, only a pulmonary overcirculation pattern is observed, characterised by an increase in the size of the pulmonary vasculature (Figure 1). However, the variability in the size of this vasculature in normal dogs makes this finding difficult to detect. Dogs with a relatively large left-to-right shunt often have a dilated left atrium and ventricle and a dilated aortic arch, giving the appearance of generalised cardiomegaly with pulmonary overcirculation, and often a venous prominence is evident.

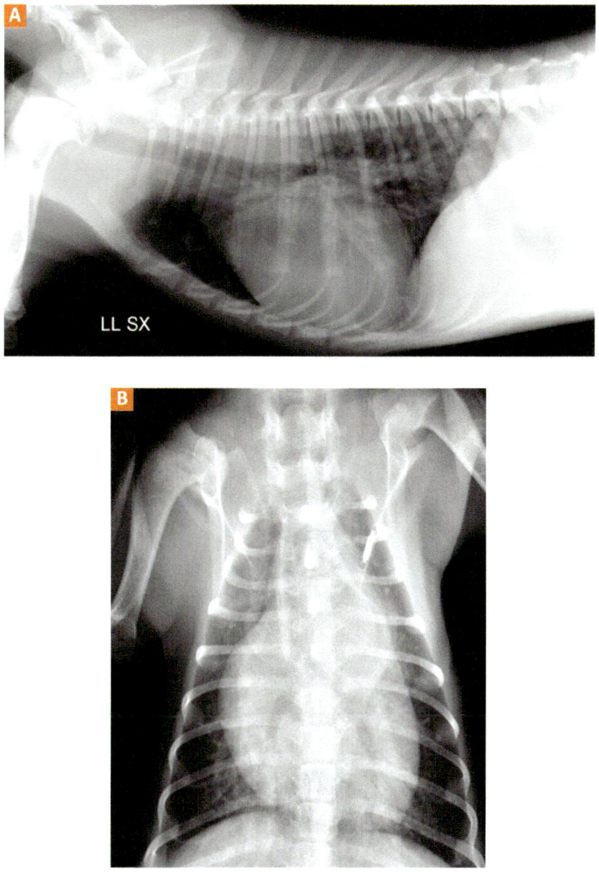

Figure 1. Left lateral (**A**) and dorsoventral (**B**) radiograph of a dog with a medium sized patent *ductus arteriosus*. In this radiographic study cardiomegaly associated with protrusion of the aortic arch and pulmonary trunk can be seen. In addition, an increase in the size of the pulmonary vessels which follow their normal path, characteristic of a pulmonary hypervascularisation pattern secondary to the presence of a patent *ductus arteriosus* can be seen: this can be confused with the presence of pulmonary infiltrate due to the increase in the radiodensity of the lung fields, caused by the prominent pulmonary vessels. The increase in size of the artery and vein to the cranial lung lobes (sign of hypervascularisation) can be seen in the lateral radiograph (A).

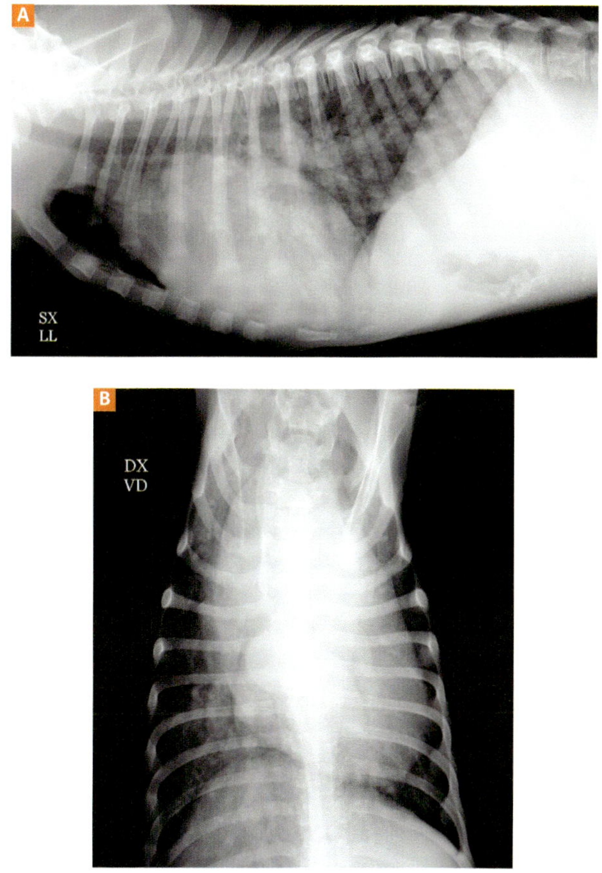

Figure 2. Left lateral (**A**) and ventrodorsal (**B**) radiograph of a dog with a large patent *ductus arteriosus*. In this radiographic study the marked left-sided cardiomegaly plus a consistent increase in radiodensity of the lung fields with the appearance of pulmonary oedema can be seen. In reality there is a marked increase in size of the pulmonary vessels, along with an increased number of vessels following their normal path, characteristic of a severe pulmonary hypervascularisation pattern secondary to the presence of a large sized patent *ductus arteriosus*. In the ventrodorsal radiograph a marked increase in size of the artery and vein to the caudal lung lobes can be seen (sign of severe hypervascularisation).

Increased size in pulmonary vasculature normally correlates with a significant increase in shunt blood volume (Figure 2). On dorsoventral or ventrodorsal radiographs, **an aneurysmal bulge** can be seen in the descending aorta in the region of the PDA (Figure 3). In cases where the main pulmonary artery is enlarged, a bulge can be seen at the 2 o'clock position on the dorsoventral or ventrodorsal radiograph. In dogs with left-sided heart failure, pulmonary venous enlargement, and pulmonary oedema may be visible.

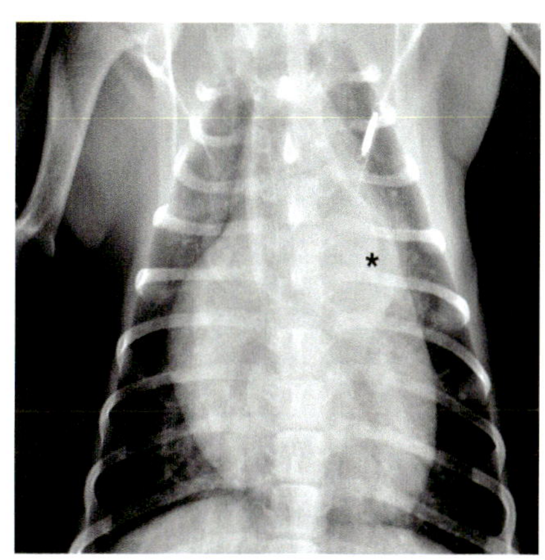

Figure 3. Dorsoventral radiograph where the descending aorta can be seen protruding in the area of the PDA and pulmonary artery (asterisk), level with the corresponding projection area at the 2 o'clock position.

Electrocardiography

The most frequent abnormality on the electrocardiogram is the **increase in the amplitude of the R wave on lead II** as a result of left ventricular enlargement (Figure 4). This finding is present in approximately 50% of cases with an enlarged left ventricle. Deep S waves can be seen in patients with right cardiac hypertrophy with pulmonary hypertension (Figure 5).

Supraventricular and ventricular arrhythmias can also occur. In a preliminary study an increased risk of sudden death in patients with ventricular arrhythmias is seen, which is a negative prognostic factor. Further research is needed to confirm these preliminary results.

Clinical Classification of PDA

The history and clinical characteristics of PDA depend on **the size and duration of the shunt**. Based on the patient's history, clinical signs, radiography, and electrocardiography, a clinical classification of PDA can be made based on **four types** (Box 2) as an anatomical and functional diagnosis, without resorting to angiography and echocardiography.

Echocardiography

Transthoracic echocardiography (TTE) provides a non-invasive examination technique which allows diagnosis of PDA by visualizing the duct, as well as evaluating its haemodynamic repercussions.

With PDA from left to right, the end-diastolic diameter of the left ventricle is increased and, generally, the degree of ventricular dilation corresponds to the size of the PDA (Figure 6).

The end-diastolic diameter of the left ventricle can be normal in very young dogs (when the pathology is detected during the first few months of life) and is often increased in adult dogs. In the author's experience, an increase in the end-diastolic diameter of the left ventricle can already be found in puppies. The shortening fraction is usually within the normal range, but in severe and advanced cases it is decreased.

Evidence of systolic dysfunction (internal diameter of the left ventricle increased in systole, reduced ejection and shortening

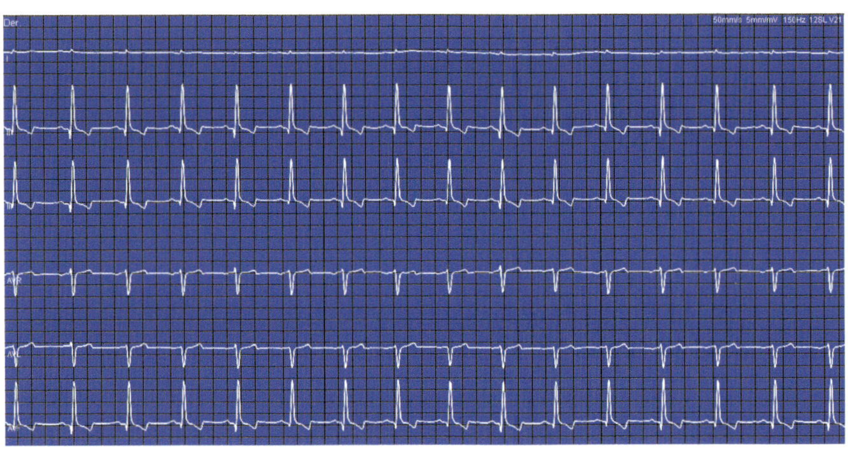

Figure 4. Six lead electrocardiogram where the increase in the amplitude of the R wave by 3.5 mV can be seen (paper speed 50 mm/s and sensitivity 5 mm/mV).

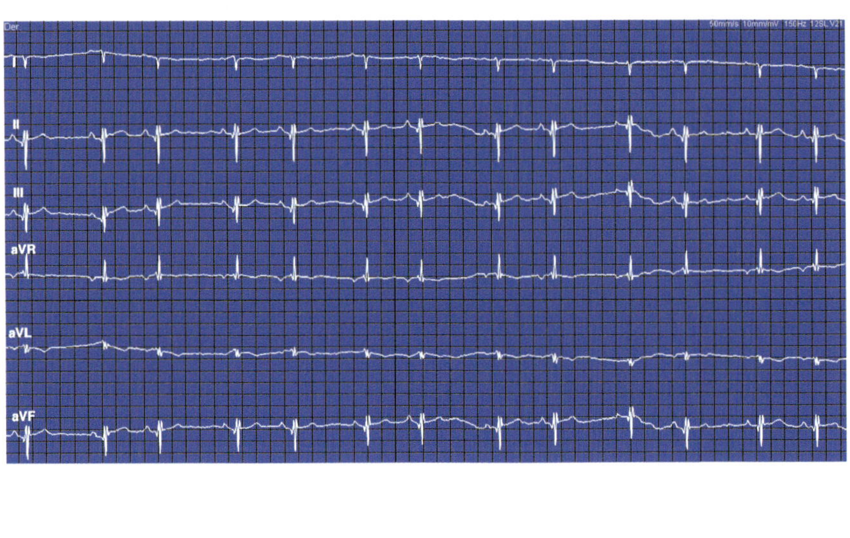

Figure 5. Six lead electrocardiogram where the electrical axis can be seen deviating to the right. Negative QRS complexes on DI, DII, DII and aVF with maximum positivity on the aVR lead (paper speed 50 mm/s and sensitivity 10 mm/mV).

Box 2. Four Types of PDA Classification

- **Type 1 (small PDA)**
  - Asymptomatic left-right shunt.
  - Continuous high-frequency murmur over the left heart base only (location of the PDA, more cranial than the base).
  - Absent or weak precordial thrill over the left heart base.
  - Normal heart rate and pulse.
  - Normal radiographs and ECG even at 1–2 years of age.
  - Surgery is not urgent but is recommended for a normal life expectancy.

- **Type 2 (moderate PDA)**
  - Asymptomatic left-right shunt.
  - Harsh continuous murmur over the area of the PDA (left cranial heart base) and slightly audible over the cardiac apex.
  - Continuous palpable thrill over the PDA area.
  - Normal or slightly increased pulse.
  - Mild to moderate left heart enlargement before 1 year of age.
  - Small to moderate PDA size.
  - Slight increase in pulmonary vascularization.
  - ECG lead II: R wave exceeds 3 mV, indicating left ventricular hypertrophy.

- **Type 3a (large PDA, before CHF)**
  - Typically shows reduced exercise capacity.
  - Harsh continuous murmur and thrill.
  - A systolic murmur due to mitral regurgitation is often present over the left apex.
  - There is usually a medium to large ductal aneurysm.
  - Marked enlargement of the left heart before 6 months of age.
  - Significant increase in the pulmonary vascular network.
  - Hammer pulse.
  - ECG lead II: R waves can exceed 5 mV.
  - Surgery is recommended without delay.

- **Type 3b (large PDA, with CHF)**
  - All the characteristics of type 3a plus dyspnoea due to pulmonary oedema.
  - Normally the animal is in poor physical condition (cachexia).
  - Sometimes atrial fibrillation is present on ECG.
  - Pulmonary oedema should be eliminated as soon as possible with cage rest, oxygen, and diuresis, before surgery is performed (see CHF treatment).

- **Type 4 (large PDA, with pulmonary hypertension)**
  - Right to left shunt or balanced.
  - From 2 weeks to 12 years of age.
  - Hindlimb weakness or collapse with exercise.
  - Usually, cyanosis is limited to the caudal part of the body.
  - Normal or weak pulse.
  - Polycythaemia (haematocrit elevation up to 80%).
  - There is usually no murmur or thrill after 1 month of age.
  - A prominent or split, second heart sound is often detected.
  - Point of impact stronger on the right side than on the left.
  - Deviation to the right on electrocardiogram due to right ventricular hypertrophy.
  - Enlarged right heart and pulmonary artery on radiographs.
  - Peripheral pulmonary arteries may be normal or diminished in size and slightly tortuous.
  - Surgery is contraindicated due to severe pulmonary vascular disease.
  - Treat polycythaemia with periodic phlebotomy or chemotherapy.

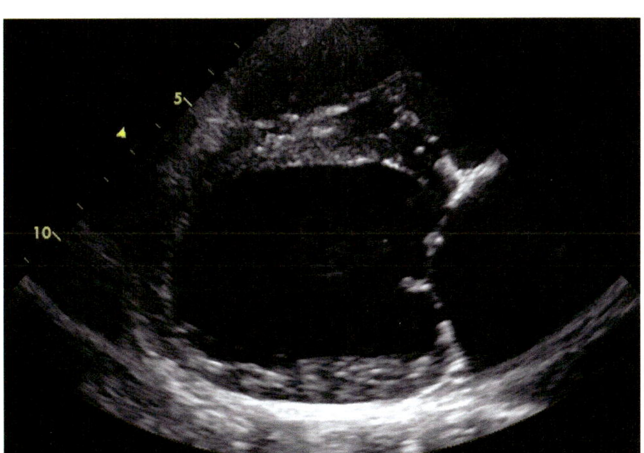

Figure 6. 2D image from a right long axis parasternal echocardiographic projection where dilatation of the left atrium and ventricle is seen.

fraction) is seen in dogs with large volumetric shunts, this dysfunction persists or appears to worsen immediately after ligation or occlusion. The left atrium is normally dilated to a degree similar to the left ventricle. **Identification of a continuous turbulent flow** with spectral (Figure 7 A) or colour (Figure 7 B) Doppler **in the pulmonary artery is characteristic of PDA**. The same PDA can be visualised from a right parasternal short axis projection (Figure 8) and from a left cranial parasternal projection (Figure 9): it presents as a hypoechoic space between the pulmonary artery trunk and the aorta. Normally, the **left cranial short axis projection** provides an optimal image.

Spectral Doppler allows the **Qp/Qs ratio** to be evaluated, providing information regarding the shunt fraction.

- A Qp/Qs ≥2 means the dimension of the PDA is moderate to large.
- The peak velocity through the PDA, when there is no increase in resistance in the pulmonary artery, is between 4 and 6 m/s.
- Peak aortic velocity is frequently increased due to volume overload and low pulmonary resistance.
- Transaortic flow velocity can be as high as 3.75 m/s with large ducts. This can lead to a misdiagnosis of concomitant subaortic stenosis. **Therefore, caution is necessary when interpreting aortic flow in patients with large shunts**.

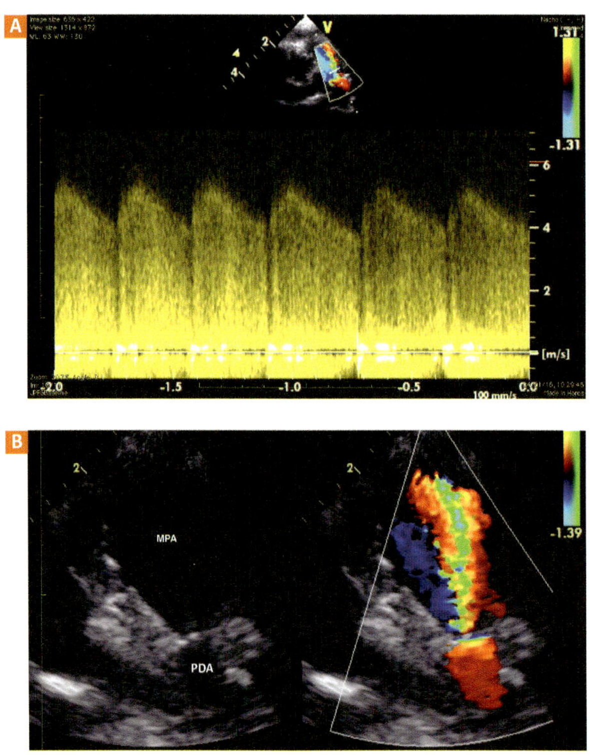

Figure 7. Continuous spectral Doppler (**A**) and colour Doppler (**B**) images from a left cranial parasternal projection. The continuous high speed (5.5 m/s) turbulent flow in the main pulmonary artery (MPA) originating from the PDA can be appreciated.

Although PDA can be seen using transthoracic echocardiography, this technique may not be sufficient for the evaluation of its morphology in dogs. To obtain comprehensive information on the morphology of the PDA, integration of measurements of the minimum diameter, the diameter of the ampulla and the length of the ampulla are necessary. **Transoesophageal echocardiology (TTE)** shows limitations for correct measurement of the ductal ampulla of the PDA. Furthermore, the length of the PDA ampulla cannot be measured using TTE because of the position of the PDA and the descending aorta, as it is generally difficult or impossible to see the confluence of the two vessels. The diameter and length of the PDA ampulla can be correctly visualised and measured using angiography, as well as by TEE (Figure 10).

TEE uses a two-dimensional transducer at the end of a flexible endoscope that is introduced through the oesophagus, providing high-quality images due to its closer proximity to the heart, with better visualization of the PDA. This contributes to a better understanding of the anatomical structure as demonstrated by angiography and postmortem studies.

The author has observed that TEE provides accurate anatomical information on the morphology of the PDA and in some cases is superior to angiography. Optimal positioning of the patient does not always occur for visualisation of the PDA by angiography and, furthermore, the superimposed structures do not give a clear image.

Angiography is also a radiological method with which the shadow of the heart is evaluated and it can sometimes be difficult to determine the actual size and morphology of the PDA. Therefore, TEE may be an echocardiographic method that overcomes angiographic limitations.

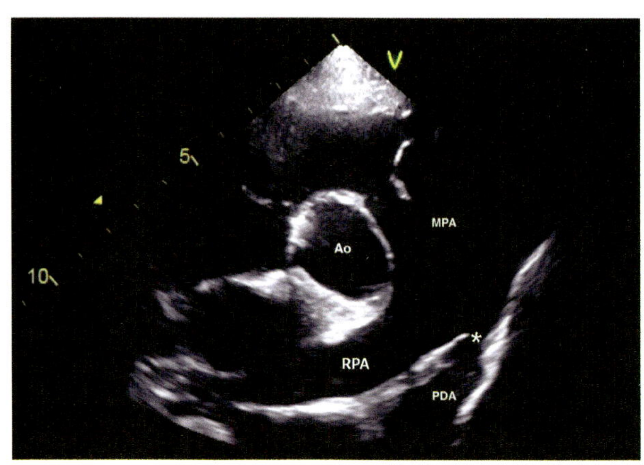

Figure 8. Magnified 2D image of a right short axis parasternal echocardiographic projection of the pulmonary artery where the PDA can be seen with its outflow, PDA *ostium* (asterisk) and the main pulmonary artery (MPA). RPA: right pulmonary artery.

Right-to-left PDA can be documented with **echocardiography** (Figure 11) by injecting a microbubble contrast preparation (saline mixed with colloidal solution) into the cephalic vein. In a right to left shunt bubbles will be seen in the abdominal aorta which should not be seen due to pulmonary entrapment, so if they are present, it means they have passed from the pulmonary artery to the aorta artery through a reverse PDA.

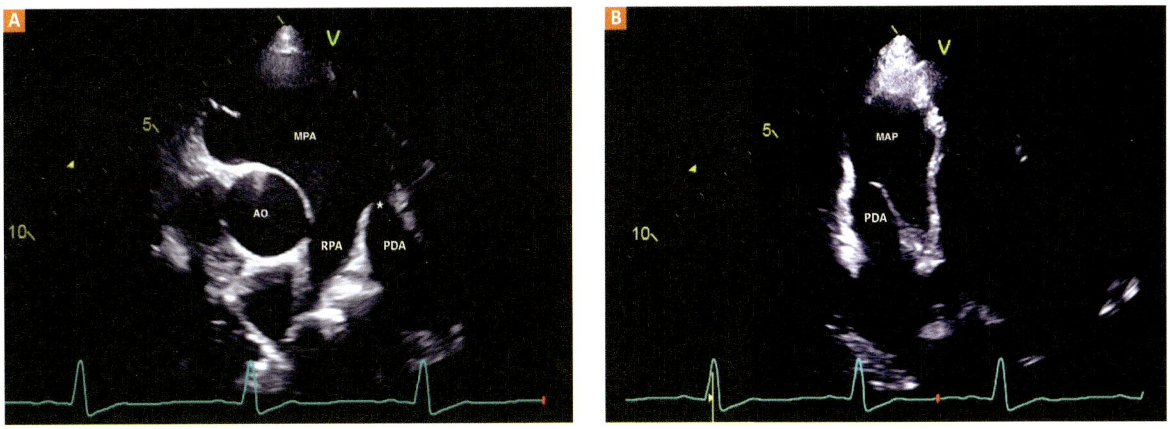

Figure 9. 2D image from a left short axis (**A**) and long axis (**B**) cranial parasternal echocardiographic projection where the PDA can be seen with its outflow, PDA *ostium* (asterisk) in the main pulmonary artery (MPA). RPA: right pulmonary artery. Ao: Aorta.

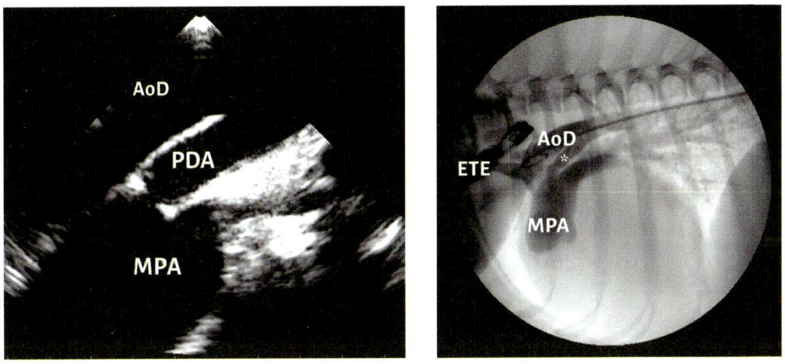

Figure 10. Combined images obtained via transoesophageal echocardiography (TEE) and selective angiography of a PDA with type IIA morphology. AoD: descending aorta. MPA: main pulmonary artery. (*):PDA. ETE: echocardiographic transoesophageal catheter.

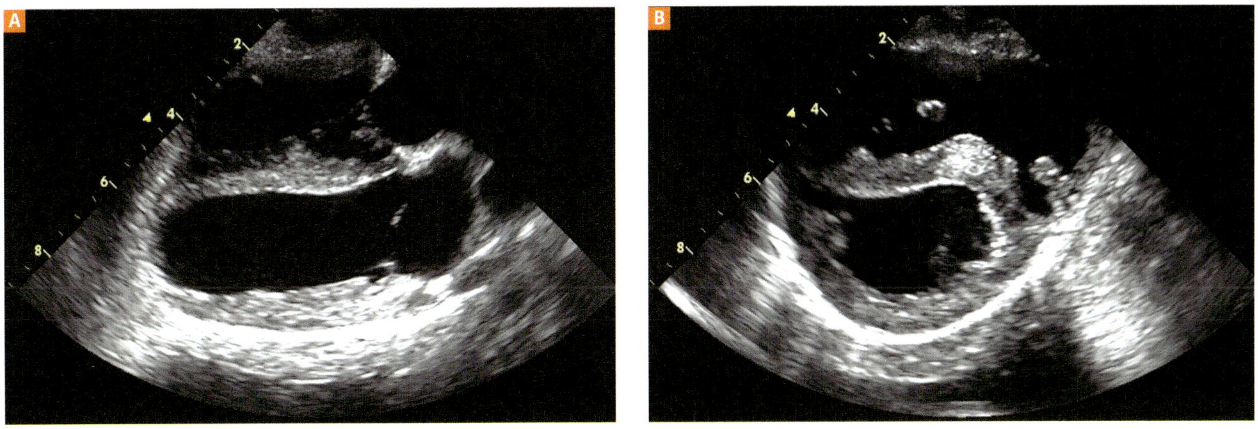

Figure 11. Right long axis (**A**) and short axis (**B**) parasternal 2D projections at the levels of the left ventricle in a dog with reverse PDA. An increase in the size of the right ventricle with flattening of the interventricular septum can be seen, which is displaced to the left, a sign of a significant increase in pressure in the right ventricle due to serious signs of pulmonary hypertension.

Treatment

Uncorrected PDAs usually end in left-sided CHF, with a mortality rate greater than 60% in the first year of life. In some dogs with PDA the clinical signs do not appear until they are adults, but are usually present before 3–5 years of age. In dogs older than 24 months of age, almost 50% have clinical signs such as tachypnoea, collapse, exercise intolerance, lethargy, and syncope. Therefore, **closing a PDA is always recommended**.

Pharmacology

In human medicine, the use of aspirin or indomethacin is described to induce the closure of the PDA in the neonatal period. To be effective, this technique requires a normal duct muscle morphology. In dogs, the persistence of DA is related to abnormalities in their musculature, so this treatment is not effective. As a consequence, the "wait until closed" approach is equally ineffective.

All patients with PDA should undergo curative closure. Given the evolution of shunt physiology, which leads to cardiac and pulmonary vasculature damage, delaying the procedure is also contraindicated. **The medical treatment of a left-to-right PDA is focused on the treatment of heart failure**. Medical treatment of right-to-left PDA aims to lower haematocrit levels.

Surgery

While surgical closure has historically been the most widely used technique, intervention or **minimally invasive catheter-based procedure** has become common. Various devices have been used and published in veterinary medicine such as coil occluders, Amplatzer ductal occluder (ADO), Amplatzer vascular plug, and Amplatz canine ductal occluder.

The Amplatz canine ductal occluder (ACDO) is a nitinol mesh device with a short waist for closure of PDA in the dog which has rapidly gained popularity since becoming commercially available.

Designed especially for this purpose, this self-expanding device makes it possible to treat PDA's of different sizes and morphologies, in dogs of a wide range of weights and somatotypes. The minimum patient weight required to use this device is approximately 4 kg. Its deployment is simple and followed by few complications if the size of the device is selected carefully, according to the size and shape of the PDA.

Briefly, the selection of the device size and therefore the viability of the patient mainly depend on the minimum ductal diameter (MD) and ductal morphology. Given the current availability of ACDO sizes, it is possible to use this device to close a PDA with a MD of 2 to 9 mm, considering that an oversize factor of 1.5 to 2 is recommended between the diameter of the device's waist and the MD. Ductal morphology is another important aspect to take into account when evaluating the feasibility of this technique.

Miller's classification describes the following types of PDA based on their morphology.

1. **Type I**: PDA diameter progressively decreases in size from the aorta to the pulmonary artery.
2. **Type IIA**: both walls of the PDA are parallel, and its diameter decreases sharply at the point of insertion in the pulmonary artery (Figure 10 A).
3. **Type IIB**: the diameter of the PDA decreases progressively and markedly from the aortic part to the pulmonary part with the narrowest part at the pulmonary insertion (Figure 10 B).
4. **Type III**: in which the diameter of the PDA does not change along its length, producing a tubular appearance.

According to the Miller classification, successful ACDO deployment has been described for PDA types IIA, IIB, and III However, **experience with PDA type III is limited and caution is advised**. Its tubular conformation and the probable lack of support for the device can produce instability and embolization. From the aforementioned, it is understood a precise study of the anatomical characteristics of the PDA is extremely important when considering percutaneous treatment with ACDO. Inaccurate selection of device size can lead to adverse events including systemic or pulmonary embolization, incomplete ductal closure, and haemolysis. Traditionally, angiography has been the method recommended for correct evaluation of the characteristics of the PDA and selection of the ACDO size, but TEE can also contribute to this purpose. In a study the author has shown that TEE can be used as a valuable alternative to angiography in evaluation of the dimensions of PDA in dogs, allowing for correct selection of ACDO size.

Finally, the author routinely uses TEE in all patients during the ACDO procedure with good results (Figure 12). The use of TEE during the procedure facilitates placement of the device through the PDA *ostium* and allows improved evaluation of its stability once placed. The decrease in ductal flow associated with plug formation can be visualised in real time with a final quantifiable assessment of the amount of residual flow. TEE may be advantageous during these procedures as it provides superior anatomical information regarding PDA morphology, dimensions, ACDO placement, and ductal closure.

Similar results have been observed by other authors using PDA coil embolization. Consequently, TEE is an important instrument for the correct placement of ACDO and intraoperative confirmation of canal closure. Furthermore, in the author's experience TEE reduces the number of contrast injections required and decreases anaesthesia and fluoroscopy time, producing a reduction in radiation exposure and costs.

Echocardiographic Changes After PDA Closure

Changes in cardiovascular haemodynamics have been observed after PDA closure (Figure 13). The presence of a left-to-right PDA is associated with an increase in left ventricular preload. Afterload plays a relative role in haemodynamics before closure, but gains importance in the postclosure phase, because preload decreases and afterload increases due to closure of the PDA.

Therefore, a decrease in preload with decreased end-diastolic dimensions (EDVI) of the left ventricle is observed.

In general, there is a more pronounced decrease in diastolic dimensions, while systolic dimensions appear to decrease to a lesser extent, and in some cases may even increase compared to diastolic dimensions before PDA closure.

All this reflects a **greater postoperative afterload**, which may determine that the SF% and EF% values tend to decrease after closure compared to when evaluated before closure. The decrease in SF% and EF% implies the presence of left ventricular systolic dysfunction after closure, an expression of the changes observed in preload (decrease) and afterload (increase).

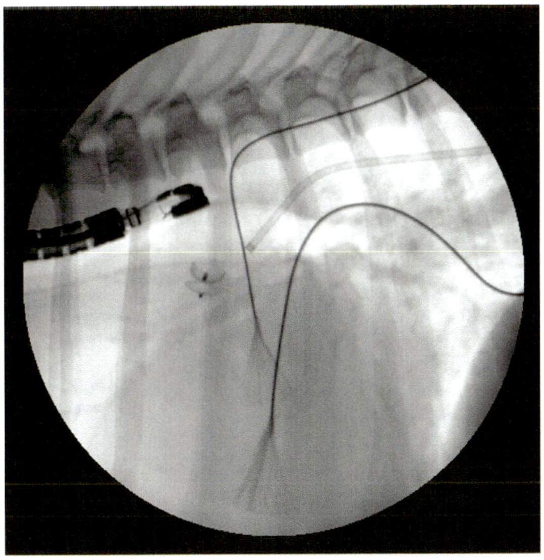

Figure 12. Fluoroscopic image with a C arch after PDA closure using an ACDO device. The ACDO device can be appreciated at the level of the PDA *ostium*. The catheter used for positioning and liberation of the ACDO device can be seen in the descending aorta. To the left of the image the probe for transoesophageal echocardiography can be seen.

Therefore, a medium- or long-term follow-up should be carried out to evaluate the recovery of left ventricular systolic dysfunction, which is generally transient, by means of serial echocardiographic check-ups.

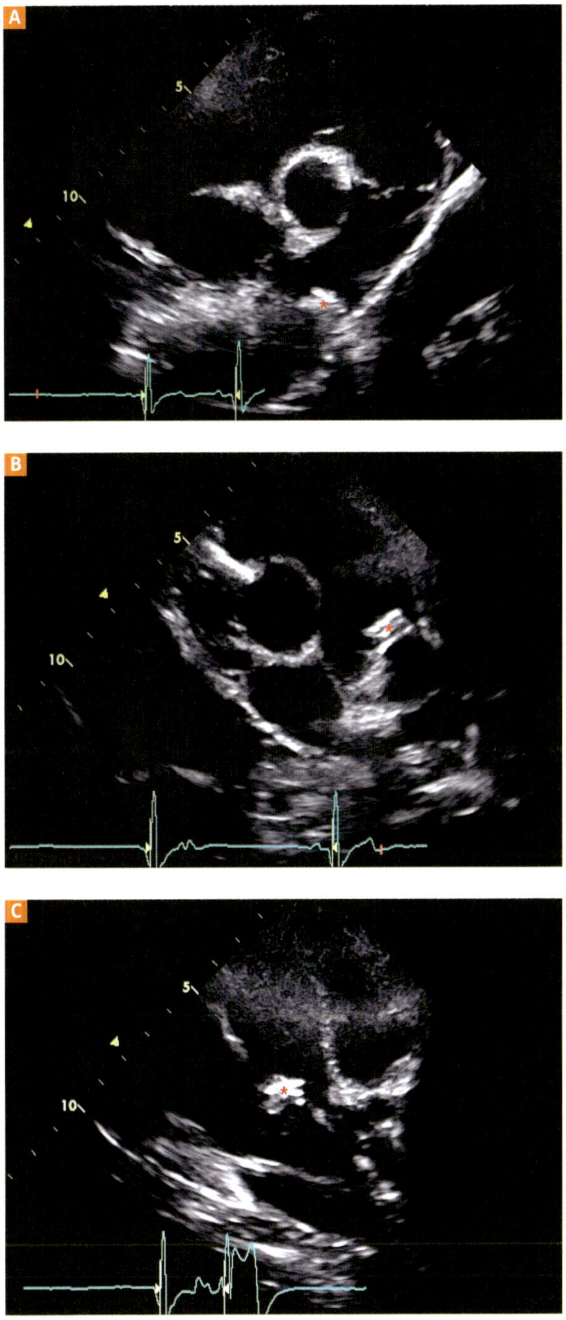

Figure 13. 2D image from a right short axis parasternal projection at the cardiac base (**A**), left short axis cranial parasternal projection (**B**) and left long axis parasternal projection (**C**), where the ACDO device can be seen at the level of the PDA *ostium* (red asterisk).

Pulmonary Stenosis (PS)

In the author's experience **pulmonary stenosis is one of the most common congenital heart defects in dogs**, representing an incidence of 32.1% of congenital heart diseases.

Pulmonary stenosis can be **classified into three types** according to the lesion's location along the right ventricular outflow tract (RVOT):

- subvalvular:
  - primary
  - secondary
- valvular:
  - type A
  - type B
  - mixed
  - hourglass
- supravalvular.

The most common type is valvular pulmonary stenosis, which can also be divided into four types: type A, type B, mixed, and hour-glass (Box 3). **Type A pulmonary stenosis is the most frequent type** observed in the authors clinic.

Depending on the cause, **subvalvular stenosis can be divided into primary and secondary**.

Anatomy and Function

In contrast to subaortic stenosis, in affected puppies **pulmonary stenosis usually presents its full severity at an early age**. However, pressure gradients can increase during the growth period, so mild pulmonary stenosis in a 4-month old dog usually progresses to moderate or severe stenosis in the first year (based on pressure gradients). In people, individuals with valvular stenosis may develop dysplastic leaflets with

Box 3. Types of Valvular Pulmonary Stenosis

Type A (Figure 14 A)

- **The *annulus* size is normal.**
- **There are various degrees of valve thickening with incomplete separation of the commissures through to almost complete fusion.**
- **There is systolic doming of the valve (windsock type image), which is more frequent with an eccentric valve opening with several degrees of reduction in transverse cross-sectional area.**
- **Poststenotic dilation of the pulmonary trunk is present with varying degrees of severity.**

Type B (Figure 14 B)

- **The pulmonary *ostium* is hypoplastic.**
- **There are various degrees of valve leaf thickening and immobility, but little commissural fusion.**
- **The common pulmonary trunk is often hypoplastic and poststenotic dilation is rarely seen.**

Mixed type

- **This type is when echocardiographic characteristics of type A and type B coexist.**

Hour-glass type (Figure 14 C)

- **Obstruction of blood flow out of the right ventricle into the pulmonary artery is due to an hourglass-like narrowing with a component of supravalvular stenosis.**

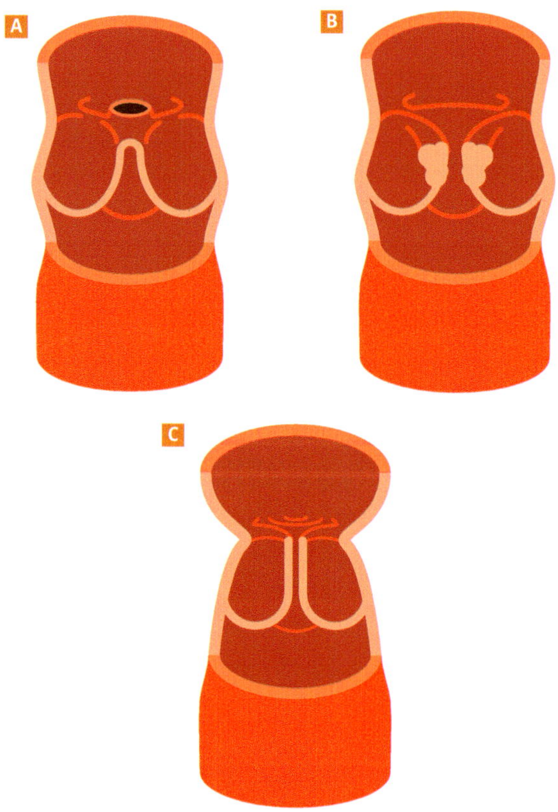

Figure 14. Schematic representation of the three types of valvular pulmonary stenosis (PS): **A, B** and hour-glass (**C**) (based on: MILO et al. Hour-glass deformity of the pulmonary valve: a third type of pulmonary valve stenosis. Br. Heart J. 1988; 60: 128–33). The original article is available via the following link: https://heart.bmj.com/content/.

annular hypoplasia and no poststenotic dilation and, in other cases, non-dysplastic valves and fused leaflets. In veterinary medicine, similar criteria for subdivision have been published, dividing PS into two main types (type A and type B).

In the author's experience, **Type A pulmonary stenosis is the most common**.

Secondary stenosis of the infundibulum is well described and the most common form of subvalvular PS. This involves various degrees of fibromuscular infundibular hypertrophy as a consequence of pressure overload hypertrophy induced by pulmonary stenosis. It is likely to have a dynamic component and leads to worsening of the stenosis with exercise or stress. **Primary subvalvular obstruction** by an infundibular fibrous ring (analogous to SAS) appears to be rare in dogs.

Primary infundibular stenosis has been described sporadically in people, dogs, and cats. This rare form of stenosis divides the right ventricle into a high-pressure proximal chamber and a low-pressure distal chamber. It is attributed to abnormal muscle bands and described as a double chambered right ventricle (DCRV), fibrous diaphragm or fibrous band of tissue obstructing the infundibulum, described as infundibular pulmonary stenosis.

In some breeds, especially the English Bulldog and Boxer, the anomalous left coronary artery type R2A surrounds the right ventricular outflow tract. This anomaly represents an exclusion criterion for any valvuloplasty procedure, since dilation of the infundibulum would cause severe coronary ischaemia and death of the patient.

Isolated supravalvular PS appears to be extremely rare. Attention should be paid during echocardiographic examination to the systolic doming of the valve in cases of type A PS, because supravalvular PS could easily be misdiagnosed.

The combination of SAS and PS occurs in a considerable number of Boxers. In a retrospective study of 500 dogs of this breed, the association of SAS and PS occurred in 24% of patients with heart disease.

In a recent study, associated congenital heart defects have been observed in 25% of dogs with pulmonary stenosis. The most frequent congenital anomaly association was subaortic stenosis, followed by ventricular septal defects and patent *ductus arteriosus*.

Genetics and Breed

Breed studies in Beagles and Keeshonds has demonstrated a hereditary basis for pulmonary stenosis. In the Beagle the heritability pattern is believed to be polygenic (several genes involved) and no specific genetic mutation has been identified. Other breeds at increased risk of pulmonary stenosis include:

- English Bulldog
- French Bulldog
- American Staffordshire Terrier
- Fox Terrier
- Pitbull Terrier
- West Highland White Terrier
- Scottish Terrier
- Miniature Schnauzer
- Chihuahua
- Beagle
- Samoyed
- Boxer
- Bull mastiff
- American Cocker Spaniel
- Boykin Spaniel.

In the author's experience, **the breed most commonly affected is the Boxer** making up 38% of cases of PS, followed by the English Bulldog (9%), mixed-breed dogs (7%), French Bulldog (6%) and Beagle (4%). Multiple other breeds made up ≤3% of dogs.

Although both sexes are considered to be equally affected, a **male predominance** has been described in the English Bulldog and the Bull Mastiff.

Pathophysiology

Regardless of the location, the main haemodynamic consequence of pulmonary stenosis is an increase in systolic pressure and parietal stress of the right ventricle, which causes hypertrophy of this cardiac chamber. There is a left septal systolic shift or flattening and an increased pressure gradient across the pulmonary valve. The magnitude of the resulting pressure gradient is directly related to the speed and amount of blood flow through the obstruction and to the stenotic region (CSA, cross sectional area). **The pressure gradient is used as an index of severity of the lesion**. Distal to the obstruction, the speed of blood flow increases and becomes turbulent. In some cases, this causes a dilation of the pulmonary artery also called poststenotic dilation.

The right ventricle becomes hypertrophic in an attempt to normalize the increased wall stress (following Laplace's law) and to preserve right ventricular systolic function and try to maintain cardiac output within the normal range. This hypertrophy of the right ventricle causes a reduction in its ability to fill properly, leading to **diastolic dysfunction**.

Progressive right atrial enlargement is the consequence of several factors including:

- elevated right ventricular diastolic pressure
- secondary tricuspid regurgitation caused by elevated systolic pressure
- changes in geometry within the right ventricle
- right ventricular hypokinesia: right ventricle loses force of contraction in a similar way to what happens in the left ventricle in cases of advanced subaortic stenosis
- decrease in cardiac output with compensatory retention of water and salt.

When high peak velocities are present in the outflow tract, the values can be converted into pressure gradients estimated by the simplified Bernoulli equation ($\Delta P = 4v^2$).

- **Mild stenosis**: gradient below 50 mmHg.
- **Moderate stenosis**: gradient between 50–80 mmHg.
- **Severe stenosis**: gradient greater than 80 mmHg.

The prognosis depends on the severity of the injury. Dogs affected with mild and even moderate PS can live normally. Animals with moderate to severe stenosis may develop complications including exertional syncope, cardiac arrhythmias, secondary tricuspid regurgitation, atrial fibrillation, right-sided CHF, and sudden death. Systolic pressure gradients are not always predictive of clinical evolution, but a general correlation between gradient and survival is observed.

Diagnosis

Clinical Presentation

Dogs are usually asymptomatic, displaying only a left heart base ejection murmur over the pulmonary valve, which radiates to the left craniodorsal heart base and in some cases radiates to the right craniodorsal base. In general, **the intensity of the murmur increases with the severity of the obstruction** and it is a harsh ejection murmur, with a crescendo-decrescendo character on the phonocardiographic image. In rare cases, a diastolic murmur due to pulmonary insufficiency may be heard. It is not uncommon to hear a holosystolic murmur due to tricuspid regurgitation over the right hemithorax.

Some cases present with ascites, exercise intolerance, and syncope related to right CHF and low cardiac output. **Arrhythmias and reflex-mediated syncope** are other causes of collapse. Sudden death without premonitory signs is rare, but can occur.

Clinical signs are more common in dogs over one year of age. Symptoms in puppies can be seen in cases of severe stenosis or with the presence of other congenital cardiac abnormalities such as SAS, ventricular septal defects and PDA.

Radiography

Thoracic radiography provides little information regarding the severity of the stenosis, with normal images in animals affected with mild to moderate PS, although right-sided cardiomegaly may be present. In patients with moderate to severe PS, prominent right heart enlargement can be seen, and in dogs with type A pulmonary stenosis, a poststenotic dilation of the main pulmonary artery can be seen (Figure 15). Pulmonary hypoperfusion can be observed depending on the severity of the stenosis.

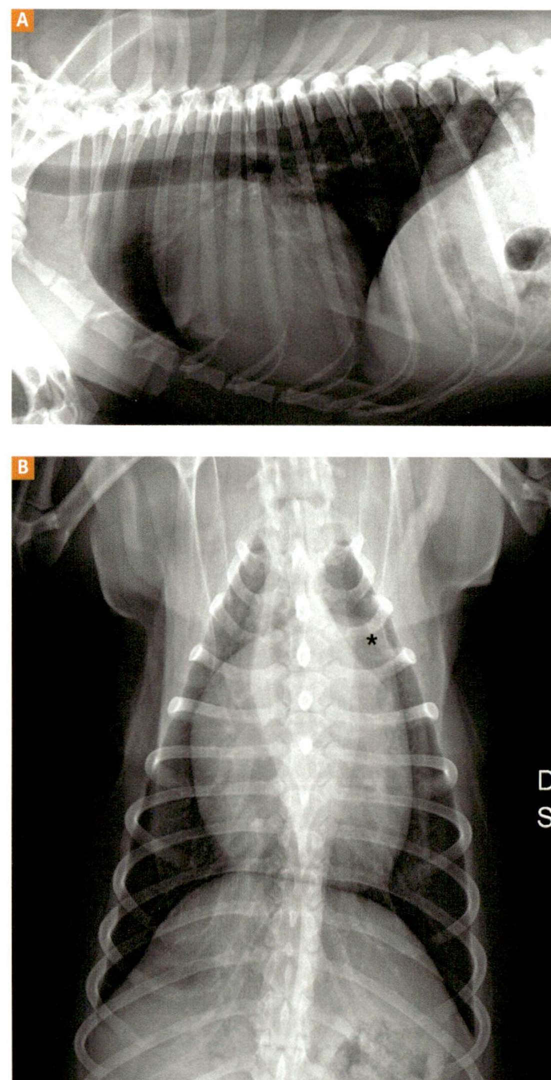

Figure 15. Left lateral (**A**) and dorsoventral (**B**) radiographs of a dog with severe pulmonary stenosis. A predominantly right-sided cardiomegaly can be seen, with increased sternal contact in A and protrusion of the main pulmonary artery in B (asterisk) at the level of the projection area corresponding to 1 to 2 o'clock. The pulmonary vessels are small in size with a normal course indicative of pulmonary hypoperfusion.

Electrocardiography

Electrocardiography may be **normal or show a right-sided enlargement pattern**, especially in severe cases with marked right ventricular hypertrophy (Figure 16). Ventricular and supraventricular arrhythmias can also occur. In some cases, 24-hour electrocardiographic monitoring (Holter study) is useful.

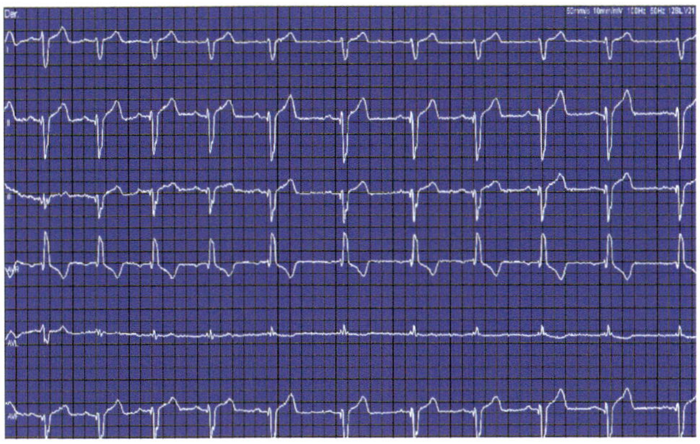

Figure 16. Six lead electrocardiogram where the electrical axis can be seen deviating to the right. Wide and negative QRS complexes can be seen on DI, DII, DII and aVF with maximum positivity on the aVR lead, indicative of a complete right branch block present in some cases with severe pulmonary stenosis (paper speed 50 mm/s and sensitivity 10 mm/mV).

Echocardiography

Echocardiographic examination is the most appropriate non-invasive diagnostic method to identify the presence of congenital heart defects, in addition to allowing classification of the type and severity of pulmonary stenosis. The right ventricular outflow tract (RVOT) has to be viewed along its entire length with a perfect long-axis view, although this can be difficult due to its curved shape.

Initially, an oblique, somewhat tangential view of the RVOT is seen in all dogs from the right parasternal short-axis projection, which allows the pulmonary *annulus* to be measured. This projection is optimised by moving the transducer towards the sternum, maintaining the same angle, trying to visualize the maximum length of the RVOT, pulmonary *annulus*, and main pulmonary artery (Figure 17). This last projection allows better alignment to register flow with colour (Figure 18) and spectral (Figure 19) Doppler.

In patients with subvalvular PS, these views are sufficient to visualize the subvalvular narrowing produced by muscular infundibular hypertrophy, a fibrous diaphragm, or fibromuscular band, as well as to observe the presence of a dynamic stenosis (which is uncommon).

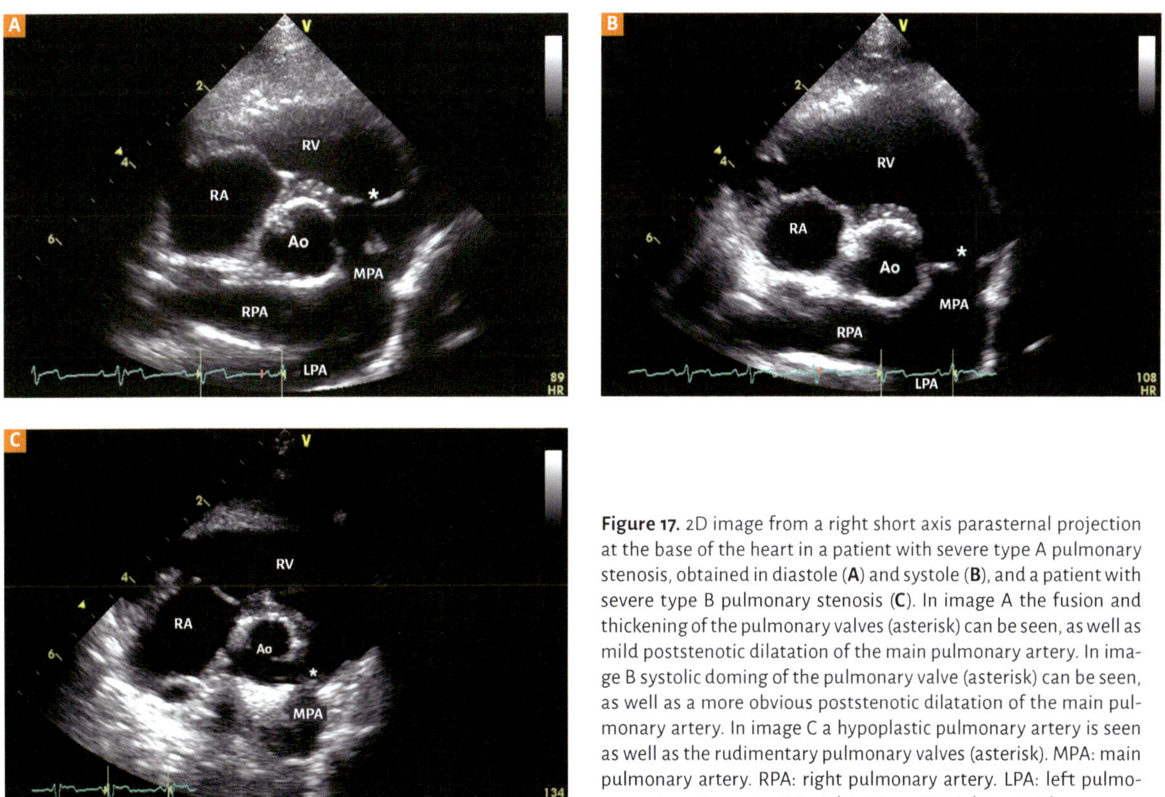

Figure 17. 2D image from a right short axis parasternal projection at the base of the heart in a patient with severe type A pulmonary stenosis, obtained in diastole (**A**) and systole (**B**), and a patient with severe type B pulmonary stenosis (**C**). In image A the fusion and thickening of the pulmonary valves (asterisk) can be seen, as well as mild poststenotic dilatation of the main pulmonary artery. In image B systolic doming of the pulmonary valve (asterisk) can be seen, as well as a more obvious poststenotic dilatation of the main pulmonary artery. In image C a hypoplastic pulmonary artery is seen as well as the rudimentary pulmonary valves (asterisk). MPA: main pulmonary artery. RPA: right pulmonary artery. LPA: left pulmonary artery. Ao: aorta. RA: right atrium. RV: right ventricle.

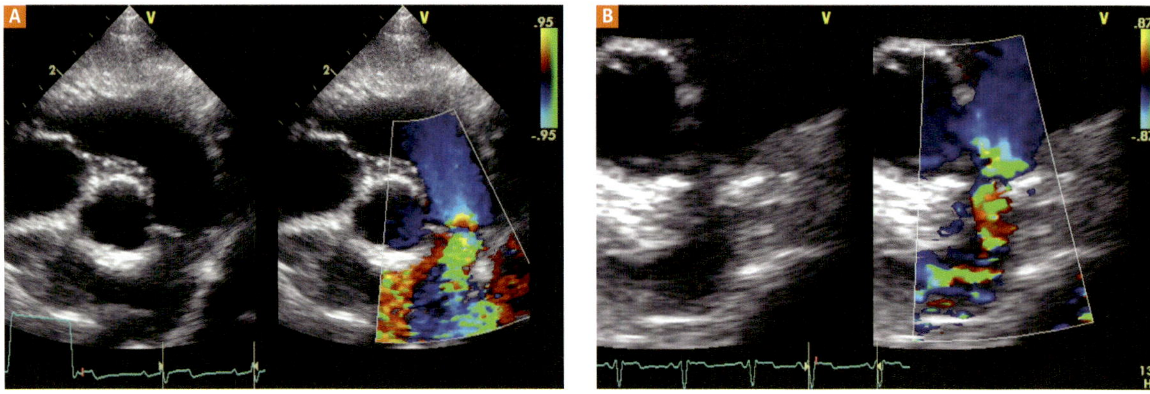

Figure 18. Duplex 2D and colour Doppler echocardiographic image of a right short axis parasternal projection at the level of the base of the heart (pulmonary artery) in a patient with type A pulmonary stenosis (**A**) and type B (**B**). The origin of the turbulent blood flow in both cases can be seen as the *annulus* or pulmonary *annulus*, which indicates valvular pulmonary stenosis and excludes a type of subvalvular stenosis.

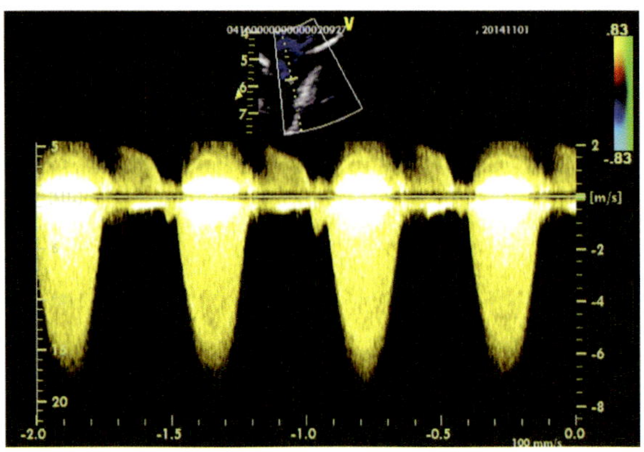

Figure 19. Continuous spectral Doppler image from a right short axis parasternal projection where high speed (6.5 m/s) turbulent systolic flow can be appreciated through the pulmonary valve.

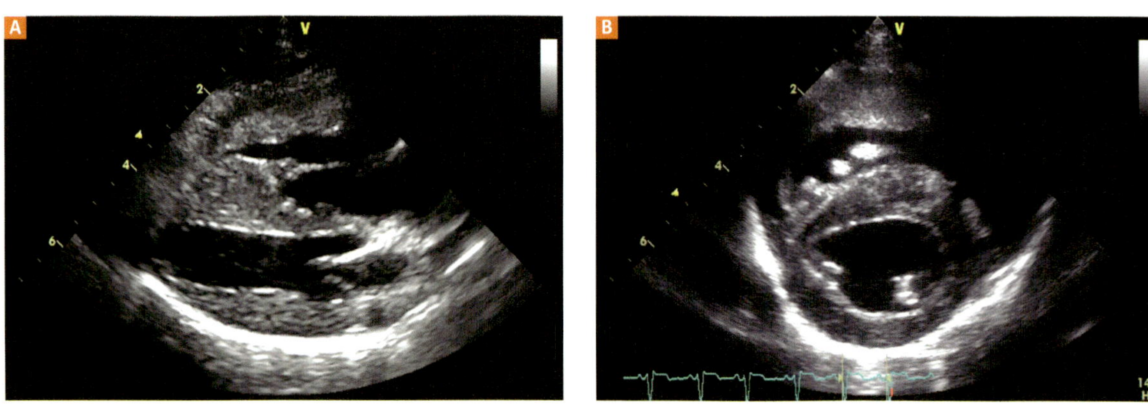

Figure 20. 2D image from a right long axis (**A**) and short axis (**B**) parasternal projection at the level of the insertion of the cordae tendineae to the papillary muscles. The marked hypertrophy of the right ventricle (RV) can be appreciated as well as that of the interventricular septum and free wall of the RV, with a reduction in size of the left-sided chambers, particularly visible in A.

Dynamic stenosis is visualised using spectral Doppler and **characterised by a "knife" flow pattern**. A differential diagnosis between a double-chambered right ventricle and anomalous left coronary artery R2A should be made in all patients with subvalvular PS. Normally, cases of valvular PS are studied using this right-sided projection, which also shows thickening and hypertrophy of the right septum and RV free wall (Figure 20), with some hyperechoic areas related to endomyocardial fibrosis, especially in severe cases. Left-sided views are essential to complete the echocardiographic examination.

The left parasternal short axis projection can be optimised for visualisation of the pulmonary artery and also the pulmonary trunk with its bifurcation. Another useful view is obtained by visualizing the long axis of the aortic root by inclining the probe dorsally with a slightly more cranial angle. This projection shows the RVOT with the main pulmonary artery at its longest point.

Another finding that **is suggestive of pulmonary stenosis is the presence of poststenotic dilations**, although this trait is not present in type B phenotypes. Echocardiography also enables determination of the severity of right ventricular hypertrophy or altered kinetics such as the presence of paradoxical movement or flattening of the septum. These findings are highly suggestive of an increase in RV pressure. However, a non-invasive estimate of the rise in pressure is only obtained by measuring the peak velocity of the pulmonary artery with the continuous Doppler beam parallel to the direction of flow. This is done through the left or right parasternal window. The values obtained are transformed into a pressure gradient estimated with the simplified Bernoulli equation. Evaluation of dilation of the tricuspid *annulus* is also important, as well as the high speed of tricuspid regurgitation. Colour Doppler also allows identification of associated congenital defects, such as ventricular muscle defects, or dynamic obstruction in the left ventricular outflow tract due to altered ventricular geometry.

In some cases, transoesophageal echocardiography (TEE) is a complementary diagnostic technique to study subvalvular, valvular, or supravalvular anatomy, especially in cases with a poor echocardiographic window or structural thoracic abnormalities.

Treatment

Special Considerations

Patients with resting gradients greater than 80 mmHg are at risk of sudden death, and balloon valvuloplasty is recommended whether the patient is symptomatic or not. Patients with intermediate pressure gradients (50–80 mmHg) often live normal lives, although long-term prognosis is uncertain. In these patients, decisions regarding treatment are determined by the clinical presentation (presence of clinical signs), degree of RV hypertrophy, and the nature of the progression. Patients with lower pressure gradients (below 40–50 mmHg) are usually asymptomatic and treatment is not necessary.

Pharmacology

The decision to treat pulmonary stenosis is based on:

- severity of clinical signs
- magnitude of the pressure gradient across the pulmonary valve
- degree of RV hypertrophy.

The pressure gradient above which medical treatment is recommended cannot be stated with certainty. Normally, with **a pressure gradient greater than 50–60 mmHg, medical treatment based on a β-blocking agent is commenced**. These substances reduce myocardial oxygen demand and increase coronary perfusion, reducing heart rate and contractility, which helps reduce the incidence of the last stage characterised by right ventricular myocardial failure.

β-blockers reduce dynamic stenosis in the RVOT, as they decrease heart rate and contractility, as well as ventricular arrhythmias, syncope events, and can even prevent sudden death. The reduction of dynamic stenosis and arrhythmias are important in cases where pulmonary balloon valvuloplasty will be performed. The recommended β-blocker is **atenolol at an initial dose of 0.2 mg/kg SID or BID** and, it is increased progressively (weekly increments) to 0.5–1 mg/kg SID or BID, always in conjunction with blood pressure monitoring and ECG.

Surgery

For pulmonic stenosis, pulmonary balloon valvuloplasty (PBV) is the treatment of choice (Figure 21). Valvuloplasty should be performed in any symptomatic patient and in any patient with a severe pressure gradient with RV hypertrophy (even if they are asymptomatic) as soon as PS is diagnosed. Delays in treatment can lead to progression of RV and infundibular hypertrophy, making the procedure more technically difficult, and reducing the immediate response to treatment.

In a retrospective study where PBV was performed in 95 dogs, a significant reduction in the pressure gradient was documented after the procedure at 24 hours and at one year, both in type A and type B pulmonary stenosis. The mean pressure gradient after the procedure at 24-hours and a year between group A and B was found to be lower in type A, suggesting better results. PBV was considered successful (reduction in pressure gradient of more than 50% from baseline) in 65 type A dogs (90%) and 7 type B dogs (54%). PBV was performed without significant complications in 93% of dogs. Based on these data, it is concluded that PBV is effective in type A and B PS but is more effective in type A. Similar results are described in human medicine literature. PBV in patients with dysplastic valves was less effective (61.11%) when compared to those with typical PS (80.59%). Even though the success rate was lower in the dysplastic group, PBV is still considered a first-line treatment for both types in human patients. In addition, PBV in type B (or dysplastic) can prevent or delay the need for surgery and provides a good long-term outcome in dogs, as it does in people.

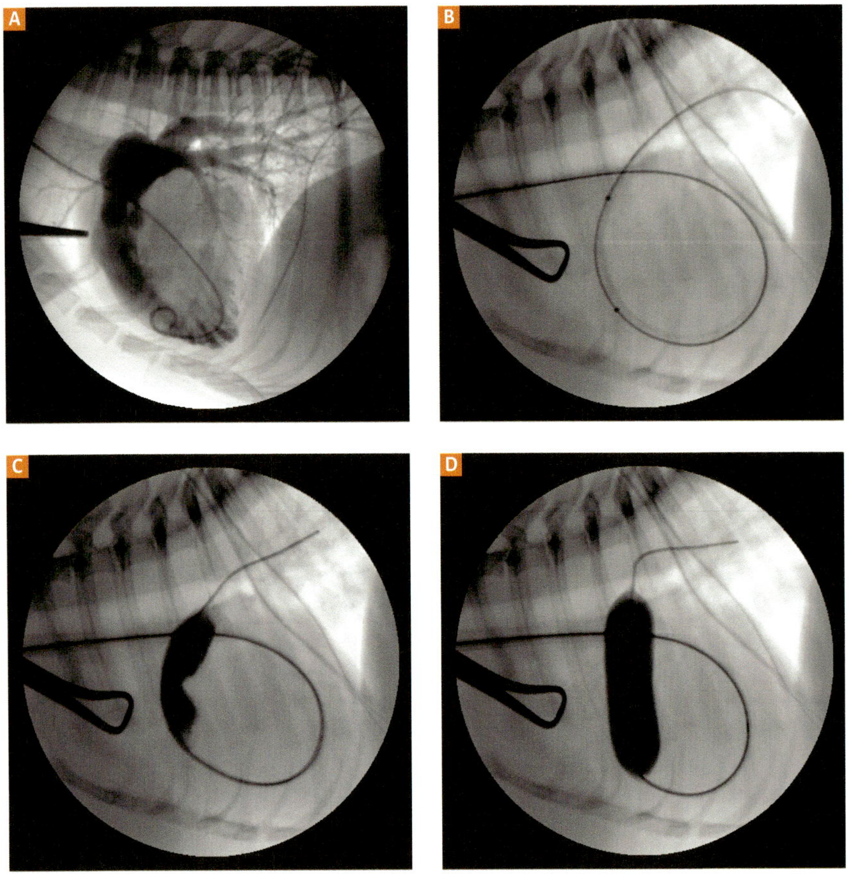

Figure 21. C-arm fluoroscopy images during a balloon pulmonary valvuloplasty in a patient with severe type A pulmonary stenosis. In **A** a selective right ventriculography with a pigtail catheter can be seen where the pulmonary valvular stenosis can be seen, as well as the poststenotic dilatation. In **B** the positioning of the balloon catheter at the level of the pulmonary valve with the help of a metallic guide which can be seen dorsally at the level of the left pulmonary artery; the length of the balloon in the catheter can be seen due to the presence of two radiopaque points which act as a guide to correctly position the balloon between the fused pulmonary valve. In **C** the initial stage of balloon dilatation is seen showing a narrowing in the area of valvular stenosis. In **D** the final stage of balloon dilatation is seen without narrowing, which indicates that there has been effective dilatation of the stenosis.

The author and their team have performed more than 120 pulmonary valvuloplasties in dogs. The major complications observed have been: right ventricular perforation, ventricular tachycardia, ventricular fibrillation and severe bradycardia with asystole. In the author's experience, the highest complication rate is around 4.8% and the mortality rate is around 2.4%. Perforation of the right ventricle with consequent pericardial effusion and presence of contrast in the pericardial space is the most dramatic complication the authors have seen, but it did not cause pericardial tamponade or death. ST-segment depression as a sign of myocardial ischaemia is of greater importance because it is associated with an increased risk of severe ventricular tachycardia.

In the author's experience, mortality during PBV was mainly due to **dangerous ventricular arrhythmias**. Ventricular tachycardia normally responds well to a lidocaine infusion unless there is severe myocardial ischaemia. These complications are related to materials, procedure technique, size of the patient, stability of the patient before the procedure, degree of RV hypertrophy with the presence of fibrosis, the type of stenosis and the experience of the operator.

The authors have also observed that **patients treated previously with β-blockers had lower incidences of malignant arrhythmias**, and a lesser degree of deterioration of dynamic pulmonary stenosis after valvular dilatation (suicidal infundibulum). This phenomenon is due to the decrease in resistance (afterload) of the RVOT which causes an exaggerated systolic movement of the infundibular area of the RVOT. This is important because it can lead to the death of the patient. This is one of the reasons why all patients should be pretreated with a β-blocker (atenolol) before performing a PBV.

In the author's experience **catheterization errors** can also complicate the procedure. The most common are contrast injections (the injected contrast enters the endocardium and appears as a spot-on fluoroscopy), air bubbles, inappropriate location of the contrast during injection, and loop formation in the guidewire in the right atrium or right ventricle. In some affected dogs, especially the English Bulldog and Boxer breeds, an abnormal left coronary artery (originating from a single right coronary artery) is present surrounding the stenotic RVOT, therefore, examination of the coronary anatomy by transoesophageal echocardiography or selective coronary angiography is essential.

Recently, the use of computed tomography angiography (or angiotomography) combined with ECG (ECG gated CT angiography) has been used for the anatomical study of the coronary arteries, as well as the pulmonary and systemic circulation. This technique can detect aberrant coronary artery abnormalities quickly and is minimally invasive, allowing better and faster patient selection for the pulmonary valvuloplasty procedure. In these patients, balloon dilation has been reported to cause rupture of the artery and sudden death.

Check-ups are usually at 3, 6, and 12 months after the procedure and then annually. Gradients may continue to decrease in the first 3 to 6 months, when compared with the gradient 24-hours after the procedure, probably due to resolution of the valvular oedema and the regression of the infundibular and RV hypertrophy. Therefore, the success of a PBV should not be confirmed until several months after the procedure. Normally, β-blocker administration is continued in dogs with a residual pressure gradient ≥60–80 mmHg, RV hypertrophy, and dynamic residual RV outlet obstruction.

Aortic Stenosis (AS)

Aortic stenosis (AS) is classified into three types, depending on the lesion's location along the left ventricular outflow tract (LVOT):

- subvalvular
- valvular
- supravalvular.

The most common form is subvalvular, commonly referred to as subaortic stenosis (SAS), which can be subdivided into three different types: type 1, type 2 and type 3.

Canine SAS is the second most common congenital heart defect, with an incidence of 21.3% of congenital heart diseases, although geographic variation in prevalence is an important factor.

Anatomy and Function

Subvalvular lesions can present at birth or develop during the first weeks or months of life. In pathology studies in the Newfoundland, subvalvular lesions were only detected in puppies aged three weeks or older. Based on these findings, SAS is not strictly congenital, but rather develops very early in the animal's life. This observation has also been described in humans. It has been seen that **lesions arise due to morphological abnormalities in the LVOT** which increase frictional stress and induce the proliferation of cells. This proliferation can be derived from the persistence of embryological endocardial tissue which maintains its proliferative capacity.

The anatomical and morphological changes to the LVOT include an increase in mitral-aortic separation, decreased aortoseptal angle (AoSA), and a small aortic ring causing cellular proliferation of endocardial tissue in the LVOT, which causes the subaortic stenotic lesion.

In dogs, the obstruction progresses during the first 12 months of life. It is important to consider this progression in puppies of predisposed breeds and it is appropriate that breeds prone to subaortic stenosis are not used for breeding until they are fully grown. **A full certification of phenotypically normal dogs can only be issued after 12 months of age**. Additionally, pressure gradients can also increase during the growth period such that mild aortic stenosis at the age of four months usually progresses to severe aortic stenosis within the first year. Therefore, when a mild to moderate SAS is diagnosed in a puppy, **a prognosis should not be given until one year of age**, because the obstruction can progress (and often does) to become more severe.

As previously indicated, **three different types of subaortic stenosis** have been described based on postmortem findings, with an increase in the severity of the disease from type 1 to 3 (Figures 22, 23 and 24, Box 4). Ventricular aortic valve leaflets may be thickened, which can lead to a misdiagnosis of aortic valve stenosis, therefore, it is important to carefully evaluate the LVOT. The most frequent types, in our experience, are types 1 and 2, which make up more than 85% of SAS cases.

In addition to the fixed subaortic lesion, a dynamic (labile) component can affect the behaviour of the SAS. In the fixed stenotic lesion, the severity of the stenosis does not change from beat to beat or during the systolic phase.

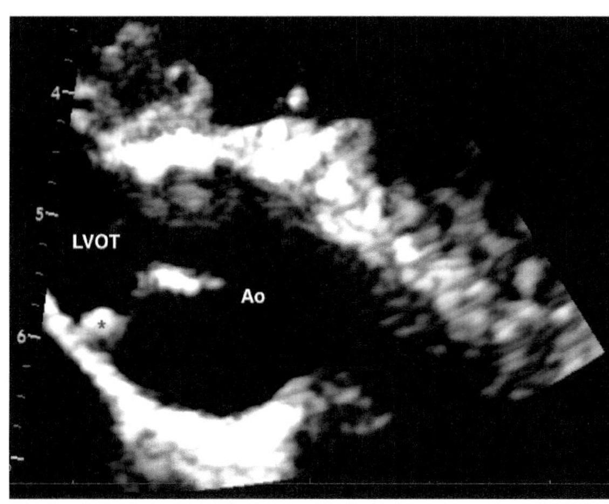

Figure 22. Magnified 2D image from a right long axis parasternal projection optimised for the LVOT in a patient with type 1 subaortic stenosis. At the level of the LVOT a nodule of about 2.5mm (asterisk) in size can be seen, just below the leaflets of the aortic valve. Ao: aorta; LVOT: left ventricular outflow tract.

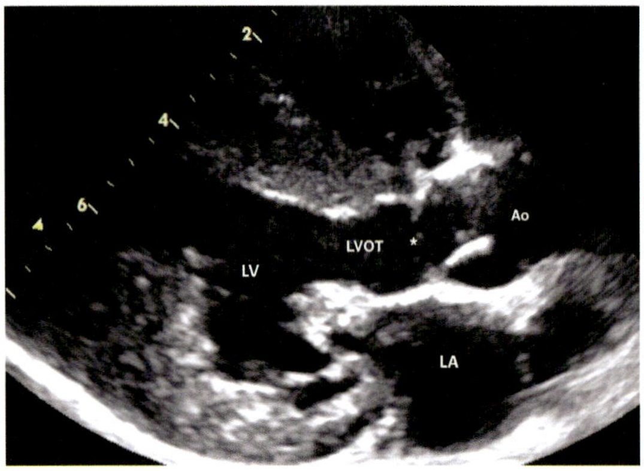

Figure 23. 2D image from a right long axis parasternal projection optimised for the left ventricular outflow tract (LVOT) in a patient with type 2 subaortic stenosis. At the level of the LVOT a ring (asterisk) can be seen passing just below the aortic valve leaflets. LA: left atrium; LV: left ventricle; LVOT: left ventricular outflow tract.

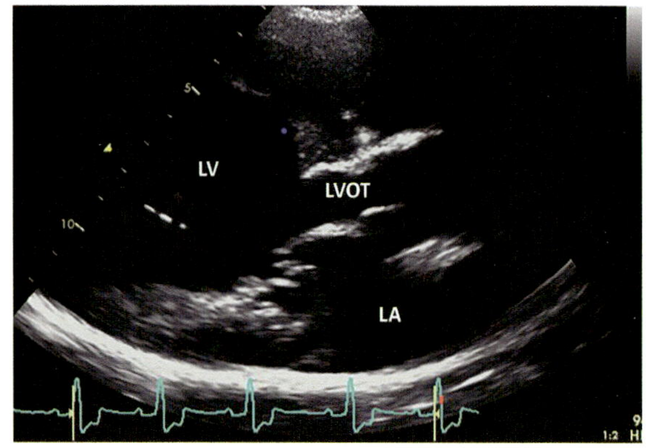

Figure 24. 2D image from a right long axis parasternal projection optimised for the left ventricular outflow tract (LVOT) in a patient with type 3 subaortic stenosis. A fibrous band can be appreciated at the level of the LVOT which causes a narrowing of the whole anatomical structure, creating a tunnel like image. LA: left atrium; LV: left ventricle; LVOT: left ventricular outflow tract.

In contrast, **the dynamic component of stenosis can change with heart rate**, state of contractility, or during the systolic phase. Muscle hypertrophy, at the level of the left ventricular outflow tract or anterior septal movement of the mitral valve are classic examples of dynamic stenosis which accompany SAS.

Box 4. Types of Subaortic Stenosis

- **Type 1. Small nodules can be seen on the endocardial surface of the ventricular septum just below the aortic valve.**
- **Type 2. Narrow thickened ridge of the endocardium that extends partially around the LVOT. The ridges are variable in location, but in most cases, they originate at the base of the anterior leaflet of the mitral valve and extend transversely through the interventricular septum below the left coronary cusp of the aortic valve.**
- **Type 3. Fibrous band or collar that surrounds the LVS, creating a tunnel-like lesion. The *annulus* often rises 1–2 mm above the endocardial surface and extends through the interventricular septum below the cusp of the aortic valve and the anterior leaflet of the mitral valve to the aortic valve. The ventricular surfaces of the aortic valve leaflets are also thickened.**

Genetics and Breed

Subaortic stenosis has been shown to be hereditary in the Newfoundland. The high prevalence of this defect in other breeds suggests heritability, but additional studies are lacking. In the Newfoundland heritability has been described as polygenic and the genetic basis is suspected to be autosomal dominant polygenic with modifier genes. Because the heritability of SAS cannot be explained by simple Mendelian genetics, dogs with mild SAS can produce severely affected offspring. As a result, detection of mild SAS is important even though mild outflow tract obstruction typically has no clinical consequences. Careful evaluation of the parents of affected puppies (including echocardiography) is therefore recommended even in the absence of a murmur. There is no sex predisposition. A breed predisposition has been identified in the following breeds:

- Newfoundland
- German Shepherd
- Boxer
- Golden Retriever
- Rottweiler
- Dogue de Bordeaux.

Pathophysiology

Regardless of the location of the obstruction, **the main haemodynamic consequence of aortic stenosis is an increase in resistance to left ventricular flow**. Increased afterload causes an increase in left ventricular systolic pressure (an increase in the pressure gradient due to stenotic lesion), an increase in the velocity of blood flow through the lesion, and **concentric hypertrophy of the left ventricle**.

Left ventricular hypertrophy is normally proportional to the severity of the obstruction (Figure 25) and attempts to normalize systolic wall stress, systolic ventricular function, and left ventricular stroke volume. Severe concentric hypertrophy can reduce end-diastolic volume and lead to increased ventricular stiffness, which can decrease the ability of the ventricle to fill properly and lead to diastolic dysfunction.

Also, chronic pressure load in the left ventricle can lead to the development of myocardial systolic dysfunction. As part of disease progression, an afterload imbalance is seen, characterised by dilation and hypocontractility of the left ventricle which also produces moderate to severe mitral regurgitation. In this situation, the peak velocity (and the aortic transvalvular gradient) are reduced due to myocardial failure and signs of left-sided CHF may occur.

SAS has been associated with intramural arteriosclerotic lesions in the coronary arteries. Abnormally narrow coronary vessels, large myocardial mass, and increased left ventricular pressure contribute to the development of myocardial ischaemia leading to a **predisposition for ventricular arrhythmias**.

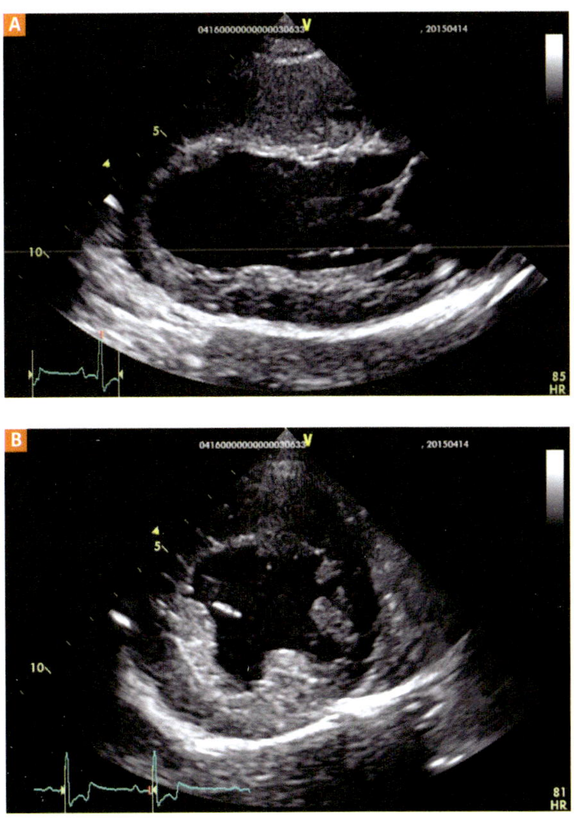

Figure 25. 2D image from a right long axis (**A**) and short axis (**B**) parasternal projection at the level of the insertion of the papillary muscles. Marked hypertrophy of the left ventricle can be seen, of both the interventricular septum and the posterior wall of the LV.

Diagnosis

Clinical Presentation

Healthy Boxers often have a 1/6 to 2/6 systolic ejection murmur without the presence of heart disease. Individuals from this breed are described as having a left ventricular outflow tract and aortic trunk which is smaller than other breeds in relation to left ventricular diameter and volume. This could lead to increased blood flow velocity and turbulence, heard as a low-intensity, short-lived heart murmur during systole.

Pathological cases present a stronger systolic ejection murmur at the left heart base, which often radiates to the right thoracic region. In mildly or moderately affected dogs, a grade 1–4/6 systolic murmur can be heard most clearly at the costochondral junction of the left 4th–5th intercostal spaces. Severely affected dogs generally have a grade 4–6/6 holosystolic murmur, often with a precordial thrill.

At the time of initial diagnosis, patients with mild or moderate SAS are usually asymptomatic and the owners describe a normal and apparently healthy individual. On physical examination, a heart murmur is the only finding. **Some severely affected animals may exhibit exercise intolerance, syncope, or signs related to left-sided CHF**. Another notable clinical finding in patients with severe SAS is a weak femoral pulse, due to a decreased and delayed left ventricular ejection volume (*parvus et tardus*). In some cases, arrhythmias are also detected at the time of the examination. **Sudden death can occur** without premonitory signs.

Radiography

Thoracic radiographs are usually normal in animals with mild to moderate SAS, because the concentric hypertrophy pattern does not increase the dimensions of the cardiac silhouette. The most common finding in severely affected dogs is an enlarged aortic root (poststenotic dilation). Signs of left-sided CHF can be seen in patients with afterload imbalances.

Electrocardiography

Morphological changes to the electrocardiogram are not common. Signs of left ventricular hypertrophy can be detected in severely affected animals. In **severe cases premature**

ventricular complexes or ventricular tachycardia induced or exaggerated by exercise can be seen. Holter recording may be of interest in patients with moderate to severe SAS to detect ventricular arrhythmias and ST segment changes that may suggest an increased probability of sudden death.

Echocardiography

Echocardiographic examination is the most important diagnostic tool to identify the presence of congenital heart defects, as well as to classify the different types and severity of SAS. For the detection of subaortic stenosis, a careful evaluation of LVOT morphology with 2D echocardiography must be performed. The dimension and morphology of the aortic *annulus* and valve cusps are evaluated from the standard long-axis right parasternal section, optimizing the LVOT (Figure 23) and also from the right parasternal short-axis section. In some cases, poststenotic dilation of the ascending aorta is observed and is clearly identified from the cranial left parasternal longitudinal section, optimizing the LVOT. The aortic valve often appears slightly thickened due to the ongoing trauma associated with the stenosis jet and it may also appear hypomobile due to reduced flow through the aorta.

Transvalvular aortic flow should be measured using spectral Doppler, with the transducer positioned caudal to the xiphoid process of the sternum to obtain a subcostal view. Pulsed Doppler and colour Doppler studies of the LVOT and aorta show a large turbulent systolic jet. A continuous Doppler study is important to measure the peak velocity and the transvalvular gradient of the aorta (Figure 26). The use of 3.5 MHz or lower frequency transducers is recommended to ensure sufficient tissue penetration and adequate strength of the Doppler recording signal, since in large dogs there is a considerable distance between the probe and the aortic valve in the subcostal view.

The standard apical five-chamber view is also a good alternative but should only be used if imaging and subcostal measurements are not feasible. This is because the alignment of the ultrasound beam and the aortic flow is lesser in the apical view, but can be completely parallel in the subcostal view.

Box 5. Criteria for Correct Identification of Dogs with Aortic Stenosis

- **Heart murmur on auscultation.**
- **Ultrasonographic image (in 2D mode) of obstructive anatomical lesions.**
  - **Type 1: small nodules (Figure 22).**
  - **Type 2: fibrous ring (Figure 23).**
  - **Type 3: narrow concentric tunnel (Figure 24).**
- **Identification of turbulent aortic flow with pulsed Doppler using high pulse repetition frequency at the highest velocity, with mean peak velocity with continuous Doppler >2 m/s during three cardiac cycles in periods of stable sinus rhythm. It has recently been suggested that dogs with peak velocities between 1.9 and 2.4 m/s without 2D abnormalities are considered as doubtful; in these cases, an echocardiographic follow up is necessary after 12 months before issuing a definitive diagnosis.**

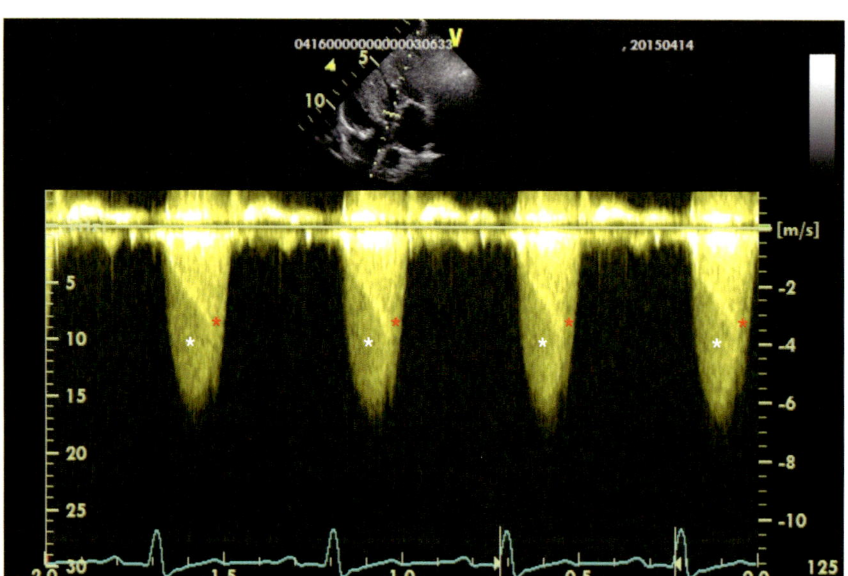

Figure 26. Continuous spectral Doppler image from a subcostal projection where high speed (6.4 m/s) turbulent systolic blood flow is seen in the LVOT. A fixed component of the subaortic stenosis (white asterisk), as well as a dynamic component which is acquired in the Doppler profile with a knife edge morphology (red asterisk).

Spectral Doppler allows assessment of a fixed or dynamic stenotic component. **Continuous Doppler enables the highest velocity peak to be measured** and the values to be calculated as a pressure gradient using the simplified Bernoulli equation ($\Delta P = 4v^2$). The values obtained are used to classify the severity of the stenosis.

- Mild stenosis: gradient below 50 mmHg.
- Moderate stenosis: gradient between 50–80 mmHg.
- Severe stenosis: gradient above 80 mmHg.

It is important to recognize that **the pressure gradient across the lesion is flow-dependent**, meaning the pressure gradient depends not only on the cross-sectional area of the stenotic orifice, but also on cardiac output. Sympathetic activation associated with clamping and disorders such as aortic valve regurgitation, patent *ductus arteriosus*, or marked bradycardia increase cardiac output and thus peak velocity in the aorta.

On the other hand, factors that decrease cardiac output, such as myocardial dysfunction, sedatives, anaesthetics, and mitral regurgitation can decrease aortic velocity. Therefore, peak aortic velocity is flow dependent, **limiting the usefulness of the pressure gradient as the sole index of severity of stenosis**.

Aortoseptal Angle (AoSA)

The aortoseptal angle (AoSA) is formed by the long axis of the ascending aorta and the longitudinal plane of the interventricular septum (Figure 27). The midline axis of the aortic root is constructed by drawing the bisector of the aortic root at the level of the *annulus* and the sinotubular junction. The midline axis of the interventricular septum is constructed by performing the same operation for the septum at the tips of the mitral valve and from that point 2 cm towards the apex. Subsequently, a line is drawn that cuts the perpendicular lines drawn in the aorta in half and another that intersects with the perpendicular lines drawn in the interventricular septum. **The angle formed by the intersection of these two lines is the aortoseptal angle**, which helps when classifying dogs at risk of developing SAS.

Dogs classified as free of SAS have an AoSA greater than 130°, while dogs affected with SAS have an AoSA less than 125°. The AoSA has been observed to be significantly smaller in dogs with SAS compared to dogs free of SAS, so a more acute AoSA may be a risk factor for the development or progression of SAS.

Treatment

Medical

Medical treatment is based mainly on the use of **β-blocking agents**, although there is a lack of data comparing treated versus untreated patients. The presumed effect of β-blocking agents is related to a **decrease in myocardial oxygen demand** and an increase in coronary perfusion, through a decrease in heart rate and contractility. These effects can prevent myocardial ischaemia associated with left ventricular hypertrophy, increased systolic wall stress, and improve coronary flow dynamics, as well as reduce the incidence of fatal ventricular arrhythmias. It is possible β-blocking agents reduce the arrhythmogenic effects of catecholamines in the diseased myocardium, reduce their frequency and, potentially, the occurrence of fatal arrhythmias. However, evidence to support this argument is lacking.

Atenolol at a starting dose of 0.25 mg/kg SID or BID is used and the dose progressively increased until its effects are seen,

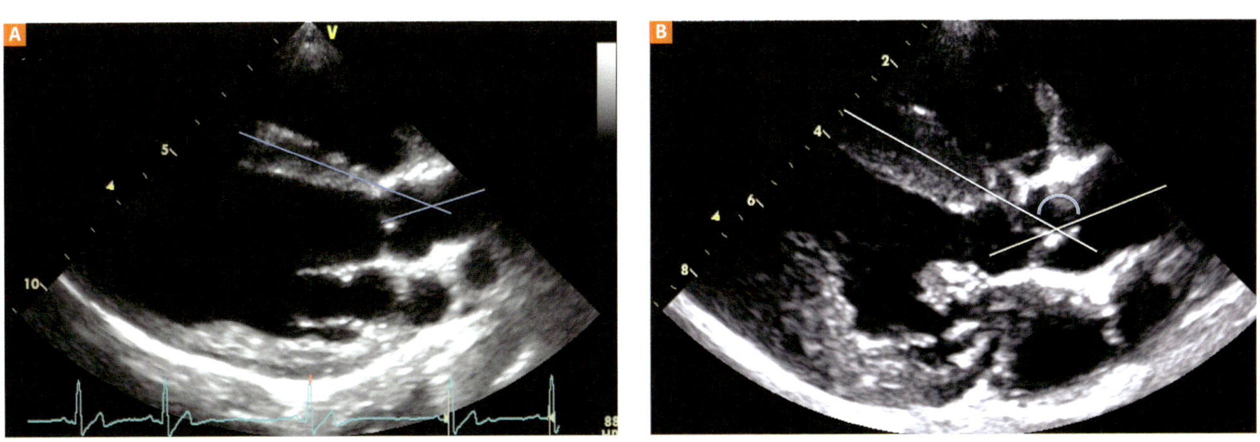

Figure 27. 2D image of a long axis right parasternal projection optimised for the LVOT in a healthy patient with an aortoseptal angle of 140° (**A**) and in a patient with type 2 subaortic stenosis with an aortoseptal angle of 122°.

always in conjunction with electrocardiogram and blood pressure monitoring before any increase in dosage.

Occasionally, medical treatment for CHF is necessary. If this is the case, diuretic treatment with ACE inhibitors is indicated.

Surgery

Initial studies for low pressure balloon catheter valvuloplasty showed short-term reduction in the systolic pressure gradient, but no long-term benefit in survival times when compared to dogs receiving atenolol. These disappointing results obtained by low pressure balloon dilation occur because of the location and nature of the stenotic lesion. Based on these data, **percutaneous balloon valvuloplasty is not indicated for SAS**.

Recently, a new technique based on the combination of a cutting balloon catheter and a high-pressure balloon catheter is being used for SAS valvuloplasty (Figure 28).

This technique involves the use of a balloon with longitudinally mounted microblades which are exposed when the balloon is inflated. These blades produce longitudinal cuts in the subaortic lesion so that it is dilated more effectively and ruptured during subsequent high-pressure balloon valvuloplasty.

Dogs with an AoSA >160° have been seen to respond to cutting balloon valvuloplasty with a greater and more favourable decrease in pressure gradient and this difference will remain, or could even decrease further, over time. In contrast, those dogs with an AoSA <160° respond with a smaller and shorter lasting decrease in aortic gradient.

On the other hand, in dogs with a more acute AoSA, the problem is not easily corrected by balloon valvuloplasty, because this technique is not designed to alter the spatial alignment between the interventricular septum and the aorta. Therefore, it is possible the presence of an abnormally acute AoSA and the resulting turbulent blood flow may contribute to the recurrence of stenosis after valvuloplasty.

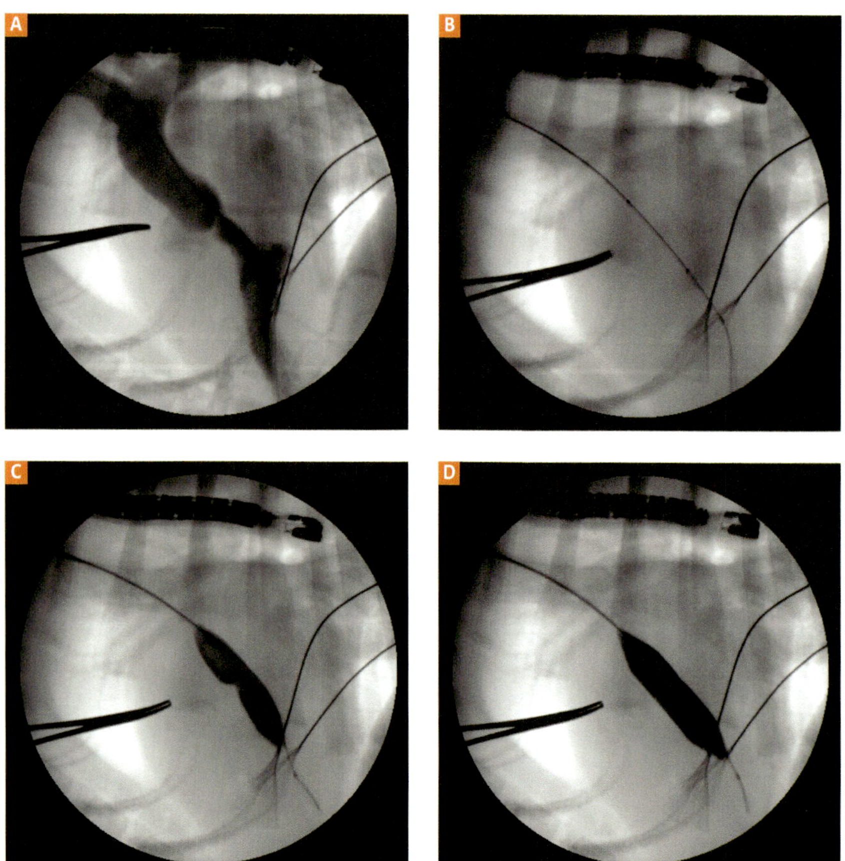

Figure 28. C-arm fluoroscopy images during a balloon aortic valvuloplasty procedure in a patient with severe type 2 subaortic stenosis. In **A** a selective left ventriculography with a pigtail catheter is seen showing the subaortic stenosis. In **B** the positioning of the balloon catheter at the level of the LVOT can be seen with the help of a metallic guide which is seen ventrally at the level of the left ventricular apex; the length of the balloon in the catheter is defined thanks to the presence of two radiopaque points, which act as a guide for correct positioning of the balloon in the LVOT. In **C** the initial stage of balloon dilatation is seen with a narrowing of the area of subaortic stenosis. In **D** the final stage of balloon dilatation can be seen, which has lost the appearance of the previous image, indicating that there has been an effective dilatation of the stenosis.

Ventricular Septal Defect (VSD)

A ventricular septal defect is a hole in the interventricular septum which allows the passage of blood between the left and right ventricles. The direction of flow depends on the pressure gradient. The blood normally flows from the left ventricle to the right, unless another congenital heart disease, such as pulmonary stenosis, is present or if pulmonary hypertension is present.

Anatomy and Function

Defects in the interventricular septum are classified according to where they are located. Thus, the following can be found (Figure 29):

- perimembranous (most common)
  - inlet (endocardial cushion defect, seen more frequently in cats)
  - trabecular (typical perimembranous), situated high up in the interventricular septum
  - infundibular (tetralogy of Fallot type defect)
  - outlet or supracristal (also called subarterial)
- muscular (rare)
  - inlet
  - trabecular
  - outlet.

The muscular portion of the ventricular septum grows from the apex towards the base (trabecular muscular septum) and from the sides towards the centre (muscular inlet septum and muscular outlet or infundibular septum). The membranous septum grows from the endocardial cushions (at the level of the atrioventricular valves) downwards, until it meets the muscular septum. The membranous and muscular septa unite just below the aortic valve: a failure in this union results in a VSD. The author has seen some patients with severe pulmonary stenosis associated with VSD. All of these patients had a muscular VSD, mainly in the inlet septum.

Genetics and Breed

Predisposition to VSD has been described in several breeds: English Springer Spaniel, Beagle, Basset Hound, West Highland White Terrier, and Lakeland Terrier among others. In addition, heritability has been described in the English Springer Spaniel and Beagle. In the Beagle, VSD has been described as an autosomal recessive trait. In the English Springer Spaniel, it has been suggested as being autosomal dominant with incomplete penetrance or possibly as a polygenic trait. No sex predisposition has been observed in the development of VSD.

Pathophysiology

Isolated VSD's produce left-to-right shunts: blood flows at high velocity through the defect from the high-pressure LV to the low-pressure RV. The shunt volume depends on the size of the defect since, in uncomplicated situations, the pressure in the left ventricle is always higher than the pressure in the right ventricle.

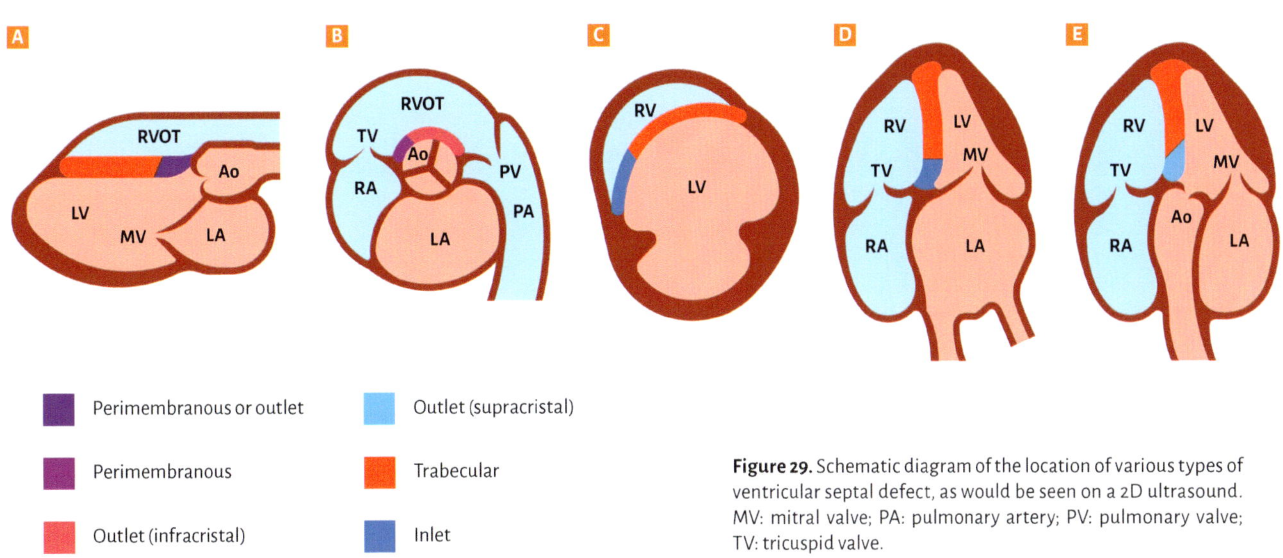

Figure 29. Schematic diagram of the location of various types of ventricular septal defect, as would be seen on a 2D ultrasound. MV: mitral valve; PA: pulmonary artery; PV: pulmonary valve; TV: tricuspid valve.

Small and medium defects usually create a high flow resistance and only allow the passage of a small volume of blood, so the systolic pressures of the right ventricle and the pulmonary artery remain normal. These small or medium-sized VSDs are commonly referred to as **restrictive**.

Large septal defects offer little resistance to blood flow and consequently a large volume of blood passes through them, which increases the pressure on the right side of the heart. As the lesion is normally located in the right ventricular outflow tract, blood is injected directly into the pulmonary circulation, so the right ventricle only acts as a conduit for shunt communication and no dilation occurs due to volume overload.

The shunt volume that passes through the RVOT into the pulmonary artery is an extra volume of blood which flows to the lungs and returns to the left ventricle, producing volume overload on the left side. Small to moderate VSDs can create some degree of cardiomegaly but left-sided volume overload is usually haemodynamically and clinically insignificant.

However, large defects produce a considerably high recirculation volume which increase diastolic volumes and pressures of the left atrium and ventricle, causing dilation of the left-side of the heart and, occasionally, left-sided heart failure. As already discussed in the section on PDA, this LV volume overload increases diastolic volume and wall tension, thus producing compensatory eccentric hypertrophy to reduce wall stress over time.

A VSD is haemodynamically significant when:

- the diameter of the VSD is greater than 60–70% of the diameter of the aorta;
- the shunt rate is high (Qp/Qs >2–2.5);
- LV volume indices are elevated (end-diastolic volume index;
- the velocity of blood flow through the shunt is low (the velocity of blood at the level of the shunt is less in a large defect than in a small or restrictive defect, because the pressure difference between the ventricles is smaller).

It is risky to measure the severity and size of the defect considering only peak communication speed, as it is difficult to perfectly align with the shunt flow and false low velocities are measured. On the other hand, it should be remembered that dogs with VSD sometimes present with high velocities which are haemodynamically significant. In addition, a large perimembranous or subarterial VSD can allow the aortic cusp to prolapse, resulting in aortic regurgitation. Aortic regurgitation can be mild or severe enough to cause additional volume overload in the left ventricle which can predispose to CHF.

In some perimembranous defects there is proliferation of the tissue of the septal leaflet of the tricuspid valve, called a **pseudoaneurysm**, which can partially or completely close the VSD. In animals with large communications, increased pulmonary blood flow can damage the vasculature, significantly increasing pulmonary vascular resistance (Eisenmenger syndrome physiology). This causes high-resistance pulmonary hypertension, which increases pressure on the right ventricle and causes RV hypertrophy.

There are three obstructive conditions affecting the right ventricle that can be associated with a VSD and complicate it.

- Tetralogy of Fallot, in which a large non-restrictive VSD is complicated by RVOT obstruction and severe concentric RV hypertrophy.
- A double-chambered right ventricle, characterised by a fibromuscular band within the cavity that creates an obstruction in the middle ventricle.
- Severe pulmonary stenosis.

In these cases, a right-to-left or biventricular shunt may predominate due to increased RV pressure. Secondary hypoxaemia and polycythaemia can develop as a result of right-to-left shunts.

Diagnosis

Clinical Presentation

Small Septal Defects

Due to the low haemodynamic impact of the lesion, patients are **usually asymptomatic**. As blood is forced through a small defect during systole, the velocity of the blood at that level is high and the flow is turbulent, resulting in a **harsh high-intensity systolic murmur over the right sternal border, often associated with a precordial thrill**. The murmur may radiate into the mitral area.

Medium Septal Defects

Depending on the haemodynamic consequences, patients often show no clinical signs or develop mild to moderate left-sided heart failure.

Large Septal Defects

Large septal defects are rare in veterinary medicine due to their haemodynamic effects and serious complications. Most puppies and kittens usually die during the first weeks of life from left-sided heart failure when pulmonary vascular resistance falls to normal limits. Surviving patients can present in CHF or with Eisenmenger syndrome physiology.

Heart murmurs tend not to be as evident as in small defects, since there is less resistance to flow, pressures are balanced, and flow velocity is decreased. A diastolic murmur over the left heart base indicates aortic regurgitation caused by aortic valve prolapse.

Radiography

Small Septal Defect

This is not usually remarkable, but in some cases there may be mild enlargement of the left atrium and ventricle with some pulmonary over-circulation.

Medium to Large Septal Defects

Cardiomegaly and pulmonary over-circulation (increased diameter of arteries and veins) can be identified as a consequence of the reported volume. Pulmonary oedema may be present.

Electrocardiography

It is usually not relevant. In haemodynamically significant VSDs, a pattern of left ventricular enlargement and arrhythmias may occur.

Echocardiography

Echocardiographic abnormalities depend on the location and size of the VSD, the pulmonary vascular resistance, and concomitant lesions (as previously discussed). A small VSD can be difficult to visualize using two-dimensional echocardiography, but it can be easily **confirmed using colour Doppler**. In large defects, the hole can be clearly seen using 2D echocardiography as an echo absent image, and the edges of the defect can sometimes be quite bright. To prevent misinterpretation of the echo absent image, Doppler studies (colour and spectral) should be used.

The echocardiographic views commonly used to identify VSD's are:

- right parasternal long axis view with the LVOT for typical perimembranous defect (Figures 30 and 31) and some muscular defects;

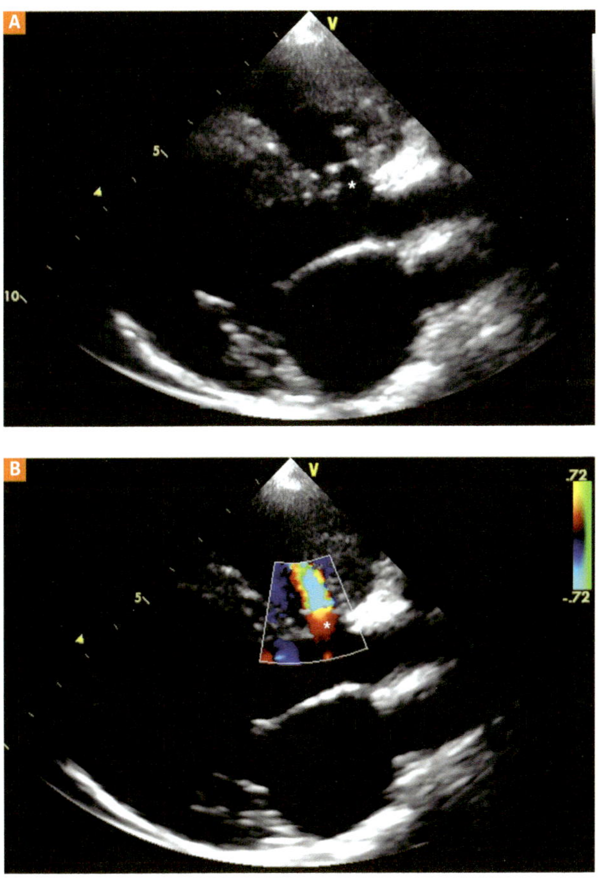

Figure 30. 2D images without (**A**) and with (**B**) colour Doppler from a right long axis parasternal projection optimised for the LVOT. In A the loss of continuity can be seen in the basal portion of the interventricular septum, where the orifice is seen in the image as a loss of echo (asterisk). In B the presence of blood flow through the defect (asterisk) from the left to right ventricle.

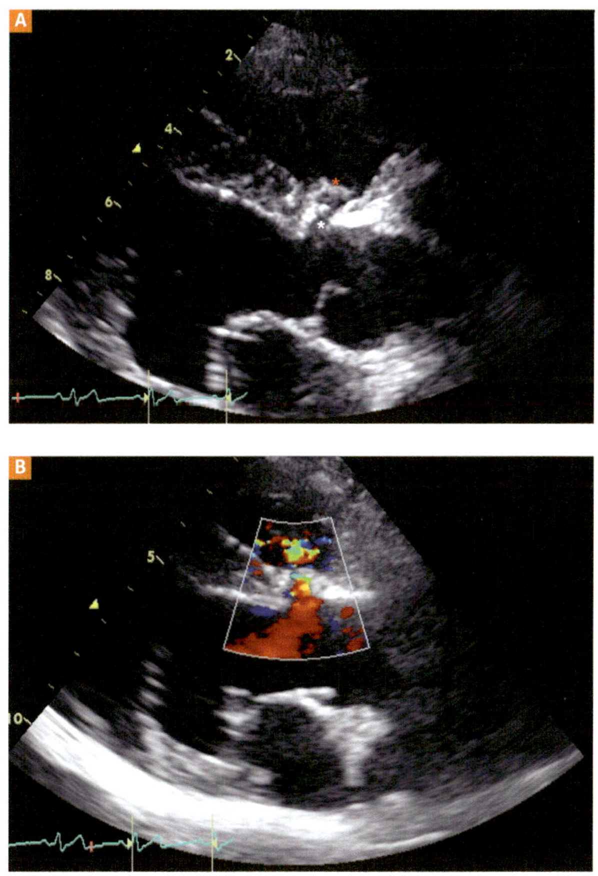

Figure 31. Magnified 2D images without (**A**) and with (**B**) colour Doppler from a right long axis parasternal projection optimised for the LVOT. In A the defect (white asterisk) can be seen associated with the presence of an echogenic membrane on the right side of the defect, attributed to the formation of a pseudoaneurysm (red asterisk). In B the presence of blood flow through the pseudoaneurysm from the left to right ventricle can be seen. Note how the blood flow appears broken through the defect, which indicates the pseudoaneurysm effect in the reduction of shunt volume.

- right parasternal short-axis view at the level of the cardiac base (aortic valve) for the typical perimembranous defect (Figure 32) and subarterial VSD;
- right parasternal short-axis projection at the level of the papillary muscles, where the interventricular septum is well appreciated, for muscle defects (Figure 33).

Continuous Doppler studies measure the velocity of blood flow through the VSD (Figure 34). The typical pressure gradient between the two ventricles in a small defect is approximately 100 mm Hg, therefore, the velocity is about 5 m/s (between 4.5–5 m/s). The larger the VSD, the smaller the pressure difference between the ventricles and, therefore,

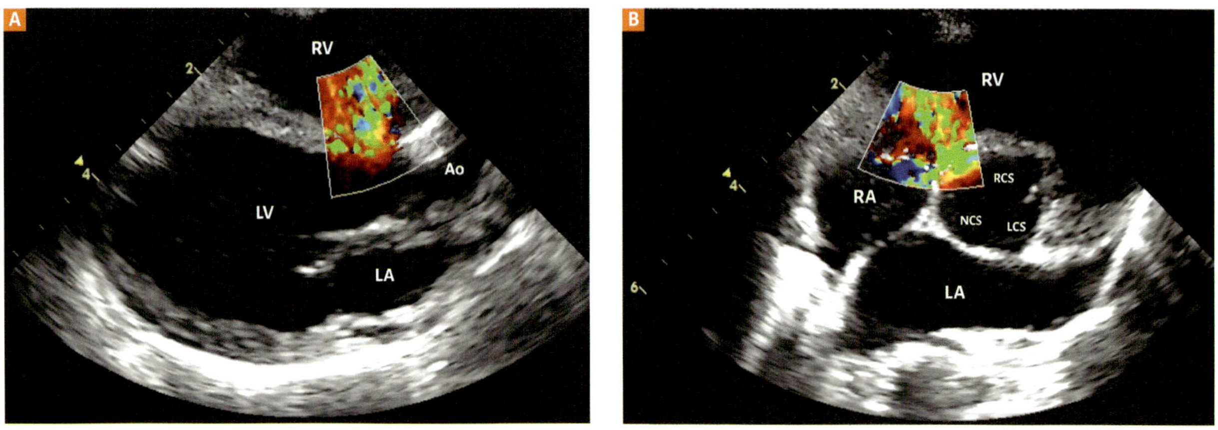

Figure 32. 2D image with colour Doppler from a right long axis parasternal projection optimised for the LVOT (**A**) and from a right short axis parasternal projection at the heart base (**B**) in a patient with a characteristic perimembranous VSD. The turbulent blood flow through the defect from the left to right ventricle can be seen. In B the turbulent flow can be seen localised between the aortic coronary Valsalva sinus and the non-coronary Valsalva sinus corresponding to the location of the characteristic perimembranous VSD. LV: left ventricle; RV: right ventricle; LA: left atrium; RA: right atrium; Ao: aorta; LCS: left coronary sinus; RCS: right coronary sinus; NCS: non-coronary sinus.

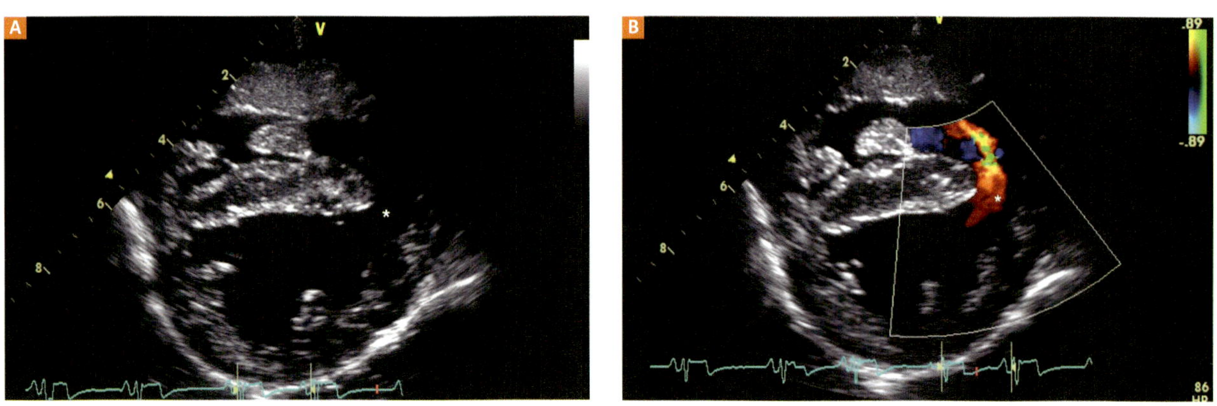

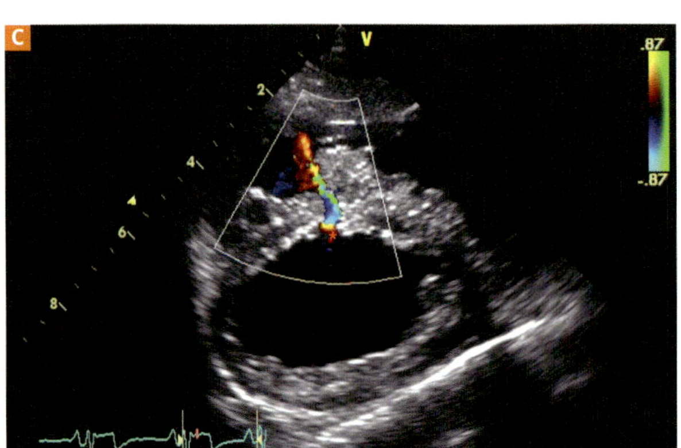

Figure 33. 2D image without (**A**) and with (**B** and **C**) colour Doppler from a right short axis parasternal view at the level of the papillary muscles where two interventricular muscular type defects in two different locations (white and red asterisks) can be seen, through which blood flows from the left to the right ventricle.

the lower the peak velocity of continuous Doppler through the shunt.

The relationship between pulmonary blood flow and systemic flow (Qp/Qs) is calculated using the pulsed Doppler method. The Qp/Qs is obtained by measuring aortic and pulmonary output, considering Qp as the volume measured at the level of the pulmonary *annulus* and Qs as the volume measured in the aortic *annulus*. Thus, the VSD defect can be considered as one of the following:

- small: Qp/Qs ≤1.5
- medium: Qp/Qs of 1.5–2.5
- large: Qp/Qs ≥2.5.

Typical **left-to-right shunts in moderate to large defects** can produce the following echocardiographic abnormalities in the left-sided chambers:

- dilation of the left ventricle in diastole (EDVI (end-diastolic volume index) increase);
- left atrial dilation (increase in the LA/Ao ratio);
- shortening fraction (SF): may increase initially, but severe chronic volume overload can result in a decreased SF due to LV dysfunction;
- left ventricular dilation in systole (ESVI (end-systolic volume index) increase).

With a large VSD the degree of pulmonary hypertension is estimated by calculating the difference between the systemic pressure gradient and that calculated via the VSD (in the absence of pulmonary stenosis). **Pressures between 50–80 mmHg indicate moderate pulmonary hypertension**, while pressures greater than 80 mmHg indicate severe pulmonary hypertension.

A 2D echocardiographic study and full Doppler examination must always be performed to identify obstructive conditions affecting the right ventricle which can cause a complicated VSD, since, **it is common to find more than one congenital pathology in the same patient**.

The author has seen some cases with moderate to large VSD's associated with pulmonary stenosis with significant right ventricular hypertrophy (Figure 35) and a low degree of aortic dextroposition. This can lead to a misdiagnosis of tetralogy of Fallot.

In **tetralogy of Fallot there is an anomalous formation of the conotruncal septum which forms the upper portion of the interventricular septum**. This portion of the septum is formed too far cranially, causing a misalignment with the lower portion of the septum and, consequently, a large interventricular septal defect is present, along with marked dextroposition of the aorta, together with a narrow RVOT and pulmonary artery. Therefore, in tetralogy of Fallot, a hypoplastic or underdeveloped pulmonary artery is the expected finding, not pulmonary stenosis in a pulmonary artery of normal size. In this disease there is also a loss of the formation of the normal angle between the aorta and the pulmonary artery, with both large arteries appearing more parallel.

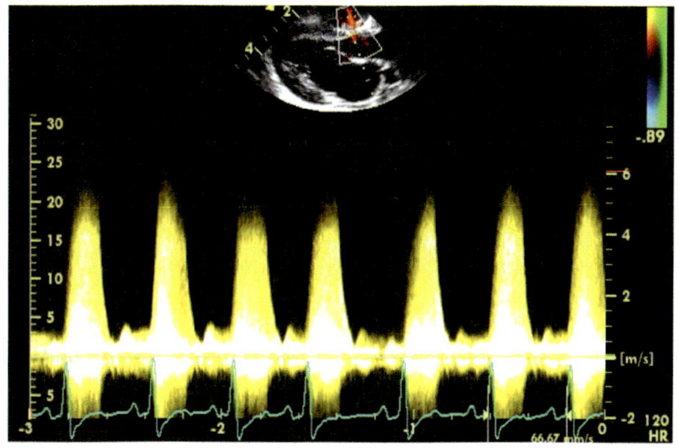

Figure 34. Continuous spectral Doppler image from a right long axis parasternal projection optimised for the LVOT and aligned as well as possible with the turbulent flow through the VSD, where a high velocity systolic flow (nearly 6 m/s) which goes from the left to right ventricle can be seen.

Treatment

Treatment of VSD should be considered carefully. In the case of a **small defect, the shunt volume tends to be small and no treatment is necessary**. In large defects, left-sided volume overload frequently causes left-sided CHF which may require treatment. For moderate-sized septal defects the clinical course is hard to predict: some dogs may not develop clinically significant consequences, others may develop heart failure, and some may develop right-to-left shunts.

Based on the author's experience, the vast majority of dogs and cats examined do not usually develop CHF or pulmonary vascular disease. Some VSDs can spontaneously close due to the development of adhesions and proliferation of tissue from the tricuspid septal leaflet. This closure creates a ventricular septal pseudoaneurysm that generally has no clinical consequences.

Medical

Small VSDs do not require treatment. Patients with left-sided heart failure should be treated as for any other heart disease causing volume-overload.

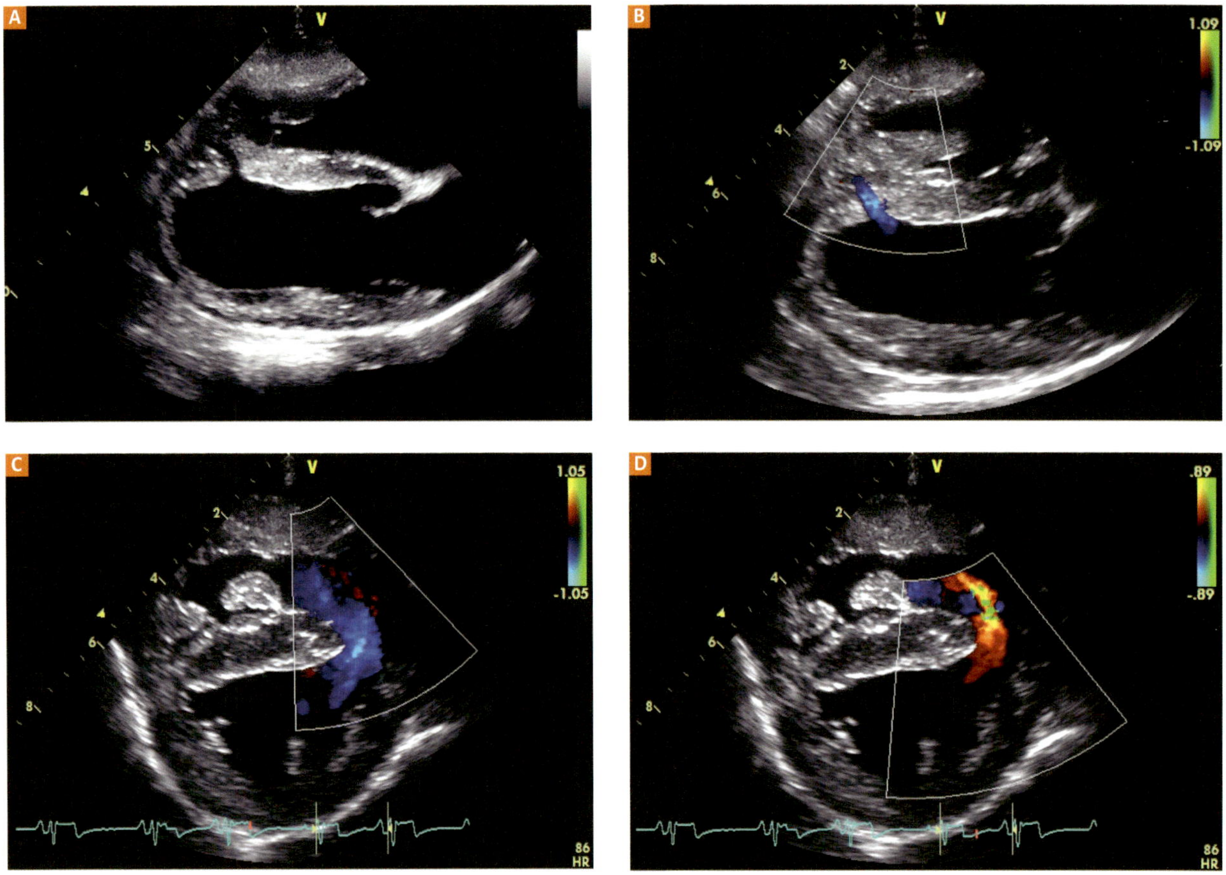

Figure 35. 2D images without (**A**) and with (**B, C** and **D**) colour Doppler from a right-sided long axis parasternal view (A and B) and a short axis view at the level of the papillary muscles (C and D), in a patient with a trabecular muscular VSD associated with severe pulmonary valve stenosis. The blood flow through the VSD in both directions right to left, as well as left to right can be appreciated depending on the point in the cardiac cycle. In images B and C a flow with a laminar tendency through the VSD right to left during systole can be seen, which is the point at which the pressure in the right ventricle exceeds that of the left ventricle due to pulmonary stenosis. To the contrary in image D blood flow from the left to right ventricle during diastole can be seen. In these images hypertrophy of the ventricular wall secondary to pulmonary stenosis can be seen.

Surgery

Before considering any surgical options, consulting a cardiologist to define whether it is a large communication or not is imperative, and to assess the possible presence of CHF. The two surgical options that are available to treat VSD are pulmonary artery banding and permanent closure of the defect. The latter option requires open heart surgery and is only performed in a few referral centres.

Closure by catheterization of ventricular septal defects may be possible. Some articles have detailed the successful closure of small to moderate perimembranous VSDs using coils. Recently, two cases have been published describing the successful percutaneous closure of a perimembranous and muscular VSD, respectively, using the muscular Amplatzer VSD Occluder.

Atrial Septal Defect (ASD)

Atrial septal defect (ASD) is a communication between the right and left atria due to a hole in the interatrial septum. Atrial septal defects are considered rare in veterinary medicine, although the incidence of small defects may be underestimated, as they do not cause a heart murmur or haemodynamic consequences.

Anatomy and Function

Embryological septation that results in the formation of a separation of the left and right atria is dependent on the development of the *septum primum* and *septum secundum*.

Initially, the *septum primum* is the first structure to develop and grow from the roof of the primitive atrium towards the atrioventricular cushions (primitive valves).

The defect that exists between the *septum primum* and the floor of the atrium is the *ostium primum*. Proliferations of this septal tissue, as well as the endocardial tissue from the atrioventricular cushion, normally ensures closure of the *ostium primum*. If this closure does not occur, the resulting defect is called ***ostium primum* ASD**, which is generally the result of an endocardial cushion defect, which is located towards the bottom of the atrium, often involving the atrioventricular leaflets. Before closure of the *ostium primum*, the reabsorption of the tissue in the dorsal portion of the *septum primum* forms a second opening, creating the *ostium secundum* of the *septum primum*.

A second septum, the *septum secundum*, develops from the roof of the right atrium and is made up of two parts, the caudal and the cranial part. The caudal part fuses with the interatrial septum along the floor of the atrium, while the cranial part grows caudally, superimposing the *septum primum* and closing the *ostium secundum*. Failure of the *septum secundum* to grow normally results in a defect called the *ostium secundum* ASD. This defect of variable size is the most common.

At the end of embryonic development, the *septum secundum* leaves a defect in the middle portion between the *septum primum* and the *secundum*. This opening is the *foramen ovale*, which is the last foetal communication between the left and right atrium and allows the passage of blood from the right atrium to the left in the foetus. At birth, the increase in volume and pressure in the left atrium (due to increased pulmonary venous return) causes the apposition of these two sheets of tissue and the foramen closes.

If this closure does not occur, a defect called *patent foramen ovale* (PFO) occurs. In addition to the types of *ostium primum* ASD, *ostium secundum* ASD and PFO there are two other types of ASD which have been described: venous sinus and coronary sinus. *Sinus venosus* defects are very close to the roof of the atrium and are believed to be caused by an abnormal union of the right pulmonary veins to either the cranial or caudal vena cava. Coronary sinus defects occur when the development of the wall between the coronary sinus and the left atrium fails (Figure 36).

Genetics and Breed

ASD has been associated with a **strong breed predisposition** in several breeds, including Boxers, Dobermanns, Samoyed, and Poodles.

In the Poodle (and less extensively in the Dobermanns) the pedigree has been evaluated demonstrating the familial nature of the disease. ASD in the Poodle is an *ostium secundum* defect. The initial evaluation of the pedigree suggests that it is probably an autosomal dominant trait, although to date not enough animals have been evaluated to confirm this definitively. In the Dobermann it is also an *ostium secundum* defect, but the pattern of heritability has yet to be established.

Septum primum defects appear to be more common in cats than in dogs.

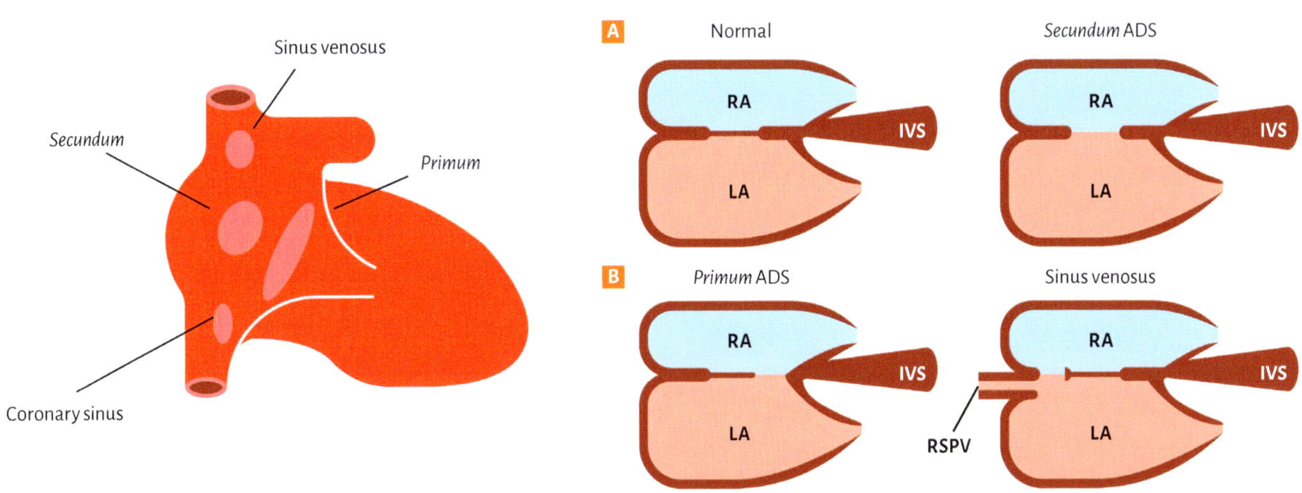

Figure 36. Schematic representation of the different types of atrial septal defects. In **A** the relationship between the different types of septal defects seen from the right side of the heart are illustrated. In **B** the differences between the different types of atrial septal defect from a four-chamber subcostal view are shown. RA: right atrium; LA: left atrium; IVS: interventricular septum; RSPV: right superior pulmonary vein.

Pathophysiology

As the pressure gradient between the atria is small, the determining factor for shunt volume is the size of the defect and the distension capacity of both ventricles. Small defects provide resistance to flow, allowing only a small shunt volume, this means they are not usually haemodynamically significant. Large defects do not provide resistance to flow, and the shunt volume depends entirely on the relationship between the distension capacity of the left and right ventricle.

Since the right ventricle is approximately two to three times more compliant than the left, the right ventricle can fill with two to three times the amount of blood as the left ventricle if there is no interatrial septum. Consequently, flow through the right heart encounters less resistance, which also determines the direction of the shunt from left to right. In conditions associated with lower right ventricular distention, such as pulmonary stenosis or pulmonary hypertension, the flow will be from right to left and hypoxaemia may occur.

In the absence of right-sided disease, the ASD produces left-to-right communication and right-side overload, which causes dilation of the right chambers.

Diagnosis

Clinical Presentation

Typically, atrial defects are not associated with velocities high enough to cause a diastolic murmur. Audible murmurs are associated with large septal defects and are a consequence of increased flow through the pulmonary valve, resulting in relative pulmonary stenosis. These are **soft, systolic murmurs** and are heard at the left base in the thoracic wall, corresponding with the location of the pulmonary valve.

The increased ejection volume is also associated with an increased ejection time and, therefore, a **splitting of the second heart sound** which can be detected as a consequence of delayed closure of the pulmonary valve. Patients with large ASDs may show signs of right-sided heart failure. Patients who have concomitant right-sided abnormalities that cause right-to-left communication through the ASD may present with exercise intolerance or cyanosis.

Radiography

Signs of right-sided enlargement and pulmonary over-circulation is found in patients with large defects and a high shunt volume.

Electrocardiography

The ECG may show evidence of **an enlarged right ventricle**.

Echocardiography

The defect can be visualised using 2D echocardiography and Doppler. The right-sided four-chamber long axis parasternal projection will position the ultrasound beam perpendicular to the interatrial septum, providing an optimal 2D ultrasound signal for inspection of the septum (Figure 37). From this view the flow will

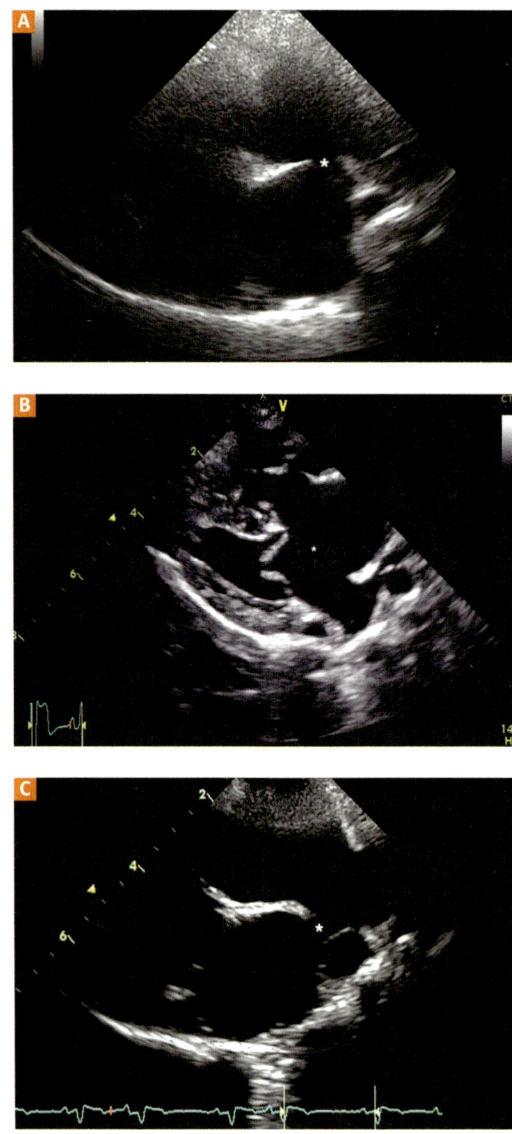

Figure 37. 2D image from a right long axis parasternal view of three dogs with an interatrial septal defect (ASD): *ostium secundum* (**A**), *ostium primum* (**B**) and sinus venosus (**C**) types, where the defect can be seen as the absence of echo at the different levels of the interatrial septum (asterisks).

be parallel to the ultrasound beam, which allows for an adequate spectral and colour Doppler flow examination. Caution should be exercised with this projection in the two-dimensional study, since, a lack of echo at the level of the septum where the *foramen ovale* is frequently seen, which can simulate a real defect.

Colour and spectral Doppler should be used to confirm the permeability of a suspicious lack of continuity of the septum, which allows the shunt jet to be identified and the direction of flow to be determined (Figure 38). Another useful ultrasound view is the **right parasternal short axis projection** at the level of the cardiac base (Figure 39).

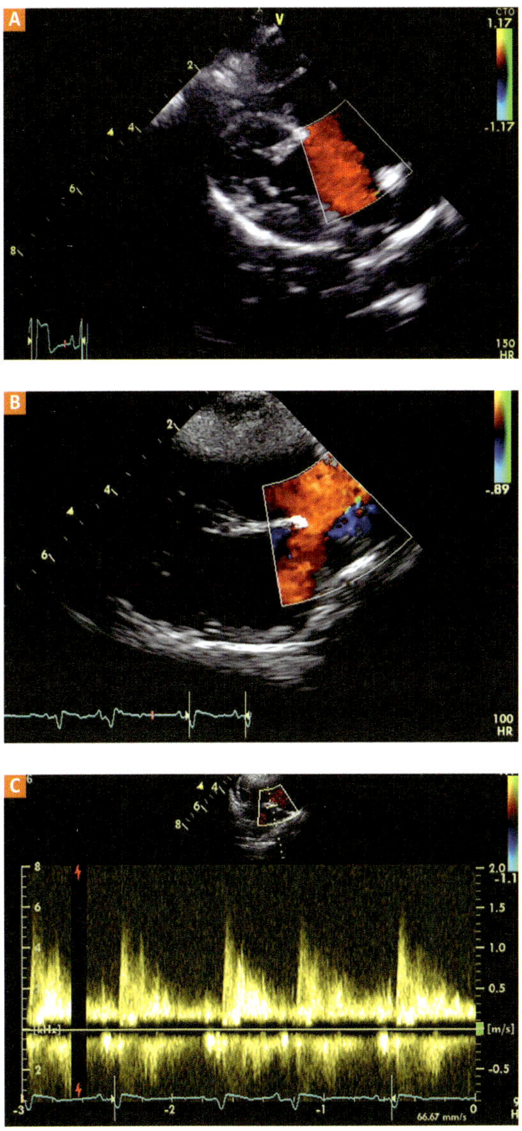

Figure 38. 2D colour Doppler (**A** and **B**) images corresponding to images B and C from Figure 37, where the presence of laminar blood flow can be seen which passes through the ASD from the left to the right atrium during diastole. In image **C** continuous Doppler shows a predominantly left-right diastolic flow with a velocity of nearly 1.5 m/s through the ASD.

The left apical parasternal four-chamber view should not be used for the 2D inspection of septum continuity because the septum is parallel to the ultrasound beam in this projection and artefacts are frequently seen. In addition, blood flow is

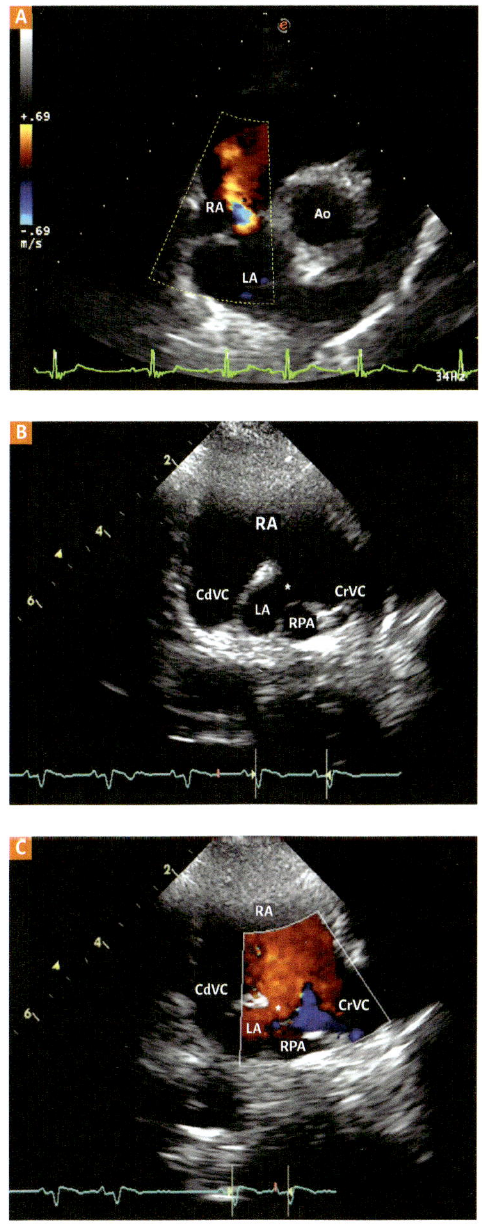

Figure 39. 2D images with colour Doppler (**A** and **C**) and without colour Doppler (**B**) of two patients, one with an *ostium secundum* type ASD (A) and the other with a sinus venosus type ASD (B and C). Image A was obtained from a right short axis parasternal projection at the level of the base of the heart, and blood flow through the ASD in a left-right direction can be seen. Images B and C were obtained from a right short axis parasternal projection at the level of the venae cavae and show the ASD (asterisk) at the level of the roof of the left atrium, through which a left-right diastolic laminar flow can be seen. Ao: aorta; LA: left atrium; RA: right atrium; CrVC: cranial vena cava; CdVC: caudal vena cava; RPA: right pulmonary artery.

perpendicular to the ultrasound beam, which is not optimal for Doppler studies.

In the absence of abnormalities associated with the right-side, the direction of the ASD shunt is left to right: therefore, right-sided chamber dilation will be seen on 2D echocardiography (Figure 40). Large ASDs cause an increase in peak pulmonary flow velocity as a consequence of increased pulmonary cardiac output.

Treatment

Medical

Small defects associated with a small shunt volume do not require treatment.

For patients with signs of right-sided failure due to large defects, standard CHF medical treatment is recommended.

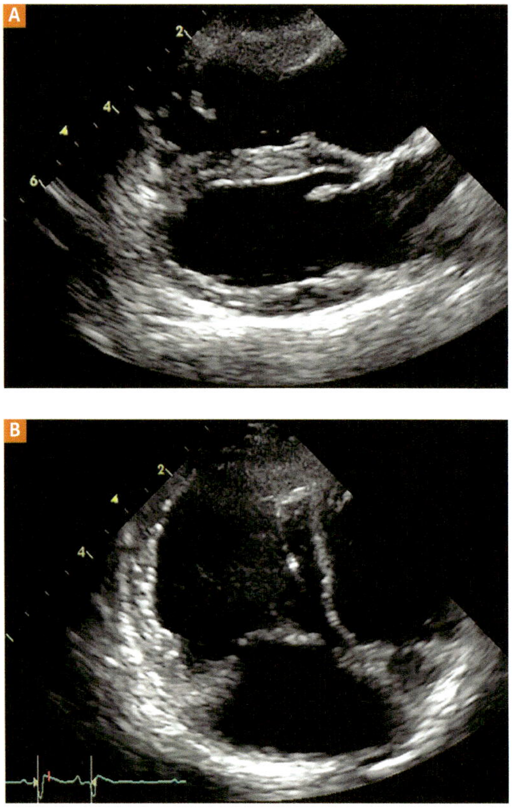

Figure 40. 2D image from right long axis parasternal (A) and left apical parasternal (B) projections optimised for the right-sided chambers, where right ventricular and atrial dilatation can be seen.

Surgery

Closure of a haemodynamically significant ASD should be accomplished by surgery or interventional cardiology.

Mitral Valve Dysplasia (MVD)

MVD is a malformation of the mitral valve leaflets, *chordae tendineae*, mitral *annulus*, or papillary muscles which alters the function of the valve causing stenosis or mitral regurgitation.

Anatomy and Function

As in the case of tricuspid dysplasia, mitral dysplasia consists of the malformation of some of its structures:

- short, thickened or notched valve leaflets that may be adhered to the septum
- short and thick, long and thin tendinous cords or the absence thereof
- poorly positioned, atrophied or hypertrophied papillary muscles.

These abnormalities compromise valve function, resulting in valvular insufficiency or stenosis.

Prevalence

The highest incidence has been observed in large breed dogs:

- Great Dane
- German Shepherd
- Bull Terrier
- Golden Retriever
- Newfoundland
- Dalmatian
- Mastiffs.

Pathophysiology

Mitral valve regurgitation is one of the most common abnormalities in mitral dysplasia, but others can be found, and their presence coexist:

- difficulty in diastolic filling of the left ventricle through a stenotic mitral valve

– left ventricular outflow tract obstruction due to systolic anterior motion of mitral valve (SAM).

The volume overload associated with mitral dysplasia has the same haemodynamic consequences as in patients with chronic degenerative mitral disease. As the disease progresses, the eccentric hypertrophy of the left ventricle allows adaptation to the increased volume overload. However, over time these adaptive mechanisms are not sufficient to compensate for the haemodynamic abnormality and **left-sided CHF occurs**.

Mitral dysplasia can manifest as stenosis. In this case, there is an increase in resistance to blood flow which overloads the left atrial and pulmonary vein circulation. As a consequence, the left atrium enlarges and pulmonary venous pressure increases, producing pulmonary oedema.

Malformation of the mitral complex can also lead to obstruction of the left ventricular outflow tract through displacement of the mitral leaflets, *chordae tendineae*, or papillary muscles. Systolic anterior motion of the mitral valve (SAM) can occur even in the absence of septal hypertrophy.

Diagnosis

Clinical Presentation

As in tricuspid dysplasia, patients may present with a murmur but are **asymptomatic, or suffering from left-sided CHF**. Animals with mitral valve stenosis may also occasionally develop evidence of right CHF due to secondary pulmonary hypertension (chronic pulmonary venous congestion leading to postcapillary pulmonary hypertension). Another cause of right-sided CHF may be the association with tricuspid dysplasia.

On auscultation, the most common finding is a **left apical systolic murmur** due to mitral valve regurgitation. Careful auscultation can be used to identify a left apical diastolic murmur in mitral valve stenosis. Patients with SAM often have a left-sided systolic murmur which varies in intensity with heart rate.

Radiography

Radiographic signs of an **enlarged cardiac silhouette** depend on the severity of the mitral dysplasia and range from moderate to severe dilation of the left atrium and ventricle. Signs of left-sided CHF may not occur until adulthood.

In cases where pulmonary hypertension has developed, varying degrees of **pulmonary artery and right ventricular enlargement are found**. All three forms of mitral dysplasia (mitral regurgitation, mitral stenosis, and SAM) can contribute to left-sided heart failure with pulmonary venous congestion and interstitial oedema eventually leading to an alveolar pattern (Figure 41).

Electrocardiogram

The tall and wide P waves, plus an increase in the amplitude of the R wave and prolongation of the duration of the QRS

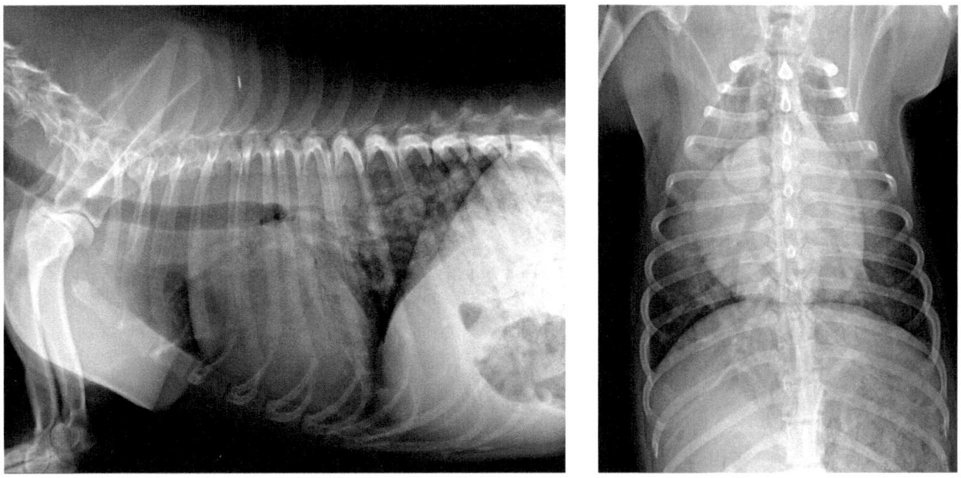

Figure 41. Left lateral and dorsoventral radiograph in a patient with mitral valve dysplasia caused by mitral insufficiency, as well as mitral valve stenosis. Generalised cardiomegaly can be seen with an interstitial-alveolar pulmonary infiltrate compatible with cardiogenic pulmonary oedema.

complex can accompany atrial and left ventricular enlargement, respectively. There may also be abnormalities that suggest an enlarged right heart, with deep S waves on leads I, II, and aVF, as a result of mitral stenosis and pulmonary hypertension. Supraventricular arrhythmias are the most common, although premature ventricular complexes can also occur.

Echocardiography

The most frequent findings are: **severe dilation of the left atrium and ventricle, massive regurgitation by the mitral valve**, and alterations in the morphology and kinetics of the mitral valve (Figure 42).

The systolic turbulent regurgitation jet is visualised by colour Doppler. Continuous Doppler allows measurement of the peak velocity of mitral regurgitation and the morphology of the mitral regurgitant flow to be studied (Figure 43).

In the case of mitral stenosis, a turbulent diastolic jet is seen which is directed from the left atrium towards the left ventricle (Figure 44). Whilst continuous Doppler aids study of the morphology of the flow and its velocity (Figure 45).

As a consequence of the regurgitation volume, the **left atrium is dilated** more frequently than the left ventricle (Figure 46). Despite severe chamber dilation due to eccentric hypertrophy, the left ventricle maintains fairly normal kinetics.

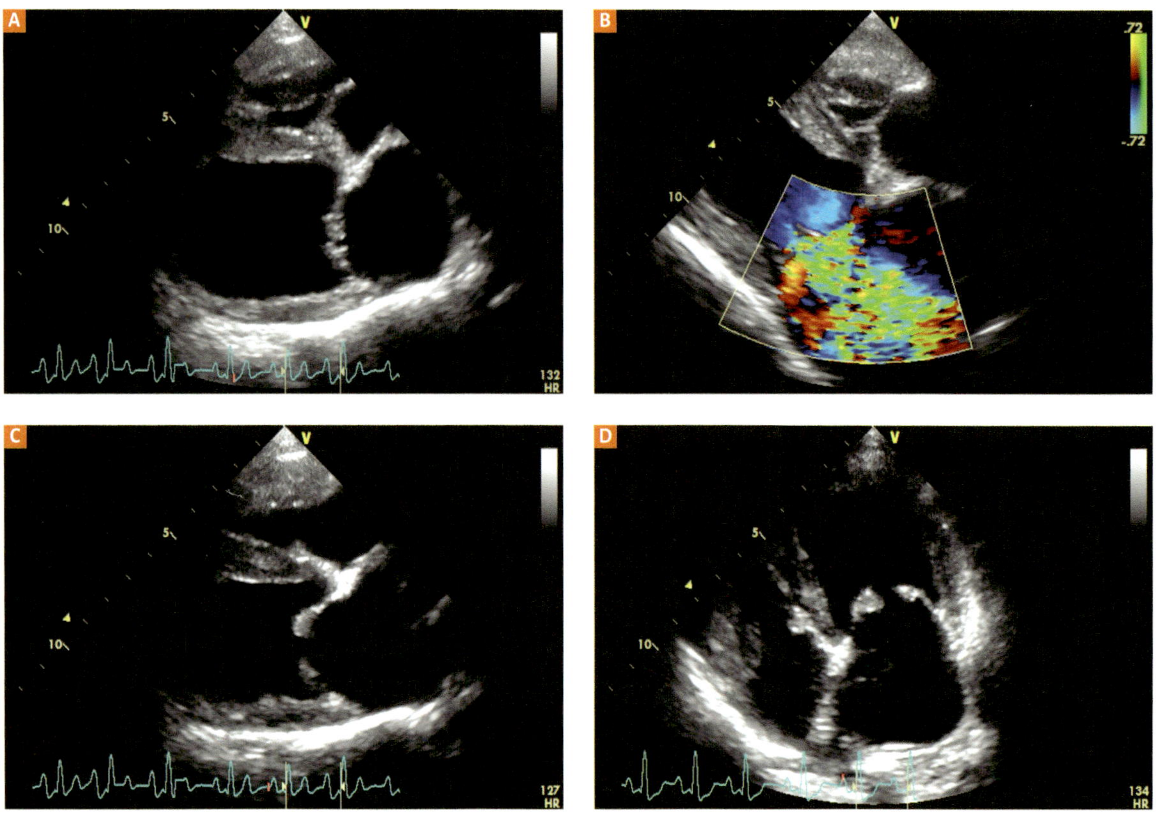

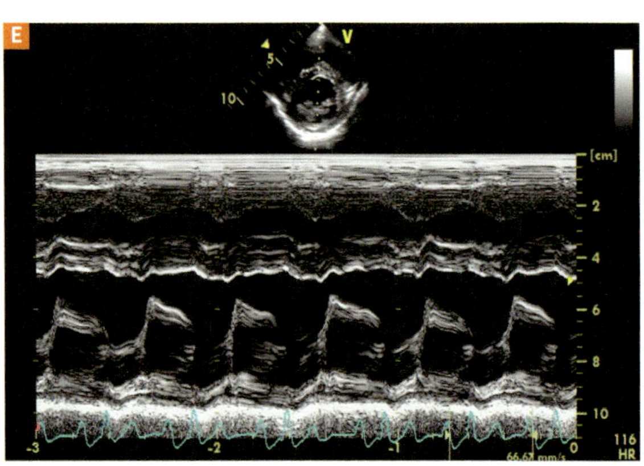

Figure 42. 2D images obtained from right long axis parasternal (**A, B, C**), left apical parasternal (**D**) projections and a right short axis parasternal view in M-mode at the level of the papillary muscles (**E**). In images A, B and C thickening of the leaflets of the mitral valve can be seen causing large scale mitral regurgitation. In images C and D a reduction in opening of the mitral valve in telediastole can be seen, showing diastolic doming. The reduced opening of the mitral valve can also be seen in the image in M-mode (E) where an increase in the EPSS (E-point to septal separation) can be seen, as well as thickening of the leaflets.

Additional echocardiographic findings include concentric hypertrophy of the left ventricle of varying degrees in cases of MVD associated with SAM.

Treatment

Medical

Treatment strategies depend on the type and severity of valve dysfunction. Patients with mitral regurgitation that develop CHF are treated with **diuretics and ACE inhibitors**. In patients with mitral stenosis, high doses of diuretics should be avoided, since cardiac output is dependent on preload.

β-blockers have been shown to alleviate dynamic left ventricular obstructions and concentric hypertrophy of the left ventricle in dogs with SAM. Antiarrhythmic drugs may be necessary to treat ventricular or supraventricular arrhythmias.

Surgical

Mitral valve repair and replacement using cardiopulmonary bypass has been described to alleviate or resolve clinical signs in dogs, although to date more data is required.

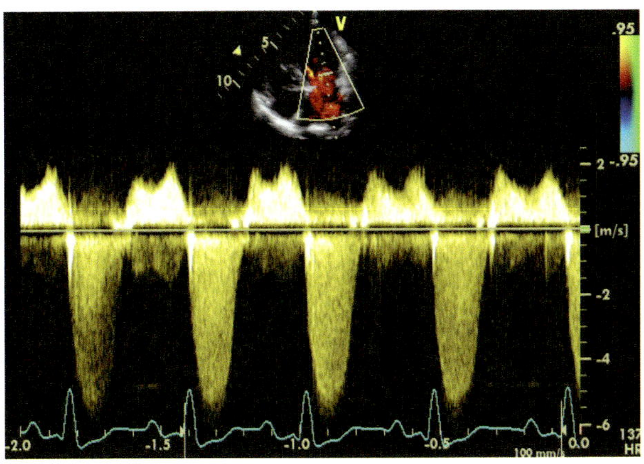

Figure 43. Continuous spectral Doppler image from a left apical parasternal projection where mitral valve regurgitation can be appreciated during systole, as well as (although less clearly) transmitral diastolic flow with a pattern showing mitral valve stenosis.

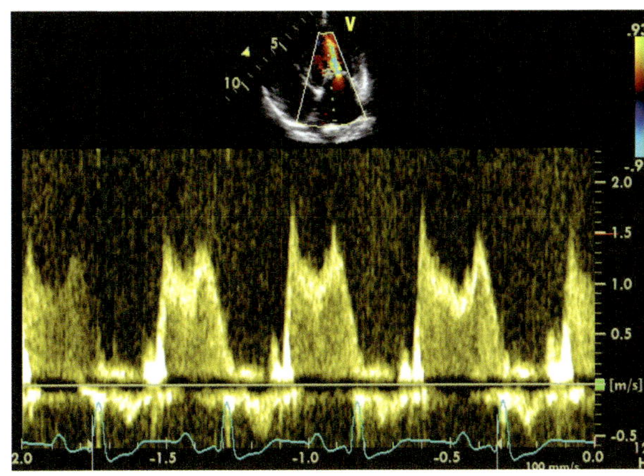

Figure 45. Pulsed spectral Doppler image from a left apical parasternal projection where transmitral diastolic flow can be appreciated, characterised by an increase in E and A wave velocity, as well as a marked increase in deceleration time of the E wave indicative of a pattern of mitral valve stenosis.

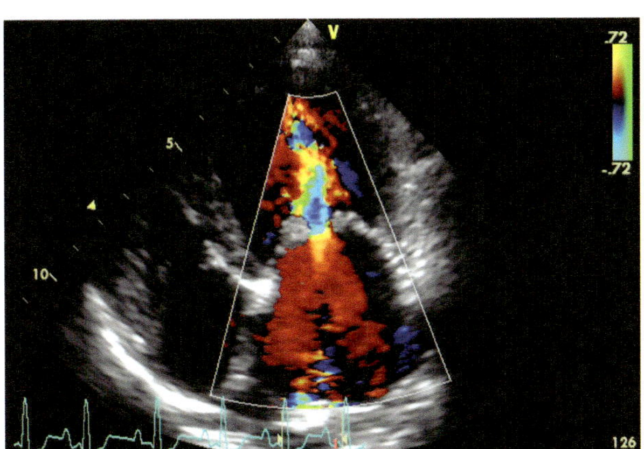

Figure 44. 2D colour Doppler image from a left apical parasternal projection where a telediastolic mitral flow can be seen which tends to be turbulent. Together with the reduced opening of the mitral valve with diastolic doming this flow is indicative of mitral valve stenosis.

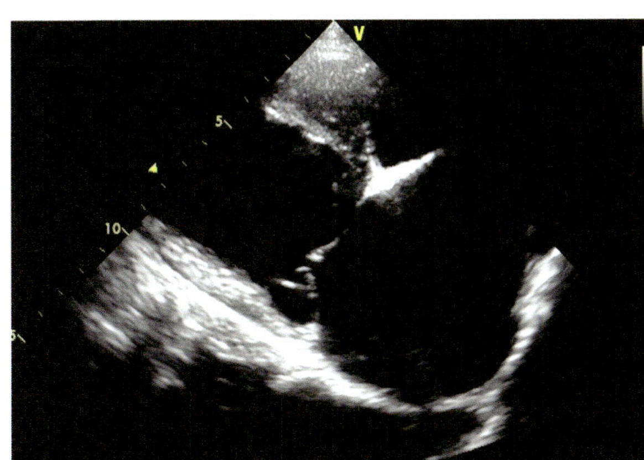

Figure 46. 2D image from a right long axis parasternal view of a patient with mitral valve dysplasia mainly caused by mitral-valve insufficiency. A marked increase in the size of the left atrium can be appreciated.

Tricuspid Valve Dysplasia (TVD)

TVD is a rare congenital heart disease in dogs and cats. It consists of a malformation of the tricuspid valve which can affect the valve leaflets, *chordae tendineae*, or papillary muscles. TVD alters the valve function, producing stenosis (occasionally) or insufficiency (more frequently). A specific type has been described in dogs due to apical displacement of the valve leaflet insertion, referred to as Ebstein's anomaly in human medicine.

Anatomy and Function

The valve apparatus is composed of the valve leaflets, *annulus*, *chordae tendineae*, and papillary muscles. Changes in any one of these components can cause valve dysfunction despite the normality of the rest of the components of the valve complex. In human medicine, several abnormalities are described:

- diffuse or focal thickening of the leaves
- underdeveloped *chordae tendineae*
- underdeveloped papillary muscles
- incomplete separation of valvular components from the ventricular wall
- focal agenesis of valvular tissue.

The common presentation in dogs and cats is the absence or reduction in length of the *chordae tendineae* and abnormal papillary muscles which insert directly into the tricuspid leaflets. The valve leaflets tend to be thickened and may contain fenestrations, and they may also be shortened or elongated. By compromising valvular function, these abnormalities frequently result in valvular regurgitation or, occasionally, stenosis.

Genetics and Breed

Tricuspid dysplasia is a rare defect that accounts for approximately 7% of congenital malformations. It has been described in several breeds and typically affects **large breed pedigree dogs**:

- Labrador Retriever
- Irish Shepherd
- Great Dane
- German Shepherd
- English Sheepdog/Bobtail
- Boxer
- Golden Retriever
- Irish Setter.

Pathophysiology

Tricuspid valve regurgitation associated with the dysplastic valve produces a volume overload of the right ventricle. To adapt to this condition, the ventricle undergoes eccentric hypertrophy and the size of the chamber increases.

As the condition progresses and the ventricle dilates, the size of the tricuspid *annulus* also increases. As a consequence, the surface area of the leaflets is not sufficient to cover the surface of the *annulus*, producing an increase in the regurgitation volume, **ending in right-sided CHF**.

Right-sided CHF also develops in tricuspid stenosis as a consequence of resistance to diastolic filling due to thickened, fused leaflets. This causes right atrial dilation, although the morphology of the right ventricle is preserved.

Diagnosis

Clinical Presentation

Dogs and cats with tricuspid dysplasia may be clinically asymptomatic, simply presenting with a heart murmur or showing signs of right-sided CHF. A right apical systolic murmur ranges from very soft to loud with a precordial thrill, depending on the amount of regurgitation and the flow rate through the valve.

Severe cases may present with a soft murmur, or sometimes no murmur is appreciated, as a consequence of a large regurgitation volume that balances the pressures between the right atrium and ventricle, causing an almost laminar regurgitation flow.

Radiography

Severe dilation of the right atrium and ventricle results in cardiomegaly and, in the dorsoventral view, **displacement of the cardiac apex to the left** (Figures 47 and 48). The apex may also be displaced dorsally in the lateral view as a consequence of severe right-sided cardiac enlargement. In some patients, the increase in cardiac silhouette size is limited to a large right atrium.

Patients with right-sided CHF present with an **increase in the diameter of the caudal vena cava due to congestion**. The main pulmonary artery is normal, and pulmonary vascularization may be normal or suggest hypoperfusion.

Electrocardiogram

One of the most common findings is a right axis deviation as a result of deep S waves on leads I, II, and aVF. Another common finding is a fragmented QRS complex (Figure 49). There may also be high P waves that suggest right atrial enlargement, although their absence does not eliminate the presence of

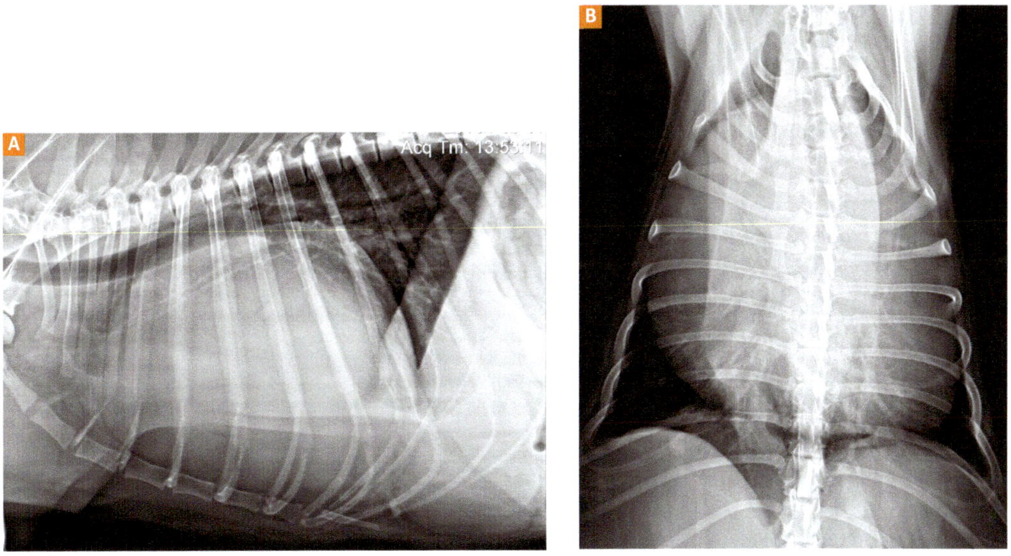

Figure 47. Right lateral (**A**) and ventrodorsal (**B**) radiograph of a patient with severe tricuspid valve dysplasia. Significant generalised cardiomegaly can be seen with a "balloon or ball" type shape, which could be confused with a radiographic image of pericardial effusion. This is one of the radiographic characteristics which should always be kept in mind when there is significant dilation of one of the right-sided chambers. In addition, the small diameter pulmonary vessels can also be appreciated as they also would in a case of significant pericardial effusion. This patient did not present pericardial effusion, the image of such visible cardiomegaly was simply caused by marked dilation of the right-sided chambers which can be appreciated in the echocardiographic image shown in Figure 53.

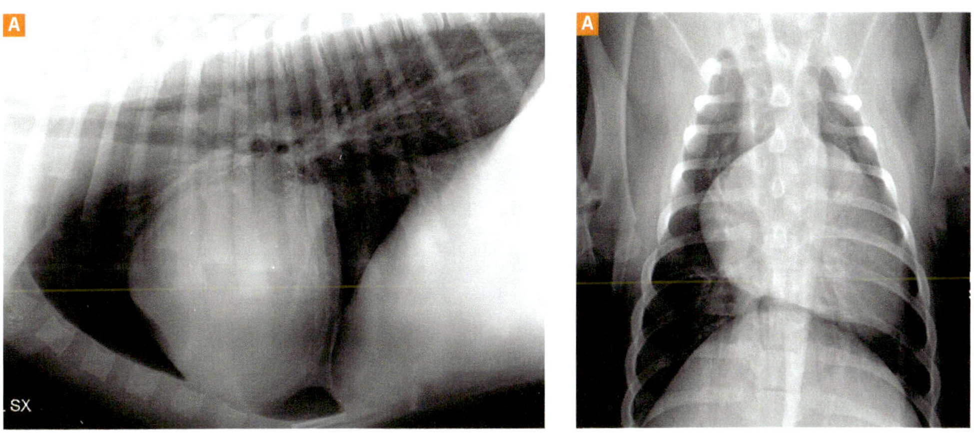

Figure 48. Left lateral (**A**) and dorsoventral (**B**) radiographs of a patient with an Ebstein type tricuspid valve dysplasia, where right-sided cardiomegaly, mainly atriomegaly can be seen.

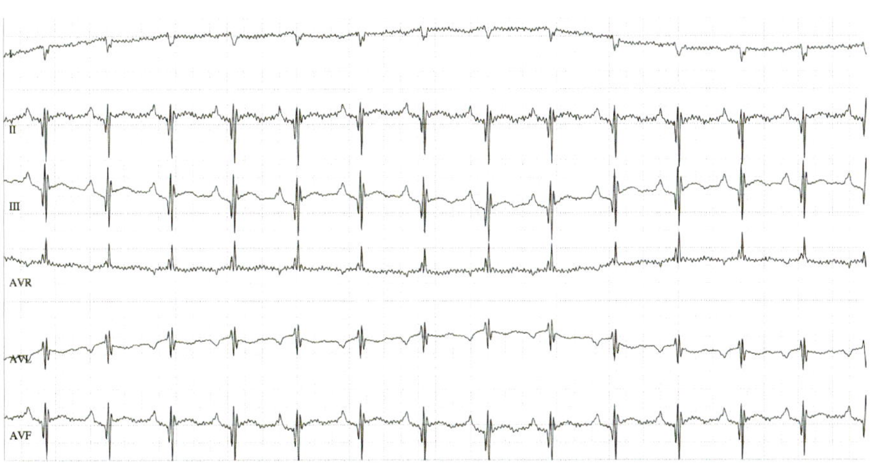

Figure 49. Six lead electrocardiogram where a conformational anomaly can be seen in the QRS complex which appears to have a notch, giving it an "M" shape, an appearance also known as a splintered QRS.

right atrial dilation. Marked enlargement of the right atrium can lead to supraventricular tachyarrhythmias, most commonly atrial fibrillation.

Echocardiography

Echocardiography provides a definitive diagnosis. Various abnormalities in the tricuspid valve can be seen on 2D echocardiography. The valve leaflets may be thickened or have abnormal mobility, due to abnormalities of the papillary muscles or adherence of the septal leaflet to the septal wall (Figure 50).

Generally in the dog, the septal leaflet of the tricuspid valve appears attached with short *chordae tendineae*. The posterior leaflet is usually very long but displays abnormal movement.

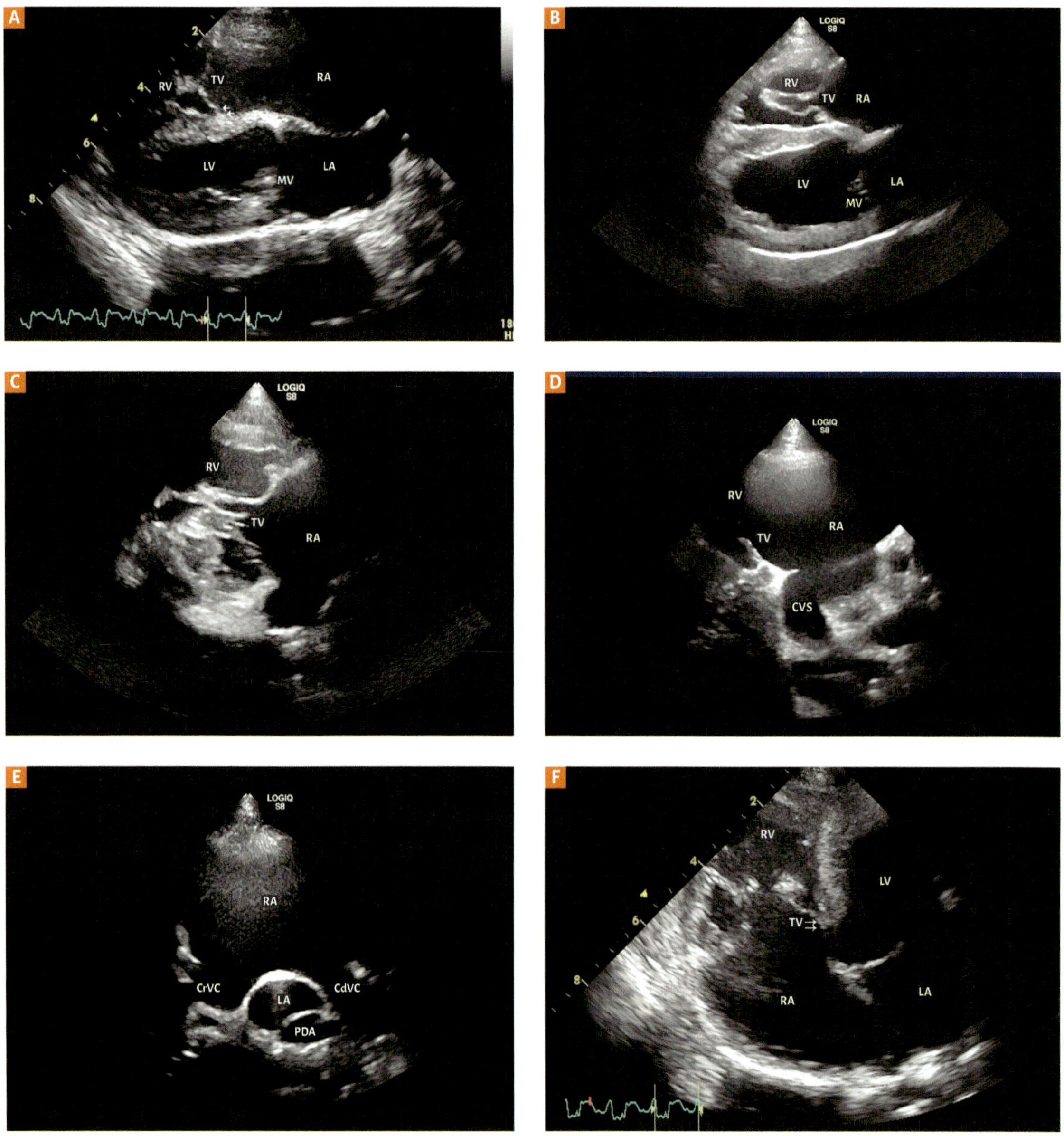

Figure 50. 2D echocardiographic image from a right long-axis parasternal projection (**A, B**), right oblique long axis parasternal projection optimised for the tricuspid valve and right atrium (**C, D**), right short axis parasternal projection at the level of the vena cavae (**E**) and left apical parasternal projection (**F**). In these images a clear malformation of the tricuspid valve apparatus is seen, with a lack of valvular coaptation associated with a marked increase in the size of the right atrium which causes displacement of the interatrial septum towards the left side. This displacement of the interatrial septum indicates an increase in pressure in the right atrium due to the volume overload caused by tricuspid insufficiency. Dilation of the vena cavae can also be seen, as well as the coronary venous sinus (CVS). In images (A) and (F) the septal leaflet of the tricuspid valve (TV) presents with an apical implantation (arrows), towards the right ventricle, which causes the atrialisation of the right ventricle, characteristic of severe type of tricuspid dysplasia, called the Ebstein anomaly.

In some cases, lack of coaptation of the valve leaflets is seen (Figure 51). When the *chordae tendineae* are present, they are thickened and short. In some cases, dilatation of the right atrium and ventricle can be seen, but enlargement of the right atrium usually predominates (Figures 52, 53 and 54). The left ventricle is usually hypovolaemic.

Treatment

Medical

The consequences of right-sided CHF are not as dramatic as those affecting the left side. Standard treatment is based on **diuretics and ACE inhibitors** to manage volume overload. Accumulation of ascitic fluid is the most common sign and may require abdominocentesis to remove the fluid.

Excessive diuresis should be avoided, especially in cases of low cardiac output. These patients can become cachectic, so proper nutrition is important. Severe atrial tachyarrhythmias should be treated to prevent further deterioration.

Surgery

Balloon valvuloplasty has been described as a treatment for tricuspid stenosis.

Surgical repair of the tricuspid valve has also been attempted, although with poor results.

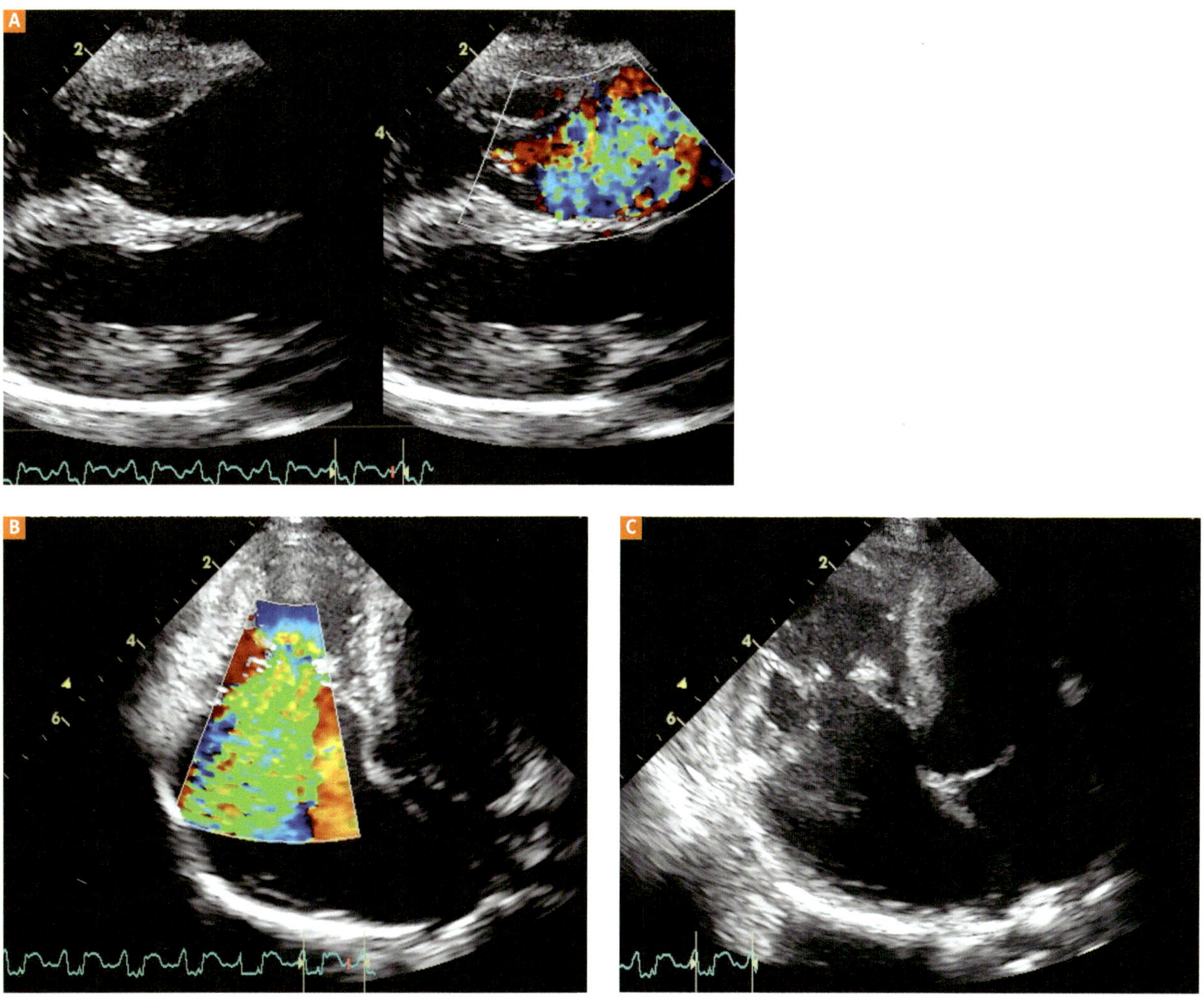

Figure 51. 2D echocardiographic and colour Doppler images obtained from a right long-axis parasternal projection (**A**) and left apical parasternal projection (**B** and **C**), where a marked lack of coaptation can be seen in the tricuspid valves causing severe tricuspid regurgitation and consequent significant dilatation of the right atrium.

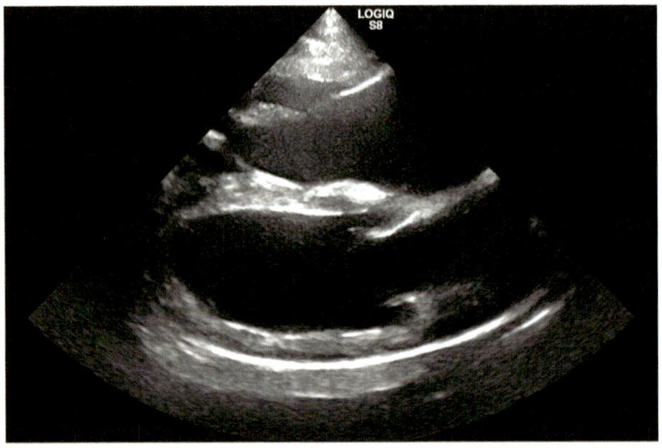

Figure 52. 2D echocardiographic image obtained from a right long-axis parasternal projection where moderate to severe dilation of the right chambers is seen. This patient was asymptomatic and did not present with an ultrasonographic signs of right-sided congestive heart failure.

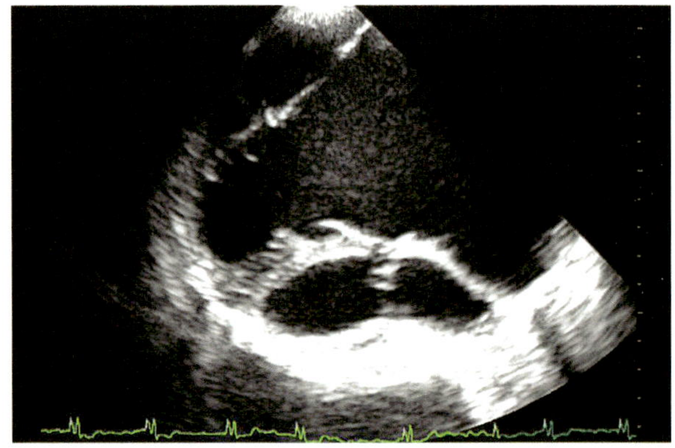

Figure 53. 2D echocardiographic image obtained from a right long-axis parasternal projection where a marked dilation of the right chambers can be seen. This patient presented with exercise intolerance, as well as clinical signs and ultrasonographic signs of right-sided congestive heart failure (ascites). Note how the ECG on this echocardiographic image appears to have an "M" morphology in the QRS complex compatible with a splintered QRS, characteristic of patients with often severe tricuspid dysplasia.

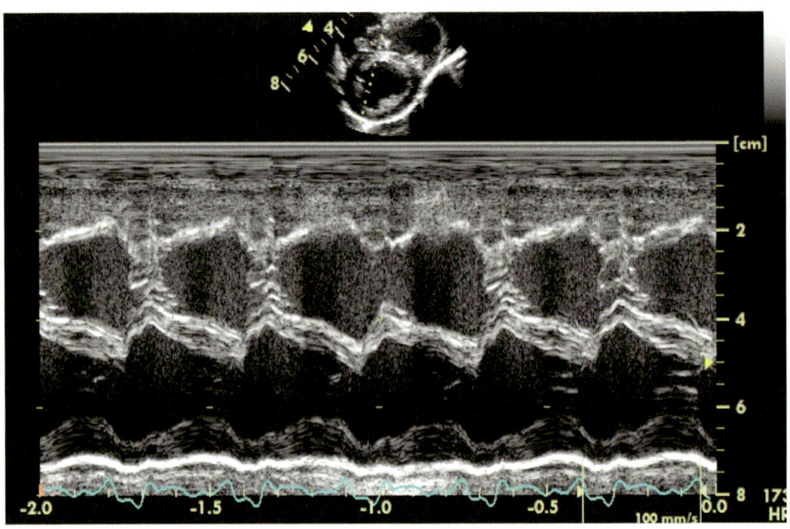

Figure 54. M-mode echocardiographic image obtained from a right short axis parasternal projection at the level of the papillary muscles where paradoxical movement of the interventricular septum (IVS) can be seen, characteristic of right-sided cardiac pathologies.

Bibliography

- Belanger, M.C., Cote, E., Beauchamp, G. (2014) Association between aortoseptal angle in Golden Retriever Puppies and subaortic stenosis in adulthood. *J Vet Intern Med*, 28, pp. 1498–503.
- Bonagura, J.D., Lehmkuhl, L.B. (1999) Congenital heart disease. In: Fox, P. *Textbook of canine and feline cardiology*, pp. 471–535.
- Bottorff, B. Sisson, D. (2012) Hypoplastic aberrant left subclavian artery in a dog with a persistent right aortic arch. *Journal of Veterinary Cardiology*, 14(2), pp. 381–85.
- Bussadori, C., Amberger, C., Le Bobinnec, G. et al (2000) Guidelines for the echocardiographic studies of suspected subaortic and pulmonic stenosis. *J Vet Cardiol*, 2, pp. 17–24.
- Bussadori, C., Carminati, M., Domenech, O. (2007)Transcatheter closure of a perimembranous ventricular septal defect in a dog. *J Vet Intern Med*, 21(6), pp. 1396–400.
- Dress, R., Francois, C.J., Saunders, J.H. (2014) Invited review-computed tomographic angiographic of the thoracic cardiovasvular system in companion animals. *Vet. Radiol. Ultrasound*, 55, pp. 229–40.
- Fujii, Y., Aoki, T., Takano, H. et al. (2009) Arteriovenous shunts resembling patent ductus arteriosus in dogs: 3 cases. *Journal of Veterinary Cardiology*, 11, pp. 147–51.
- Gordon, S.G., Miller, M.W., Roland, R.M. et al. (2009) Transcatheter atrial septal defect closure with the Amplatzer atrial septal occluder in 13 dogs: short- and mid-term outcome. *J Vet Intern Med*, 23(5), pp. 995–1002.
- Hamabe, L., Kim, S., Yoshiyuki, R. et al.(2015) Echocardiographic Evaluation of Myocardial Changes Observed. After Closure of Patent Ductus Arteriosus in Dogs. *J Vet Intern Med*, 29, pp. 126–31.
- Höllmer, M., Willesen, J.L., Jnesen, A.N. et al. 2008) Aortic stenosis in Dogue de Bordeaux. *J Vet Small Animal Practice*, 49, pp. 432–37.
- Johnson, M. S., Martin, M. et al. (2004) Pulmonic stenosis in dogs: balloon dilation improves clinical outcome. *J Vet Intern Med*, 18(5), pp. 656–62.
- Kienle, R.D., Thomas, W.P., Pion, P.D. (1994) The natural clinical history of canine congenital subaortic stenosis. *J Vet Intern Med*, 8(6):423–31.
- Kleman, M.E., Estrada, A.H., Maisenbacher, W. (2012) How to perform combined cutting balloon and high pressure balloon valvuloplasty for dogs with subaortic stenosis. *Journal of Veterinary Cardiology*, 14, pp. 351–61.
- Laborda-Vidal, P., Pedro, B., Baker, M. et al. (2016). Use of ECG-gated computed tomography, echocardiography and selective angiography in five dogs with pulmonic stenosis and one dog with pulmonic stenosis and aberrant coronary arteries. *Journal of Veterinary Cardiology*, 18, pp. 418–26.
- Meurs, K.M. (2010) Genetics of cardiac disease in the small animal patient. *Clin Vet North Am*, pp. 701–15.
- Miller, M.W., Gordon, S.G., Saunders, A.B. et al. (2006) Angiographic classification of patent ductus arteriosus morphology in the dog. *J Vet Cardiol*, 8 (2), pp. 109–114.
- Milo, S., Fiegel, A., Shem-Tov, A. et al. (1988) Hour-glass deformity of the pulmonary valve: a third type of pulmonary valve stenosis. *Br Heart J*, 60, pp. 128–33.
- Oliveira, P., Domenech, O., Silva, J. et al. (2011) Retrospective review of congenital heart disease in 976 dogs. *J Vet Intern Med*, 25(3), pp. 477–83.
- Oyama, M.A., Sisson, D., Thomas, W.P. et al. (2005) Congenital heart disease. In: Ettinger, S.J. Textbook of Veterinary Internal Medicine 6th edition, pp. 972–1021.
- Quintavalla, C., Guazzetti, S., Mavropoulou, A. et al. (2010) Aorto-septal angle in Boxer dogs with subaortic stenosis: An echocardiographic study. *The Veterinary Journal*, 185, pp. 332–37.
- Shen, L., Estrada, A.H., Cote, E. et al. (2016) Aortoseptal angle and pressure gradient reduction following balloon valvuloplasty in dogs with severe subaortic stenosis. *Journal of Veterinary Cardiology*.
- Silva, J., Domenech, O., Mavropoulou, A. et al. (2013) Transesophageal Echocardiography Guided Patent Ductus Arteriosus Occlusion with a Duct Occluder. *J Vet Intern Med*, 27, pp. 1463–70.
- Singh, M. K., Kittleson, M. D., Kass, P. H. et al. (2012) Occlusion Devices and Approaches in Canine Patent Ductus Arteriosus: Comparison of Outcomes. *J Vet Intern Med*, 26, pp. 85–92.
- Spalla, I., Locatelli, C., Zanaboni, A.M. et al. (2016) Speckle-Tracking Echocardiography in Dogs with Patent Ductus Arteriosus: Effect of Percutaneous Closure on Cardiac Mechanics. *J Vet Intern Med*, 30, pp. 714–21.
- Stern, J. A., Meurs, K. M.,. Nelson, O. L. et al. (2012) Familial subvalvular aortic stenosis in golden retrievers: inheritance and echocardiographic findings. *Journal of Small Animal Practice*, 53, pp. 213–16.

Test

Answers on Page 254

1. Which of these statements is correct?

a. Patent *ductus arteriosus* originates from the 2nd aortic arch.
b. Patent *ductus arteriosus* originates from the 4th aortic arch.
c. Patent *ductus arteriosus* originates from the 6th aortic arch.
d. Patent *ductus arteriosus* originates from the 8th aortic arch.

2. A dog with a large patent *ductus arteriosus* and a HCT of 70% is indicative of:

a. Pulmonary hypertension with flow through the PDA from right to left.
b. Systemic hypertension with flow through the PDA from left to right.
c. Association of PDA with severe pulmonary stenosis.
d. Association of PDA with severe aortic stenosis.

3. Which of the following types of pulmonary stenosis is the most common?

a. Type A.
b. Type B.
c. Mixed type.
d. Hour-glass type.

4. In a patient with severe type A valvular pulmonary stenosis with exercise intolerance, what is the treatment of choice?

a. Atenolol.
b. Diltiazem.
c. Cardiac surgery with extracorporeal circulation.
d. Pulmonary valvuloplasty.

5. Which of the following types of subaortic stenosis is the least common?

a. Type 1.
b. Type 2.
c. Type 3.
d. Type 4.

6. A non-haemodynamically significant left-to-right shunt caused by a perimembranous interventricular defect will present a maximum flow velocity through the defect of:

a. 7 m/s.
b. 5 m/s.
c. 3 m/s.
d. 1 m/s.

7. Which of the following types of interatrial defect is the most common?

a. *Ostium primum.*
b. *Ostium sinus venosus.*
c. *Ostium secundum.*
d. Patent *foramen ovale.*

8. QRS splintering is characteristic of:

a. Tricuspid dysplasia.
b. Mitral valve dysplasia.
c. Interventricular septal defect.
d. Interatrial septal defect.

Clinical Case

Signalment. 2-year-old Pinscher, 2.6 kg.

Reason for consultation. When the dog plays or runs a lot, he tires much earlier than the other two dogs in the household which are the same breed and who are approximately the same age.

Physical examination. 5/6 pansystolic murmur over the left cardiac base, radiating towards the right cardiac base. Heart rate of 120 bpm with normal femoral pulse. Pulmonary auscultation within normal limits. Respiratory rate of 20 bpm. Pink mucous membranes, with CRT <2 seconds.

Thoracic radiography. See figures below.

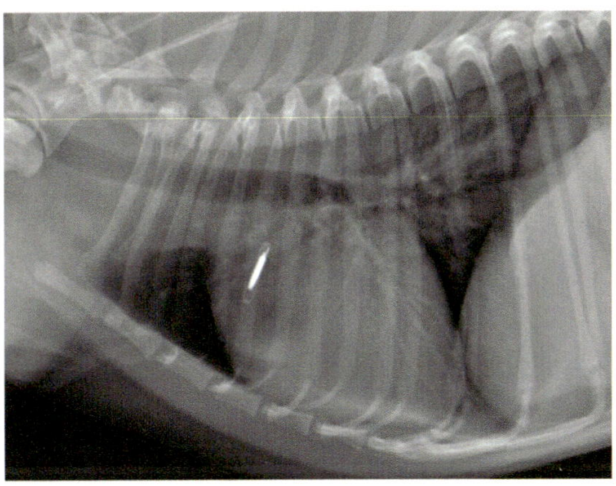

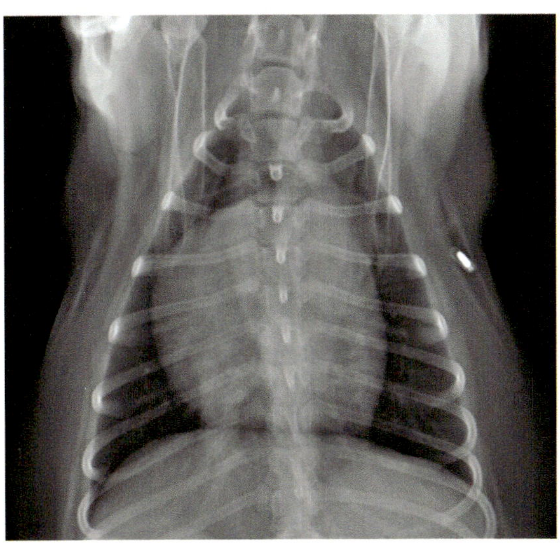

Electrocardiography. Paper speed 50 mm/s, sensitivity: 5 mm/mV. See figure below.

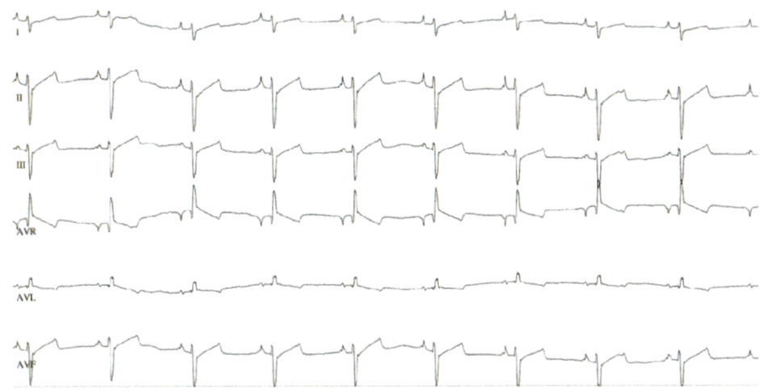

Echocardiography. See figures below (MPA: Main pulmonary artery, LV: left ventricle; RV: right ventricle).

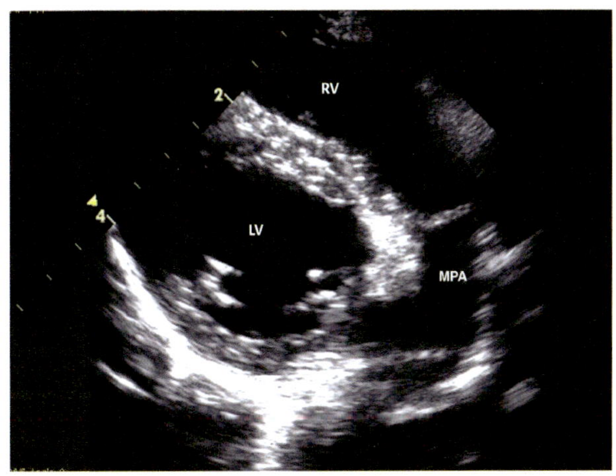

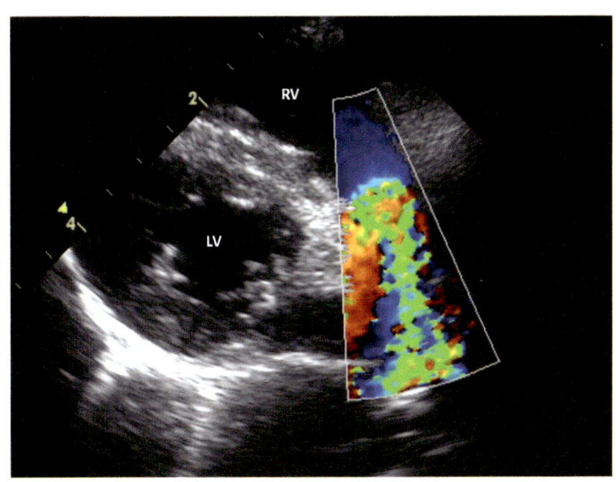

251

Questions:

1. **What is the most likely cause of the murmur in this dog?**
   a. Patent *ductus arteriosus*.
   b. Mitral valve dysplasia.
   c. Interatrial septal defect.
   d. Pulmonary stenosis.

2. **Which of these options corresponds to the radiographic abnormalities in this patient?**
   a. The radiograph shows an image of left-sided cardiomegaly with pulmonary hypoperfusion.
   b. The radiograph shows an image of left-sided cardiomegaly with a vascular pulmonary pattern.
   c. The radiograph shows an image of right-sided cardiomegaly with protrusion of the projection area of the main pulmonary artery.
   d. The radiograph shows an image of right-sided cardiomegaly with an interstitial-alveolar pulmonary infiltrate.

3. **Which of these options corresponds with the electrocardiographic abnormalities in this patient?**
   a. The mean electrical axis of the QRS complex is +30°.
   b. The ECG shows a basal sinus rhythm with an increasing pattern in the right ventricle.
   c. The mean electrical axis of the QRS complex is +150°.
   d. The ECG shows a basal sinus rhythm with an increasing left ventricular pattern.

4. **If the clinical history physical examination, radiography and electrocardiography are taken into consideration, which of these pathologies is the patient most likely to present with?**
   a. Pulmonary stenosis.
   b. Aortic stenosis.
   c. Tricuspid dysplasia.
   d. Mitral valve dysplasia.

5. **The 2D echocardiogram and colour Doppler (right parasternal short axis view) are compatible with:**
   a. Pulmonary valve stenosis.
   b. Double-chambered right ventricle.
   c. Patent *ductus arteriosus*.
   d. Pulmonary hypertension.

6. **What is the most appropriate treatment for this patient?**
   a. Spironolactone + ACEI + pimobendan.
   b. Furosemide + ACEI + pimobendan.
   c. Furosemide + ACEI + digoxin.
   d. Pulmonary valvuloplasty.

Notes

Correct Answers:

Test

1. c
2. a
3. a
4. d
5. c
6. b
7. c
8. a

Clinical Case

1. d
2. c
3. b
4. a
5. a
6. d

NOTES

Canine Myocardial Disease

Pedro Oliveira

Myocardial diseases (or cardiomyopathies) are diseases of the heart muscle, and one of the most common forms of acquired heart disease in dogs. They can be divided into **primary and secondary cardiomyopathies** depending on whether they are caused by a primary cardiac muscle disorder or are secondary to extracardiac disease. Primary cardiomyopathies include:

- dilated cardiomyopathy (DCM)
- arrhythmogenic right ventricular cardiomyopathy (ARVC)
- hypertrophic cardiomyopathy (HCM)
- restrictive cardiomyopathy (RCM).

Causes of secondary cardiomyopathies include:

- ischaemia
- valvular disease
- systemic hypertension
- inflammation
- metabolic disorders: endocrine, infiltrations, deficiencies, amyloid
- muscular dystrophies
- neuromuscular disease
- generalised systemic disease
- sensitivity and toxicity reactions, peripartal.

Cases that do not fit the criteria defined for the above groups have historically been referred to as suffering from an **unclassified cardiomyopathy (UCM)**. In this chapter, the most common myocardial diseases seen in the dog are discussed, focusing on their diagnosis and treatment.

Dilated Cardiomyopathy (DCM)

Dilated cardiomyopathy is a disease of the myocardium characterised by **impaired systolic function and dilation of either the left or both ventricles** in the absence of abnormal loading conditions (e.g. valvular disease, patent *ductus arteriosus*, hypertension, etc.).

Aetiology

It is suspected that DCM is the result of myocardial damage caused by genetic abnormalities, nutritional deficiencies, viral infections, and toxic insults amongst others.

Genetic Causes

In humans, up to 50% of cases have been shown to be familial with mutations identified in more than 40 genes. In dogs a **genetic cause** is suspected or has been identified in the following breeds:

Dobermann

There is evidence of **familial disease with an autosomal dominant mode** of inheritance with equal gender representation and male-to-male transmission. A splice-mutation in the pyruvate dehydrogenase kinase 4 (PDK4) gene has been associated with the development of DCM in Dobermanns in North America and **a genetic test is available**. This mutation shows incomplete penetrance, which means not all affected dogs develop the disease and it may show varying degrees of severity. In Europe, the PDK4 mutation has not been associated with the development of DCM and other genetic mutations are being investigated.

Irish Wolfhound

There is evidence of familial disease with an autosomal recessive mode of inheritance and sex-specific alleles. Males may be overrepresented.

Great Dane

There is evidence of familial disease with a mode **of inheritance linked to the X chromosome** in some families of dogs. This means male descendants of affected females are at high risk of developing the disease. However, a study in a different population of dogs suggested an autosomal dominant mode of inheritance. Abnormal expression of calstabin2 and triadin was documented in this breed, both of which are important for appropriate ryanodine receptor function (RyR2) and calcium flow in the myocardial cell. **Further studies are necessary** to determine the association between these findings and the development of DCM in this breed.

Newfoundland

There is evidence of familial disease with an autosomal dominant mode of inheritance, with late onset and reduced penetrance. A gender predisposition has not been identified in this breed. Several possible gene mutations have been investigated, but a causative mutation(s) has not been identified to date.

Portuguese Water Dog

There is evidence of familial disease with an autosomal recessive mode of inheritance. A mutation on the canine chromosome 8 has been identified.

Boxer

An association between a deletion in the striatin gene and the development of a DCM phenotype is suspected in this breed, particularly with the homozygous type.

Nutritional Deficiencies

An association between **low plasma levels of taurine and carnitine** and the development of DCM has been identified in some breeds of dogs such as the American Cocker Spaniel, Golden Retriever, and Newfoundland. A report looking at a family of Golden Retrievers has shown a familial taurine deficiency associated with the development of DCM. Lamb and rice only diets have also been shown to be associated with the development of DCM in some dogs.

Infectious Causes

Infectious agents may lead to development of DCM by causing myocardial inflammation and consequent damage. Some examples include parvovirus, distemper virus, canine herpesvirus, *Borrelia burgdorferi*, *Ehrlichia canis*, leishmania, rickettsia, *Trypanosoma cruzi*, *Toxoplasma gondii*.

Toxic Insults

The most common example of a toxic insult leading to myocardial damage and development of the DCM phenotype in dogs is the **administration of anthracyclines** (e.g. doxorubicin, epirubicin) to treat neoplastic disease. The cardiotoxic effect of doxorubicin is dose-dependent and irreversible. Doses exceeding 80 mg/m²/day or 25 mg/m²/week over 4–11 weeks are likely to cause myocardial damage with clinical signs (e.g. ventricular arrhythmias). Less common examples of toxic insults with the potential to lead to myocardial damage include cobalt (e.g. hip implants) and gossypol (e.g. cottonseed) poisoning.

Cardiac Arrhythmias

Rhythm disturbances that result in prolonged periods of tachycardia may result in myocardial damage and development of a DCM phenotype. This form of cardiomyopathy is described in a dedicated section on arrhythmia-induced cardiomyopathies.

Pathophysiology

As mentioned above, DCM is characterised by **cardiac chamber dilation secondary to systolic myocardial dysfunction**. Impaired ventricular contractility leads to a reduction in stroke volume and cardiac output accompanied by an increase in volume load as the ventricle is unable to pump blood effectively. **A reduction in cardiac output triggers the activation of the normal compensatory mechanisms** of the body (e.g. sympathetic activation, renin-angiotensin-aldosterone system, etc.) leading to renal sodium and water retention. This results in a **further increase in the cardiac volume load**, causing stretching of the myocardium. Eccentric hypertrophy occurs, resulting in a larger ventricle to accommodate the additional volume of blood and restore the stroke volume and cardiac output to normal. Progressive dysfunction and chamber dilation may eventually reach a stage in which compensation is no longer possible and heart failure occurs. Increased diastolic pressures lead to congestive failure (e.g. pulmonary oedema, ascites) and insufficient cardiac output may result in low-output failure and even cardiogenic shock in terminal stages.

Arrhythmias are common in this disease, particularly ventricular arrhythmias, and sudden death is often attributed to the occurrence of such arrhythmias. For more information on the pathophysiology of heart disease and heart failure see Chapter 8.

Pathology

Gross pathology typically demonstrates ventricular and atrial dilation (Figure 1). Left-sided chambers are often affected more than those on the right. The ventricular wall appears thin in comparison to the size of the ventricular chamber, but an increase in heart-to-body weight ratio demonstrates the presence of eccentric hypertrophy.

Histopathologic findings are fairly nonspecific and include attenuated wavy fibres, fibrosis, necrosis, myocyte vacuolization and in some cases fatty infiltration (Figure 2).

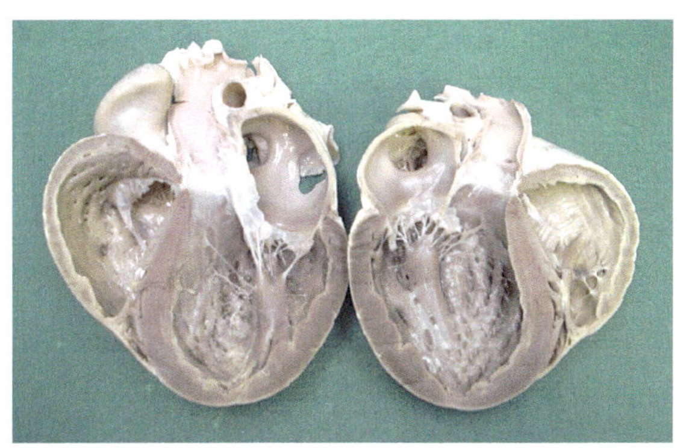

Figure 1. Heart affected by DCM. The heart is enlarged and the left ventricle in particular is affected. The wall of the left ventricle is thin compared to the size of the chamber, although it is thicker than normal due to eccentric hypertrophy. (Photo: Claudio Bussadori, Gran Sasso Veterinary Clinic, Milan, Italy).

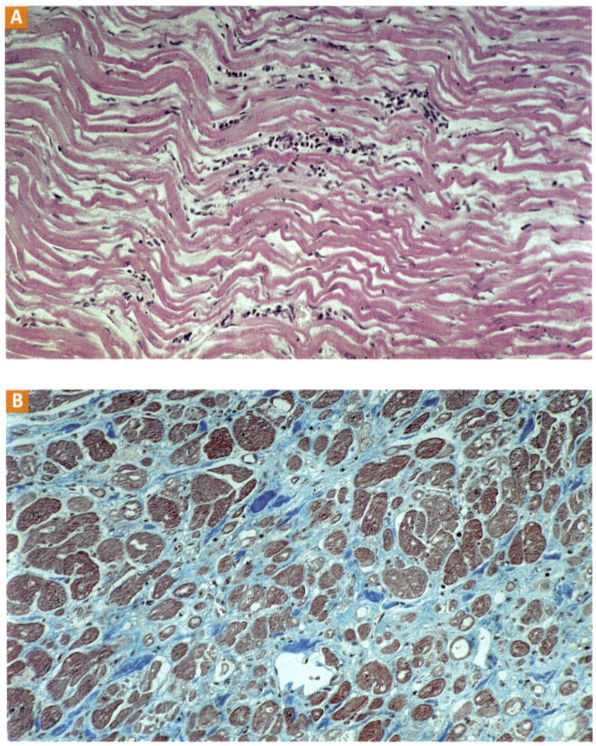

Figure 2. Histopathological changes associated with DCM. **A**. Wavy fibre pattern (Masson's trichrome stain). Myofibres are thinner than normal and have a wavy appearance. This is the most common type of DCM in dogs. **B**. Fibrosis and fat infiltration (Masson's trichrome stain). The myofibres are atrophied and show vacuolar degeneration and lipid and collagen deposits (stained blue) between them. This presentation is most often seen in Dobermanns with DCM and Boxers with DCM/RVACM. (Photos: Anna Tidholm, Albano Animal Hospital, Stockholm, Sweden).

Prevalence and Signalment

Overall, DCM is not a very common disease in dogs, with a **reported prevalence between 0.3 to 1.1%. Large and medium sized breeds** are mostly affected, with some breeds being overrepresented such as the Dobermann, Irish Wolfhound, Great Dane, Newfoundland, Airedale Terrier, and Cocker Spaniel.

There are differences in breed prevalence between different geographic locations, likely representing breed popularity and strong genetic influences of certain dogs which are popular in an area. DCM is an adult-onset disease except for in the Portuguese Water Dog and Toy Manchester Terrier, where most affected dogs are diagnosed before one year of age.

Dobermann

The prevalence of DCM in this breed is reported to be as high as 45–63% in the USA and Canada, and 58% in Europe. The mean age of **onset is five to seven years of age** although dogs as young as two years of age may be affected.

Early studies suggested a higher prevalence in male dogs although this has not been confirmed in more recent studies. In fact, an equal gender distribution has been reported in a recent European study. Females develop signs of disease at a more advanced age in comparison to males and this provides a possible explanation for this disparity in results from early studies in comparison to later studies. Earlier studies did not consistently include Holter monitoring or electrocardiography as part of the screening method. Since males are known to develop signs of disease earlier it is possible a proportion of affected females in the preclinical stage may have not been identified in earlier studies, whereas a higher proportion of males were already showing signs detectable via echocardiography.

Irish Wolfhound

The reported prevalence of DCM in this breed is approximately 30%. The mean age of onset has been estimated at **four to five years of age, with male dogs** more frequently affected and at a younger age than females.

Great Dane

The prevalence of DCM in this breed has been reported to be as high as 35.9% based on a recent study.

Clinical Presentation

Many dogs with DCM remain asymptomatic for a prolonged period before developing clinical signs of disease. Based on its natural progression, DCM is divided into three stages:

Stage 1. Healthy Dogs of a Predisposed Breed

At this stage, there is no evidence of disease in individuals of a predisposed breed. The heart appears normal from a morphological and electrical point of view and there are no clinical signs.

Stage 2. Preclinical Stage

At this stage, affected individuals appear outwardly normal and do not display any clinical signs of the disease. However, evidence of structural or electrical cardiac abnormalities is present and may be **found with the aid of diagnostic tests** (e.g. echocardiography, electrocardiography, Holter). This is an asymptomatic stage also known as the "occult" or "silent" stage of the disease. This stage may last for several years before clinical signs develop (e.g. it lasts approximately two to four years in most Dobermanns).

Stage 3. Clinical Stage

This is the symptomatic stage where signs referable to congestive heart failure (e.g. lethargy, respiratory difficulties, reduced tolerance to exercise, ascites), low output heart failure (e.g. weakness and collapse) or sudden death are seen. It is also known as the "overt" stage. It is normally of short duration with a **survival time of months** rather than years following diagnosis.

Diagnosis

Diagnosis of DCM in the preclinical stage is challenging. The identification of a soft systolic murmur most audible over the left apex (mitral regurgitation), a gallop sound (S3), or an irregular heart rhythm may be the first signs of DCM and **should not be overlooked**.

Stage 2. Preclinical Stage

Most of the information available on canine DCM derives from studies on Dobermanns. In this breed, the occult stage is reported to last two to four years. The initial clinical manifestations of the disease often consist of **ventricular arrhythmias**, even before structural cardiac changes are detected.

Electrocardiography (ECG)

A 5 minute ECG is an insensitive method to identify cardiac arrhythmias and not recommended as the sole diagnostic test. However, if at least one ventricular premature beat is identified over five minutes on a regular ECG, further investigation is warranted with a 24 hour ambulatory ECG (Holter).

Ambulatory Electrocardiography (Holter)

Holter monitoring is essential for the diagnosis of occult DCM. A recording of sufficient duration (>23h) and quality is necessary, and analysis performed or verified by an experienced veterinary cardiologist to avoid incorrect interpretation.

Ventricular arrhythmias are the hallmark of DCM although in some breeds such as the Irish Wolfhound and the Great Dane, atrial fibrillation may be an early sign of DCM instead (Figures 3 and 4). Generally, fewer than 50 ventricular ectopic beats (VPCs) in 24 hours may be found in normal dogs and values above this limit are considered suspicious of disease. However, it should be noted that many diseases may cause ventricular arrhythmias and these should be ruled out before a diagnosis is issued.

The following recommendations have been issued for the Dobermann.

- 300 VPCs/24h or 50–300 VPCs/24h in two subsequent recordings within a year are considered diagnostic of DCM regardless of the concurrent echocardiographic findings. Many studies use a cut-off of >100 VPCs/24h for the diagnosis of occult DCM, but the former are the most recent recommendations.
- 1–50 VPCs/24h with a short coupling interval (instantaneous rate beat-to-beat >250 bpm), R-on-T, and higher complexity (couplets, triplets, bigeminy, ventricular tachycardia >260 bpm/min) should raise suspicions of myocardial disease and are less likely to be seen with myocardial damage caused by systemic disease. Follow-up Holter monitoring is recommended in 3–6 months.
- >300 VPCs/24h followed by a recording with <50 VPCs/24h within 12 months remains suspicious and ongoing screening is strongly recommended.

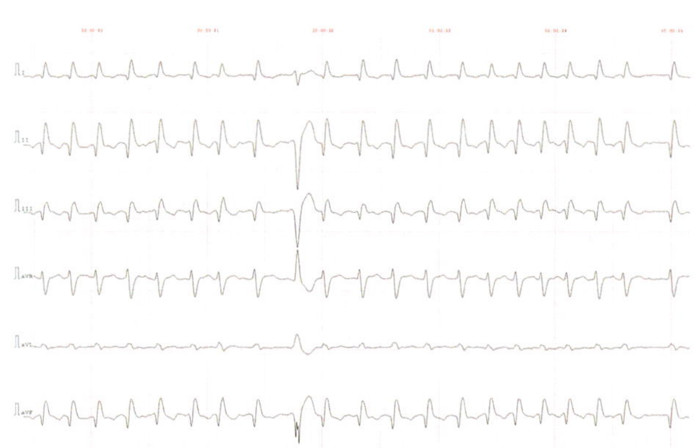

Figure 3. Atrial fibrillation in a Great Dane with DCM. The underlying rhythm is an irregular narrow QRS rhythm without visible P waves consistent with atrial fibrillation. The heart rate is approximately 200–220 bpm. An isolated ventricular ectopic beat may also be seen with a right bundle branch block conformation suggesting a left ventricular origin. (50 mm/s, 5 mm/mV) (8-year-old, male, Great Dane with a diagnosis of DCM).

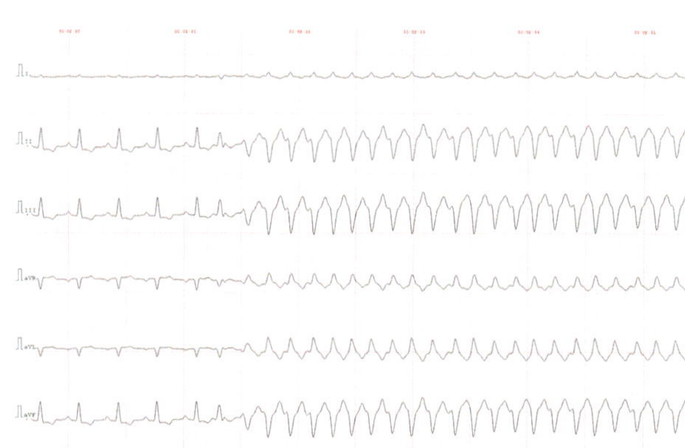

Figure 4. Ventricular tachycardia in a Doberman with DCM. On the left side of the trace a sinus rhythm is seen with a heart rate of approximately 180 bpm. A rapid monomorphic ventricular tachycardia can then be seen with a heart rate of approximately 340 bpm. The ventricular ectopic beats display a right bundle branch block conformation suggesting a likely left ventricular origin. (50 mm/s, 10 mm/mV) (8-year-old, male, Dobermann with a diagnosis of DCM).

Ventricular escape complexes or idioventricular rhythms (<160 bpm) are not considered diagnostic of DCM and possible extracardiac disease should be investigated.

Echocardiography

Echocardiographic diagnosis is challenging at this stage as the heart may appear structurally normal. A complete echocardiographic examination should be performed (2D, M-mode, Doppler) by an experienced operator. Evidence suggesting the presence of DCM includes left-sided or bilateral cardiac chamber size above the reference range (2D or M-mode derived measurements of size or volume), or systolic dysfunction in the absence of any other acquired or congenital cardiac disease which could account for volume overload and/or systolic dysfunction.

The following recommendations have been issued for the Dobermann.

- 2D derived measurements of volume indexed to body surface area have been reported to be superior to M-Mode values for early identification of DCM. These are calculated with Simpson's method of discs (see Chapter 6 for more information). The following indicate the presence of DCM:
  - left ventricular end-diastolic volume indexed to BSA (EDVI) >95 ml/m²
  - left ventricular end-systolic volume indexed to BSA (ESVI) >55 ml/m²
- M-mode derived measurements of the left ventricle:
  - left ventricular diastolic diameter (LVDd) >48 mm (male, any weight)
  - LVDd >46 mm (female, any weight)
  - left ventricular systolic diameters (LVDs) >36 mm (male or female of any weight)
  - LVDd >0.1749 x weight (kg) + 40.3 mm
  - LVDs >0.1402 x weight (kg) +26.7 mm
- Additional supportive parameters:
  - EPSS >6.5
  - sphericity index <1.6.

Cardiac Biomarkers

Cardiac Troponin-I

Cardiac troponin-I (cTnI) is a **marker of myocardial injury**. Two studies report the utility of cTnI testing for diagnosis of DCM in the occult stage. One of these reports involved a population of predisposed breeds (Great Dane, Dobermann and Boxer) compared to normal dogs. cTnI levels were significantly higher in affected dogs, however diagnosis was based on electrocardiography and echocardiographic information only and neither Holter nor a longitudinal study of these dogs were performed to confirm presence of the disease. Another study involving only Dobermanns which were followed throughout an 18-month period, with a complete diagnostic workup, found higher levels of cTnI in all disease stages. It concluded that **cTnI is valuable for detection of DCM in otherwise clinically normal Dobermanns**. A cut-off value of 0.22 ng/ml was proposed. Identification of elevated plasma cTnI should always prompt a full investigation including echocardiography and Holter monitoring.

Natriuretic Peptides

Natriuretic peptides (e.g. NT-proBNP) are **peptides released from the myocardium in response to stimuli including volume overload, hypoxia, ischaemia and neurohormonal upregulation**. They counteract the effects of the renin-angiotensin-aldosterone system to protect the heart from excessive volume overload. NT-proBNP levels are increased in dogs with congestive heart failure in comparison to dogs with primary respiratory disease. In dogs with DCM, NT-proBNP levels are higher than unaffected dogs, even in the occult stage. **A value above 500 pmol/l is suspicious and should prompt further investigation** with echocardiography, Holter monitoring and thoracic radiographs to assess for the presence of signs of congestive heart failure. However, NT-proBNP is most useful in predicting the presence of echocardiographic changes of DCM but not useful in cases that present with ventricular arrhythmias only.

Breed Screening Recommendations

Breed screening is recommended in Dobermanns from as young as two years of age in both males and females. Annual Holter monitoring and echocardiographic examinations should ideally be performed in all Dobermanns. However, if this is not possible, males being used for breeding should be screened yearly whereas females used for breeding and non-breeding dogs may be screened every two years. A one-off screening is not sufficient as the disease is detected with increasing age in most dogs.

Stage 3. Clinical Stage

Unfortunately, the **first clinical sign of DCM may be sudden death**. For this reason, significant effort is put into identifying the disease in the occult stage and the cases at risk of sudden death which is usually **attributed to ventricular arrhythmias**.

Dobermanns with significant ventricular dilation (LVDd >55 mm, LVDs >45 mm, fractional shortening <23%) with rapid sustained ventricular tachycardia are at higher risk of sudden death. Curiously, progression of left ventricular dysfunction is associated with a lower incidence of sudden death.

Haematology and Serum Biochemistry

Full complete blood count and biochemistry including thyroid function analysis and taurine/carnitine level assessment should be considered in all suspected cases of DCM. **A higher risk of hypothyroidism** is reported in Dobermanns with DCM although it does not seem to play a role in its aetiology or progression. Thyroid supplementation should be considered in case of hypothyroidism.

Electrocardiography

Many dogs with DCM have normal electrocardiograms. Evidence of chamber enlargement (e.g. tall/wide P waves, wide QRS) may be seen (see Chapter 4). Sinus tachycardia or tachyarrhythmia's such as atrial fibrillation (Figure 3) and/or ventricular arrhythmias are common (Figure 4).

Radiography

Radiographic findings are subtle in initial stages and consist of several degrees of cardiomegaly (typically left chamber enlargement) (Figure 5). **A definitive diagnosis of DCM cannot be obtained from the analysis of thoracic radiographs**, although these are particularly useful for identifying signs of congestive heart failure (e.g. pulmonary venous congestion, pulmonary oedema).

Echocardiography

Echocardiography is the diagnostic test of choice for the diagnosis of DCM in the overt stage. Left or bilateral chamber enlargement with documented reduction of systolic function are the hallmarks of DCM (Figure 6). However, echocardiographic diagnosis of DCM is not always easy and straightforward. For this reason, a scoring system has been proposed in which points are attributed to different echocardiographic parameters (Table 1). **A score of at least 6 or higher is necessary for the diagnosis of DCM**.

Table 1. Scoring system for the diagnosis of dilated cardiomyopathy in the overt stage.

Parameter	Points
Left ventricular dilation	3
Increased left ventricular sphericity <1.65	3
Fractional shortening <20–25%	3
Ejection fraction <40%	3
Ventricular arrhythmias	1
Atrial fibrillation	1
EPSS <7 mm	1
PEP/LVET >0.4	1
Fractional shortening 20–30%	1
Atrial dilation	1

Cardiac Biomarkers

Cardiac Troponin-I (cTnI)

Plasma cTnI levels are higher in dogs with overt DCM in comparison to normal dogs. **cTnI levels >0.22 ng/ml suggest the presence of DCM and should prompt further investigation with echocardiography and Holter monitoring**. Furthermore, cTnI levels >0.34 ng/ml are a predictor for the risk of sudden cardiac death in Dobermanns. With ultrasensitive cTnI assays a cut-off of >0.139 ng/ml was shown to predict morphological echocardiographic changes due to DCM with 100% sensitivity and 79% specificity. It is important to notecTnI levels may increase with various diseases that can cause myocardial damage is not exclusive to DCM. Additional cardiac or systemic diseases should be investigated in cases of elevated cTnI levels.

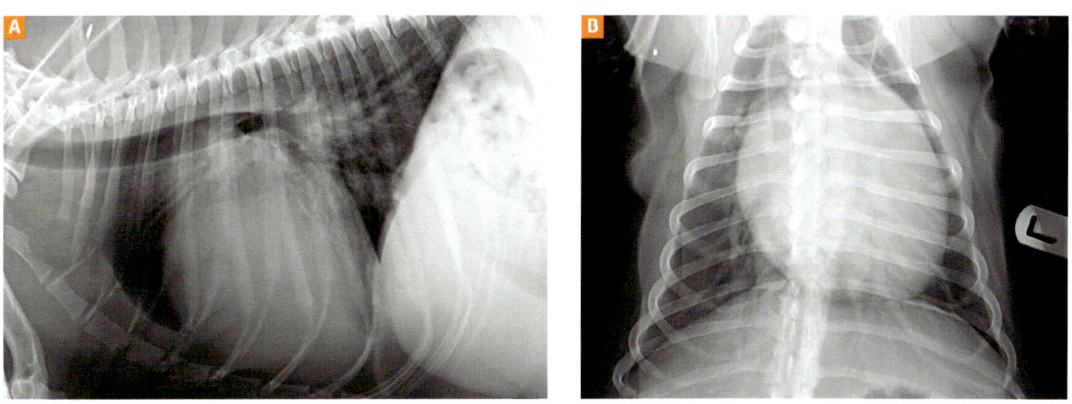

Figure 5. Radiographic findings in a dog with DCM. **A**. Right lateral view of the thorax. Significant cardiomegaly is seen with an estimated vertebral heart score of 15 (normal <10.5). The trachea is elevated, and the vena cava is directed upwards suggesting left-sided enlargement (atrial and ventricular). Some degree of peri-hilar and caudal infiltrate is apparent, suggesting possible pulmonary oedema although a significant part of this appearance may be the result of left atrial enlargement and superimposition of all the different structures present in this area as well as the respiratory phase. The visible cranial lung lobe vessels appear small and do not suggest obvious venous congestion. **B**. Dorsoventral view of the thorax. Significant cardiomegaly with evidence to suggest enlargement of the left-sided chambers: the left border of the cardiac silhouette and apex of the heart are closer to the left thoracic wall suggesting left ventricular enlargement; the main bronchi/vessels appear separated as a result of left atrial enlargement. The visible main pulmonary vessels appear slightly larger than would be expected, however the appearance of the visible pulmonary parenchyma does not suggest the presence of pulmonary oedema, supporting the hypothesis that the peri-hilar/caudal lung infiltrate seen on the lateral view may have been the result of structure superimposition and possibly a slightly expiratory view. The respiratory rate and pattern were normal at the time these radiographs were taken, also supporting this interpretation. (9-year-old, male neutered, English Cocker Spaniel with suspicion of DCM).

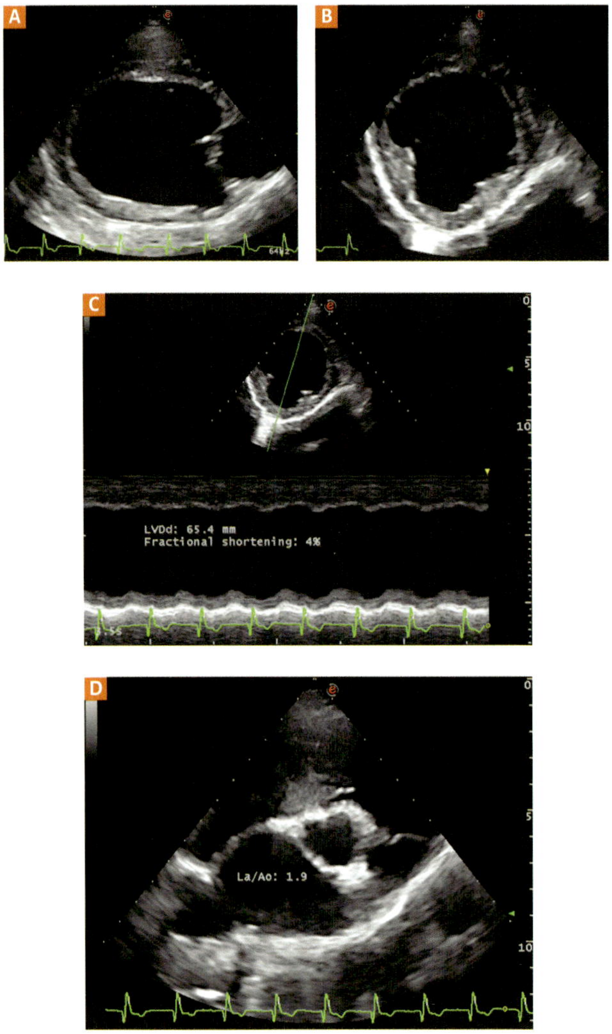

Figure 6. Echocardiographic findings in a dog with a DCM phenotype. **A**. Long-axis right parasternal view. The left ventricle is visibly enlarged with a rounder appearance (sphericity index: 1.17; normal >1.65). This view is used to determine the diastolic and systolic volumes with Simpson's method of discs and subsequently calculate the ejection fraction. In this case, the ejection fraction was 12% (normal >40%) with an end-diastolic volume index (EDVI) of 217 ml/m² (expected <109 for this breed), signalling significant volume overload and an end-systolic volume index (ESVI) of 191 ml/m² (expected <66.3 for this breed), signalling significant systolic dysfunction. **B**. Short-axis right parasternal view of the left ventricle. This view is used to perform visualisation in M-mode of the left ventricle. Visualising the left ventricle whilst paying attention to the direction of contraction is also useful. **C**. M-mode study of the left ventricle. The internal diastolic and systolic diameters of the left ventricle are determined and used to subsequently calculate fractional shortening. In this dog, a fractional shortening of 4% was estimated (normal >20%) with an internal diastolic diameter of 65.4 mm (expected <47.7 for this breed), signalling significant volume overload and an internal systolic diameter of 62.7 mm (expected <37.1 for this breed), signalling significant systolic dysfunction. **D**. Short-axis right parasternal view at the level of the left atrium and aorta showing left atrial enlargement (La:Ao – 1.9; normal <1.6). (4-year-old, male, English Springer Spaniel with suspicion of DCM).

Natriuretic Peptides (e.g. NT-proBNP)

Elevated NT-proBNP levels suggest possible cardiac remodelling and congestive heart failure in patients showing clinical signs such as respiratory difficulties. **They are more useful in asymptomatic patients as a screening method as described above**. In symptomatic patients, thoracic radiographs are more useful to confirm the presence of congestive heart failure.

Treatment

Ideally, an underlying cause should be identified in every patient and treatment aimed at the primary insult to the myocardium.

Stage 2. Preclinical Stage

Treatment of the disease at this stage should theoretically result in a longer survival time and time free of congestive heart failure. Unfortunately, clinical studies are lacking, except for one study that showed that the use of pimobendan at this stage prolongs the time to onset of clinical signs and extends survival. This study was performed in Dobermanns and may not apply to other breeds, although most clinicians have started using this drug in dogs of any breed with suspicion of DCM. An earlier study suggested treatment with benazepril hydrochloride might delay progression of occult DCM although further studies are necessary to confirm this.

Treatment of Arrhythmias

Ventricular Arrhythmias

Significant ventricular arrhythmias (e.g. rapid sustained ventricular tachycardia) which occur during Holter monitoring require medical treatment as they **may result in sudden death**. Patients experiencing episodes of collapse and that display evidence of "malignant" ventricular ectopy on ECG/Holter such as R-on-T, organised ventricular beats (couplets, triplets, bigeminy), episodes of ventricular tachycardia with an instantaneous rate >280 bpm are normally considered candidates for **antiarrhythmic treatment**. Commonly used drugs include sotalol, mexiletine or amiodarone.

Given that systolic function is an issue in this disease sotalol should be used with care and is avoided by many clinicians. Mexiletine is often the first choice as it is safe in these cases, although it does not always achieve optimal control of arrhythmias. Better control of ventricular arrhythmias is achieved when mexiletine is combined with another anti-arrhythmics such as sotalol or amiodarone. **Amiodarone is efficacious as an antiarrhythmic drug due to its multiple anti-arrhythmic properties and has the advantage of a relatively low impact on systolic function. It is the drug of choice when other antiarrhythmic drugs have failed**.

Unfortunately, **long-term administration of this drug carries the risk of hepatopathy and liver failure**. Several studies have investigated the efficacy and toxicity of this drug, particularly in the Dobermann. It should be noted this breed is predisposed to hepatopathy and hypothyroidism, both of which can occur with long-term administration of amiodarone. In one study, almost half of Dobermanns (10/22 dogs) showed signs of toxicity both with loading and maintenance doses of amiodarone.

These signs included anorexia, vomiting and diarrhoea with accompanying increases in liver enzymes. In all but one case these changes were reversible with discontinuation of the drug or reduction of the dosage. Hepatopathy is reported 1.5 to 8 months after starting treatment in most cases. If this drug is chosen, baseline blood tests should be performed including a complete blood count and serum biochemistry with bile acid and thyroid status assessment. These should be repeated at 1–3 monthly intervals to monitor any increase in serum liver enzymes and decrease in thyroid hormone levels. The drug should be discontinued if hepatopathy is suspected.

Haematological abnormalities such as neutropenia and a positive Coomb's test have also been reported with amiodarone administration. It is important to note that although antiarrhythmic treatment is aimed at reducing the frequency and severity of ventricular arrhythmias hopefully preventing sudden death, the ability of any antiarrhythmic drug to achieve these goals has not been studied.

Supraventricular Arrhythmias

The significance of supraventricular arrhythmias (if present) should be assessed in each case. In some breeds, atrial fibrillation is found at stage 2 of DCM and rate control may be necessary. Treatment with digoxin, digoxin combined with diltiazem, or sotalol are the most commonly used options for rate control in atrial fibrillation. If concomitant ventricular arrhythmias are present, digoxin should be used with care or avoided as ventricular arrhythmias are a possible side-effect. More information about the use of antiarrhythmic drugs can be found in Chapter 12.

Overt Stage

Treatment of clinical DCM is similar to the treatment of congestive heart failure caused by other diseases (e.g. valvular disease). A combination of furosemide, ACE-inhibitors (e.g. benazepril) and pimobendan are used. There is evidence that both ACE-inhibitors and pimobendan contribute to an increase in survival time and time free of congestive heart failure. Nonspecific treatments including nutritional supplementation (e.g. taurine, carnitine, fatty acids) may also be considered, especially if low levels are confirmed or suspected.

Prognosis

Prognosis varies depending on the underlying cause of DCM. For example, dogs with DCM due to taurine deficiency have a good prognosis with dietary taurine supplementation. Unfortunately, in most cases the underlying cause is not identified. Certain negative predictors of survival have been identified and include age of onset of clinical signs, pleural effusion, pulmonary oedema, ascites, atrial fibrillation, end-systolic volume index, ejection fraction, and a restrictive transmitral flow pattern.

Monitoring every six months with repeat Holter and echocardiography is recommended.

Tachycardia-Induced Cardiomyopathy

Aetiology and Pathophsyiology

Tachycardia-induced cardiomyopathy (TICM) is often considered a form of DCM and is unknown to many veterinary clinicians. Abnormal calcium handling, reduced cellular energy storing, and abnormal energy use have been proposed as the underlying mechanisms responsible for this syndrome. These mechanisms determine myocardial remodelling. Cellular changes include loss of myocytes, cellular elongation, myofibril misalignment, and loss of sarcomere register, which may be due to derangement of the extracellular matrix.

In humans, similar changes have been reported with **frequent ventricular ectopic beats in the absence of prolonged tachycardia**. For this reason, the term arrhythmia-induced cardiomyopathy has been suggested instead of TICM.

As the name suggests, this form of cardiomyopathy is induced by tachycardia. Prolonged tachycardia such as may occur with atrial fibrillation, ventricular or supraventricular arrhythmias, results in reduced contractility, cardiac dilation, elevated filling pressures and heart failure, much like in DCM. This has been demonstrated in experimental models and is well described in human medicine. In experimental models, changes can be seen as early as 24–48 hours after rapid cardiac pacing with continuing deterioration in ventricular function for up to 3–5 weeks.

Diagnosis

TICM is similar to DCM in every aspect and should always be considered in any case of unexplained DCM in which tachyarrhythmias are identified (Box 1). Echocardiographic diagnosis is as described above.

Naturally, identification of tachyarrhythmias is paramount for suspicion of this disease and this is mainly achieved by **Holter monitoring** (Figure 7).

Box 1. Arrhythmias That May Cause TICM

Supraventricular:

- **atrial fibrillation**
- **atrial flutter**
- **accessory-pathway mediated tachycardias**
- **focal/multifocal atrial tachycardia.**

Ventricular:

- **ventricular tachycardia**
- **bundle-branch reentry tachycardia**
- **high rate ventricular pacing.**

Treatment and Prognosis

The significance of this disease lies in that **complete recovery is possible after appropriate control of heart rhythm**. Naturally, this depends on the chronicity of the disease and severity of the resulting structural changes, but prognosis is generally good.

Treatment is aimed at controlling the underlying tachyarrhythmia. Medical treatment or invasive treatment with radiocatheter ablation are used.

Arrhythmogenic Right Ventricular Cardiomyopathy

This type of cardiomyopathy is characterised by progressive replacement of the myocardium with fibro-fatty tissue leading to ventricular arrhythmias and in some cases systolic dysfunction. It mainly affects the right ventricle, and the left ventricle only occasionally, hence the name arrhythmogenic right ventricular cardiomyopathy (ARVC). It is **common in the Boxer** and was described as Boxer cardiomyopathy for many years until similarities were found with human ARVC.

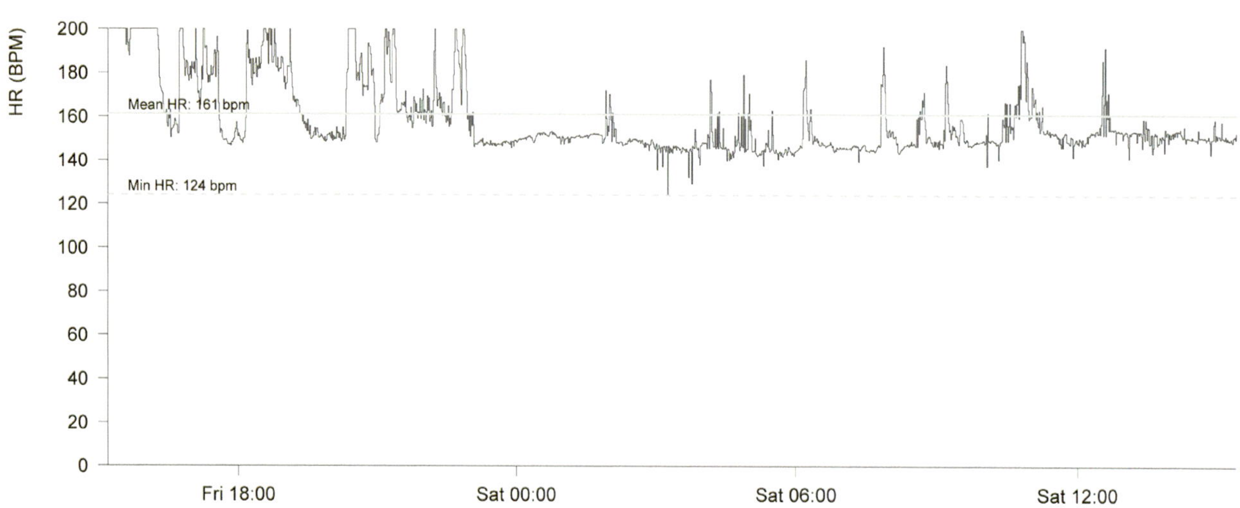

Figure 7. Elevated average heart rate in a dog with a tachyarrhythmia and a DCM phenotype. A tachogram is seen showing the heart rate recorded over a 24-hour period with a Holter monitor. The minimum heart rate was 124 bpm (normally 30–40 bpm) with an average heart rate of 161 bpm (normally 65–90 bpm). The underlying rhythm in this dog was an incessant junctional tachycardia confirmed with an electrophysiology study that lead to TICM.

It has also been reported in cats and other breeds of dogs such as English Bulldogs, Labrador Retrievers, Siberian Huskies, Bullmastiffs, Dachshund, Weimaraner, Dalmatians, and Shetland Sheepdogs. Boxer ARVC is used as a model for the study of human ARVC which has contributed significantly to advances in our knowledge of this disease in veterinary medicine.

Aetiology and Pathophysiology

ARVC is an adult-onset familial disease in the Boxer. It is inherited as an autosomal dominant trait with variable genetic penetrance. This means affected dogs can manifest varying degrees of severity and different clinical presentations ranging from being asymptomatic to syncope, sudden death, and systolic dysfunction with congestive heart failure.

ARVC is thought to be a disease of the desmossome, a structure involved in adhesion between myocardial cells. A reduction of the number of desmosomes and other structures of the intercalated disk involved in cell-to-cell adhesion and communication (gap junctions, adherens junctions) was demonstrated in Boxers with ARVC.

A deletion mutation in the 3' untranslated region of striatin, a gene which encodes for a desmosomal protein, has been identified in Boxers. This mutation shows a 70% genetic penetrance which means that 70% of dogs with the mutation develop the disease and the remaining 30% do not.

A reduction of the expression of cardiac ryanodine receptor (RyR2) in the myocardium of Boxers with ARVC has also been reported. The RyR2 is a channel that controls the flow of calcium to the sarcoplasmic reticulum, and plays a major role in excitation-contraction coupling. These changes are thought to contribute to electrical instability and arrhythmias.

Structural changes may be absent or subtle and confined to a localised region of the right ventricle. A segmental form of ARVC in which regional dilation of the right ventricular outflow tract has been described in English Bulldogs. Progression to more diffuse right ventricular disease may occur and involve the left ventricle. The level of structural change depends on the degree of replacement of myocardial cells with non-contractile fibro-fatty tissue.

Clinical Presentation

ARVC manifests itself in one of three forms or stages.

- **Stage I**: asymptomatic dogs with frequent ventricular ectopic beats.
- **Stage II**: dogs with syncope due to ventricular tachyarrhythmias.
- **Stage III**: cardiac enlargement and systolic dysfunction.

The most common presenting complaint with ARVC is syncope, secondary to haemodynamically significant arrhythmias. Syncope is commonly associated with excitement or exercise, likely due to sympathetic tone surges, but this is not always the case. Sudden death may be the first and only clinical sign. Occasionally, lethargy and exercise intolerance are reported, and rarely biventricular failure and congestive heart failure occur.

Diagnosis

Physical examination is unremarkable in most dogs although a cardiac rhythm disturbance may be identified. In dogs in stage three a heart murmur and signs of congestive heart failure (e.g. ascites, respiratory signs) may be seen.

Electrocardiogram

Identification of arrhythmias of right ventricular origin (Figure 8) is essential if there is suspicion of ARVC. The identification of at least one VPC during a 5-minute electrocardiogram is indicative of ARVC in Boxers. However, a normal electrocardiogram is not sufficient to rule out the disease as it is not sensitive enough for the identification of intermittent arrhythmias.

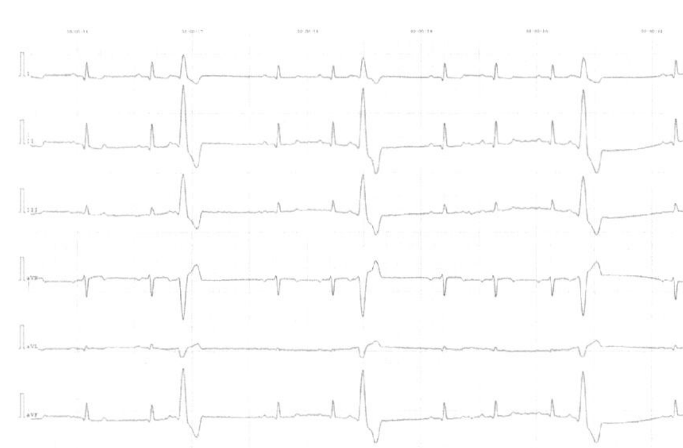

Figure 8. Ventricular arrhythmias in a dog with suspicion of ARVC. The underlying rhythm is a normal sinus rhythm with a heart rate of approximately 120 bpm. Beats 3, 6 and 10 are premature and display a wide QRS with a left bundle branch block conformation. These characteristics are suggestive of ventricular premature ectopic beats originating from the right ventricle. (50 mm/s, 10 mm/mV) (8-year-old, male, Boxer dog with suspicion of ARVC).

24h Holter Monitoring

Holter monitoring is the gold-standard for diagnosis of ARVC and is indicated in all suspected cases. It is also useful to assess treatment efficacy and document the cardiac rhythm during syncopal episodes whenever possible as some dogs may experience syncope due to bradycardia (e.g. vasovagal syncope) and this may have an influence on the choice of treatment.

The occurrence of >100 VPC over 24 hours, ventricular couplets/triplets, or runs of tachycardia are suggestive of ARVC (Figure 9). However, it is important to consider that a **significant day-to-day variation** has been reported in dogs (as high as 83% in Boxers). This means a dog may experience frequent ventricular ectopy one day and not at all on the following day. This illustrates the usefulness of serial or multiple day Holter recordings in these cases. A classification system has been proposed for the diagnosis of ARVC in Boxers based on Holter monitoring and can be found in Table 2.

Echocardiography

Echocardiography is often normal in these cases but it is an important part of the diagnostic investigation as it **allows exclusion of possible structural diseases**. Right ventricular enlargement, either generalised or segmental, is indicative of ARVC. Left ventricular enlargement and systolic dysfunction may also be present.

Total normal beats:	134 253
Normal premature:	1
Supraventricular tachycardias:	0
Bradycardia:	0
Dropped beats:	1
Pauses:	0

Total aberrant beats:	28 867 (average 1160 per hour) 17.7% of total
Premature aberrant beats:	14 590 (average 586 per hour) 8.9% of the total
Couplets:	1273
Triplets:	126
Salvos (3–5 rapid beats):	14, longest 4 beats at 18:52
Ventricular tachycardia:	15, longest 14 beats at 14:11
Fastest heart rate:	292 bpm at 19:08
Maximum heart rate:	157 bpm at 10:28 (1 minute on average)
Minimum heart rate:	87 bpm at 13:11 (1 minute on average)
Total QRS complexes:	163 247
Stimulated heartbeats:	0

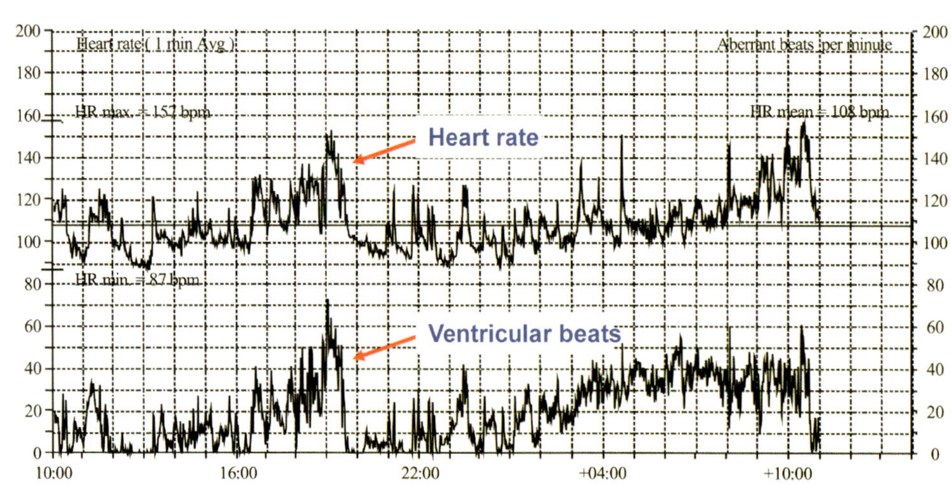

Figure 9. Ventricular arrhythmias in a dog with suspicion of ARVC. Holter results from the same dog as in Figure 8. Top. In the upper right box the number of ventricular ectopic beats are displayed. This dog experienced 28867 ventricular ectopic beats in 12 hours (17.7% of the total beats) with several examples of organization into couplets, triplets, and ventricular tachycardia. Bottom. Tachogram: the left-hand y-axis shows the average heart rate plotted against time using the 24-hour clock on the x-axis. The right-hand y-axis shows the number of ventricular beats per minute. The upper line shows the average heart rate and the lower line shows the frequency of ventricular ectopy. The lines are parallel which suggests that sympathetic tone influences the occurrence of ventricular arrhythmia. (8-year-old, male, Boxer dog with suspicion of ARVC).

Table 2. Classification system and recommendations for the diagnosis of ARVC in asymptomatic Boxers based on Holter monitoring.

Diagnosis of ARVC in asymptomatic Boxers based on Holter monitoring		
Grade 1	0–50 VPCs/24h	Results within normal limits
Grade 2	51–100 VPCs/24h	Repeat Holter in 6–12 months
Grade 3	100–300 VPCs/24h	Suspicious
Grade 4	100–300 VPCs/24h with increased complexity (e.g. couplets, triplets) and/or ventricular tachycardia or 300–1000 VPCs/24h	Likely affected
Grade 5	>1000 VPCs/24h	Affected. Start treatment

Thoracic Radiographs

Thoracic radiographs are often normal in ARVC.

Cardiac Biomarkers

Cardiac troponin I (cTnI) plasma levels have been shown to be elevated in Boxers with ARVC and correlate with the frequency and severity of the arrhythmias. However, **overlap with levels in unaffected dogs limits its usefulness for diagnosis**. In conclusion, elevated cTnI supports diagnostic suspicions, but normal levels are not sufficient for exclusion of the disease from a diagnosis.

Natriuretic peptide levels seem to be normal in dogs with ARVC and are therefore not useful for diagnosis.

Histopathology

Definitive diagnosis of ARVC requires histopathology to show the characteristic fibro-fatty **replacement of the myocardium** affecting right or both ventricles.

Treatment

Treatment is aimed at the **control of ventricular arrhythmias**. In asymptomatic patients, the decision to treat may be difficult but **treatment is usually started in cases with >1000 VPC in 24 hours, runs of ventricular tachycardia or R on T phenomenon**. Symptomatic patients (e.g. weakness, syncope) are generally also started on treatment. Unfortunately, although treatment is effective in reducing the number and severity of the arrhythmias, prevention of sudden death has not been demonstrated.

Sotalol, mexiletine, or a combination of both is the treatment of choice for most cardiologists. Amiodarone may also be considered in refractory cases. Treatment with atenolol or procainamide monotherapy may also be effective. **Fish oil supplementation** may also contribute to a reduction in arrhythmias.

Holter studies are necessary to assess treatment efficacy. Ideally, a baseline Holter should be performed before treatment, and repeated two to three weeks after the start of treatment. Given the high day-to-day variation in VPC numbers demonstrated in dogs, a reduction of more than 85% of ventricular ectopy should be documented with treatment.

Cases with biventricular enlargement, systolic dysfunction and congestive heart failure benefit from treatment with furosemide, ACE-inhibitors, and pimobendan. Improvement in systolic function has also been noticed with L-carnitine supplementation in some affected Boxers.

Prognosis

Dogs with ARVC are at risk of sudden death but many dogs live for many years without manifesting symptoms of the disease. **Monitoring every six months** with repeat Holter and echocardiography is recommended.

Myocarditis

Myocarditis is a form of myocardial disease in which a certain agent causes myocardial inflammation and possibly necrosis or degeneration. Physical trauma, chemical agents, and several infectious diseases may cause myocardial inflammation and lead to severe myocardial impairment. Box 2 lists some causative agents of myocarditis. The resulting clinical condition may be similar to dilated cardiomyopathy with significant ventricular enlargement, systolic dysfunction and congestive heart failure. A variety of tachy- or bradyarrhythmias (e.g. atrioventricular block) are frequently seen.

Clinical Presentation

Clinical signs vary according to the underlying cause. The history is often useful in determining the possible underlying cause (e.g. doxorubicin administration, trauma, etc.) as is the presence of concomitant clinical signs (e.g. fever).

Box 2. Causative Agents of Myocarditis

- Physical injury:
  - — trauma
  - — electric shock
  - — heat stroke
  - — migrating foreign body.
- Drugs or toxins:
  - — doxorubicin
  - — cobalt
  - — gossypol.
- Infectious:
  - — parvovirus
  - — distemper virus
  - — canine herpesvirus
  - — *Leishmania*
  - — *Ehrlichia canis*
  - — *Rickettsia rickettsi*
  - — *Borrelia burgdorferi*
  - — *Trypanossoma cruzi*
  - — *Toxoplasma gondii*.

Diagnosis

Cardiac rhythm disturbances are frequently the first sign of myocarditis, although some cases present with severe myocardial failure and congestive heart failure.

Electrocardiogram and Holter Monitoring

An electrocardiogram often discloses the **presence of arrhythmias**. Ventricular arrhythmias are most common, although supraventricular arrhythmias may also be identified if the atrial myocardium is affected. Conduction system involvement may be present (e.g. atrioventricular block). Continuous ECG monitoring is useful in most cases during hospitalization. **Holter monitoring** is useful particularly to assess the frequency and severity of intermittent arrhythmias and determine the efficacy of antiarrhythmic treatment.

Echocardiography

An **echocardiographic examination is warranted** in all cases. Findings are often similar to DCM although abnormal areas of myocardium (e.g. hyper- or hypoechoic) are suggestive of local inflammation, infiltration, or fibrosis. Systolic function assessment and risk of congestive heart failure is important to determine whether supportive treatment with inotropes or other drugs is necessary.

Cardiac Biomarkers

Cardiac troponin I (cTnI) is extremely useful as it confirms the presence of myocardial injury. Serial measurements are also useful to determine whether inflammation is ongoing, and whether there is improvement with treatment or not.

Complete Blood Count, Serum Biochemistry and Serological Analysis

A complete blood count and biochemistry, as well as serological tests to disclose the underlying causative agent are warranted.

Other Diagnostic Tests

Other tests such as thoracic or abdominal imaging (radiographs, CT scan, ultrasound) may be indicated depending on the underlying cause. **Blood cultures** should be considered where bacterial infection is suspected.

Treatment and Prognosis

Treatment is aimed at resolution of the underlying cause of myocarditis. Supportive treatment (e.g. inotropes, antiarrhythmic drugs, etc.) may be necessary.

The prognosis will depend on successful treatment and on the amount of damage sustained by the myocardium.

Atrial Standstill Due to Myocarditis or Cardiomyopathy

A particular form of cardiomyopathy or myocarditis that destroys the atrial myocardium has been described in some breeds of dogs (English Springer Spaniel, Old-English Sheepdog, Shih-Tzu, etc.). The destruction of the atrial myocardium, including the sinus node and internodal tracts, results in loss of normal sinus node activity leading to bradycardia.

The electrocardiographic features include absent or very small P waves and bradycardia (40–60 bpm). Atrial contraction cannot be documented on echocardiography, confirming atrial standstill and the atria are often enlarged. Clinical signs secondary to bradycardia are seen (e.g. lethargy, weakness, syncope) and progression to congestive heart failure may occur. Ventricular involvement may follow, and prognosis is poor in these cases.

Artificial pacing usually results in a temporary improvement of clinical signs but unfortunately most cases eventually die suddenly or of heart failure.

RECOMMENDED READING

- Basso, C., Fox, P.R., Meurs, K.M. et al. (2004) Arrhythmogenic right ventricular cardiomyopathy causing sudden cardiac-death in boxer dogs: a new animal model of human disease. *Circulation*, 109(9), pp. 1180–5. Epub 2004 Mar 1.
- Baumwart, R.D., Meurs, K.M. (2005) Assessment of plasma brain natriuretic peptide concentration in Boxers with arrhythmogenic right ventricular cardiomyopathy. *Am J Vet Res*, 66(12), pp. 2086–9.
- Baumwart, R.D., Orvalho, J., Meurs, K.M. (2007) Evaluation of serum cardiac troponin I concentration in Boxers with arrhythmogenic right ventricular cardiomyopathy. *Am J Vet Res*, 68(5):524–8.
- Boon, J.A. (2011) Myocardial diseases, In: *Veterinary Echocardiography*, Second ed. Wiley-Blackwell. Capítulo 7. pp. 381–396.
- Dukes-McEwan, J., Borgarelli, M., Tidholm, A. (2003) ESVC Taskforce for Canine Dilated Cardiomyopathy. Proposed guidelines for the diagnosis of canine idiopathic dilated cardiomyopathy. *J Vet Cardiol*, 5(2), pp. 7–19.
- Holler, P.J., Wess, G. (2014) Sphericity index and E-point-to-septal-separation (EPSS) to diagnose dilated cardiomyopathy in Doberman Pinschers. *J Vet Intern Med*, 28(1), pp. 123–9.
- Kienle, R.D., Kittleson, M.D. (2005) Primary myocardial disease, In: *Small animal cardiovascular medicine textbook*. VIN.com. Capítulo 20.
- Meurs, K.M., Ederer, M.M., Stern, J.A. (2007) Desmosomal gene evaluation in Boxers with arrhythmogenic right ventricular cardiomyopathy. *Am J Vet Res*, 68(12):1338–41.
- Meurs, K.M., Lacombe, V.A., Dryburgh, K. et al. (2006) Differential expression of the cardiacryanodine receptor in normal and arrhythmogenic right ventricular cardiomyopathy canine hearts. *Hum Genet*, 120(1), pp. 111–8.
- Meurs, K.M., Stern, J.A., Reina-Doreste, Y. et al. (2014) Natural history of arrhythmogenic right ventricular cardiomyopathy in the boxer dog: a prospective study. *J Vet Intern Med*, 28(4), pp. 1214–20.
- Meurs, K.M., Stern, J.A., Sisson, D.D. et al. (2013) Association of dilated cardiomyopathy with the striatin mutation genotype in boxer dogs. *J Vet Intern Med*, 27(6), pp. 1437–40.
- Meurs, K.M. (2004) Boxer dog cardiomyopathy: an update. *Vet Clin North Am Small Anim Pract*, 34(5), pp. 1235–44, viii.
- Meurs, KM. (2010) Myocardial disease: Canine, In: Ettinger, S.J., Feldman, E.C., *Textbook of Veterinary Internal Medicine*, 7th Edition. Saunders Elsevier. Capítulo 251. pp. 1320–1328.
- O'Grady, M.R., O'Sullivan, M.L. (2004) Dilated cardiomyopathy: an update. *Vet Clin North Am Small Anim Pract*, 34(5), pp. 1187–207.
- Oxford, E.M. et al. (2011) Ultrastructural changes in cardiacmyocytes from Boxer dogs with arrhythmogenic right ventricular cardiomyopathy. *J Vet Cardiol*, 13(2), pp. 101–13.
- Oyama, M.A., Reiken, S., Lehnart, S.E. et al. (2008) Arrhythmogenic right ventricular cardiomyopathy in Boxer dogs is associated with calstabin2 deficiency. *J Vet Cardiol*, 10(1), pp. 1–10.
- Pérez-Silva, A., Merino, J.L. (2009) Tachycardia-induced cardiomyopathy. E-Journal of the ESC Council for Cardiology Practice Vol7 N°16 13 Enero 2009. (www.escardio.org).
- Scansen, B.A., Meurs, K.M., Spier, A.W. et al. (2009) Temporal variability of ventricular arrhythmias in Boxer dogs with arrhythmogenic right ventricular cardiomyopathy. *J Vet Intern Med*, 23(5), pp. 1020–4.
- Spier, A.W., Meurs, K.M. (2004) Assessment of heart rate variability in Boxers with arrhythmogenic right ventricular cardiomyopathy. *J Am Vet Med Assoc*, 224(4), pp. 534–7.
- Spier, A.W., Meurs, K.M. (2004) Evaluation of spontaneous variability in the frequency of ventricular arrhythmias in Boxers with arrhythmogenic right ventricular cardiomyopathy. *J Am Vet Med Assoc*, 224(4), pp. 538–41.
- Summerfield, N.J., Boswood, A., O'Grady, M.R. (2012) Efficacy of pimobendan in the prevention of congestive heart failure or sudden death in Doberman Pinschers with preclinical dilated cardiomyopathy (the PROTECT Study). *J Vet Intern Med*, 26(6), pp. 1337–49.
- Wess, G., Butz, V., Mahling, M. et al. (2011) Evaluation of N-terminal pro-B-type natriuretic peptide as a diagnostic marker of various stages of cardiomyopathy in Doberman Pinschers. *Am J Vet Res*, 72(5), pp. 642–9.
- Wess, G., Mäurer, J., Simak, J. et al. (2010) Use of Simpson's method of disc to detect early echocardiographic changes in Doberman Pinschers with dilated cardiomyopathy. *J Vet Intern Med*, 24(5), pp. 1069–76.
- Wess, G., Schulze, A., Butz, V. et al. (2010) Prevalence of dilated cardiomyopathy in Doberman Pinschers in various age groups. *J Vet Intern Med*, 24(3), pp. 533–8.
- Wess, G., Schulze, A., Geraghty, N. et al. (2010) Ability of a 5-minute electrocardiography (ECG) for predicting arrhythmias in Doberman Pinschers with cardiomyopathy in comparison with a 24-hour ambulatory ECG. *J Vet Intern Med*, 24(2), pp. 367–71.
- Wess, G., Simak, J., Mahling, M. et al. (2010) Cardiactroponin I in Doberman Pinschers with cardiomyopathy. *J Vet Intern Med*, 24(4), pp. 843–9.

TEST

1. The prevalence of dilated cardiomyopathy in dogs is around:
- a. 5–10%.
- b. <1.5%.
- c. 15%.
- d. 20–30%.

2. There is a risk of sudden death in:
- a. Dilated cardiomyopathy in the asymptomatic stage.
- b. Dilated cardiomyopathy in the symptomatic stage.
- c. Right ventricular arrhythmogenic cardiomyopathy.
- d. All of the above.

3. The asymptomatic stage of dilated cardiomyopathy in the Dobermann has been identified as lasting:
- a. 6 months – 1 year.
- b. <2 years.
- c. 2–4 years.
- d. >5 years.

4. Which drug administered in the asymptomatic stage delays the onset of clinical signs and prolongs the life expectancy in cases of DCM?
- a. Furosemide.
- b. Pimobendan.
- c. Spironolactone.
- d. None of the above.

5. Regarding tachycardia-induced cardiomyopathy, which statement is correct?
- a. The prognosis is always unfavorable with risk of sudden death.
- b. The mere existence of atrial fibrillation with an average rate of 110 bpm may be the cause.
- c. Full recovery is possible once proper control of heart rhythm is achieved.
- d. Atropine is used to prevent syncope.

6. A definitive diagnosis of dilated cardiomyopathy can be obtained in a Dobermann with:
- a. Shortening fraction <20%.
- b. Shortening fraction <25%.
- c. 50–100 premature ventricular complexes/24 h.
- d. >300 premature ventricular complexes/24 h.

ANSWERS ON PAGE 272

7. Atrial fibrillation can be an early sign of dilated cardiomyopathy in which of the following breeds?
- a. Boxer.
- b. Dalmatian.
- c. American Cocker Spaniel.
- d. Irish Wolfhound.

CLINICAL CASE

Patient. 6-year-old male Boxer.

Clinical history. One episode of collapse. No further symptoms are described.

Physical exam. Conscious and alert. Respiratory rate of 20 bpm with a normal respiratory pattern. Heart rate of 90 bpm with irregular rhythm. Normal peripheral pulse along with pinkish mucous membranes and a normal capillary refill time.

No abnormal findings on auscultation.

1. What steps should be followed to study this case?

Electrocardiogram:

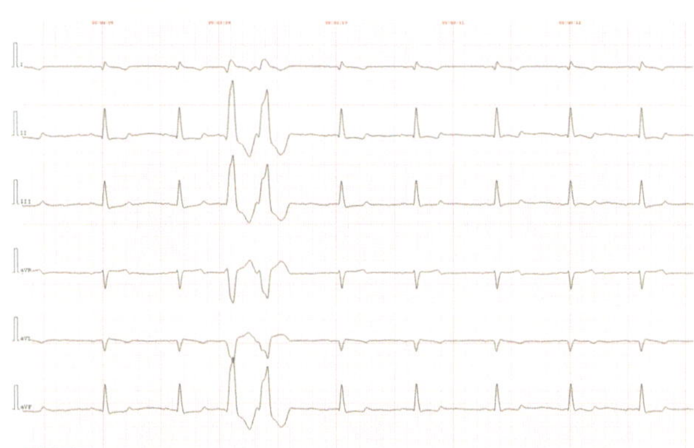

2. What would the electrocardiographic diagnosis be?

Echocardiography. Normal size, structure, and function. No evidence of structural disorders or anatomical defects.

Holter monitoring (no collapse periods are recorded):

Quantification of beats			
Normal heartbeats	**Ectopic ventricular beats**	**Ectopic supraventricular beats**	**Sinus beats**
Number: 113 009 Percentage: 68% Maximum: 8312 (Monday 13:00)	Number: 52 670 Percentage: 32% Maximum: 3448 (Monday 19:00)	Number: 0 Percentage: 0% Maximum: 0	Number: 0 Percentage: 0% Maximum: 0

Rhythm-related events		
Heart rhythms (average in 1 minute)	**Bradycardia: 66**	**Tachycardia: 516**
Maximum heart rate: 203 bpm (Monday 13:06) Average heart rate: 113 bpm Minimum heart rate: 51 bpm (Tuesday 06:21)	Total: 10 min, 48 s, 0.7% Longest: 32 beats (Tuesday 12:25) Minimum heart rate: 31 bpm (Tuesday 00:02)	Total: 1 h, 2 min, 45 s, 4.1% Longest: 537 beats (Monday 13:07) Maximum heart rate: 222 bpm (Monday 13:10)

Ventricular arrhythmias	Supraventricular arrythmias
Ventricular tachycardia	**Atrial fibrillation**
38 (0.1% of total beats) Longest: 6 beats (Tuesday 10:52) Maximum heart rate: 225 bpm (Tuesday 10:52)	0 episodes Total duration: - Maximum heart rate: -
(Accelerated) Idioventricular rhythm	**SV tachycardias**
78 (0.4% of all beats) Longest: 33 beats (Tuesday 12:25) Maximum heart rate: 89 bpm (Tuesday 14:25)	0 Longest: - Maximum heart rate: -
Couplets	**SV ectopic beats**
1389 (1.7% of total beats)	0 (0.0% of all beats)
Triplets	
272 (0.5% of all beats)	
Ectopic beats	
11 061 (6.7% of all beats)	

3. What would the interpretation of the Holter monitoring results be?

Blood tests. Results normal.

4. What would the presumptive diagnosis be?

5. How would this patient be treated and monitored?

6. What would the prognosis be?

Correct Answers:

Test

1. b
2. d
3. c
4. b
5. c
6. d
7. d

Clinical Case

1. Which steps should be followed to work up this case?
The problem list for this case includes collapse and irregular heart rhythm. The diagnostic tests which should be considered include the following.

- An electrocardiogram to investigate the irregular heart rhythm observed during the physical examination.
- An echocardiographic examination to evaluate structure and function of the heart and the possible presence of an underlying structural cardiopathy.
- Blood tests (complete blood count and biochemistry, including electrolytes) to investigate the possibility of a non-cardiac disease which could cause cardiac arrythmia. If abnormalities are detected, additional tests may be necessary (for example, abdominal ultrasound).
- Holter monitoring for 24–48 h to investigate intermittent cardiac arrythmias, determine their frequency and severity, the risk of ventricular fibrillation and death and document the rate and heart rhythm during the episode of collapse, if this occurs during the period of monitoring.
- Additional useful information when investigating collapse in a dog includes a neurological examination and video of the episode to distinguish syncope from convulsions or movement disorders.

2. What would the electrocardiographic diagnosis be?
Sinus rhythm with a heart rate of approximately 100 beats per minute, interrupted by a pair of ventricular ectopic beats (beats 3 and 4). Ectopic beats display a left branch block conformation (wide QRS with positive deflexion on leads II, III and aVF) which suggests right ventricular origin. Holter monitoring was recommended to evaluate the frequency and severity of ventricular arrhythmias.

3. What would interpretation of results from the Holter monitoring indicate?
Presence of ventricular arrythmias with various episodes of ventricular tachycardia at a maximum rate of 225 bpm. No episodes of collapse are recorded during monitoring. Although a transitory bradyarrhythmia cannot completely be ruled out, it is reasonable to attribute the episode described to a ventricular arrythmia.

4. What is the presumptive diagnosis?
In a dog of this breed and age these findings are highly indicative of arrhythmogenic right ventricular myocardiopathy (stage 2).

5. How should this patient be treated and monitored?
Based on the findings from Holter monitoring (grade 5: >1000 VPC/24 h) and the episodes of collapse described, an antiarrhythmic treatment should be considered. Monotherapy with sotalol (1–3 mg/kg), mexiletine (5 mg/kg two or three times a day) or both drugs combined, would be a good starting point. Amiodarone could also be considered if the previous treatment proposal failed. Holter monitoring should be repeated 2–3 weeks after to evaluate the effectiveness of treatment and after that every 6 months. Echocardiography should be considered every 6 months or at least once a year to evaluate any structural changes.

6. What is the prognosis?
Dogs with right ventricular arrhythmogenic cardiopathy are at risk of sudden death, but the majority live for many years without clinical signs of the disease.

NOTES

Feline Cardiomyopathies

Mª Josefa Fernández-del Palacio, Giorgia Santarelli

Cardiomyopathies represent a **heterogeneous group of myocardial diseases**, associated with mechanical (systolic or diastolic dysfunction) or electrical (predisposition to arrhythmias) dysfunction.

Cardiomyopathies are classified into two groups, which are further subdivided:

- **primary cardiomyopathies**: this group mainly or only affects the myocardium, and is divided into:
  - **genetic**: hypertrophic cardiomyopathy and arrhythmogenic right ventricular cardiomyopathy
  - **mixed**: dilated cardiomyopathy and restrictive cardiomyopathy (neither dilated nor hypertrophic)
  - **acquired**: myocarditis, tachycardiomyopathy
- **secondary cardiomyopathies**: pathological involvement of the myocardium is part of a generalised systemic (multi-organ) condition such as systemic arterial hypertension or hyperthyroidism.

Recently, the American College of Veterinary Internal Medicine Consensus statement has proposed a classification of feline cardiomyopathies based on phenotype, which should be used until an underlying cause has not been identified. This chapter addresses primary feline cardiomyopathies.

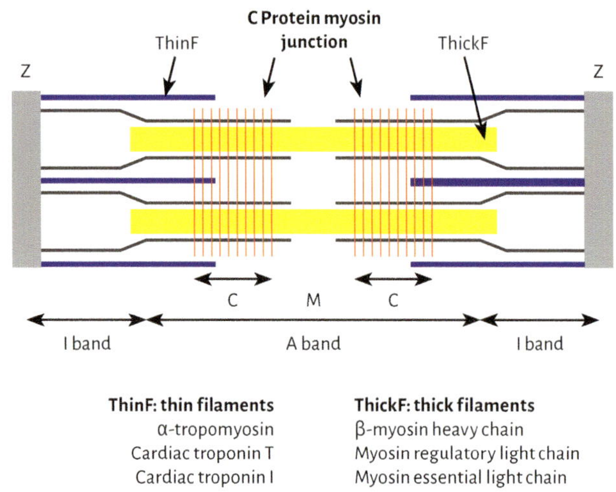

Figure 1. Diagram of the sarcomeric proteins associated with familial hypertrophic myopathy in human patients. HCM genes code for contractile proteins in the thick filaments (yellow), proteins associated with the thin filaments (blue) and the myosin junction protein (red). The Z-lines and the titin filaments appear in grey and black, respectively. C and M correspond with the C and M zones of the A band of the sarcomere respectively. (Modified from Bonne et al., 1998).

Hypertrophic Cardiomyopathy

Hypertrophic cardiomyopathy (HCM) is the most common feline heart disease. It is a **primary disease of the myocardium**, which is hereditary but not congenital. The condition is characterised by thickening of the LV walls in the absence of pressure overload or metabolic stimulus (e.g. aortic stenosis, systemic arterial hypertension, or hyperthyroidism, amongst others).

HCM was first described in human medicine by Teare et al. in 1958 in several young individuals who died suddenly. Later, in 1990, the same research group established its familial nature and described the first sarcomeric mutation associated with HCM in the gene that encodes the heavy chain of β-myosin (MYH7). Currently, more than 140 variants in at least 14 genes that encode sarcomeric proteins are known to cause HCM in human patients (Figure 1).

In 1995, Fox et al. described a primary cardiomyopathy in cats with echocardiographic and pathological phenotypes similar to human HCM. Later, in 1999 Kittleson et al. revealed the familial character of HCM in the Maine Coon breed. Following this, causal mutations in the gene encoding myosin-binding protein C (MYBPC3) in Maine Coons and Ragdolls were identified by Meurs et al. in 2005 and 2007, respectively.

Although the current mutations may have existed for centuries, HCM is considered a relatively new disease in terms of clinical recognition.

Pathology

Postmortem examination of HCM cats shows variable degrees **of left ventricular hypertrophy** (Figure 2) and highly heterogeneous patterns. In addition, the ventricular chamber is significantly reduced in size, the papillary muscles are hypertrophic, and the left atrium can be dilated. Some **cats present with pulmonary oedema and aortic thromboembolism** (Figure 3).

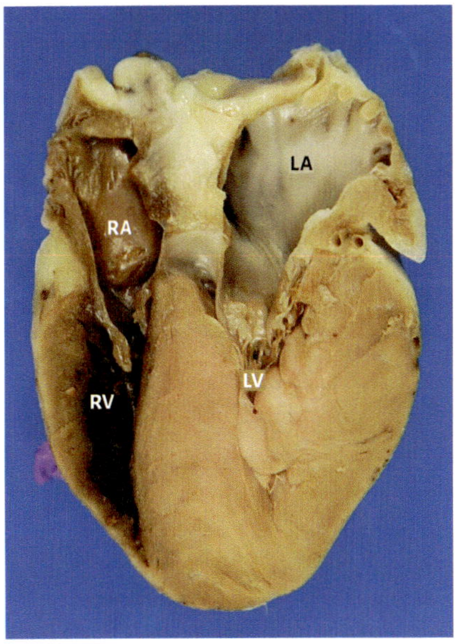

Figure 2. Macroscopic image of the heart of a cat with HCM, which shows severe hypertrophy of the walls of the left ventricle (LV) and reduced chamber size. LA: left atrium, RV: right ventricle, RA: right atrium.

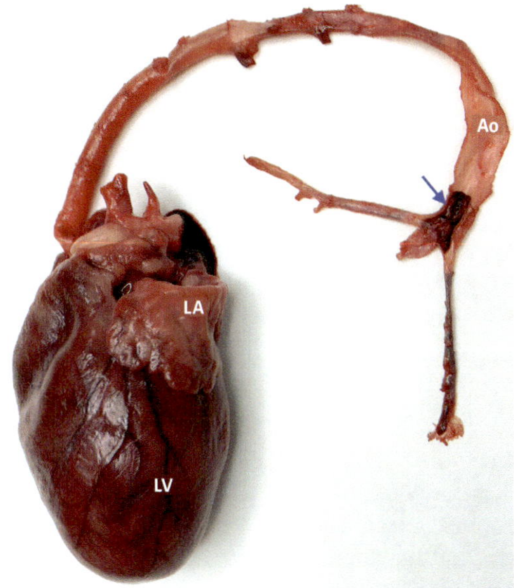

Figure 3. Macroscopic image of the heart, descending aorta (Ao) and iliac arteries in a cat with thromboembolism where dilation of the left atrium (LA) and thrombus in the distal aorta and iliac arteries (arrow) can be seen. LV: left ventricle.

Histological examination is typified by **myofibrillar disorientation** (disarray) and the loss of normal parallel alignment of myocardial fibres. The random orientation of hypertrophic myocytes gives the myocardial architecture a swirling appearance. Additional findings include arteriosclerosis of the intramural coronary arteries and an increase in the interstitial matrix, with substitution of the myocardium with fibrosis. These lesions are responsible for **diastolic dysfunction, myocardial ischaemia, and arrhythmias**. In the final stages of the disease, myocardial ischaemia affects different parts of the ventricular myocardium and can cause parietal thinning, chamber dilation, and systolic dysfunction.

Aetiology

As in human medicine, HCM seems to be a genetic disease in cats, with an autosomal mode of inheritance, incomplete penetrance and variable expression. Two sarcomeric mutations have been discovered in the gene encoding myosin-binding protein C (MYBPC3):

- A31P, associated with HCM in Maine Coon cats
- R820W, in Ragdoll cats.

In other cat breeds, such as the Sphynx, Norwegian Forest Cat, or British Shorthair, the heritable nature of the disease has been demonstrated, but the causal mutations not yet identified. Therefore, more genetic studies are needed in cats applying the new high-throughput sequencing techniques used in human medicine.

Since the causal mutation has only been identified in 34% of Maine Coon cats and 17–23% of Ragdoll cats, it is believed other factors may contribute to the HCM phenotype, as is the case for certain polymorphisms (SRRA), epigenetic factors (DNA methylation, histone acetylation, micro-RNA) or the environment (sex, obesity, systemic arterial hypertension, etc.). These aspects are still being researched.

Physiopathology

There is consensus in the literature that the initial defects caused by the mutated proteins converge in a common pathway of abnormal cardiac function, with the following characteristics:

- increased myocyte stress and hypercontractility;
- increased energy consumption;
- alterations in the sensitivity and reuptake of cytosolic Ca^{2+};
- subsequent activation of intracellular kinase signals and trophic factors, which activate the transcriptional machinery, inducing cardiac hypertrophy;
- appearance of histological phenotypes : disorganization of myocytes, interstitial fibrosis, arteriosclerosis of intramural arteries and mitral valve abnormalities in some cases;
- myocardial ischaemia;
- decreased myocardial relaxation;
- appearance of clinical phenotypes: diastolic dysfunction, left ventricular outflow tract obstruction, arrhythmias, and congestive heart failure (CHF).

One of the notable early haemodynamic abnormalities in HCM is **diastolic dysfunction**. This is characterised by slow relaxation caused by a difficulty in the reuptake of cytosolic Ca^{2+} by the sarcoplasmic reticulum system calcium pump, which is further accentuated as hypertrophy and fibrosis appears. Secondarily, there is an **increase in left atrial dimensions**, an indirect indicator of diastolic pressure and predictor of CHF.

Dynamic left ventricular outflow tract obstruction is common in cats (67%) with HCM. Changes that occur within the architecture of the LV, such as septal narrowing of the LV outflow tract (LVOT) or an abnormal mitral subvalvular apparatus, result in **anterior systolic anterior movement (SAM) of the mitral valve and dynamic LVOT obstruction** (LVOT pressure gradient ≥30 mmHg). In cats, the presence of SAM at diagnosis has not been associated with a higher risk of CHF, but with a lower risk of death according to studies published so far by Payne et al. (2015).

In some cats with HCM, **thrombus formation** is common in the left atrial appendage, and may detach to cause obstruction in the distal aorta and/or iliac arteries **resulting in paralysis of the hindlimbs**. Other arteries in the forelimbs and other organs (mesentery, kidneys, brain) may also be affected. Thrombus formation is classically attributable to Virchow's triad (endothelial damage, blood stasis, and hypercoagulability). In cats with HCM all the factors of this triad may be present:

- diastolic dysfunction, left atrial dilation, and decreased flow in the atrial appendage **predispose to blood stasis** due to lack of clearance of activated clotting factors and increased interactions of platelets with the endothelium;
- many cats with HCM manifest a state of hypercoagulability;
- at necropsy, patches of endomyocardial necrosis have been observed, which could initiate thrombus formation due to exposure of subendothelial tissue factor.

Epidemiology and Clinical Presentation

The prevalence of HCM in felines is higher than in humans, estimated at around 15% in the general population (<5% in very young cats and up to **30% in cats over nine years of age**). As in humans, many of these animals appear to have a favourable clinical progression and, therefore, the prevalence could be even higher as they can remain asymptomatic for years. **Others develop CHF, arterial thromboembolism, or suffer sudden death**. The disease affects all breeds of cats (not just pedigree cats) and ages, with a higher prevalence in males.

Although **older, obese, and male animals** appear more prone to this disease than other cats, these are not specific risk factors for cardiac mortality within the general feline population.

The physical examination of cats with HCM may be normal but in other cases **abnormalities in cardiac auscultation** are detected in routine examinations, e.g. murmurs, arrhythmia, gallop sounds or signs of CHF and/or aortic thromboembolism. In exceptional cases, **sudden death** is the first clinical sign, with the diagnosis made at postmortem.

Murmurs in cats with HCM are often related to LVOT obstruction and mitral regurgitation due to distortion of the valvular apparatus, but they are **not specific** and a differential diagnosis with other heart diseases must be made. **Gallop sounds (S3 or S4) are more specific for cardiomyopathy** than murmurs, they suggest diastolic dysfunction, elevated left atrial pressure, and ventricular rigidity, although they can also be detected in geriatric, anaemic, and hyperthyroid cats. **Auscultation of arrhythmias in cats suggests structural cardiac involvement that should be investigated**.

The main clinical sign in cats that develop CHF is **recent onset of respiratory distress, related to pulmonary oedema and/or pleural effusion**. Tachycardia is common (although not always present) and coughing rare; chronic cough in a cat with respiratory distress often suggests bronchial disease. Recently, the RAPID CAT study has demonstrated that tachycardia, gallop sounds, profound tachypnoea and hypothermia generally indicate dyspnoea of cardiac origin in cats.

Some cats with HCM (also with other cardiomyopathies) develop **thromboembolic events**, the most characteristic of which cause the obstruction of the distal aorta and iliac arteries, causing sudden-onset hindlimb paralysis (lower motor neuron signs). **The absence of femoral pulse, cold extremities, and discoloration of the pads of the hindlimbs compared to the forelimbs is characteristic**.

Diagnosis

Clinical signs and physical examination can raise the suspicion of HCM in cats. However, it is essential to **rule out the presence of non-cardiac conditions** such as anaemia, hyperthyroidism, and systemic arterial hypertension, especially in older cats.

Echocardiography

Echocardiography is the standard non-invasive technique for diagnosing cats with HCM and ruling out other forms of heart disease. It should be remembered that ultrasound is an operator-dependent technique, which requires experience since the hypertrophy patterns in cats with HCM are highly variable and the management of these cats is not always easy.

The diagnosis of HCM is based on demonstrating an **increase in the thickness of the interventricular septum and/or the LV free wall in diastole** (IVSd, FWd). Due to the heterogeneous distribution of ventricular hypertrophy, measurements are taken from several echocardiographic views (right parasternal long axis with four and five chambers and short axis at the level of the papillary muscles and *chordae tendineae* of the mitral valve), in M and 2D modes (Figures 4 and 5).

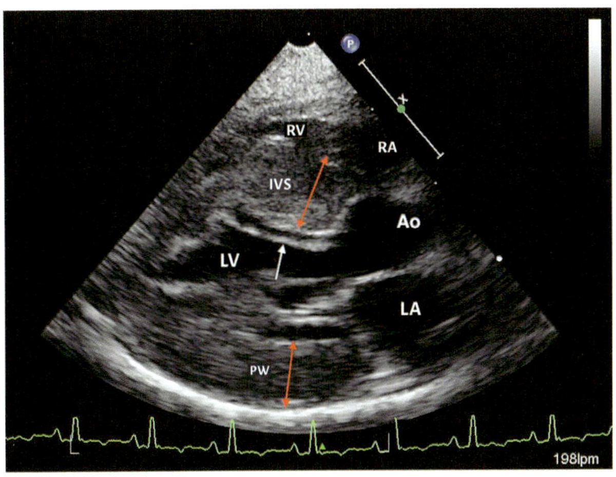

Figure 4. 2D echocardiogram obtained via a right parasternal long axis five chamber view in a cat with HCM phenotype. Hypertrophy of the interventricular septum (IVS) and posterior wall (PW) of the left ventricle (LV) and a "false tendon" which runs from the apical ventricular area to the interventricular septum (white arrow) are observed. The red arrows show the locations for measurements of IVS and free wall (FW) thickness of the LV. LA: left atrium, Ao: aorta.

In order to obtain accurate measurements, the endocardial border must be accurately identified, especially on the right ventricular side of the IVS as the *chordae tendineae* and papillary muscles can cause erroneous measurements. Although there is no consensus on how to measure septal and parietal thickness in 2D mode, the authors of this chapter do so by measuring the walls using the **leading-edge-to-leading-edge technique**, that is, including an endocardial border and excluding the other (Figure 5).

The upper limit of normal values for both IVSd and FWd is 5 mm, even though the classic cut-off value for a cat considered as having ventricular hypertrophy is ≥6 mm. Therefore, cats with ventricular myocardial measurements between 5 and 6 mm can be considered doubtful and repeating the echocardiographic examination in 6–12 months is recommended.

Papillary muscles can also appear hypertrophic (even before the IVS and FW), although there are no reliable methods for measurement due to the variability in their morphology (Figure 4). Alterations in the morphology of the mitral valve may also occur, such as elongated and thickened leaflets, similar to those that occur in human patients with HCM.

The presence of false tendons (cord-like structures which cross the LV and insert into the interventricular septum or papillary muscles) is common in cats with HCM (Figure 5) but also found in normal cats that do not develop HCM.

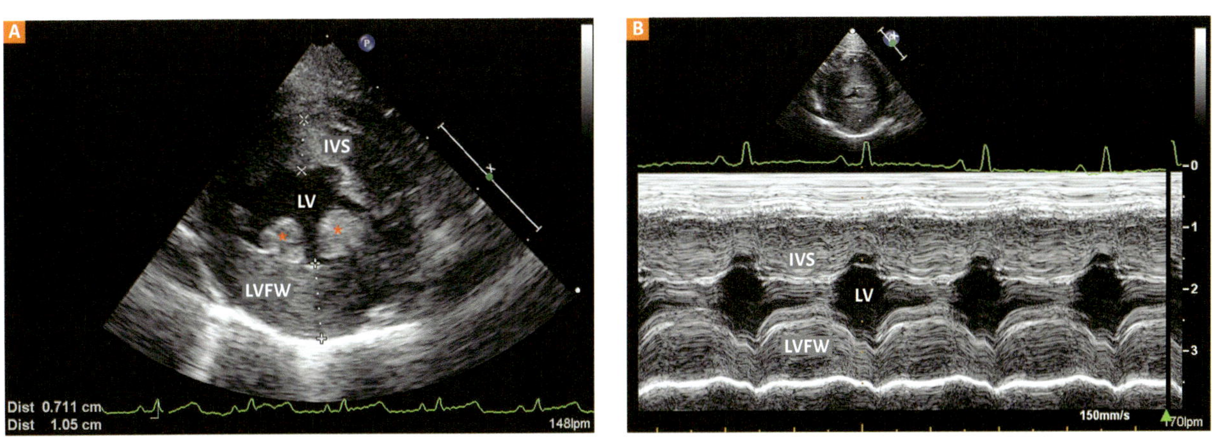

Figure 5. 2D (**A**) and M-mode (**B**) echocardiogram of a cat with HCM phenotype, obtained via a right short axis parasternal view of the left ventricle where marked hypertrophy of the interventricular septum (IVS), left ventricular (LV) free wall (FW) and papillary muscles (*) can be seen. In A, measurements of the IVS and FW can be visualised.

At least a third of the cats with HCM presents with dynamic LVOT obstruction due to the systolic anterior movement (SAM) of the mitral valve, i.e. the anterior leaflet shifts towards the ventricular outflow tract during systole, causing it to narrow (Figure 6), with increased blood flow velocity and mitral regurgitation (Figure 7). Valve displacement can be observed in both M and 2D modes. It can be present at rest or appear only when cats are stressed. Due to the obstruction, the flow velocity in the LVOT increases and the Doppler spectrum shows a dagger shape (Figure 8). The transmitral flow pattern can be normal, show an abnormal relaxation pattern with peak A velocity higher than that of peak E (Figure 9) or a restrictive type pattern with an E/A ratio >2.

In cats with atrial dilation, spontaneous contrast and even the presence of a thrombus can be observed within the left atrium or auricle (Figure 10).

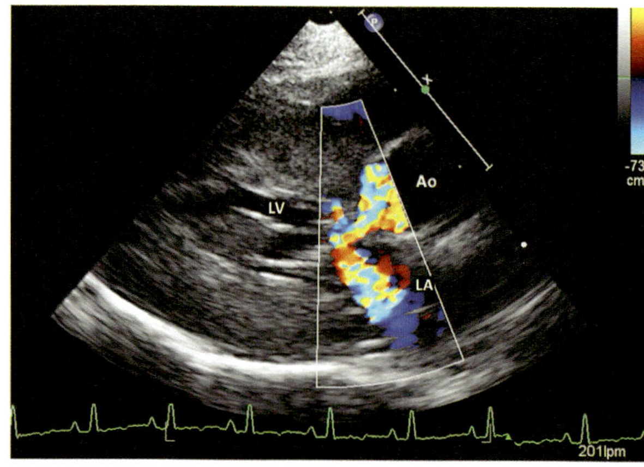

Figure 7. Colour Doppler echocardiogram of a cat with obstructive HCM phenotype, obtained via a right long axis parasternal view, where turbulent flow in the left ventricular (LV) outflow tract and ascending aorta (Ao) can be seen as well as mitral regurgitation due to anterior systolic movement of the mitral valve. LA: left atrium.

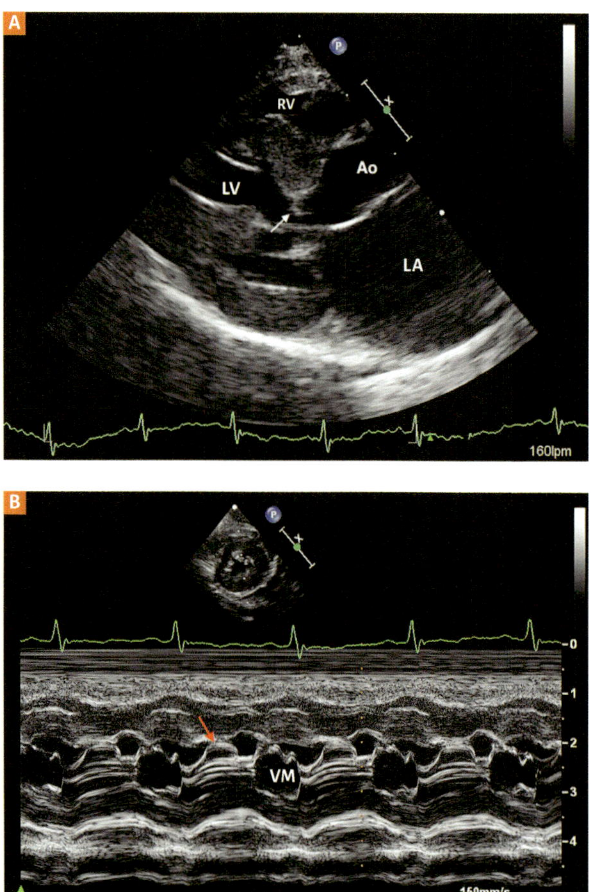

Figure 6. 2D (**A**) and M-mode (**B**) echocardiogram of a cat with obstructive HCM phenotype, obtained via a right long axis (**A**) parasternal view and a short axis view at the level of the mitral valve (MV) (**B**). **A.** Hypertrophy of the left ventricular (LV) walls can be seen, which is more severe in the basal segment of the interventricular septum, next to dilation of the left atrium (LA). In both images the anterior systolic movement of the mitral valve (arrows) can be seen. Ao: ascending aorta, RV: right ventricle.

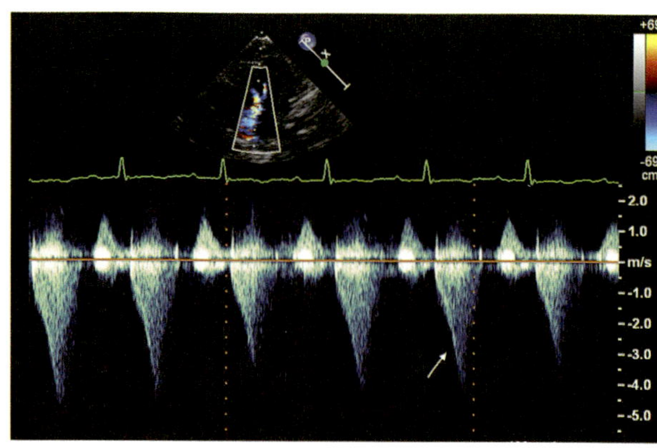

Figure 8. Continuous-wave Doppler interrogation of the left ventricular outflow tract and ascending aorta in a cat with obstructive HCM phenotype, obtained via a left apical five chamber view. An elevated end-systolic velocity (Vmax = 5 m/s and GPD 100 mmHg) and a dagger shape profile can be observed, due to dynamic obstruction.

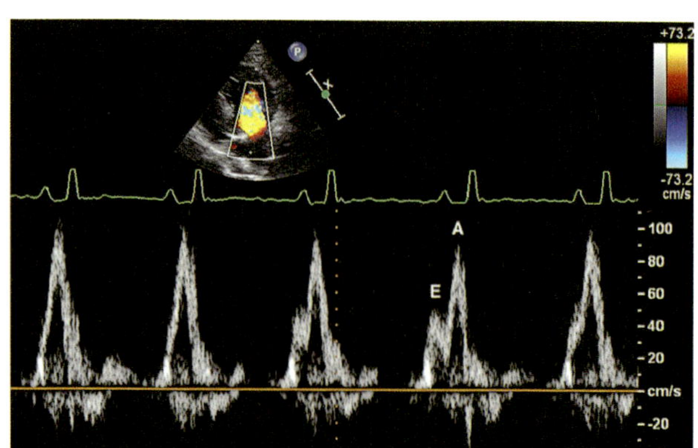

Figure 9. Pulsed-wave Doppler interrogation of mitral inflow in a cat with HCM phenotype, obtained via a left apical four chamber view. A delayed relaxation pattern characterised by an E/A ratio <1 is observed, indicating diastolic dysfunction.

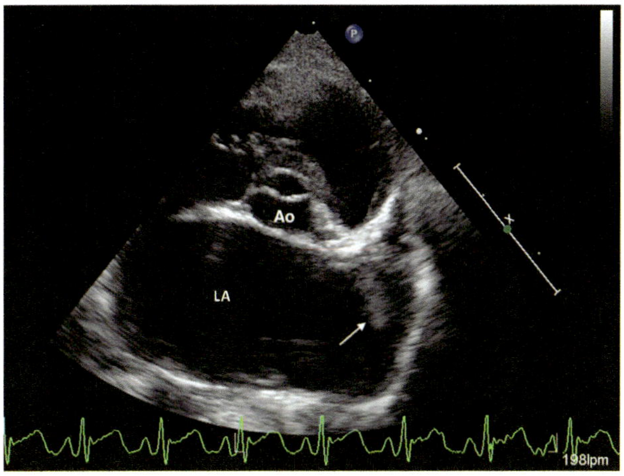

Figure 10. Right parasternal short axis 2D image of a cat with HCM phenotype, obtained at the level of the aorta (Ao) and left atrium (LA), showing LA dilation and a thrombus in the left auricular appendage (arrow).

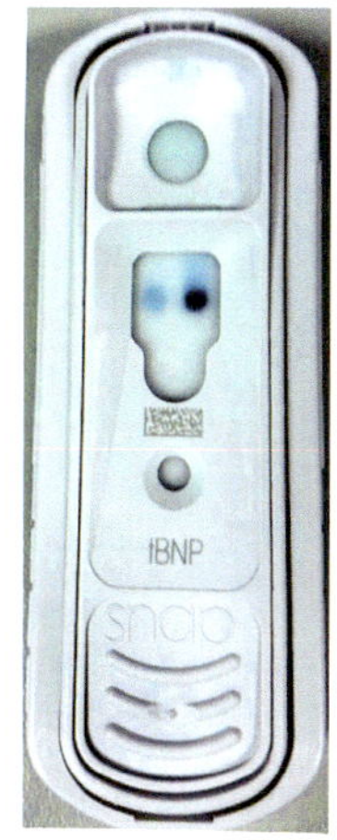

Figure 11. Image of a snap test for measurement of NTProBNP obtained in a cat presenting with respiratory distress to the emergency service. A positive result can be seen.

The main echocardiographic findings associated with a high risk of CHF or aortic thromboembolism are the following:

- severe hypertrophy of the IVS and left ventricular FW (>9 mm)
- regional hypokinesia and/or signs of infarction (advanced stages of the disease due to myocardial ischaemia)
- left atrial dilation: >16 mm in the long-axis 4-chamber view (ventricular systole) or a LA/Ao ratio >1.5 (Figure 10)
- spontaneous echocardiographic constrast in the left atrium
- reduced left ventricular shortening fraction (<30%)
- reduced left atrial shortening fraction (<12%)
- restrictive transmitral flow pattern (E/A >2)
- reduced left atrial appendage velocity (<0.25 m/s).

Biomarkers

Cardiac biomarkers measured in blood can be used as an aid to the diagnosis of HCM, especially for veterinarians in general practice and in emergency clinics since these tests do not require special training and are relatively inexpensive. The most widely used biomarkers are **NT-proBNP and cardiac troponin I (cTnI)**.

In cats with HCM, myocytes release NT-proBNP as a consequence of cardiomegaly and wall distension; a marker used as a screening parameter for HCM in asymptomatic cats. **Several studies indicate a cut-off value for NT-proBNP >270 pmol/l in a dyspnoeic cat allows differentiation of CHF from a respiratory disease** as the cause of respiratory distress. The problem is that results are not immediate because the samples must be sent to a laboratory. In emergency situations, a commercial rapid test (SNAP® Feline proBNP, IDEXX Laboratories) can be used to differentiate between high and low risk cats (Figure 11).

Recent studies have shown that cut-off values for NT-proBNP >100 pmol/l, have a sensitivity of 93.9% and a specificity of 92.4% for differentiating healthy cats from those with HCM. If the NT-proBNP cut-off is increased to >150 pmol/l, the specificity increases to 100%.

Despite the advantages of an objective test, it should be considered that measurement of NT-proBNP cannot detect cats with mild or moderate HCM, especially in young animals, so the results should be confirmed with echocardiography.

cTnI is released into the circulation as a consequence of myocardial damage. Recent studies show increased cTnI concentrations reflect the severity of HCM in cats and cut-off values >0.7 ng/l are associated with increased risk of cardiac mortality. A more recent study has shown a cut-off value for cTnI = 0.234 ng/ml has a sensitivity of 95.0% and a specificity of 77.8% for ruling out congestive heart failure. However, as myocardial damage can be intermittent, some cats may show low plasma concentrations, so this is **not a sensitive marker for HCM**.

Thoracic Radiology

Thoracic radiographs may appear normal in cats with HCM, especially in the preclinical phase. In symptomatic animals, cardiomegaly may appear with elongation of the cardiac silhouette and prominent **left atrial silhouette in the lateral projection and with the characteristic "Valentine" heart shape** (due to atrial dilation) in the dorsoventral projection (Figure 12).

Interstitial and alveolar oedema may be observed, the latter appearing diffusely in patches or located in the caudal or accessory lobes, which may be difficult to differentiate from a primary respiratory disease. Pleural effusion secondary to cardiomyopathies also commonly causes respiratory distress in cats with HCM (Figure 13).

Radiography is not considered a sensitive or specific technique for the diagnosis of cardiomyopathies in cats.

Electrocardiogram

The electrocardiogram may be normal or show an increased R-wave voltage, left axis deviation, premature ventricular or supraventricular arrhythmias, and even atrial fibrillation when the left atrium is severely dilated.

Genetic Tests

Commercial genetic tests are available to identify mutations in Maine Coon and Ragdoll cats. One published study has shown only 34% of Maine Coon cats had the mutation (positive genotype) and, of these, 88% had a negative echocardiographic phenotype at an age of 5.4 years. Therefore, **echocardiographic examination continues to be the technique of choice for the diagnosis of HCM**, even in genotype-positive cats.

Screening Programmes in Cats with HCM

Due to breeder and veterinary demand, screening programmes have been implemented in several breeds of cat (e.g. Maine Coon, Norwegian Forest, Siberian, British Shorthair, Ragdoll, Sphynx and Devon Rex) based on **echocardiographic examination**.

In general, it is recommended that cats intended for breeding are **evaluated from one to three-years of age**. Echocardiographic examination should then be repeated later in life, such as at five and eight-years of age. Even for experts it can be **difficult to differentiate normal cats from cats with mild hypertrophy**, due to the highly variable echocardiographic phenotypes that cats with HCM present and the lack of consensus on normal measurement technique and reference ranges.

Animals with equivocal hypertrophy should not be used for breeding until their phenotype has been ascertained using further diagnostic tests. In fact, even mildly affected parents can generate offsprings that might develop severe forms of HCM.

Genetic tests must be interpreted with caution, since there are cats with a positive genotype which never develop the disease and others with a negative genotype that present hypertrophy.

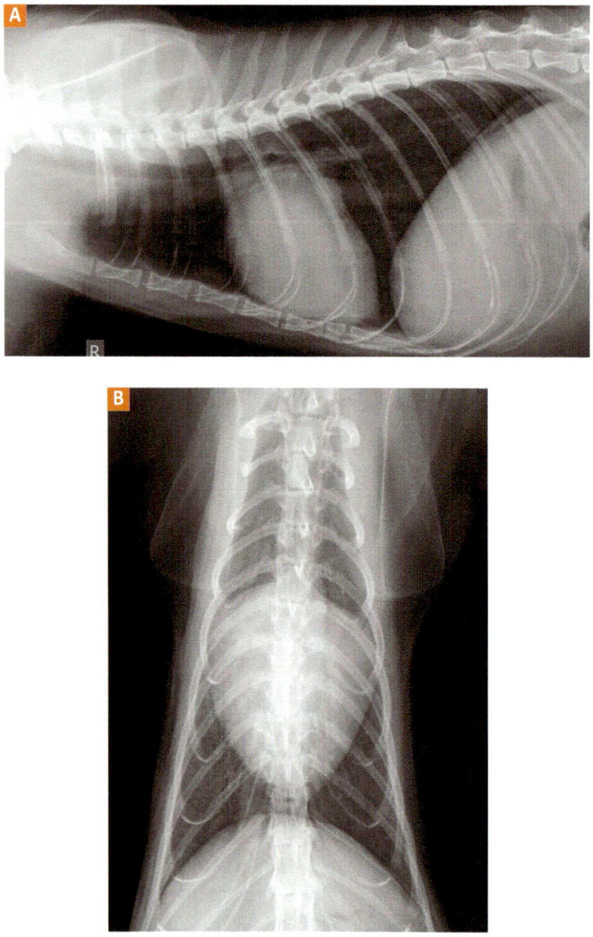

Figure 12. Right lateral (**A**) and ventrodorsal (**B**) radiograph of a cat with HCM phenotype on echocardiography, where an increase in size of the left atrial and ventricular silhouettes, plus an interstitial pattern can be seen. In **B** a characteristic image of a "Valentine" heart is seen, due to atrial dilation.

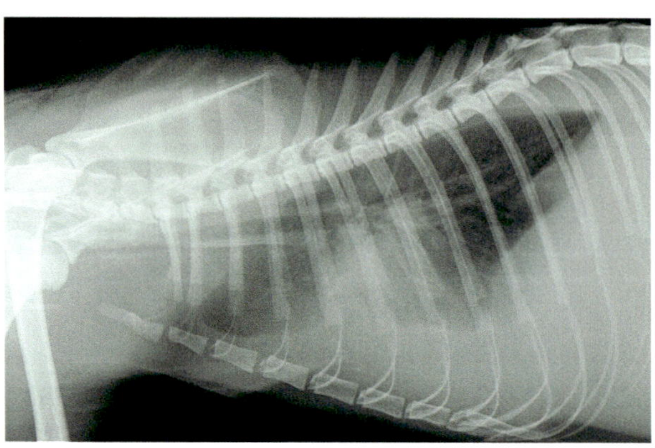

Figure 13. Lateral thoracic radiograph of a cat with HCM phenotype on echocardiography, and CHF where pleural effusion can be seen.

Treatment

Asymptomatic Cats

In this phase, no medication has demonstrated to improve survival or quality of life. Despite this, in cats with **severe LVOT obstruction, atenolol can be considered at a dose of 6.25–12.5 mg in total every 12–24 hours**, since it can reduce the pressure gradient. However, a positive impact on 5-year survival has not been demonstrated in cats receiving this medication, nor has an improvement in their quality of life as perceived by their owners. Recent studies in mice, cats and people have shown the **MYK-461 molecule** to be a promising drug because it decreases sarcomeric contractility, reducing the pressure gradient of the ventricular outflow tract and myocardial hypertrophy.

In cats with significant LA dilation and/or spontaneous **echocardiographic contrast**, anticoagulant therapy is recommended. In a recent study, **clopidogrel (18.75 mg/cat PO every 24 hours)** was found to be more effective than aspirin (81 mg/cat PO every 72 hours) in preventing recurrence of thromboembolism in cats, so it is considered the first option for prevention of thrombus formation.

Cats with CHF

Treatment of cats with CHF is similar as for the different types of cardiomyopathies and discussed at the end of this chapter.

Prognosis

The data from the recent REVEAL study (Fox et al. 2018) carried out in cats with preclinical HCM showed that **cardiovascular morbidity occurred in 30%** of the animals and there were no differences between obstructive and non-obstructive forms or with survival, regardless of the time of diagnosis. In cats that developed cardiovascular morbidity, survival was 1.3 ± 1.7 years. Few cats (10%) with preclinical HCM reached 9–15 years of age.

Other studies have shown that in cats with HCM that survived 24-hours of hospitalization after an episode of CHF, survival has ranged from 596 to 732 days.

The presence of aortic thromboembolism is associated with a poor prognosis and mortality is high. Among those who survive and overcome an episode, survival is estimated at 184 days. Other signs such as syncope and arrhythmias indicate a poor prognosis.

Restrictive Cardiomyopathies

Restrictive cardiomyopathy (RCM) is a **disease of the ventricular myocardium characterised by diastolic dysfunction** and variable phenotypic expression, **without thickening of the walls**. Systolic function is generally preserved or slightly reduced.

Pathology

RCM has been morphologically subclassified into two forms:

- **endomyocardial**
  - Macroscopically this is characterised by endomyocardial fibrosis, appearing as defined lesions which cross the left ventricle or as a diffuse scarring process which causes obliteration of the cavity (Figure 14).
- **myocardial**
  - In cases of myocardial RCM there is an increase in cardiac mass with minimal or no hypertrophy of the left ventricle.

In both forms, **severe biatrial dilatation is common**, sometimes with the volume of the atrial chambers significantly exceeding that of the ventricles.

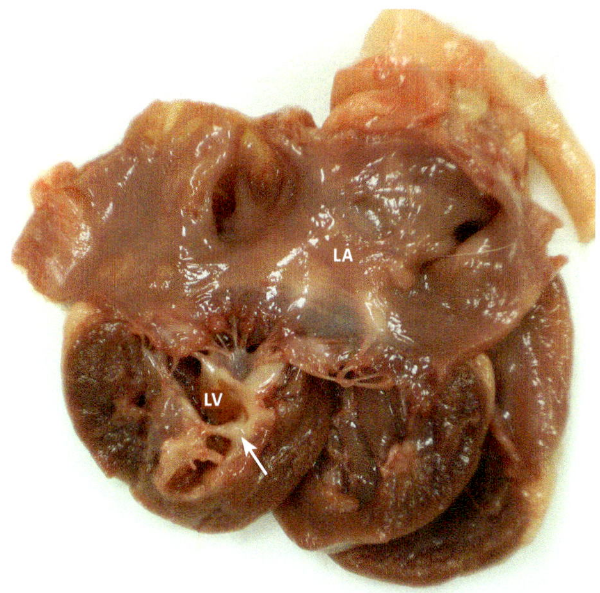

Figure 14. Macroscopic image of the heart of a cat with restrictive cardiomyopathy with the presence of left atrial (LA) dilation, and the left ventricle (LV) appears "lined" with fibrous tissue (endomyocardial type) connecting the interventricular septum with the free wall (arrow).

Histopathologically, typical **endomyocardial type lesions** include endocardial thickening, fibrosis, and accumulation of granulation and hyaline tissue which extends to the subendocardial myocardium. Inflammatory cells may also be seen.

In **myocardial RCM**, there is myofibre disorganization, replacement fibrosis, and vascular abnormalities. Some of these microscopic features are found in HCM, so the distinction between HCM and RCM may be unclear. At present, there is little consensus on the histopathological diagnosis of feline RCM.

Aetiology

The origin of this condition is not yet fully understood. Fibrosis could be the result of scarring, secondary to an immune, inflammatory or infectious process. In some cases of endomyocardial fibrosis, signs of endomyocarditis have been found, and parvoviral genetic material has been isolated in cats affected by cardiomyopathies, although a clear causal relationship has not been established.

It has been suggested that RCM may represent the end-stage of other cardiomyopathies. Furthermore, familial forms secondary to genetic mutations found in humans have not yet been identified in cats.

Physiopathology

The **progressive alteration of diastolic function**, which is usually biventricular, causes a disproportionate increase in ventricular end-diastolic pressure in response to small volumes of blood, which in turn causes **atrial dilation**. Increased ventricular filling pressures can result in **venous congestion and left and/or right CHF**.

Epidemiology and Clinical Presentation

This is a relatively rare condition, representing between 15 and 20% of all feline cardiomyopathies according to studies undertaken in populations examined at referral centres. In the general population, forms of cardiomyopathy other than the hypertrophic type are uncommon.

The disease appears in adulthood, with a **mean age at diagnosis of around 7–10 years**. No breed predisposition has been identified, although the condition has been described in Burmese, Siamese, Persian and Maine Coon cats, and in domestic short- and long-haired cats. Concomitant histopathological features of restrictive and hypertrophic cardiomyopathies have been found in Norwegian Forest cats, and it is suggested this breed may suffer from a mixed form, also described in human medicine.

At the time of diagnosis, clinical signs are frequently present although these are nonspecific and generally related to the presence of CHF and include **tachypnoea, dyspnoea, and anorexia**. Due to the high incidence of **aortic thromboembolism**, an affected animal may be referred for hindlimb paralysis.

On physical examination, gallop sounds are relatively common, with tachyarrhythmias and mild murmurs also described. However, it should be noted that in some cases of RCM, no abnormalities are present on cardiac auscultation.

Diagnosis

As with other cardiomyopathies, thoracic radiography and electrocardiography often show nonspecific abnormalities. Of these, arrhythmias are common, in **particular ventricular premature complexes and supraventricular tachycardias** (Figure 15).

By definition, the presence of RCM is demonstrated by confirming a restrictive left ventricular diastolic filling pattern through Doppler echocardiography. However, restrictive physiology related to decreased ventricular compliance is also seen in other pathologies such as HCM and DCM. In addition, fusion of the early (E) and late (A) diastolic filling waves of transmitral flow is common in cats due to high heart rates, and diastolic dysfunction can be difficult to demonstrate.

The **echocardiographic diagnostic criteria** for RCM are not uniformly accepted: the most frequent findings are not consistent in all patients and are common to other cardiomyopathies. These findings include:

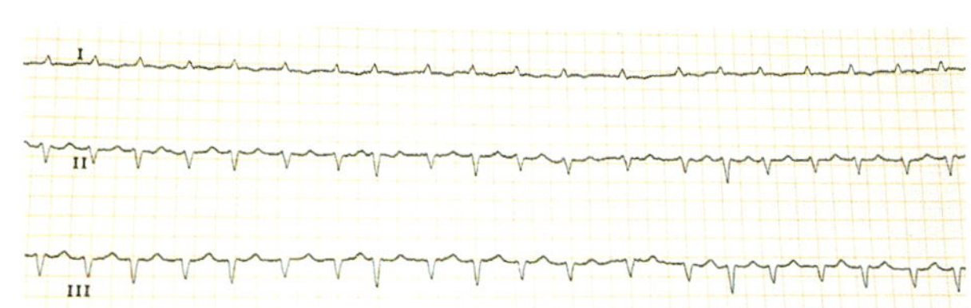

Figure 15. Surface electrocardiogram, obtained in lateral recumbency, of a cat with restrictive cardiomyopathy where the P waves cannot be identified, and the rhythm is irregularly irregular, compatible with atrial fibrillation. The electrical axis deviates to the left (-45°), compatible with an anterior left fascicular hemiblock (50 mm/s; 1 cm = 1 mV).

- **dilation of the left atrium or both atria**, which is usually severe;
- spontaneous contrast or **thrombi in the left atrium**;
- normal or enlarged ventricular chamber and walls on two-dimensional and M-mode echocardiography, and a normal or decreased shortening fraction;
- asymmetrical appearance of the left ventricular myocardium with areas of both thinning and thickening, and in cases of myocardial infarction hypokinetic or akinetic areas;
- right ventricular abnormalities, although less frequently;
- in the endomyocardial form, hyperechogenic endocardium and connections between the interventricular septum and the free wall of the left ventricle (Figure 16);
- valves which generally appear normal; systolic anterior motion of the mitral valve is uncommon;
- pleural and pericardial effusion in decompensated cats.

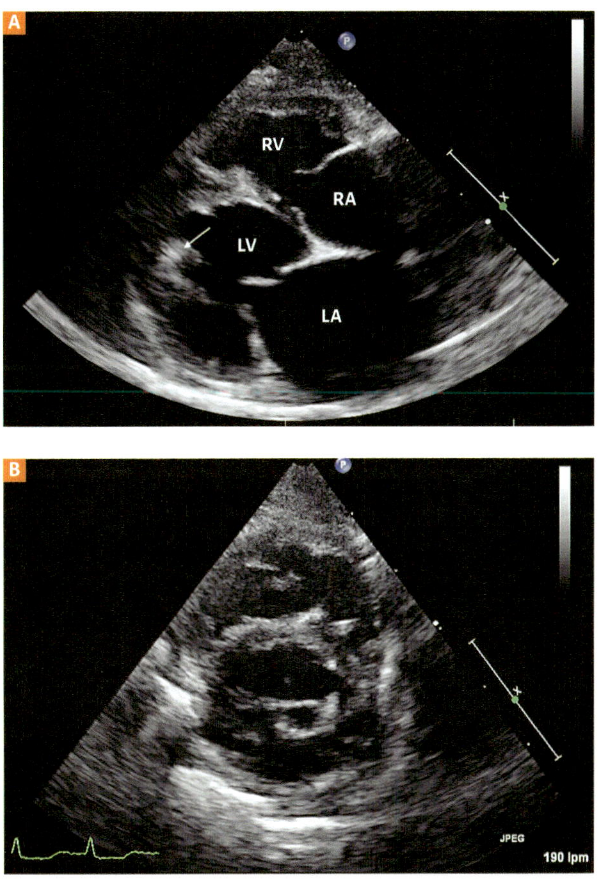

Figure 16. 2D mode echocardiogram of the cat in Figure 14 with a restrictive cardiomyopathy phenotype, obtained via a right parasternal view. **A**. A long axis image, which shows dilation of the four chambers and hyperechogenic endocardium in the ventricular apical area (arrow). **B**. Short axis view at the level of the ventricles where hyperechogenic tissue between the papillary muscles can be seen. LA: left atrium, RA: right atrium, LV: left ventricle, RV: right ventricle.

Doppler echocardiography may reveal mitral regurgitation, which is usually mild, and an absence of anterior systolic movement of the mitral valve. **Diastolic dysfunction is the predominant feature** of the disease, and transmitral flow shows a restrictive filling pattern, due to high left atrial pressure, characterised by an increased E wave velocity with rapid deceleration, and a low A wave velocity (Figure 17). However, in early RCM there may be an abnormal relaxation pattern, characterised by an E:A ratio <1. The isovolumetric relaxation time is usually reduced by the early equalization of the atrial and ventricular pressures. Pulmonary vein flow reflects elevated left atrial pressure with a decreased S wave velocity, and tissue Doppler often shows an E/E' ratio >12, suggesting elevated ventricular filling pressures.

Treatment

There is no consensus on the treatment of RCM in the preclinical stage. However, the administration of anticoagulants in the presence of left atrial dilation, spontaneous echocardiographic contrast, or thrombi is common practice.

The management of CHF is similar for all cardiomyopathies.

Prognosis

The prognosis is usually poor and the majority of affected animals (60–86%) die from cardiac causes. Average survival

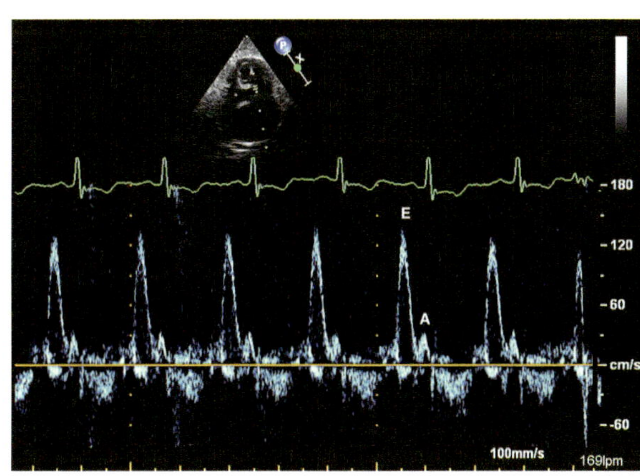

Figure 17. Pulsed Doppler echocardiogram of a cat with restrictive cardiomyopathy, obtained via a left apical four chamber view. The transmitral flow shows a restrictive pattern. The E peak (initial phase of diastole) shows a rapid filling phase of short duration and the A peak (atrial systole), a very low velocity, reflecting the severe diastolic dysfunction due to ventricular rigidity. The E/A ratio = 4.16 (reference range E/A = 1.1-2.9).

times of 3–24 months have been reported, although death in the first 24–48 hours after diagnosis is not uncommon. Cardiac causes of death include spontaneous or sudden death or euthanasia in animals with CHF or aortic thromboembolism.

Dilated Cardiomyopathy

Dilated cardiomyopathy (DCM) is a **disease of the ventricular myocardium characterised by systolic dysfunction and dilation of the cardiac chambers** in the absence of congenital heart disease and valvular or vascular disease.

Pathology

Macroscopically, the DCM phenotype is characterised by the presence of **severe and generalised dilation of both ventricles**, often accompanied by biatrial dilation. Cardiac weight is usually increased. There is thinning of the ventricular walls, along with flattening and atrophy of the papillary muscles and myocardial trabeculae. These changes may be accompanied by fibrosis.

The histopathological findings are variable. Classically, myofibers are thin, with nuclear hypertrophy and pleomorphism, and in some areas may have a corrugated appearance. However, cardiomyocytes may be normal in size, except in areas of interstitial fibrosis where they are atrophic. There may be foci of coagulative necrosis, granulation, and myocytolysis.

Aetiology

This condition may be primary or secondary. The secondary form may be due to:

- toxic causes e.g. anthracycline administration
- a sequelae of myocarditis
- immune-mediated or metabolic diseases
- chronic tachyarrhythmias
- chronic volume overload (as in severe mitral regurgitation)
- end-stage HCM
- taurine deficiency.

Cardiomyopathy due to taurine deficiency is now rare because commercial foods are supplemented with this amino acid. Currently, animals at risk of DCM due to taurine deficiency are those fed unusual diets such as vegetarian or homemade foods, which are inadequately balanced. **Idiopathic DCM** is referred to when other causes of secondary myocardial failure, such as taurine deficiency, have been ruled out.

In humans, numerous genetic causes of DCM have been identified and in Doberman Pinschers with DCM, a genetic mutation has been recognised. To date, no causal genetic mutations have been described in cats with DCM, although a complex pattern of inheritance has been observed in a colony of domestic short-haired cats.

Physiopathology

Systolic dysfunction of the left or both ventricles continues with both systolic and diastolic dilation of the ventricular chambers. As a consequence, there is a widening of the atrioventricular valvular annuli and secondary valvular regurgitation, potentially contributing to atrial dilation secondary to the progression of myocardial failure and the development of CHF.

Epidemiology and Clinical Presentation

This condition is rarely diagnosed since commercial foods are adequately supplemented with taurine.

There is no clear breed predisposition in cats for the development of DCM, although the most frequently affected cats are the domestic shorthair, Burmese, Siamese, Persian, Himalayan and Abyssinian. The disease affects adult cats, with an average age of onset of 9 years old.

The presence of clinical signs such as **dyspnoea and ascites** is common at presentation; these are nonspecific but due to CHF. The presence of hypotension is not uncommon. Finding hindlimb paralysis secondary to aortic thromboembolism and episodes of collapse is less common.

Physical examination may detect ascites, muffled heart sounds, gallop sounds, tachyarrhythmias, and low-intensity systolic murmurs. In cases of taurine deficiency, there may be **degenerative changes in the retina**, although these are inconsistent.

Diagnosis

The main differential diagnoses include unclassified cardiomyopathy and HCM accompanied by myocardial infarctions.

Radiography and electrocardiography are relatively nonspecific tests for the detection of feline cardiomyopathies, and the findings detailed in the section on HCM are found in all conditions described in this chapter (Figure 18). However, DCM can sometimes be accompanied by severe eccentric remodelling which is rare in HCM.

Echocardiographic findings are more specific and include systolic dysfunction and ventricular dilation (Figure 19). Systolic dysfunction may precede dilation, which generally affects the left ventricle, while the right may or may not be involved. The **shortening fraction is less than 20%** and often much lower; however, this parameter should not be the only one used to analyse systolic function, due to its dependence on preload and afterload. Ventricular walls may be normal in size but are often thin (Figure 20). The E point to septal separation is usually increased.

The left atrium or both atria dilate as myocardial dysfunction progresses. Occasionally, spontaneous echocardiographic contrast or thrombi can be seen in the left atrium.

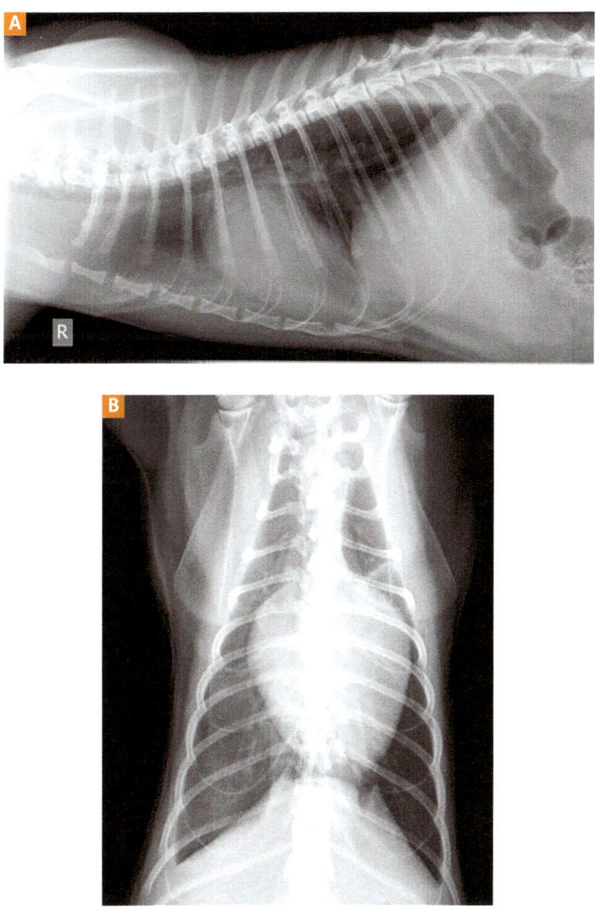

Figure 18. Right lateral and dorsoventral thoracic radiographs of a cat with a dilated cardiomyopathy phenotype, which shows an enlarged left atrial and ventricular silhouette, interstitial and alveolar pattern in the right caudal lobe and pleural effusion. **B**. The characteristic "Valentine" heart seen in the image is due to biatrial dilation.

Doppler echocardiography often shows mitral regurgitation, and the transmitral flow pattern may indicate the presence of diastolic dysfunction.

In cases of suspected DCM secondary to taurine deficiency, it is advisable to **measure taurine levels**. Measurement in whole blood appears to be more reliable than in plasma. False positives can be obtained from prolonged fasting or anorexia and false negatives from artefacts (sample not rapidly processed), postprandial sampling, recent dietary changes, or thromboembolism.

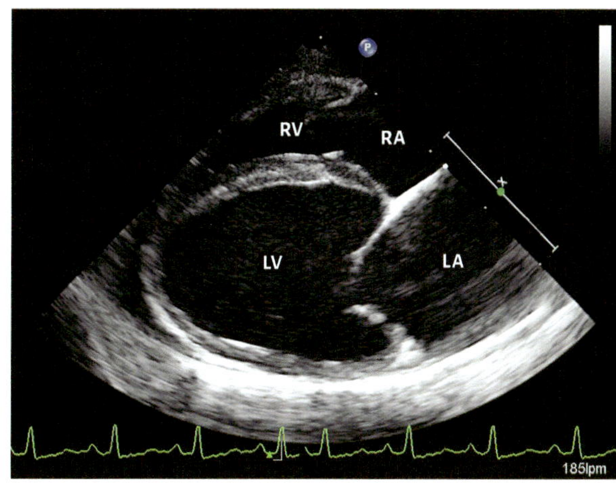

Figure 19. 2D echocardiogram of a cat with a dilated cardiomyopathy phenotype, obtained using a right, long axis, four chamber parasternal view. Marked dilation of the four chambers and thin walls can be seen. LV: left ventricle, LA: left atrium, RV: right ventricle, RA: right atrium.

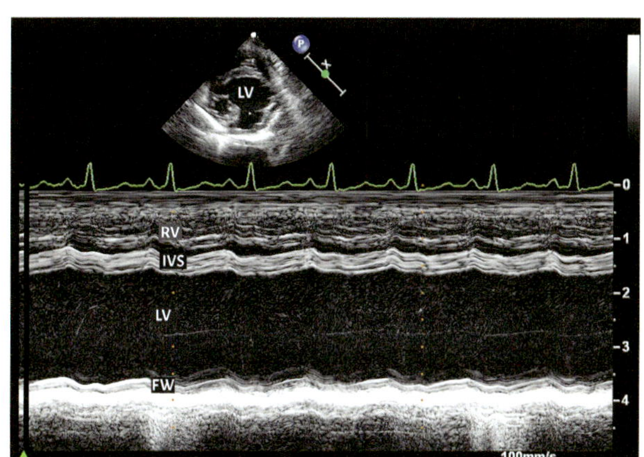

Figure 20. M-mode echocardiogram of the cat in Figure 19 with a dilated cardiomyopathy phenotype, obtained using a right, short axis parasternal view at the ventricular level. Dilation of both ventricles and reduced fractional shortening can be seen. RV: right ventricle, LV: left ventricle, IVS: interventricular septum, FW: free wall of the ventricle.

An eye examination may reveal the presence of retinal degeneration in cases of taurine deficiency, although the finding is not consistent.

Treatment

The management of DCM **includes treatment of CHF and supplementation with taurine**. The administration of taurine is recommended even in the presence of normal blood levels, due to the extremely favourable response to treatment and the possibility of false negatives. Cats that survive CHF and receive adequate supplementation generally demonstrate echocardiographic improvement within 3–6 weeks.

A **positive inotrope** could improve ventricular systolic function, and pimobendan administration appears to improve survival in cats that do not respond to taurine supplementation. Therefore, its administration may be recommended, although it should be noted that pimobendan is not currently approved for use in cats and the prescription of this drug requires the consent of the owner.

The use of **antiarrhythmic drugs** could be indicated in cases of atrial fibrillation or other haemodynamically significant arrhythmias or those with malignant characteristics.

The management of CHF is similar in all cardiomyopathies.

Prognosis

In general, **the prognosis for patients with DCM is poor** if there is no response to taurine supplementation. The median survival time reported in cats that did not respond to taurine supplementation in a study that included 32 patients was 49 days if they were treated with pimobendan and 12 days if they did not receive inodilators.

Arrhythmogenic Cardiomyopathy

This condition is a rare, spontaneous cardiomyopathy, described in cats, dogs and humans. It is characterised by **marked intramyocardial fibrous-fat infiltration, which causes dilation and ventricular dysfunction** (primarily on the right-side) and is associated with **ventricular arrhythmias, CHF, and/or sudden death**. Due to the possible involvement of other chambers, the previous designation right ventricular arrhythmogenic cardiomyopathy is being abandoned in favour of the more generic term **arrhythmogenic cardiomyopathy**.

Pathology

Macroscopically, cats with arrhythmogenic cardiomyopathy may have **normal or dilated right ventricles with thin walls**. Ventricular wall thinning can be diffuse or segmental, and translucent and aneurysmal areas can be seen, often located in the apical, infundibular, or sub tricuspid regions. Right atrial dilation may be seen, and the left ventricle may occasionally be affected. Lymphocytic infiltration is not uncommon.

Histopathological examination generally shows substitution of the myocardium with adipose and fibrous tissue, with the lesions extending from the epicardium to the endocardium.

Aetiology

In humans and **Boxer dogs,** it is recognised as a familial disease, while the aetiology in cats is unknown.

Physiopathology

It is a disease in which cell adhesion is affected, leading to cell separation, inflammation, death of myocytes, and fibrolipomatous repair. Apoptosis and myocarditis appear to contribute to the damage and repair of myocytes. Alteration of the electromechanical coupling due to the ultrastructural abnormalities described can promote arrhythmogenesis.

Progressive atrophy of the right ventricular myocardium is associated with chamber dilation and secondary tricuspid regurgitation. Ventricle function is compromised and can result in **right-sided CHF**.

Epidemiology and Clinical Presentation

The exact prevalence of the disease is unknown, although at referral centres it is reported to represent 1–4% of feline cardiomyopathy cases.

No breed, sex or age predisposition has been identified. The clinical signs are not specific and **generally associated with CHF, including tachypnoea and dyspnoea, lethargy and anorexia**, although many cats are asymptomatic at diagnosis. Murmurs and arrhythmias may be detected on physical examination. Respiratory distress, abdominal distention, jugular distention, and muffled heart sounds may also be seen in cats with CHF.

Diagnosis

Differential diagnoses include other myocardial disorders and congenital or acquired heart disease affecting the right-side of the heart, such as tricuspid dysplasia and Uhl's anomaly.

Currently, diagnosis is based on the combination of a familial history, marked dilation of the right ventricular chamber on echocardiography, ventricular or supraventricular arrhythmias, and compatible pathological findings including right ventricular dilation and fibrofatty replacement.

Treatment

Although there are no studies on treatment in cats with this cardiomyopathy, arrhythmias can be treated with **sotalol at a dose of 2–4 mg/kg/12h orally**.

The management of CHF is similar in all cardiomyopathies.

Cardiomyopathies with a Nonspecific Phenotype

The terminology unclassified cardiomyopathies, recently replaced by **cardiomyopathies with a nonspecific phenotype**, brings together the set of myocardial modifications that are not strictly hypertrophic, dilated, or restrictive. It can be difficult to distinguish between RCM, a cardiomyopathy with a nonspecific phenotype and end-stage HCM. Clinical signs cannot be differentiated from other cardiomyopathies; however, treatment and prognosis are similar.

Myocarditis

Myocarditis refers to **inflammation of the myocardium**, which can lead to cardiac dysfunction. It is a **rare condition in cats**, which generally affects animals under 8-years of age, although it is also diagnosed in older cats.

The main cause in cats is infection, which can be:

- viral (i.e. feline immunodeficiency virus)
- bacterial (i.e. *Streptococcus*)
- protozoal (i.e. *Toxoplasma gondii*).

Predisposing factors include congenital heart abnormalities, anaemia, diabetes mellitus, hyperthyroidism, or trauma. In other cases the cause cannot be identified.

The inflammation, myocardial necrosis, degeneration and even fibrosis caused by the aetiological agents can cause **ventricular systolic and/or diastolic dysfunction with atrial dilation and development of tachyarrhythmias**.

The disease can develop in days or weeks, with inconspicuous and nonspecific clinical signs such as apathy, respiratory distress, fever, weakness, anorexia, and even sudden death due to ventricular arrhythmias.

Diagnostic work-up includes echocardiographic examination, laboratory analysis (complete blood count, biochemistry, urinalysis, and TnIc), electrocardiogram, and thoracic radiographs.

Treatment includes correcting the cause if known, and treating tachyarrhythmias (atenolol or sotalol) as well as CHF if present (see the end of the chapter).

Treatment of Cats with Cardiomyopathies and CHF

Identifying the type of cardiomyopathy in a cat with respiratory distress is not of great importance, but what is important is determining whether or not CHF (pulmonary oedema and/or pleural effusion) is present. Treatment should be tailored to each animal.

Treatment guidelines are detailed below.

Emergency Treatment: Decompensated Cats

- **Oxygen therapy**: oxygen cages are a good option.
- **Sedation**: can be necessary to avoid stress. Butorphanol (0.25 mg/kg IM) can be employed in these cases.
- **Thoracentesis**: of pleural effusion greatly improves dyspnoea.
- **Furosemide**: IV boluses (for example 1–2 mg/kg IV and repeat after one hour at a dose of 1 mg/kg until dyspnoea

is controlled) or by continuous infusion.

- **Pimobendan** (the suggested dose in cats is 0.625–1.25 mg/PO and in dogs 0.15 mg/kg IV or 0.2–0.3 mg/kg PO): may be a good option in cases of systolic dysfunction and without significant LVOT obstruction.
- **Dobutamine** (1.25 µg/kg/min): if there are signs of systolic dysfunction and low cardiac output, such as apathy, low body temperature and blood pressure, and azotaemia, and no improvement is observed after administration of pimobendan.

Fluid therapy should be avoided in cats with CHF.

Treatment guidelines for **aortic thromboembolism** include analgesia (opioids), monitoring and correction of electrolyte and acid-base abnormalities. Prevention of new thrombi formation and extension of these can be attempted using heparin (100-200 IU/kg, then 100 IU/kg/6 h) and clopidogrel.

Maintenance Therapy: Cats with Cardiomyopathy

- **Elimination of abnormal fluid retention** and modulation of neurohormonal activity.
  - **Oral furosemide** (0.5–2 mg/kg/12–24 h) to control oedema.
  - **ACEIs** (benazepril) have not been shown to be effective at delaying treatment failure in cats with cardiomyopathies with or without CHF, but are still used by some cardiologists.
- **Optimization of haemodynamic function**
  - Studies in both cats and humans suggest **diltiazem** *retard* (30 mg/12–24 h PO) could improve diastolic function in cases of HCM by relaxing the ventricle, but there is currently no consensus on its use.
  - In cats with dynamic obstruction, **atenolol** (6.25–12.5 mg/12–24 h PO) should be considered for its theoretically beneficial effects, although it should not be used in cats with unstable CHF and no significant improvement in survival time and quality of life have been demonstrated.
- **Prevention of thromboembolism**: aspirin (81 mg total/72 h) or clopidogrel (18.75 mg total/24 h). The latter has shown a better effect than aspirin in preventing relapses.
- **Taurine supplementation** (250–500 mg/12 h PO) in cats with DCM secondary to a deficiency of this amino acid.
- **Treatment of ventricular arrhythmias** in cats with arrhythmogenic cardiomyopathy: sotalol at a dose of 2–4 mg/kg/12 h PO (or atenolol) can be used.

There is no evidence that treatment of asymptomatic cats with HCM delays the appearance of clinical signs.

Bibliography

- Biasato, I., Francescone, L., La Rosa, G. et al. (2015) Anatomopathological staging of feline hypertrophic cardiomyopathy through quantitative evaluation based on morphometric and histopathological data. *Res Vet Sci*, 102:, pp. 136–41.
- Bonne, G., Carrier, L., Richard, P. et al. (1998) Familial Hypertrophic Cardiomyopathy: From Mutations to Functional Defects. *Circ Res*, 83, pp. 580–593 .
- Boon, J. (2011) Myocardial diseases. In: Boon, J. ed. *Veterinary echocardiography*, 2nd edition. Oxford: Blackwell Publishing, pp. 359–410.
- Borgeat, K., Sherwood, K., Payne, J.R. et al. (2014) Plasma cardiac troponin I concentration and cardiac death in cats with hypertrophic cardiomyopathy. *Vet Intern Med*, 28, pp. 1731–7.
- Chetboul, V. (2017) Feline myocardial disease. In: Ettinger, S.J., Feldman, E.C. eds. *Textbook of veterinary internal medicine*, 8th ed. St.Louis: Saunders Elsevier, pp. 1278–1305.
- Chetboul, V., Passavin, P., Trehiou-Sechi, E. et al.(2019) Clinical, epidemiological and echocardiographic features and prognostic factors in cats with restrictive cardiomyopathy: A retrospective study of 92 cases (2001–2015). *J Vet Intern Med*, 33, pp. 1222–1231.
- Ciaramella, P., Basso, C., Di Loria, A. et al. (2009) Arrhythmogenic right ventricular cardiomyopathy associated with severe left ventricular involvement in a cat. *J Vet Cardiol*, 11, pp. 41–45.
- Coleman, A.E., DeFrancesco, T.C., Griffiths, E.H. et al. (2020) Atenolol in cats with subclinical hypertrophic cardiomyopathy: a double-blind, placebo-controlled, randomized clinical trial of effect on quality of life, activity and cardiac biomarkers. *J Vet Cardiol*, 30, pp. 77–91.
- Côté, E., MacDonald, K.A., Meurs, K.M. et al. (2011) Restrictive/Unclassified Cardiomyopathy. In: Côté, E., MacDonald, K.A., Meurs, K.M., Sleeper, M.M. *Feline Cardiology*, first edition. John Wiley & Sons, Inc.
- Dickson, D., Little, C.J.L., Harris, J., et al. (2018) Rapid assessment with physical examination in dyspnoeic cats: the RAPID CAT study. J Small Anim Pract, 59, pp. 75-84.
- Elliott, P.M., Anastasakis, A., Borger, M.A. et al. (2014) ESC Guidelines on diagnosis and management of hypertrophic cardiomyopathy. The Task Force for the Diagnosis and Management of Hypertrophic Cardiomyopathy of the European Society of Cardiology (ESC). *Eur Heart J*, 35.pp. 2733–79.
- Ferasin, L., Sturgess, C.P., Cannon, M.J. et al. (2003) Feline idiopathic cardiomyopathy: a retrospective study of 106 cats (1994–2001). *J Fel Med Surg*, 5, pp. 151–159.
- Fox, P.R. (2004) Endomyocardial fibrosis and restrictive cardiomyopathy: pathologic and clinical features. *J Vet Cardiol*, 6, pp. 25–31.
- Fox, P.R. (2014) Arrhythmogenic right ventricular cardiomyopathy in cats. In: Bonagura, J.D., Twedt, D.C. eds. *Kirk´s current veterinary therapy XV*. St.Louis: Elsevier Saunders, pp. 277–281.
- Fox, P.R., Basso, C., Thiene, G. et al. (2014) Spontaneously occurring restrictive nonhypertrophied cardiomyopathy in domestic cats: a new animal model of human disease. *Cardiovasc Pathol*, 23, pp. 28–34.
- Fox, P.R., Keene, B.W., Lamb, K. et al. (2018) International collaborative study to assess cardiovascular risk and evaluate long-term health in cats with preclinical hypertrophic cardiomyopathy and apparently healthy cats: The REVEAL Study. *J Vet Intern Med*, 32, pp. 930–943.
- Fox, P.R., Keene, B.W., Lamb, K. et al. (2019) Long-term incidence and risk of noncardiovascular and all-cause mortality in apparently healthy cats and cats with preclinical hypertrophic cardiomyopathy. *J Vet Intern Med*, 33, pp. 2572–2586.
- Fox, P.R., Liu, S.K., Maron, B.J. (1995) Echocardiographic assessment of spontaneously occurring feline hypertrophic cardiomyopathy. An animal model of human disease. *Circulation*, 92, pp. 2645–51.
- Fries, R., Heaney, A.M., Meurs, K.M. (2008) Prevalence of the myosin binding protein C mutation in Maine Coon cats. *J Vet Intern Med*, 22, pp. 893–896.
- Guglielmini, C., Diana, A. (2015) Thoracic radiography in the cat: identification of cardiomegaly and congestive heart failure. *J Vet Cardiol*, 17, pp. S87–S101.
- Häggström, J., Luis Fuentes, V., Wess, G. (2015) Screening for hypertrophic cardiomyopathy in cats. *J Vet Cardiol*, 17Suppl 1:S134–S149.
- Hambrook, L.E., Bennett, P.F. (2012) Effect of pimobendan on the clinical outcome and survival of cats with non-taurine responsive dilated cardiomyopathy. *J Fel Med Surg*, 14:233–239.
- Hogan, D.F., Fox, P.R., Jacob, K. et al. (2015) Secondary prevention of cardiogenic arterial thromboembolism in the cat: The double-blind, randomized, positive-controlled feline arterial thromboembolism; clopidogrel vs. aspirin trial (FAT CAT). *J Vet Cardiol*, 17 Suppl 1, pp. 306–17.
- Hori, Y., Iguchi, M., Heishima, Y. et al. (2018) Diagnostic utility of cardiac troponin I in cats with hypertrophic cardiomyopathy. *J Vet Intern Med*, 32, pp. 922–929.
- King, J.N., Martin, M., Chetboul, V. et al. (2019) Evaluation of benazepril in cats with heart disease in a prospective, randomized, blinded, placebo-controlled clinical trial. *J Vet Intern Med*, 33, pp. 2559–71.
- Kittleson, M.D., Meurs, K.M., Munro, M.J. et al. (1999) Familial Hypertrophic Cardiomyopathy in Maine Coon Cats An Animal Model of Human Disease. *Circulation*, 99, pp. 3172–80.
- Luis Fuentes, V., Abbot, J., Chetboul, V. et al. (2020) ACVIM Consensus statement guidelines for the classification, diagnosis and management of cardiomyopathies in cats. *J Vet Intern Med*, 34, pp. 1062–77.
- Luis Fuentes, V., Wilkie, L.J. (2017) Asymptomatic Hypertrophic Cardiomyopathy: Diagnosis and Therapy. *Vet Clin Small Anim*, 47, pp. 1041–54.

■ März, I., Wilkie, L.J., Harrington, N. et al. (2015) Familial cardiomyopathy in Norwegian Forest cats. *J Fel Med Surg*, 17, pp. 681–691.

■ Meurs, K.M., Norgard, M.M., Ederer, M.M. et al. (2007) A substitution mutation in the myosin binding protein C gene in ragdoll hypertrophic cardiomyopathy. *Genomics*, 90, pp. 261–64.

■ Meurs, K.M., Sanchez, X., David, R.M. et al. (2005) A cardiac myosin binding protein C mutation in the Maine Coon cat with familial hypertrophic cardiomyopathy. *Hum Mol Genet*, 14, pp. 3587–93.

■ Paige, C.F., Abbott, J.A., Elvinger, F. et al. (2009) Prevalence of cardiomyopathy in apparently healthy cats. *J Am Vet Med Assoc*, 234, pp. 1398–1403.

■ Payne, J.R., Borgeat, K., Brodbelt, D.C. et al. (2015) Risk factors associated with sudden death vs. congestive heart failure or arterial thromboembolism in cats with hypertrophic cardiomyopathy. *J Vet Cardiol*, 17 Suppl 1, pp. S318–28.

■ Payne, J.R., Brodbelt, D.C., Luis Fuentes, V. (2015) Cardiomyopathy prevalence in 780 apparently healthy cats in rehoming centres (the CatScan study). *J Vet Cardiol*, 17 Suppl 1, pp. S244–57.

■ Pion, P.D., Kittleson, M.D., Rogers, Q.R. et al. (1987) Myocardial failure in cats associated with low plasma taurine: a reversible cardiomyopathy. *Science*, 237, pp. 764–68.

■ Rolim, V.M., Casagrande, R.A., Wouters, A.T. et al. (2016) Myocarditis caused by Feline Immunodeficiency Virus in Five Cats with Hypertrophic Cardiomyopathy. *J Comp Pathol*, 154, pp. 3–8.

■ Schober, K.E., Zientek, J., Li X. et al. (2014) Effect of treatment with atenolol on 5-year survival in cats with preclinical (asymptomatic) hypertrophic cardiomyopathy. *J Vet Intern Med*, 28, pp. 838–46.

■ Silverman, S.J. (2012) Hypertrophic cardiomyopathy in the Sphynx cat: a retrospective evaluation of clinical presentation and heritable etiology. *J Feline Med Surg*, 14, pp. 246–49

■ Spalla, I., Locatelli, C., Riscazzi, G. et al. (2016) Survival in cats with primary and secondary cardiomyopathies. *J Fel Med Surg*, 18, pp. 501–509.

■ Stepien, R.L. (2007) Specific feline cardiopulmonary conditions. In: Luis Fuentes, V., Swift, S. *BSAVA manual of small animal cardiorespiratory medicine and surgery*. Shurdington: British Small Animal Veterinary Association, pp. 45–261.

■ Stern, J.A., Markova, S., Ueda, Y. et al. (2016) A small molecule inhibitor of sarcomere contractility acutely relieves left ventricular outflow tract obstruction in feline hypertrophic cardiomyopathy. *PLos One*, 11:e0168407.

■ Teare, D. (1958) Asymmetrical Hypertrophy cardiomyopathy of the heart in young adults. *Br Heart J*, 20, pp. 1–8.

■ Wess, G., Schinner, C., Weber, K. et al. (2010) Association of A31P and A74T polymorphisms in the myosin binding protein C3 gene and hypertrophic cardiomyopathy in Maine Coon and other breed cats. *J Vet Intern Med*, 24, pp. 527–32.

■ Wilkie, L.J., Smith, K., Luis Fuentes, V. (2015) Cardiac pathology findings in 252 cats presented for necropsy, a comparison of cats with unexpected death versus other deaths. *J Vet Cardiol*, 17, pp. S244–S257.

TEST

ANSWERS ON PAGE 294

1. Cardiomyopathies are the most common acquired heart diseases in cats. Which is the most frequent clinical sign and its underlying cause in affected cats?

a. Ascites due to right-sided congestive heart failure.
b. Cough due to left-sided congestive heart failure.
c. Dyspnoea due to left-sided congestive heart failure.
d. Sudden death due to life-threatening arrhythmias.

2. Which medication is recommended for acute and chronic treatment of congestive heart failure in cats?

a. Atenolol.
b. Benazepril.
c. Furosemide.
d. Pimobendan.

3. Which diagnostic test is currently recommended to diagnose and stage cardiomyopathies in asymptomatic cats?

a. Echocardiography.
b. NT-proBNP.
c. Myocardial biopsy.
d. Thoracic radiography.

4. Which echocardiographic finding among the following is the most characteristic of a dilated cardiomyopathy phenotype?

a. Atrial dilation.
b. Restrictive transmitral flow pattern.
c. Systolic anterior motion of the mitral valve.
d. Ventricular dilation.

5. Thrombus formation can occur in cats with cardiomyopathies, most likely as a consequence of a combination of blood stasis, endothelial damage, and a hypercoagulable state. Which medication has shown to prevent a first episode of thromboembolism in cats?

a. Acetylsalicylic acid
b. Clopidogrel
c. Heparin
d. None

6. Cardiac biomarkers can be used as an aid to the diagnosis of cardiomyopathies. Which is the stimulus needed for the release of cardiac troponin I from myocardial cells?

a. Altered reuptake of cytosolic calcium.
b. Myocyte damage.
c. Myocyte stretch.
d. Sympathetic stimulation.

Clinical Case

Signalment. 10-year-old domestic short-haired cat, weighing 4.5 kg.

Reason for consultation. Acute onset respiratory distress, heart murmur.

History and clinical background. A heart murmur was detected four years ago, but not investigated. No clinical signs were detected before the current, acute onset, respiratory distress, which occurred a few hours ago. No relevant pathology has been diagnosed previously. Vaccinated and properly dewormed. Lives indoors. A sibling of the same litter, also in the owner's possession died suddenly two weeks ago. A month ago, the family moved house, which according to the owners was a major stressor for the cats.

Physical examination. Dyspnoea, restrictive respiratory pattern with tachypnoea (respiratory rate: 80 bpm). Slightly pale mucous membranes, with capillary refill time <2 seconds. Weak femoral pulse that matches the heartbeat. Thoracic auscultation: diffuse crackles in both hemithorax. Grade IV/VI heart murmur, with a point of maximum intensity on the sternal border, accompanied by a gallop sound. HR >200 bpm, regular rhythm.

Questions:

1. **Based on the history and physical examination, indicate the most likely cause of the respiratory problem in this cat:**
   a. Cardiogenic pulmonary oedema.
   b. Chronic bronchial disease .
   c. Pulmonary fibrosis.
   d. Pulmonary neoplasia.

2. **Which of the following is most appropriate action to stabilise the cat?**
   a. Administer corticosteroids and a bronchodilator.
   b. Administer oxygen and furosemide parenterally.
   c. Obtain thoracic radiographs and perform blood tests to guide treatment.
   d. Perform thoracentesis.

3. **Indicate what is most characteristic on thoracic radiographs performed after stabilising the cat:**
   a. Thoracic mass compatible with primary pulmonary neoplasia.
   b. Bronchial and interstitial pattern, characteristic of feline asthma.
   c. Miliary interstitial pattern compatible with metastatic lung disease.
   d. Interstitial and alveolar pattern compatible with pulmonary oedema and CHF.

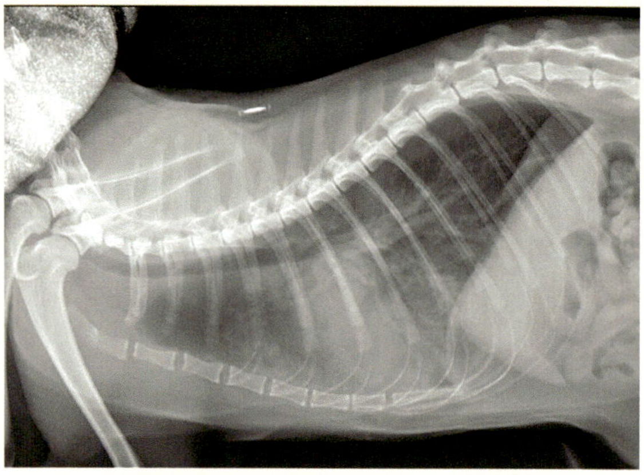

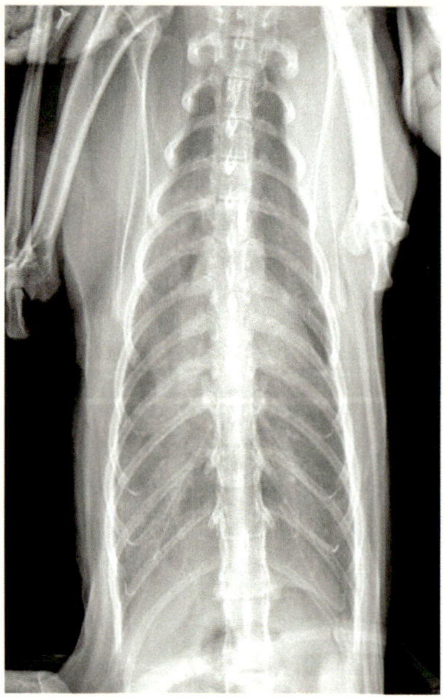

4. Indicate the most likely diagnosis based on the echocardiographic image obtained after stabilising the cat:

a. Arrhythmogenic right ventricular cardiomyopathy.
b. Dilated cardiomyopathy.
c. Obstructive hypertrophic cardiomyopathy.
d. Interventricular septal defect.

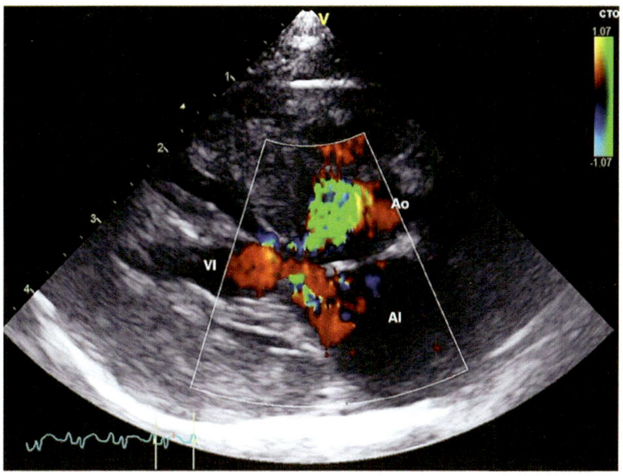

5. Which supplementary diagnostic test is least necessary for the short-term management of this case?

a. Serum biochemistry.
b. Bronchoscopy and bronchoalveolar lavage.
c. Measurement of systemic blood pressure.
d. Thyroid parameters.

6. Which drug should be prioritised, among those indicated below, for the long-term treatment of this cat once it is discharged from the hospital, since the owners have mentioned that it is difficult to medicate?

a. Atenolol.
b. Diltiazem.
c. Furosemide.
d. Prednisolone.

Correct Answers:

Test

1. c
2. c
3. a
4. d
5. d
6. b

Clinical Case

1. a
2. b
3. d
4. c
5. b
6. a

NOTES

Pericardial Diseases and Cardiac Neoplasms

Domingo Casamián Sorrosal

This chapter covers **pericardial disease and cardiac neoplasms. These two conditions are often closely linked** with many cardiac tumours presenting with pericardial effusion, and the most common cause of pericardial effusion being the presence of a cardiac neoplasm. Thus, although the chapter is divided into two sections, there are important references in one section to the other and reading the chapter in its entirety is recommended.

Pericardial Disease

Within the group of pericardial diseases the **main cause of clinical signs is pericardial effusion**, hence this process is the central topic discussed in this section. This is followed by a description of the main diseases that cause pericardial effusion (excluding neoplasms discussed in the corresponding section), and other pericardial conditions in which the presence of pericardial effusion is not the main finding.

Anatomy and Physiology

The pericardium is a sac-like structure that surrounds the heart. It is made up of two layers.

- The **outer, fibrous pericardium**:
  - the fibrous pericardium is a thick, robust tissue, which connects to the adventitia of the great vessels and veins of the heart.
- The **inner, serous pericardium**:
  - the serous pericardium forms the closed pericardial cavity, it is lined with mesothelial cells and composed of a parietal and a visceral layer:
    - the visceral layer is the portion that invaginates over the heart and forms the epicardium
    - the parietal layer is firmly attached to the fibrous pericardium.

The **normal volume of pericardial fluid is around 0.25 ml/kg in dogs and cats**, and has a lubricating function in the pericardial space. Lymphatic drainage from the pericardium occurs through lymphatic vessels which drain into the tracheal and sternal lymph nodes, or into the pleural veins which drain on the right side.

The two main functions of the pericardium are:

- **protecting the heart** from neoplasms and infections within the thorax; and
- **anchoring the heart** within the thorax to prevent dislocation.

Normally the intrapericardial pressure of the pericardial space is zero and thus has no negative effect on cardiac filling. However, due to its limited compliance, if it fills rapidly this leads to a large increase in intrapericardial pressures and alterations in ventricular filling. The pericardium is able to hypertrophy and if filling with fluid occurs over a long period it is able to progressively expand. Due to this, **the elevation of intrapericardial pressures depends not only on the volume, but also on the speed with which the volume accumulates**.

Clinical Signs

Cardiac tamponade refers to the accumulation of volume and intrapericardial pressure that causes abnormal ventricular filling and the subsequent clinical consequences. Cardiac tamponade is not all or nothing, but progresses and varies in intensity as intrapericardial pressure increases.

- Initially transmural pressure decreases, but intracardiac pressure remains higher than intrapericardial pressure, and cardiac filling decreases (according to Starling's law), but only slightly.
- As intrapericardial pressure increases, the patient enters phase 2 in which the intrapericardial pressure is equal to or greater than the pressure in the right atrium and the filling pressure of the right ventricle.
- In phase 3 the intrapericardial pressure rises above left ventricular filling pressures.

This chain of events leads to a **decrease in cardiac output and an increase in venous systemic pressure**. As previously mentionned intrapericardial pressure does not only depend on the volume of pericardial effusion, but also on how quickly this effusion forms; since the pericardium can distend if filling is gradual.

The presence of pericardial effusion produces a change in the right atrial pressure curve (obtained by catheterization), with an increase in pressure (above 10–15 mmHg) and a marked decrease in the descent of the curve and, as a result, during passive diastole this causes difficulty with ventricular filling.

Many dogs with pericardial effusion present with right-sided heart failure, due to increased right atrial and systemic venous pressure. **Tachycardia, jugular vein distention** (Figure 1), and ascites are commonly seen on physical examination. Also, right-sided heart failure may cause pleural effusion and on physical examination this presents as **dyspnoea and attenuated breath sounds**. It is also common to observe signs of circulatory collapse (obstructive shock) due to decreased cardiac output, with evidence of pale mucous membranes, weak pulses, and low body temperature (unless the effusion is due to septic pericarditis, in which case there will almost always be a high temperature).

The presence of *pulsus paradoxus* is also seen on occasion (the pulses during inspiration are weaker than during expiration). This change in systolic pressure during inspiration is normal, since during expiration there is greater venous return that leads to increased right ventricular filling, with a consequent decrease in the left ventricular filling (and of the systolic ejection volume) due to ventricular interdependence. Typically, however, this difference between systolic pressure on inspiration and expiration is slight, less than 10 mmHg, and cannot be detected by assessing the pulse (pulse pressure is the difference between systolic and diastolic pressure). However, this difference is exacerbated (to more than 10 mmHg) when there is pericardial effusion, as ventricular filling is impeded (there is less "space" for the filling of the two ventricles).

On auscultation, patients with pericardial effusion have attenuated heart sounds, and may present with both ventricular and supraventricular arrhythmias. Dogs with pericardial effusion and tamponade may also experience episodes of fainting or collapse. In one study, the prognosis was worse for dogs suffering from **fainting or collapse** than for those whose main clinical sign of pericardial effusion was ascites. This is most likely because ascites is caused by a more progressive accumulation of fluid in the pericardium (more likely to be idiopathic pericarditis, for example), while the presence of collapse can be associated with acute pericardial filling (for example, haemorrhage due to a haemangiosarcoma).

Other clinical signs seen in dogs with pericardial effusion include **cough** (due to compression of the airways), gastrointestinal signs (due to the presence of portal hypertension and/or lymphangiectasia secondary to right-sided congestive failure) and signs of general disease such as **lethargy, anorexia and weakness**. It should be remembered that, if the pericardial effusion is caused by or associated with an extracardiac disease, the clinical signs may be due in part or whole to this (for example, rupture of a splenic haemangiosarcoma).

Breed can also provide clues with regard to the underlying disease. German Shepherds are predisposed to haemangiosarcomas, brachiocephalic breeds, especially Boxers are predisposed to aortic base tumours, and Golden Retrievers, Labrador Retrievers and the Saint Bernard suffer from idiopathic pericarditis.

Diagnosis

Radiography

On radiographs (Figure 2) a **marked enlargement of the cardiac silhouette** is often observed, which becomes spherical in shape without clear definition of its edges. In cases where the effusion volume is small, these changes are more difficult to observe. The consequences of right-sided heart failure are also often observed: **dilatation of the caudal vena cava,**

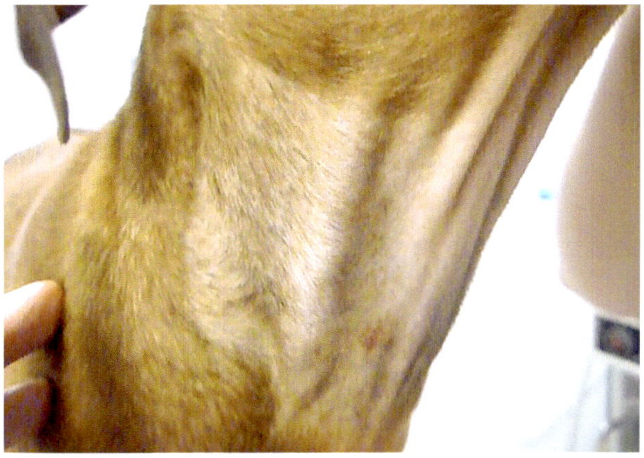

Figure 1. Photograph of a dog with jugular vein distension associated with right sided congestive heart failure secondary to cardiac tamponade due to severe pericardial effusion.

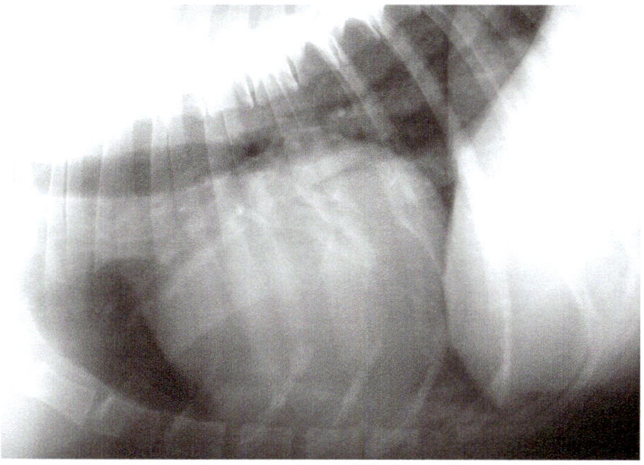

Figure 2. Lateral radiograph of a dog with moderate pericardial effusion in which a significantly enlarged cardiac silhouette is seen, which is a circular shape without well-defined edges.

pleural effusion, hepatomegaly, and loss of abdominal serous detail consistent with ascites. On occasion, the presence of masses can also be seen or suspected, for example, in the mediastinum due to an aortic-base tumour (Figure 3).

Sinus tachycardia is usually seen on the ECG, although supraventricular or ventricular tachycardias may also be present. Electrical alternation of the R wave (varying sized R wave) and a low amplitude of this wave can sometimes be seen. After draining the pericardium and resolving the tamponade, it is common for heart rate to drop rapidly. Ventricular ectopy is sometimes seen during pericardiocentesis, primarily if the myocardium is punctured.

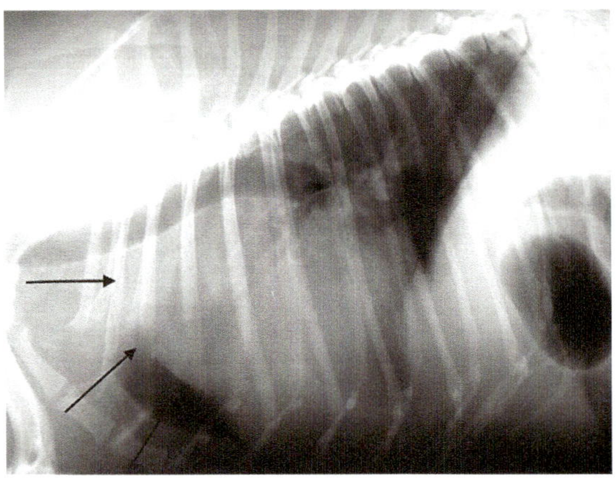

Figure 3. Lateral radiograph of a dog with a mediastinal mass level with the base of the aorta [arrows] (it was confirmed as being a chemodectoma in an exploratory thoracotomy where a pericardiectomy was performed and biopsy taken). The tumour caused elevation of the trachea at this level. In this dog pericardial effusion was also present at the time of the radiograph, but it was mild.

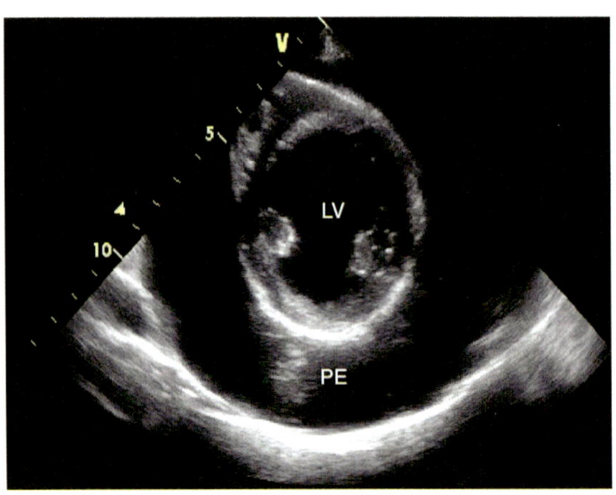

Figure 4. Right transverse parasternal view (short axis) at the height of the papillary muscles in a dog with severe pericardial effusion. The pericardial effusion can be seen as a hypoechogenic layer (PE) between the heart (LV represents the left ventricle) and the rest of the thorax.

Ultrasound

Echocardiography is the main tool for diagnosis of pericardial effusion and to evaluate the possible presence of cardiac or pericardial tumours.

When **pericardial effusion** is present (Figure 4) a hypoechoic layer is observed surrounding the heart, which appears to float in it. This layer (unlike pleural effusion) does not extend beyond the cardiac base and is restricted to the periphery of the heart. However, **pleural effusion** (both effusions at the same time) is often seen as well (Figure 5). Pericardial effusion can be seen on virtually all standard echocardiographic views. Cardiac tamponade with collapse of the right atrium (Figure 6) and sometimes the right ventricle can also be seen.

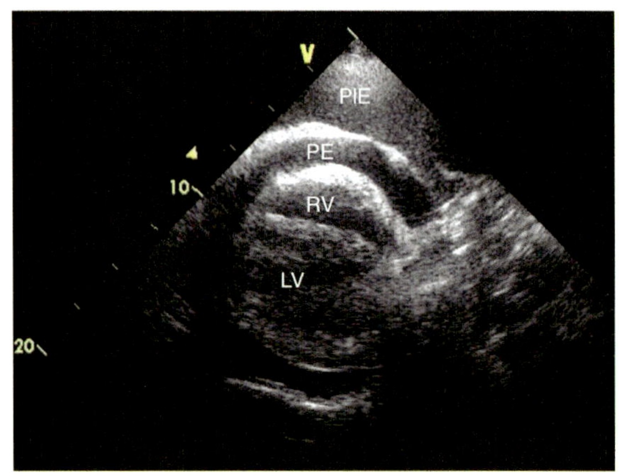

Figure 5. Right longitudinal parasternal view (long axis) of a dog with pleural effusion (PIE) secondary to right-sided heart failure due to pericardial effusion (PE). LV: left ventricule, RV: right ventricle.

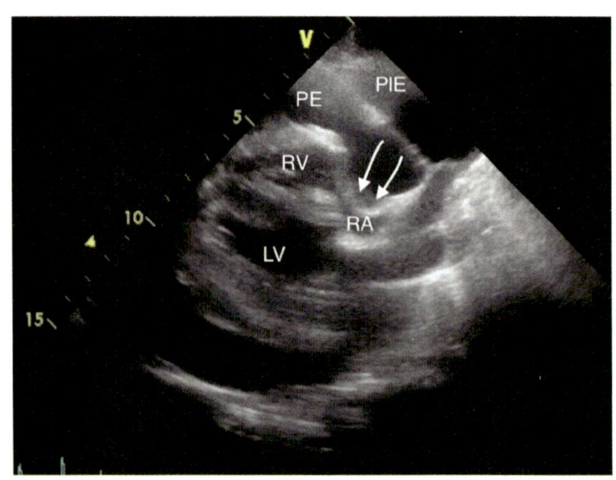

Figure 6. Right longitudinal parasternal view (long axis) of a dog with pericardial (PE) and pleural (PIE) effusion and cardiac tamponade. Right atrial (RA) collapse can be seen (arrows). LV: left ventricule, RV: right ventricle.

When evaluating the abdomen, liver congestion (Figure 7) and ascites (Figure 8) are often present.

When a diagnosis of pericardial effusion is established, the **search for neoplasia should commence**, preferably before drainage since the presence of fluid facilitates the visualization of tumours. The echocardiographic search for tumours must be exhaustive and include all existing views, including left cranial views in which the right atrial appendage is better visualised, plus non-standard views extending to the highest possible area of the heart base.

- **Haemangiosarcomas** (Figure 9) **often occur in the right atrium or ventricle** and, in particular, in the right atrial appendage. They are often heterogeneous in appearance,

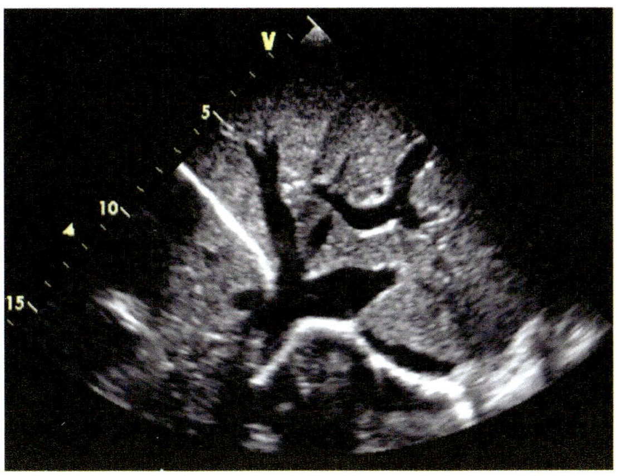

Figure 7. Hepatic congestion in a dog with right sided heart failure secondary to pericardial effusion.

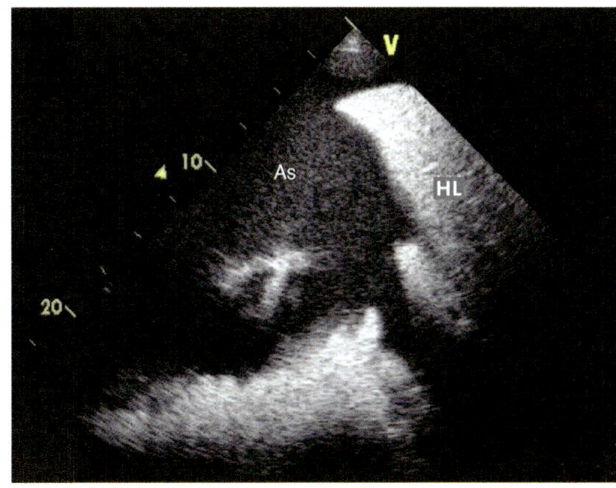

Figure 8. Ascites in a dog with right sided heart failure secondary to pericardial effusion. As: free abdominal fluid, HL: hepatic lobe.

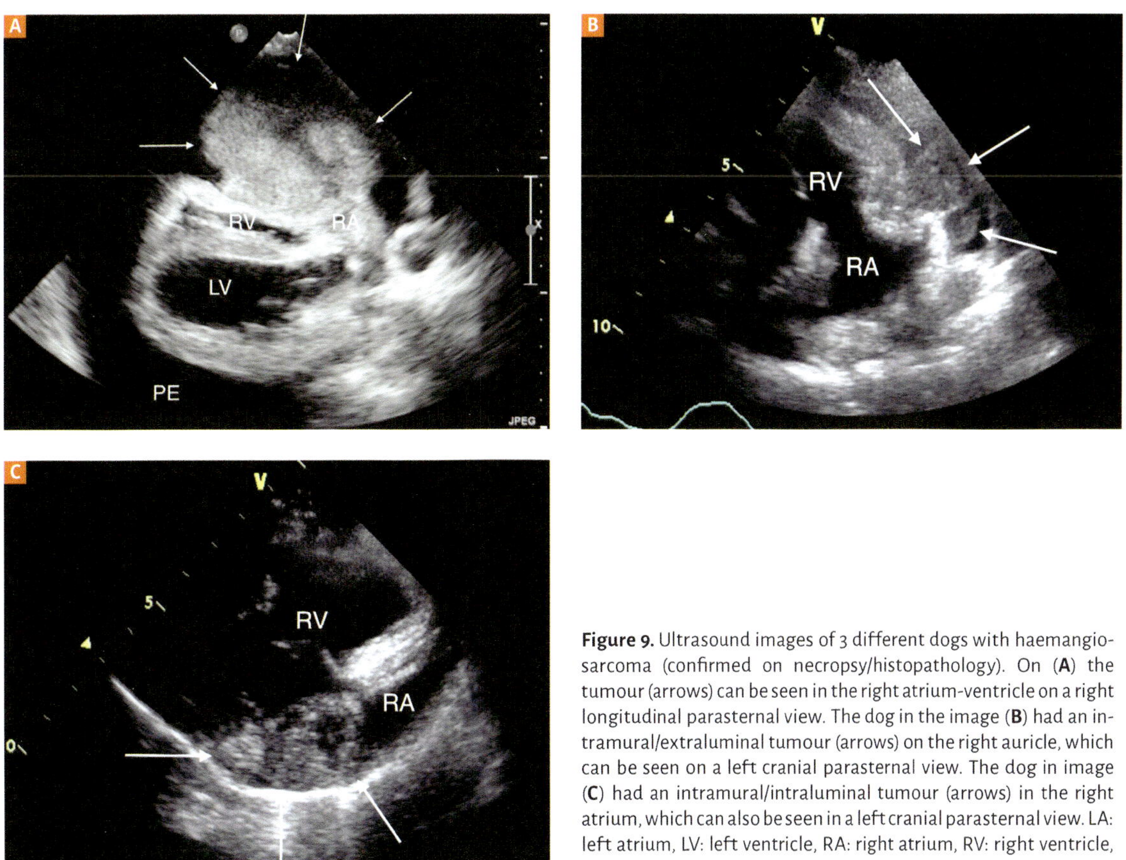

Figure 9. Ultrasound images of 3 different dogs with haemangiosarcoma (confirmed on necropsy/histopathology). On (**A**) the tumour (arrows) can be seen in the right atrium-ventricle on a right longitudinal parasternal view. The dog in the image (**B**) had an intramural/extraluminal tumour (arrows) on the right auricle, which can be seen on a left cranial parasternal view. The dog in image (**C**) had an intramural/intraluminal tumour (arrows) in the right atrium, which can also be seen in a left cranial parasternal view. LA: left atrium, LV: left ventricle, RA: right atrium, RV: right ventricle, PE: pericardial effusion.

with cavitation and poorly defined borders, and can be intraluminal, extraluminal, or intramural.
- **Aortic-base tumours** (Figure 10) often appear more homogeneous, well-defined, sometimes circular in shape, and are often adjacent to the ascending aorta.
- **Mesotheliomas** do not usually present specific echocardiographic changes and, although thickening of the pericardium and the presence of hyperechoic plaques are sometimes seen, this can also be seen in inflammatory pericarditis.

Pericardial thickening (unless extreme) is difficult to diagnose, partly because the acoustic difference of this tissue with adjacent fluids may give a false appearance of increased thickness, plus there are no specific standard measurements available in dogs.

Although there are more or less defined echocardiographic characteristics for the most common cardiac tumours, it is important to remember that it is **only possible to talk about the probability of the findings being compatible with one tumour or another**, but a final diagnosis cannot be made. In a recent study, it was observed that 25–50% of presumptive diagnoses on echocardiography did not correlate with autopsy findings. Echocardiography can also be used to perform ultrasound-guided aspirations of tumours where there is an adequate window to perform this technique.

Axial High Resolution Computerised Tomography (CT)

CT is a useful technique for evaluation of pericardial disease. It is a complementary technique and mainly used to **evaluate extracardiac tumours** (for example, thoracic base) (Figure 11) and to evaluate the presence of metastases or tumours that may have metastasised to the heart.

Cytology

In most cases **pericardial fluid cytology is not helpful** in reaching a diagnosis. A large number of effusions that cause cardiac tamponade are haemorrhagic (Figure 12), and cytology does not help differentiate those caused by neoplasms from those caused by inflammation.

In order to differentiate neoplastic effusions from inflammatory ones, the measurement of pH, electrolytes, glucose, haematocrit, urea and endothelial fluid vascular growth factor

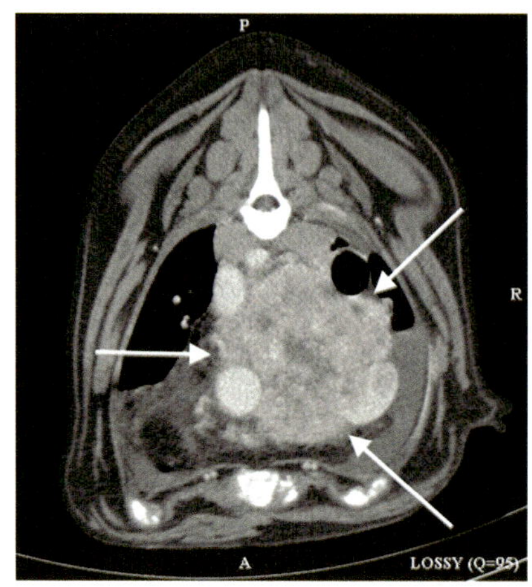

Figure 11. High resolution CT showing the presence and extent of a tumour (arrows) in a dog which was taken to a consultation for severe pericardial effusion. Due to its size, initially it was impossible to identify whether it originated from the heart or cardiac base.

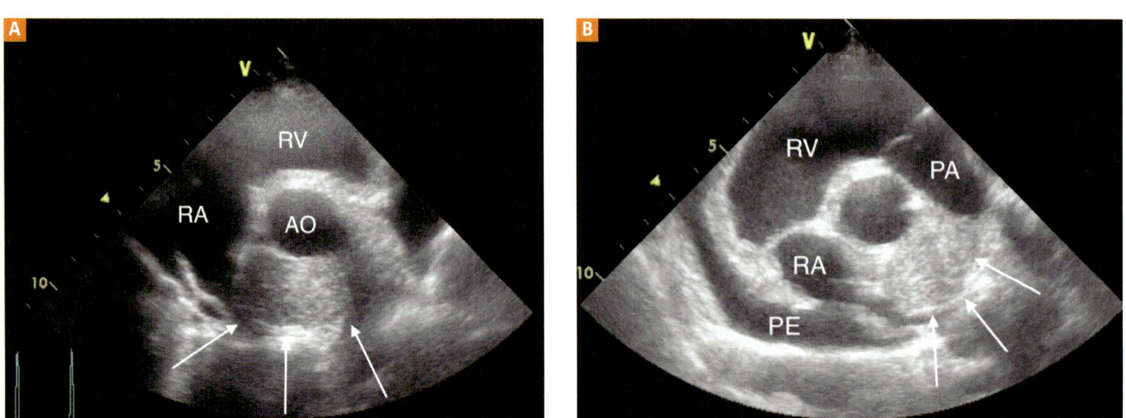

Figure 10. Two ultrasounds from dogs with chemodectomas that can be seen (confirmed on histopathology) adjacent to the ascending aorta. In image (**A**) the tumour (arrows) can be seen on a mixed right transverse/longitudinal parasternal view (short axis/long axis) at the level of the base of the aorta. In image (**B**) the tumour (arrows) can be seen in a left cranial parasternal view optimised for tumour visualisation.

has been investigated, but **none were found to be useful**. It was noted that troponin I was higher in cases of tumours (especially in haemangiosarcoma), but there is a lot of overlap and it is not usually used clinically.

Cytology is useful in cases of lymphoma (where there is a lymphoblastic effusion) and in some cases of mesotheliomas. However, there are many false positives and negatives, since there is an overlap between the reactive appearance and the neoplasms of this cell group, so the diagnosis usually requires histopathology.

Cytology is also useful in the diagnosis of septic pericarditis, in which an exudate with degenerate neutrophils and the presence of bacteria is seen (Figure 13).

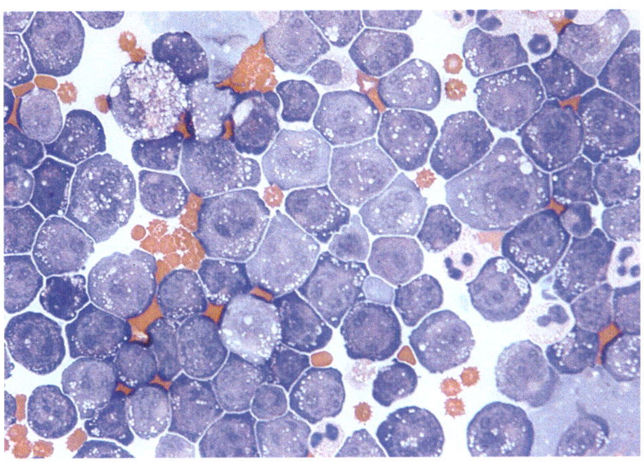

Figure 12. Cytology of a haemorrhagic effusion in a dog with idiopathic pericarditis (also typical of tumours) where abundant erythrocytes can be seen. (Image courtesy of K. Papasouliotis).

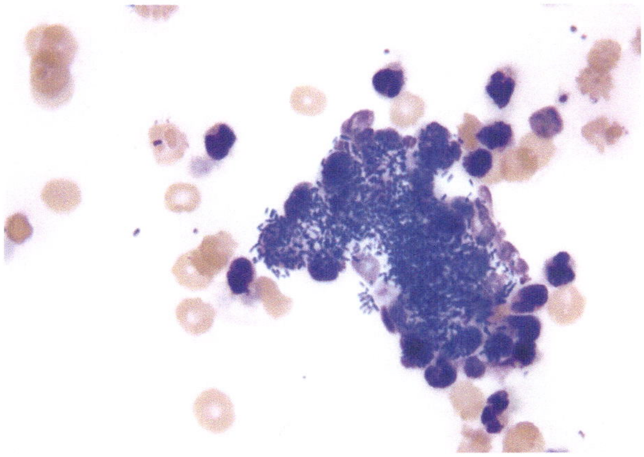

Figure 13. Cytology of septic effusion (septic pericarditis) with the presence of numerous degenerate neutrophils with intracellular bacteria. (Image courtesy of K. Papasouliotis).

Most cases with a pericardial transudate are due to various systemic causes or heart failure, as explained later in the chapter, and do not usually present with cardiac tamponade. If there is abdominal fluid, it is advisable to sample this to confirm it is a transudate if right heart failure is suspected. If the fluid were, for example, haemorrhagic, it would suggest a case of bicavitary haemorrhage with a very different prognosis, since it may be due to a coagulopathy (for example, DIC) associated with the tumour or also a bicavitary tumour.

Pericardiocentesis

Patients with cardiac tamponade are usually weak and in **circulatory collapse**, which means with the aid of local anaesthesia **pericardiocentesis** can be performed in the conscious animal. However, there are patients where this is not possible and sedation or general anaesthesia may be necessary.

It is advisable to prepare everything before sedation or anaesthesia in order to minimize the time from inducing anaesthesia until the pericardium is drained and the tamponade corrected. **Administering intravenous fluids** prior to pericardiocentesis is advisable (e.g. Lactated Ringer's at 10–20 ml/kg/h), during preparation and induction, to increase preload and intracardiac pressures. **Prior to pericardiocentesis the administration of diuretics is contraindicated** as this would create the opposite effect.

The dog is positioned in **left lateral or sternal recumbency**. Drainage is performed in the **fifth, right intercostal space at the level of the costochondral junction**. Ultrasound guidance can be used, especially in cases where there is also pleural effusion. However, in most cases this is not necessary as the effusions are large, although it may be useful to mark the incision area once the best location has been identified by echocardiography.

There are different methods (from basic to more complex) to perform a pericardial drainage.

- A simple method is to use a long, large gauge catheter (14 or 16G), inserting the catheter, and then draining with a syringe and three-way stopcock. The main problem with this method is the catheter tends to kink and the procedure repeated several times. Also once some fluid has been drained, the rest of the pericardial fluid may leak into the pleura through the open hole which can make complete drainage more difficult. Although it is advisable to perform complete drainage (for example, it is useful to monitor whether there is recurrence of the effusion) on many occasions with partial drainage and fluid that leaks into the thorax the tamponade subsequently disappears.
- Another common technique includes the use of a type

of long, multi-fenestrated catheter inserted through the pericardium in order to completely drain the fluid. There are different types of cather. Another simple way is to pass a normal (large animal) 12 or 14 G catheter and, once the catheter is in the pericardium, a urinary catheter is inserted and the pericardium is drained using a three-way tap.

- A more sophisticated and possibly the most widely used technique is to use specialised pericardiocentesis catheters with which the Seldinger or modified Seldinger technique is used. First, a needle is inserted into the pericardium, and then a small catheter through which a guidewire is inserted, mostly into the pericardium. In some kits the guide is inserted directly through the needle (without the placement of a catheter). Through this guide, a drainage tube or catheter with multiple fenestrations is then introduced, most of which is located within the pericardium.

During drainage monitoring with an ECG is advisable since ventricular arrhythmias may occur if the heart is punctured. The fluid drained is normally haemorrhagic. If there is a pleural effusion, it is common to obtain a transudate when draining the pleura and haemorrhagic fluid when draining the pericardium. **Haemorrhagic pericardial fluid**, like any haemorrhagic cavitary effusion, **does not usually clot** (as the fibrin has been consumed). If thrombi are formed, it is essential to stop the procedure and ensure everything is correctly placed as it is possible a vessel of considerable size or the heart has been punctured. Once the effusion has been drained, the signs of circulatory collapse usually improve rapidly and, as long as there is no recurrence, the accumulation of fluid in the abdomen decreases in volume until it disappears over the following days.

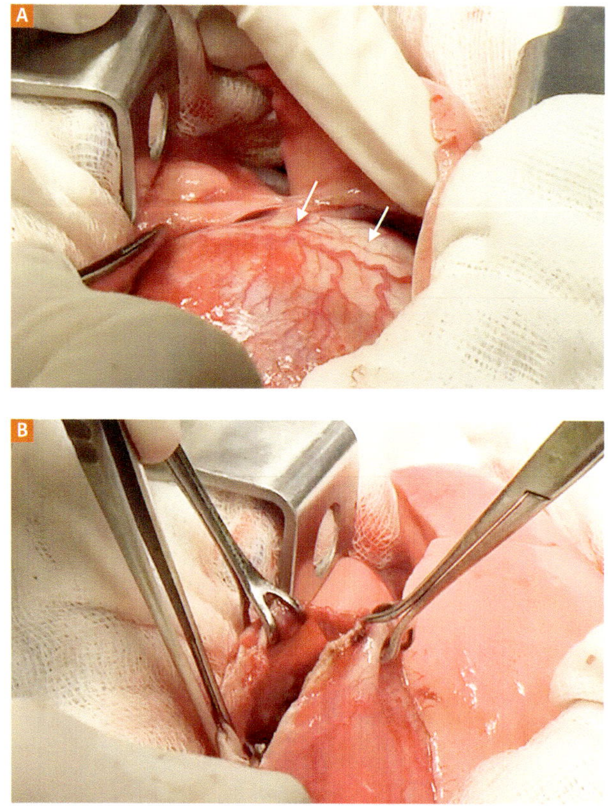

Figure 14. Images of a pericardiectomy using a right lateral approach. In the image (**A**) the exposed pericardium and phrenic nerve (arrows) are shown. In (**B**) the beginning of the pericardiectomy near the subphrenic space. (Images courtesy of Esteban González Gasch).

Surgery

The most common surgery within pericardial diseases is pericardiectomy. Sometimes cardiac (usually right base haemangiosarcomas) or cardiac base (usually thyroid chemodectomas or carcinomas) tumours can also be removed or, at least, biopsied during thoracotomy to perform pericardiectomy. Other more unusual pericardial surgeries include the repair of peritoneal-pericardial-diaphragmatic hernias (PPDH), the removal of pericardial foreign bodies, or the repair of congenital or traumatic pericardial defects.

Pericardiectomy

Pericardiectomy is usually performed in patients with recurrent effusions in whom no neoplasia has been detected, for palliative reasons in the presence of neoplasia, or patients with constrictive pericarditis.

A **subtotal pericardiectomy** (below the phrenic nerve) is usually performed (Figure 14 A), since total pericardiectomy (dissecting the phrenic nerve) does not provide major benefits and requires a more complex dissection. Subtotal pericardiectomy can be performed through a sternotomy or a right lateral thoracotomy (Figure 14 B). A mortality rate associated with surgery of 12% has been described. It can also be performed by thoracoscopy, usually through a transdiaphragmatic approach. However, it must be kept in mind that thoracoscopy achieves the resection of a pericardial window (usually not of the entire pericardium).

Diseases of the Pericardium

Idiopathic Pericarditis

Canine idiopathic pericarditis is, as the name suggests, a **disease of unknown origin**. An immunological study indicates the cause does not appear to be vasculitis or a primary immune-mediated process, but rather its appearance is that of a secondary inflammatory process. Although some studies have been carried out trying to associate it with viral or bacterial infectious agents, there are no reliable studies that demonstrate an association of the disease with any pathogen. The fact that the disease occurs frequently in some breeds such as the Golden Retriever could also indicate associated genetic factors.

Dogs with idiopathic pericarditis usually present with pericardial effusion and its classic clinical signs, referred to in the previous section. The effusion is usually haemorrhagic, although on rare occasions, non-septic or lymphocytic neutrophilic effusions have been described with an inflammatory appearance and of unknown cause. It is unknown whether these represent a disease similar to typical idiopathic pericarditis that presents with haemorrhagic effusion.

After a single pericardiocentesis, there are a number of dogs where the effusion never recurs (34% in one study) and no further treatment is necessary. For the rest, after the second or third pericardiocentesis, a surgical pericardiectomy is recommended to establish a definitive diagnosis (rule out mesothelioma or hidden tumours) and resolve the clinical signs. **Performing surgery early prevents constrictive pericarditis developing**. Normally, if the surgery is successful, the prognosis is good.

Constrictive Pericarditis

Sometimes, the pericardium is not filled with fluid but is thickened, rigid, and lacks compliance. This may be the result of ongoing severe and/or chronic inflammation or infection or of diffuse intrapericardial neoplasia. In most dogs the parietal pericardium is severely affected and not the visceral (although there are exceptions).

Dogs with constrictive pericarditis **manifest clinical signs of right-sided heart failure** and circulatory collapse similar to dogs with pericardial effusion, although the pathophysiology leading to increased pressures on the right side is slightly different. During constrictive pericarditis, unlike in dogs with pericardial effusion, there is an abrupt decrease in the curve and early diastolic filling in the pressure trace of the right atrium, but this stops rapidly (as the pericardium cannot expand further) and forms what is called the "square root sign" on the graph.

On auscultation, the presence of a **pericardial knock** (attributed to the vibration produced when the blood hits a ventricle that cannot distend) is sometimes observed. Decreased vena caval pressures and increased venous return on the right side during inspiration are not seen during constrictive pericarditis (as opposed to pericardial effusion) because intrathoracic pressure changes are not transmitted to the heart. Thus, *pulsus paradoxus* is not seen and, in severe cases, an increase in systemic venous pressures may be observed during inspiration (Kussmaul's sign). It is not uncommon for pericardial disease to be a mixture (called effusive-constrictive pericarditis) in which a small volume of fluid causes severe heart failure, which persists as the effusion drains.

Diagnosis of constrictive pericarditis is more difficult than that of pericardial effusion. The echocardiographic changes mentioned above (possible pleural effusion, hepatic distention, ascites) are observed suggesting right-sided heart failure (together with jugular distention). As previously mentioned, appreciating pericardial thickening on echocardiography is difficult, unless it is an extreme case.

Doppler echocardiography may be useful to evaluate some of the haemodynamic abnormalities as a result of constrictive pericarditis. These include variations with respiration in the isovolumic relaxation time, a marked reduction in transmitral flow during inspiration (more than 15–25% is abnormal) (Figure 15), and possible changes in left ventricular flow propagation using colour Doppler in M-mode.

On occasions when the diagnosis is unclear, it can be confirmed by cardiac catheterization. The two most classic findings are an equalization of the diastolic pressures in the four cardiac chambers and the finding of the abrupt and short-term descent of the wave and during the examination of the right atrium. It should be remembered in the case of effusive-constrictive pericarditis, all the findings described are masked, but may appear once the effusion has drained.

Treatment is surgical by pericardiectomy. If the process is limited to the parietal pericardium and there is no underlying neoplasm with a poor prognosis, the patient's prognosis is good.

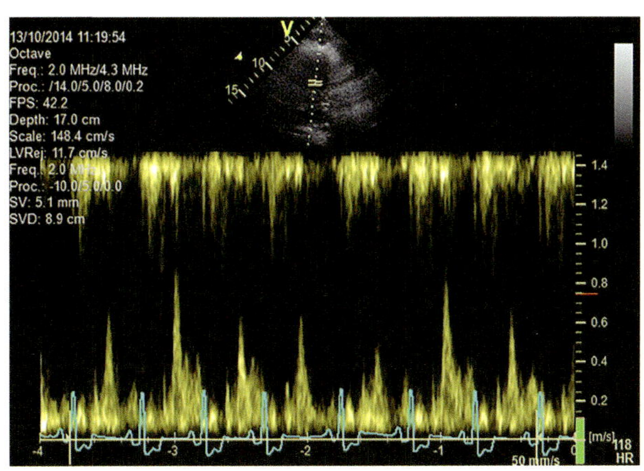

Figure 15. Echocardiographic image in pulsed Doppler mode of transmitral flow in a dog with constrictive pericarditis. A marked variation in transmitral flow on inspiration and expiration can be seen.

However, if the visceral pericardium is also affected, surgery is usually less successful as it requires decortication and removal of the visceral and fibrous pericardium, which is not always possible.

Septic Pericarditis

Septic pericarditis is caused by a **bacterial infection of the pericardium**. In many cases this is due to migration of foreign bodies in the pericardium, but it may also be due to the spread of local infections (from lung lesions) and/or potentially haematogenous.

Dogs often show signs of **sepsis and septic shock** (in addition to cardiogenic due to effusion). The cytological diagnosis of septic effusion is usually definitive, with the presence of degenerated neutrophils and bacteria. On ultrasound, in addition to pericardial effusion, the presence of a foreign body may be observed on occasion.

Treatment, after initial drainage and haemodynamic stabilization, is surgical with thoracic examination, pericardiectomy, and adequate antibiotic therapy.

The prognosis is good if there is no irreparable intrathoracic damage (for example, by a foreign body), or serious consequences of septic shock (such as irreversible organ damage). Bacterial infection can sometimes lead to a severe, abnormal granulomatous reaction called botryomycosis.

Fungal Infections

In countries like the United States, where coccidiomycosis or blastomycosis are present, they can cause pericarditis and fungal myocarditis. There may also be (in any country) fungal infections due to various agents secondary to foreign bodies, immunosuppression or occasionally, idiopathic. Treatment is a combination of surgery and specific antifungal agents and the prognosis depends on the severity.

Protozoal Infections

Leishmania infantum can cause inflammatory pericarditis. Although it is rare for this (along with cardiac tamponade) to be the main symptom in a dog with leishmaniasis.

Coagulopathies

Coagulopathies can also cause pericardial haemorrhagic effusion. Normally, this effusion is **accompanied by effusions in other cavities**.

Congenital coagulopathies, rodenticide poisoning (vitamin K antagonists such as warfarins), disseminated intravascular coagulation, and liver failure are the most common causes. It is important where a coagulopathy is suspected that a clotting time analysis is performed before pericardiocentesis. This is because performing pericardiocentesis could be fatal as in many cases the haemorrhage is contained within the pericardial sac and the introduction of a needle or catheter into the pericardium produces more bleeding.

Left Atrial Rupture in Mitral Valve Disease

The presence of atrial lesions due to atrial enlargement and continuous pounding of the regurgitant jet can cause rupture of the left atrium and severe acute pericardial haemorrhage. In these cases, severe mitral valve disease with significant enlargement of the atrium, pericardial effusion and, in many cases, a clot adjacent to the left atrium is seen. As bleeding is acute and potentially continuous, it is possible when the pericardium drains the blood does not clot.

Some of these dogs also present in left-sided congestive heart failure. Although they can survive a first episode (probably due to spontaneous closure of a small defect) the prognosis is usually poor.

Transudates

Pericardial transudates are observed with various conditions. In the vast majority of cases, these are **small to moderate in volume** and do not usually cause cardiac tamponade or associated clinical signs. In many cases, they are the consequence of systemic diseases and there are transudates in other cavities. Pure transudates can be observed in cases of hypoalbuminaemia and modified transudates secondary to right-sided congestive heart failure, vasculitis of varying aetiology, uraemia, and toxaemia.

Congenital Defects

The most common defect is **peritoneal-pericardial-diaphragmatic hernia (PPDH)**, which is easily diagnosed by radiography (Figure 16) and echocardiography. Occasionally, these defects do not cause clinical problems, or these are subtle and go unnoticed by the owner. **The clinical signs are secondary to cardiorespiratory dysfunction** or associated with the presence of abdominal organs in the pericardium, mainly intestinal loops or liver.

Some clinical signs observed include tachypnoea, dyspnoea, coughing, vomiting, diarrhoea, anorexia, circulatory weakness, and collapse. The surgical approach to correct these hernias

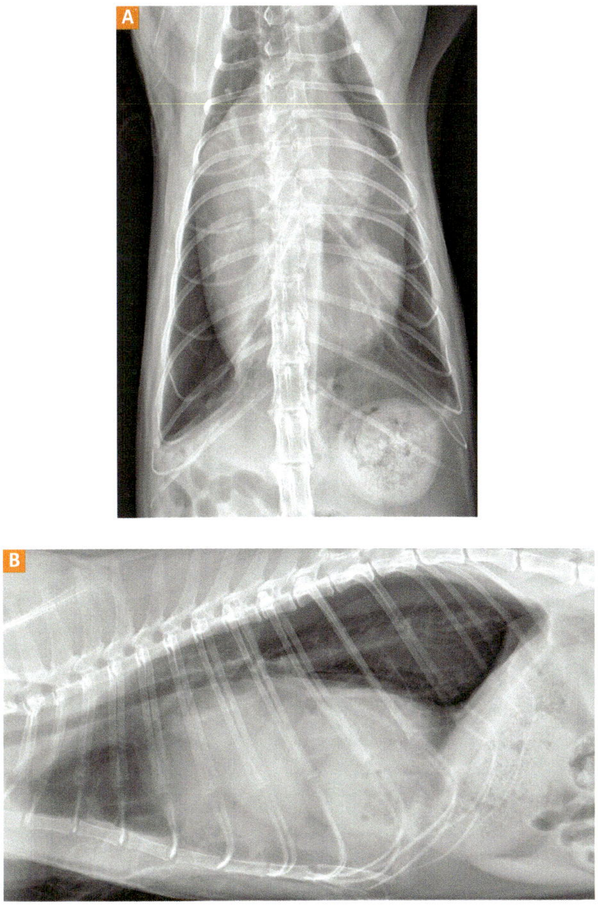

Figure 16. Dorsoventral (A) and lateral (B) radiographs of a patient with a peritoneal-pericardial-diaphragmatic hernia (PPDH). A very enlarged cardiac silhouette can be seen which is joined to the diaphragm (with loss of the diaphragmatic line). The absence of the hepatic silhouette in the abdomen (classic finding) and the presence of part of the stomach within the pericardium can be seen.

is by abdominal incision. Although there may be surgical and postsurgical complications, the prognosis is usually good.

Other pericardial birth defects include pericardial cysts and an incomplete pericardium which cause herniation of cardiac structures. Both are rare and may need surgical correction.

Pericardial Disease in the Cat

Pericardial disease in the cat is rare. The most common cause of pericardial effusion in cats is the presence of transudates due to **congestive heart failure secondary to cardiomyopathy**. Primary (such as lymphoma) or secondary (such as melanoma or carcinoma) cardiac neoplasms are the second most common cause. Most cases with an effusion do not cause cardiac tamponade and do not require treatment.

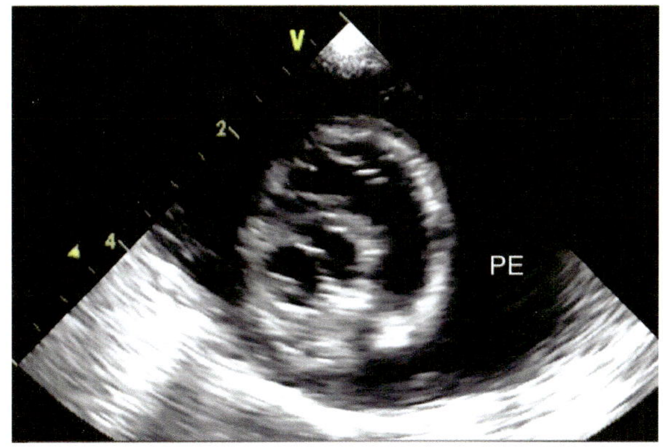

Figure 17. Echocardiographic image of a cat with feline infectious pericarditis with a severe pericardial effusion. PE: pericardial effusion.

Other important causes include infectious agents (FIP or septic pericarditis) (Figure 17), transudates from systemic diseases (uraemia, hypoalbuminaemia), coagulopathies, and congenital defects (PPDH).

Cardiac, Pericardial, and Aortic Base Neoplasms

The focus of this section is **canine neoplasms**, with feline disease considered at the end.

The prevalence of cardiac tumours in the dog varies depending on the study (0.12–4.33%). Tumours can be primary or secondary, with the proportion of the total varying significantly in different studies. The **most common tumour in dogs is haemangiosarcoma** (69%) followed by chemodectoma, thyroid carcinoma, mesothelioma, and lymphoma. However, many other tumors have been described (Figure 18), including thyroid adenoma, melanoma, mast cell tumour, blastoma, granulosa cell tumour, myxoma, myxosarcoma, sarcoma, fibroma, fibrosarcoma, rhabdomyosarcoma, leiomyoma, leiomyosarcoma, chondrosarcoma, osteosarcoma, paraganglioma, haemartoma, and lipoma.

An interesting finding is that unlike haemangiosarcomas or cardiac-base tumours, **most metastatic tumours (75%) are found in the ventricular free wall, the septum, or both**. Only 25% of metastatic tumours are found in the right atrium or ventricle.

The clinical presentation of cardiac tumours depends on their location and malignancy. Thus, they may be an incidental finding, cause pericardial effusions, arrhythmias

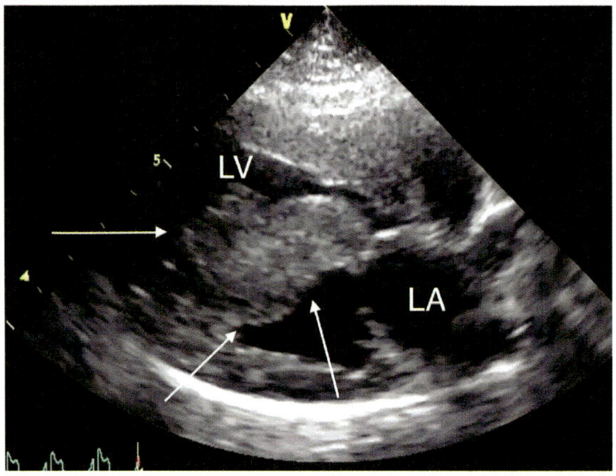

Figure 18. Echocardiographic image of a rhabdomyosarcoma (arrows) seen on a right longitudinal parasternal view (long axis). LV: left ventricle, LA: left atrium.

(supraventricular, ventricular or bradyarrhythmias), or have haemodynamic consequences with obstructions of venoatrial, atrioventricular, ventriculoaortic, or ventriculopulmonary flow.

Some tumours (such as myxomas or myxosarcomas) can affect the valves and cause incompetence of these structures with consequent cardiac remodelling. In some cases, due to these haemodynamic consequences, patients may present with left or right-sided heart failure.

For the diagnosis of neoplasms, a combination of echocardiography and CT is used to diagnose cardiac neoplasms. The CT scan mainly serves to evaluate the presence of concurrent extracardiac neoplasms. It is sometimes possible to collect samples from the heart, either by ultrasound-guided fine needle aspiration, fluoroscopy-guided myocardial biopsy and transoesophageal ultrasound, thoracoscopy, or by thoracotomy. If there are metastases or primary extracardiac neoplasms, it may be easier and more accessible in these cases to take samples of extracardiac tissues.

Treatment options in each case (surgical, radiotherapy or chemotherapy) should be made in conjunction with an oncologist and a soft tissue surgeon. Treatment and prognostic expectations described for the most common tumours are described below.

In some cases, with flow obstructions (for example, drainage of the vena cava in the atrium), minimally invasive techniques such as the implantation of stents that facilitate blood flow in that area can be helpful.

Haemangiosarcoma

Haemangiosarcoma is the most common tumour in the dog, with the German Shepherd dog predisposed. Diagnosis is often presumptive, based on the echocardiographic characteristics and location in the atrium or right ventricle. The percentage of dogs with **concurrent splenic haemangiosarcoma** varies between studies from between 8.7–25%.

In a study of untreated dogs with cardiac haemangiosarcoma, median survival was 7.1 days. **Performing palliative pericardiocentesis does not appear to improve survival**, probably because the creation of a pericardial window eliminates the possible bleeding containment function of the pericardium. Considering the low survival, many patients are euthanised when the diagnosis is confirmed or at the time of the first recurrence.

If removal of the tumour is possible (as is the case with tumours located on the right appendage), the median reported survival time is 86 days, which is extended to 189 days if chemotherapy (standard treatment with doxorubicin) is added to the surgery. A recent study opened a new line of treatment, describing fewer pericardiocentesis and a median survival time of 79 days in dogs with haemangiosarcomas treated with a single session of radiation therapy.

Aortic Base Tumours

Although there are many types of aortic base tumours, the most common are **chemodectomas followed by thyroid carcinomas**.

Chemodectomas usually appear in the wall of the ascending aorta at the level of the cardiac base, and **brachiocephalic dogs**, particularly Boxers, appear predisposed. Chemodectomas are non-functional paraganglial cell tumours and this is associated with a **benign nature and low metastatic potential**. Many chemodectomas are incidental findings during an ultrasound or CT scan performed for another reason. Most, however, present with signs associated with a pericardial effusion or signs secondary to the presence of a mass at the aortic base (cough).

Tumours that are not locally invasive can be removed. For tumours causing pericardial effusion, typically an exploratory thoracotomy is performed, and where possible the tumour removed and a pericardiectomy performed during the same surgery. If the tumour cannot be removed, a tumour biopsy is usually performed, followed by a pericardiectomy. Chemodectomas treated with pericardiectomy (without removal of the tumour) have shown a higher mean survival time (732 days) than if it is not performed (41 days).

Before surgery, a complete CT scan is advisable to evaluate the presence of metastases, although these tumours have little metastatic potential. Toceranib is frequently used for the management of this neoplasm. A recent study evaluated toceranib treatment in dogs with aortic base tumours. In these dogs there was a complete resolution of clinical signs in 81% of cases with gastrointestinal toxicity (normally well tolerated) of 54% described. The median survival of dogs without metastasis was 796 days (68–1190 days) and 532 days with metastasis (77–679 days), although there was no significant difference statistically when both groups were compared.

In a recent study, stereotactic radiation therapy was also used in six dogs with aortic-base tumours (although not all had a final diagnosis of chemodectoma). Tumour shrinkage ranged from 30–76%, with complications including cough, tachyarrhythmias, and congestive heart failure, and variable survival times (range 150–1228 days after treatment).

Mesothelioma

Mesothelioma is the result of neoplastic transformation of the mesothelial cells of the pericardium. Diagnosis is usually by histopathology, as the fluid cytology or echocardiographic and CT characteristics are usually not specific. Thus, it is common for the tumour to be **diagnosed histopathologically after pericardiectomy in dogs with recurrent pericardial effusion**. Sometimes the effusions are also pleural and/or abdominal. In the event they are also pleural (and it is suspected this is not a result of right heart failure), taking a pleural biopsy at the time of pericardiectomy is advisable. Sometimes, even in histopathology, the final diagnosis is not clear and new immunohistochemical markers have been described which can aid diagnosis.

After treatment, **chemotherapy with carboplatin, doxorubicin, or a mixture of both** is recommended. This can be administered intravenously or through a pleural port (Figure 19) which also serves for long-term intermittent drainage. Median survival times of 60 days were described in one study (range 8 to 300 days) and 4, 9 and 27 months in other individually described cases.

Lymphoma

Primary cardiac lymphoma is defined as lymphoma that affects the heart, the pericardium, or both. According to the World Health Organization classification, cardiac lymphoma with pericardial effusion is classified as stage V (extranodal outside the liver and spleen) and Substage B (with clinical signs). The largest study on lymphoma included 12 cases in

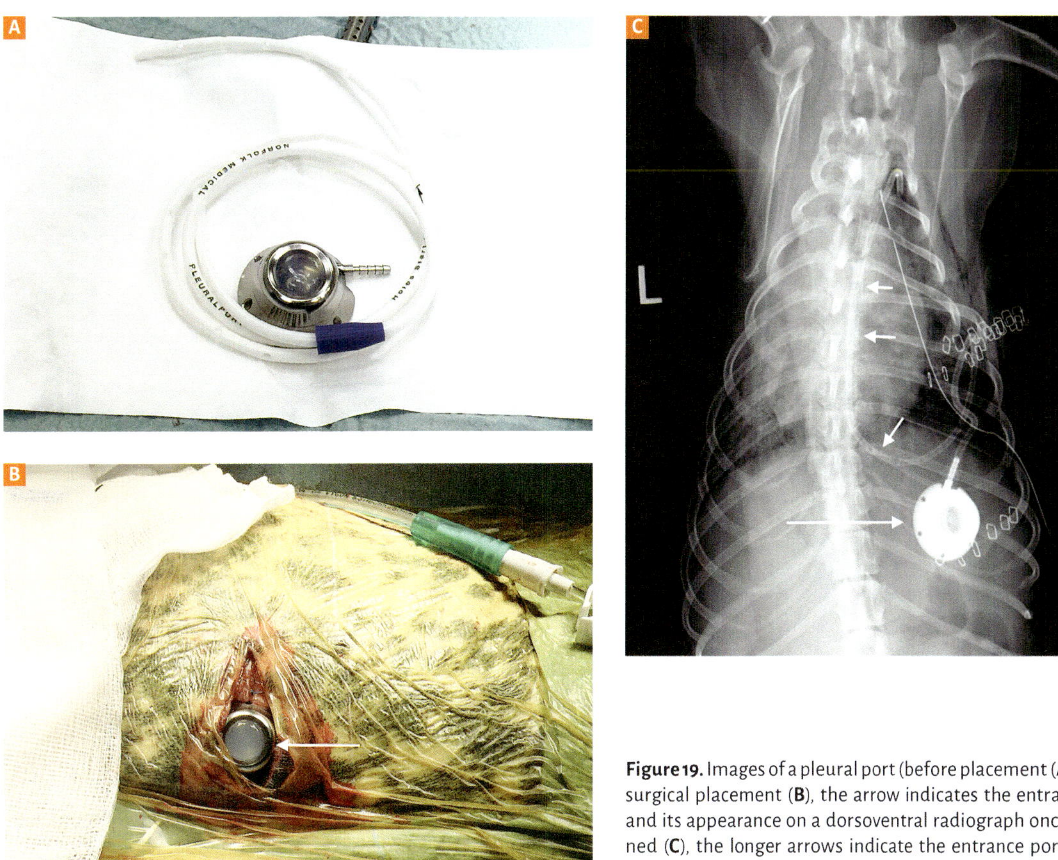

Figure 19. Images of a pleural port (before placement (**A**), during surgical placement (**B**), the arrow indicates the entrance port) and its appearance on a dorsoventral radiograph once positioned (**C**), the longer arrows indicate the entrance port and the short arrows the drainage tube).

which the majority were diagnosed by cytology of pericardial effusion or by histopathology of the pericardium. There was a variety of origins (T and B cells). Median survival of dogs treated with pericardiocentesis, and standard lymphoma chemotherapy (five animals) was 157 days.

Neoplasms in the Cat

Cardiac tumours are less common in cats than dogs and tend to be malignant. Lymphoma is the most common (40% of tumours in cats) and about 20% are secondary. Interestingly, as in the dog, these secondary tumours have been described in a study as being **mainly located in the left ventricle**. The diagnostic and clinical implications are similar to those described in the dog.

In a study of seven cats with pericardial lymphoma (one unclassified, three T-cell and three B-cell) survival was between 7 and 11 days in cats that were not given treatment or were given glucocorticoids or doxorubicin as a sole agent, but a cat administered a CHOP protocol (cyclophosphamide, doxorubicin, vincristine, prednisolone) reached complete remission and was alive at 750 days.

Bibliography

- Atencia, S., Doyle, R.S., Whitley, N.T. (2013) Thoracoscopic pericardial window for management of pericardial effusion in 15 dogs. *J Small Anim Pract*, 54(11), pp. 564–9.
- Banz, A.C., Gottfried, S.D. (2010) Peritoneopericardial diaphragmatic hernia: a retrospective study of 31 cats and eight dogs. *J Am Animal Hosp Assoc*, 46(6), pp. 398–404.
- Ben-Amotz, R., Ellison, G.W., Thompson, M.S. et al. (2007) Pericardial lipoma in a geriatric dog with an incidentally discovered thoracic mass. *J Small Anim Pract*, 3rd ed, 48(10), pp. 596–9.
- Boddy, K.N., Sleeper, M.M., Sammarco, C.D. et al. (2011) Cardiac Magnetic Resonance in the Differentiation of Neoplastic and Nonneoplastic Pericardial Effusion. *Journal of Veterinary Internal Medicine*, 25(5), pp. 1003–9.
- Brambilla, P.G., Roccabianca, P., Locatelli, C. (2006) Primary Cardiac Lipoma in a Dog. *Journal of Veterinary Internal Medicine*. Wiley/Blackwell (10.1111), 20(3), pp. 691–3.
- Cagle, L.A., Epstein, S.E., Owens, S.D. et al. (2013) Mellema MS, Hopper K, Burton AG. Diagnostic Yield of Cytologic Analysis of Pericardial Effusion in Dogs. *Journal of Veterinary Internal Medicine*. 2nd ed., 28(1), pp. 66–71.
- Casamian-Sorrosal, D., Fournier, D., Shippam, J. et al. (2008) Septic pericardial effusion associated with pulmonary and pericardial botryomycosis in a dog. *J Small Anim Pract*, 49(12), pp. 655–9.
- Case, J.B., Maxwell, M., Aman, A. et al. (2013) Outcome evaluation of a thoracoscopic pericardial window procedure or subtotal pericardectomy via thoracotomy for the treatment of pericardial effusion in dogs. *J Am Vet Med Assoc*, 242(4), pp. 493–8.
- Chapel, E., Russel, D., Schober, K. (2014) Partial pericardial defect with left auricular herniation in a dog with syncope. *J Vet Cardiol*, 16(2), pp. 133–9
- Costa, A., Lahmers, S., Barry, S.L. (2014) Fungal pericarditis and endocarditis secondary to porcupine quill migration in a dog. *J Vet Cardiol*, 16(4), pp. 283–90
- de Laforcade, A.M., Freeman, L.M., Rozanski, E.A. et al. (2005) Biochemical Analysis of Pericardial Fluid and Whole Blood in Dogs with Pericardial Effusion. *Journal of Veterinary Internal Medicine*. Wiley/Blackwell (10.1111), 19(6), pp. 833–6.
- Ehrhart, N., Ehrhart, E.J., Willis, J. et al. (2002) Analysis of factors affecting survival in dogs with aortic body tumors. *Veterinary Surgery*, 31(1), pp. 44–8.
- Fine, D.M., Tobias, A.H., Jacob, K.A. (2003) Use of pericardial fluid pH to distinguish between idiopathic and neoplastic effusions. *J Vet Intern Med*, 17(4), pp. 525–9
- Fraga Veloso, G., Fraga Manteiga, E., Trehy, M. et al. (2014) Septic pericarditis and myocardial abscess in an English Springer spaniel. *J Vet Cardiol*, 16(1), pp. 39–44
- Ghaffari, S., Pelio, D.C., Lange, A.J. et al. (2014) A retrospective evaluation of doxorubicin-based chemotherapy for dogs with right atrial masses and pericardial effusion. *J Small Anim Pract*, 55(5), pp. 254–7.

■ Hamilton-Elliott, J., Finotello, R., Murgia, D. et al. (2018) Ectopic medullary (C cell) thyroid carcinoma in a dog with pericardial effusion. *Vet Rec Case Rep*, 6(4):e000729.

■ Hodgkiss-Geere, H.M., Palermo, V., Liuti, T. (2014) Pericardial cyst in a 2-year-old Maine Coon cat following peritoneopericardial diaphragmatic hernia repair. *Journal of Feline Medicine and Surgery*, 17(4), pp. 381–6.

■ Humm, K.R., Keenaghan-Clark, E.A., Boag, A.K. (2009) Adverse events associated with pericardiocentesis in dogs: 85 cases (1999–2006). *Journal of Veterinary Emergency and Critical Care*, 19(4), pp. 352–6.

■ Johnson, M.S., Martin, M., Binns, S. et al. (2004) A retrospective study of clinical findings, treatment and outcome in 143 dogs with pericardial effusion. *J Small Anim Pract*. Wiley/Blackwell (10.1111), 45(11), pp. 546–52.

■ Lew, F. H., McQuown, B., Borrego, J., Cunningham, S., & Burgess, K. E. (2019). Retrospective evaluation of canine heart base tumours treated with toceranib phosphate (Palladia): 2011 2018. *Veterinary and comparative oncology*, 17(4), 465-471.

■ Loureiro, J., Burrow, R., Dukes-McEwan, J. (2009) Canine intrapericardial cyst – complicated surgical correction of an unusual cause of right heart failure. *J Small Anim Pract*, 50(9), pp. 492–7.

■ MacGregor, J.M., Faria, M., Moore, A.S. (2005) Cardiac lymphoma and pericardial effusion in dogs: 12 cases (1994–2004). *J Am Vet Med Assoc*, 227(9), pp. 1449–53.

■ Magestro, L.M., Gieger, T.L., Nolan, M.W. (2018) Stereotactic body radiation therapy for heart–base tumors in six dogs. *Journal of Veterinary Cardiology*, 20(3):186–97.

■ Nijs, M.I., Vink, A., Bergmann, W. et al. (2018) Left ventricular cardiac myxoma and sudden death in a dog. *Acta Vet Scand*. BioMed Central, pp. 1–4.

■ Nolan, M.W., Arkans, M.M., LaVine, D. et al. (2017) Pilot study to determine the feasibility of radiation therapy for dogs with right atrial masses and hemorrhagic pericardial effusion. *Journal of Veterinary Cardiology*, 19(2), pp. 132–43.

■ Pedro, B., Linney, C., Navarro–Cubas, X. et al. (2016) Cytological diagnosis of cardiac masses with ultrasound guided fine needle aspirates. *J Vet Cardiol*, 18(1), pp. 47–56.

■ Rajagopalan, V., Jesty, S.A., Craig, L.E. et al. (2013) Comparison of Presumptive Echocardiographic and Definitive Diagnoses of Cardiac Tumors in Dogs. *Journal of Veterinary Internal Medicine*, 27(5), pp. 1092–6.

■ Scollan, K.F., Bottorff, B., Stieger-Vanegas, S. et al. (2014) Use of Multidetector Computed Tomography in the Assessment of Dogs with Pericardial Effusion. *Journal of Veterinary Internal Medicine*, 6 ed., 29(1), pp. 79–87.

■ Shaw, S.P., Rozanski, E.A., Rush, J.E. (2004) Cardiac troponins I and T in dogs with pericardial effusion. *J Vet Intern Med*, 18(3), pp. 322–4.

■ Sims, C.S., Tobias, A.H., Hayden, D.W. et al. (2003) Pericardial effusion due to primary cardiac lymphosarcoma in a dog. *J Vet Intern Med*, 17(6), pp. 923–927

■ Treggiari, E., Pedro B, Dukes-McEwan J. et al. (2015) A descriptive review of cardiac tumours in dogs and cats. *Vet Comp Oncol*, 15(2), pp. 273–88.

■ Vicari, E.D., Brown, D.C., Holt, D.E. et al. (2001) Survival times of and prognostic indicators for dogs with heart base masses: 25 cases (1986–1999). *J Am Vet Med Assoc*, 219(4), pp. 485–7.

■ Wagner, A., MacGregor, J.M., Berg, J. et al. (2006) Septic pericarditis in a Yorkshire Terrier. *Journal of Veterinary Emergency and Critical Care*. 6 ed., 16(2), pp. 136–40.

■ Woolley, R.M., Devine, C.B., French, A.T. (2006) Left ventricular flow propagation using color M-mode echocardiography in the diagnosis of effusive-constrictive pericardial disease. *Veterinary Radiology & Ultrasound*. 3rd ed., 47(4), pp. 366–9.

■ Yamamoto, S., Hoshi, K., Hirakawa, A. et al. (2013) Epidemiological, Clinical and Pathological Features of Primary Cardiac Hemangiosarcoma in Dogs: A Review of 51 Cases. *J Vet Med Sci*, 75(11), pp. 1433–41.

■ Zini, E., Glaus, T.M., Bussadori, C. et al. (2009) Evaluation of the presence of selected viral and bacterial nucleic acids in pericardial samples from dogs with or without idiopathic pericardial effusion. *The Veterinary Journal*, 179(2), pp. 225–9.

Test

Answers on Page 312

1. Which of these neoplasms are not a common cause of pericardial effusion in dogs?
- a. Mesothelioma.
- b. Thymoma.
- c. Chemodectoma.
- d. Haemangiosarcoma.

2. Which of these aetiologies is the least common cause of pericardial effusion in cats?
- a. Congestive heart failure.
- b. Lymphoma.
- c. Idiopathic inflammatory pericarditis.
- d. Other neoplasms.

3. Which of these diseases that can cause pericardial effusion has the best prognosis?
- a. Mesothelioma.
- b. Chemodectoma.
- c. Haemangiosarcoma.
- d. DIC secondary to carcinomatosis.

4. Which of these statements is false regarding pericardial disease?
- a. Brachiocephalic dogs are predisposed to chemodectomas.
- b. The cause of idiopathic pericarditis is unknown.
- c. Pericardiocentesis is performed on the right side.
- d. Cytology of pericardial effusion is very helpful in diagnosing mesotheliomas.

5. Which of these statements is true regarding tumours in dogs?
- a. Haemangiosarcomas occur most frequently in the left atrium.
- b. Chemodectomas occur most often in the right atrium.
- c. Metastatic tumors occur most often in the left ventricle.
- d. Mesotheliomas occur most often in the right ventricle.

6. Which of these statements is correct?
- a. The presence of elevated troponin I in pericardial fluid can be used to differentiate between a haemangiosarcoma and a chemodectoma with a sensitivity of 93% and a specificity of 100%.
- b. Cytology has a specificity and sensitivity of more than 95% for the diagnosis of mesothelioma.
- c. Cytology is especially useful in cases of septic pericarditis or lymphoma.
- d. Cytology is especially useful in cases of chemodectomas and metastatic tumours.

7. Which of these statements is false?
- a. Pericardiocentesis is performed on the right side of the thorax.
- b. It is advisable not to completely empty the pericardium as tissue reperfusion could occur.
- c. If haemorrhagic pericardial effusion is seen, it should not clot once the fluid is removed from the pericardium.
- d. Ventricular premature complexes can occur during pericardiocentesis due to, among other causes, puncture of the heart.

8. Which of these statements is true?
- a. In constrictive pericarditis, thickening of the pericardium is always seen on echocardiography.
- b. In constrictive pericarditis, an increase in transmitral flow on inspiration and a decrease on expiration can be observed on echocardiography.
- c. When a dog with constrictive pericarditis is catheterised, the diastolic pressures of the right ventricle and the right atrium, but not the left ventricle, can be seen equalizing.
- d. When a dog with constrictive pericarditis is catheterised, the diastolic pressures of the right ventricle and left ventricle can be seen equalizing, but not that of the right atrium.

9. Which of these statements is correct?
- a. Dogs with pericardial effusion often have pulsus alternans on auscultation, characterised by a stronger pulse during inspiration.
- b. Dogs with ascites have a worse prognosis than dogs presenting with collapse.
- c. In dogs with pericardial effusion, an abrupt decrease in the curve, also called the square root sign, is observed on the pressure traces from the right atrium obtained by catheterization.
- d. During pericardial effusion, but not during constrictive pericarditis, a difference between inspiratory and expiratory pulse pressures of more than 10 mmHg can be observed.

10. Which of these statements is false?
- a. Idiopathic pericarditis usually has a good prognosis after pericardiectomy.
- b. In 50% of cases, cardiac haemangiosarcomas are associated with splenic haemangiosarcomas.
- c. The median survival time of dogs with chemodectomas is higher than that of haemangiosarcomas.
- d. Haemangiosarcomas treated with surgery and chemotherapy have a better prognosis than those which are not treated.

Clinical Case

An eight-year-old neutered male Labrador cross presents at the practice with severe lethargy, an episode of collapse and an enlarged abdomen. On physical examination the following are detected: jugular distention, tachycardia (heart rate 160 bpm), slight tachypnoea (35 rpm), pale mucous membranes, weak pulse, a temperature of 37.5 °C, attenuated heart sounds, and abdominal ascites.

1. How should these findings be interpreted?

An IV catheter is placed, oxygen given, and an initial thoracic echocardiogram/ultrasound performed (image below). Ascites is also seen on a FAST abdominal ultrasound, and when aspirated and analysed, this effusion was a modified transudate.

2. Interpret the echocardiographic image and outline the next steps.

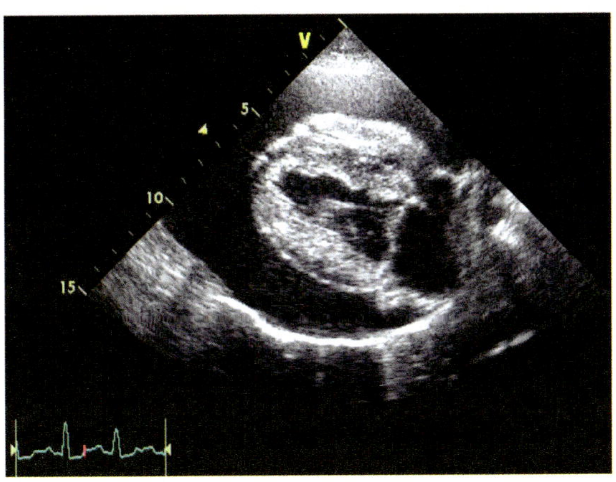

Pericardiocentesis is performed and 600 ml of haemorrhagic fluid obtained. Vital parameters gradually improve after drainage, although ascites persists. Pericardial fluid is haemorrhagic when tested (no tumour cells are present).

3. What would an appropriate course of action be?

After four months the patient returns with the same clinical signs. The same steps described above are performed again and the effusion is drained. Masses are still not seen on echocardiography.

4. What recommendations could be made at this point in time?

Correct Answers:

Test

1. b
2. c
3. b
4. d
5. c
6. c
7. b
8. b
9. d
10. b

Clinical Case

1. **How should these findings be interpreted?**
   The presence of a weak pulse, tachycardia, and pale mucous membranes indicates circulatory collapse. This could be due to hypovolaemic, cardiogenic, or obstructive (less likely septic, due to the appearance of the mucous membranes and the low temperature) shock. There could also be a combination of both. Jugular distention and ascites (along with tachycardia) indicate right-sided heart failure is likely, suggesting the shock is likely cardiogenic, obstructive, or mixed (for example, combined with acute haemorrhage causing hypovolaemia). The presence of attenuated heart sounds indicates a pericardial effusion may be the cause of the suspected heart failure, although it cannot be ruled out that this attenuation of heart sounds is due to a pleural effusion or a thoracic mass.

2. **Interpret the echocardiographic image and outline the next steps.**
   A right longitudinal parasternal view (long axis) shows the heart surrounded by a hypoechoic layer which extends to the cardiac base. This image indicates a severe pericardial effusion. This finding, together with the evidence of jugular distension and ascites (modified transudate) suggests right-sided congestive heart failure secondary to a severe pericardial effusion. The severe pericardial effusion would also explain the circulatory collapse (obstructive shock).

   The next step is to administer fluids at high volumes to increase blood volume (eg. 10 ml/kg in 20–30 minutes) while the equipment is urgently prepared for pericardiocentesis. If there is suspicion of coagulopathy (there is not in this case), a complete blood count and an analysis of clotting times should be performed prior to pericardiocentesis. While the material is being prepared, an echocardiogram is performed (since masses are better seen when there is fluid) and no cardiac, pericardial or base mass is observed.

3. **What would an appropriate course of action be?**
   The patient is kept hospitalised for 24 hours to assess whether the effusion rapidly recurs. Ascites gradually disappears (furosemide could be given at this time to accelerate its disappearance but is not necessary) over the next few days if there is no recurrence of effusion and cardiac tamponade. The vital parameters have been normalised. On repeating full echocardiography, (which must be performed by an experienced cardiologist) after 24 hours there is no recurrence of the effusion and no cardiac, pericardial or cardiac base masses are observed. The patient is discharged. The working diagnosis is idiopathic pericarditis, but a very small neoplasm or pericardial mesothelioma cannot be ruled out.

4. **What recommendations could be made at this point in time?**
   Subtotal pericardiectomy is recommended after the second or third episode of pericardial effusion. In this case, the procedure is done after the second episode. A thoracic and abdominal CT scan is also done before pericardiectomy. This is not essential, but evaluates the possible presence of metastasis (in case a cardiac or pericardial tumour has not been observed on echocardiography) and the possible presence of an aortic-base tumour in an area too high and therefore difficult to access with ultrasound. The pericardiectomy is successful, the histopathology confirms inflammatory pericarditis and the dog progresses favourably, with no further recurrences, and leads a completely normal life after the operation.

Notes

Arrhythmias: Cardiac Rhythm Anomalies and Treatment

Gemma Fraga Veloso and Dolores Porteiro Vázquez

Both **sinus rhythm** and **sinus (or respiratory) arrythmia** are considered **normal cardiac rhythms in the dog** (Figures 1 and 2). In both rhythms, a P wave precedes the QRS complex.

Sinus arrhythmia most commonly occurs due to **high vagal tone** but can also result from **wandering pacemaker**. The latter occurs due to the changes in the origin of the impulse generated within the sinus node, and the morphology of the P wave may vary (Figure 2). This is considered a **normal finding in the dog**, usually associated with sinus arrhythmia due to increased vagal tone.

Unlike dogs, **cats do not usually present sinus arrhythmia** in the consult room, although they can manifest it at home in a quiet environment. If a feline patient is found to have sinus arrhythmia, this could indicate an underlying disease which increases vagal tone (for example, respiratory or gastrointestinal disease).

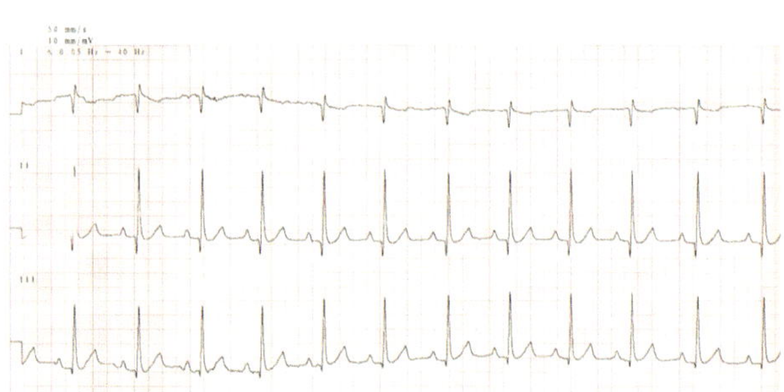

Figure 1. ECG including leads I, II and III showing a normal sinus rhythm (50 mm/s and 10 mm/mV).

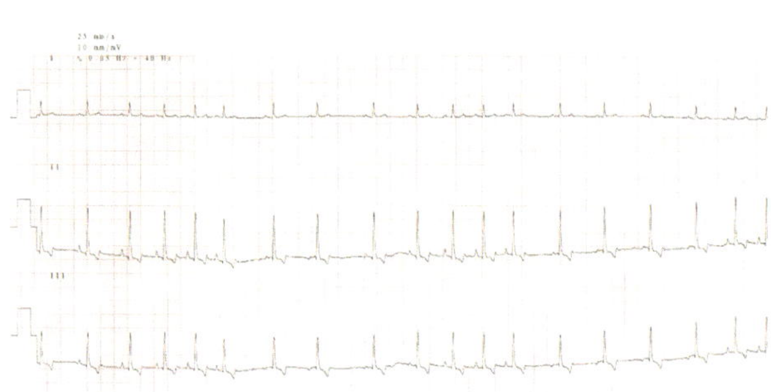

Figure 2. ECG including leads I, II and III showing normal sinus arrhythmia (25 mm/s and 10 mm/mV). A regularly irregular rhythm is present. A wandering pacemaker is also present (slight change in P wave morphology).

Arrhythmias are classified into:

- **bradyarrhythmias** (low heart rate)
- **tachyarrhythmias** (high heart rate)
- **conduction disturbances**.

Bradyarrhythmias

Sinus Bradycardia

This rhythm is when the sinus node generates an impulse and depolarizes slower than normal.

The ECG shows a normal cardiac rhythm, but with a slower than normal heart rate (heart rate in adult dogs <60–70 bpm, heart rate in cats <120 bpm) (Figure 3).

Causes

This can be **a normal and appropriate response** (for example, when the animal is sleeping or resting), secondary to **elevated vagal tone** (respiratory, abdominal, or intracranial diseases or

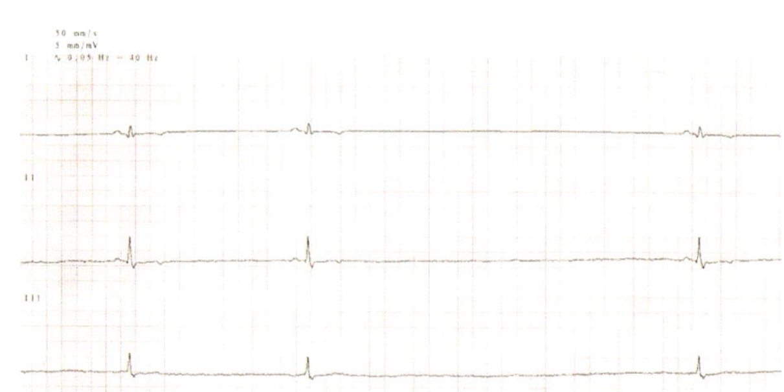

Figure 3. ECG including leads I, II and III showing sinus bradycardia (50 mm/s and 5 mm/mV). A sinus rhythm with a heart rate of 36 beats/minute is present.

pressure on the carotids or eyeballs), **drug use** (β-blockers, calcium channel blockers, morphine, etc.), **hyperkalaemia** (Addison's disease), hypothyroidism, hypothermia, or conditions such as sick sinus syndrome.

Treatment

When bradycardia is an appropriate physiological response then no treatment is necessary. When there is a primary cause, treatment consists of **resolving/treating the primary cause**.

The use of antiarrhythmic drugs is not usually necessary, but if required the following agents are used.

- **Anticholinergics**: atropine (injectable), glycopyrrolate (injectable, but with a longer duration than atropine), propantheline (oral).
- **Sympathomimetics**: isoproterenol (injectable), terbutaline (injectable, oral).
- **Xanthine** derivatives: theophylline (injectable, oral), pentoxifylline (oral).

Escape Rhythms

Escape rhythms appear when the **dominant pacemaker (usually the sinus node) stops generating an impulse** for a prolonged period and pacemaker tissue with a slower discharge rate (junctional or ventricular) takes over (Figure 4). Therefore, complexes or escape rhythms are often associated with bradyarrhythmias and no attempt should be made to suppress them. Treatment is directed at correcting the underlying bradyarrhythmia.

Junctional escape rhythms are generated near the atrioventricular (AV) node and are characterised by **narrow QRS complexes** with a normal appearance with a heart rate of 60–70 bpm. However, the ventricular escape rhythm is characterised by wide and bizarre QRS complexes with a heart rate of 30–50 bpm.

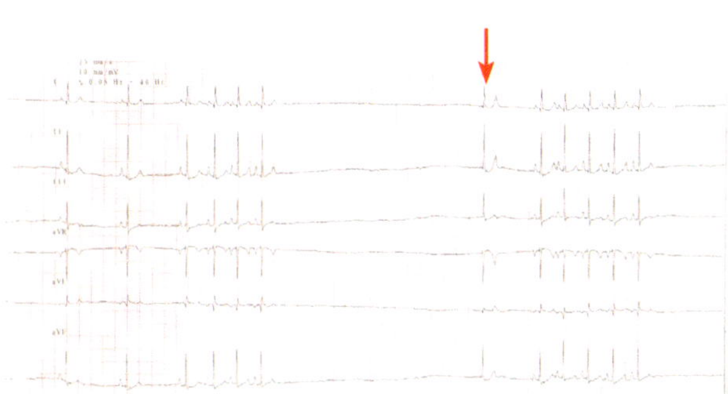

Figure 4. Six lead ECG including leads I, II, III, aVR, aVL and aVF showing sinus arrest followed by an escape complex with supraventricular morphology (red arrow) (25 mm/s and 10 mm/mV).

Sinus Arrest or Block

Transient arrest of the sinus node is known as sinus arrest. However, if an impulse generated in the sinus node is blocked and not conducted to the atrial myocardium, it is called **a sinus block**. The ECG shows an **absence of the P wave** due to an occasional arrest or blockage of the sinus node (Figure 4). In both cases there are no P waves or QRST complex, but they differ because in the case of sinus block the RR interval is equal to double or multiple of the preceding RR interval (Figure 5).

Causes

A brief pause may be normal in dogs during respiratory sinus arrhythmia. The causes of sinus arrest or block are the same as those of sinus bradycardia.

Atrioventricular (AV) Blocks

AV blocks are due to **the lack of conduction of an impulse through the AV node**. AV blocks are classified as explained below.

First-degree AV Block

There is a delay in conduction through the AV node; **on its own this does not cause clinical problems**. **It can be normal in animals with low heart rates** and is caused by high vagal stimulation, the use of antiarrhythmic agents that delay AV node conduction (such as digoxin and β-blockers), or degenerative changes in the AV node. The ECG shows a prolongation of the PR interval (Figure 6).

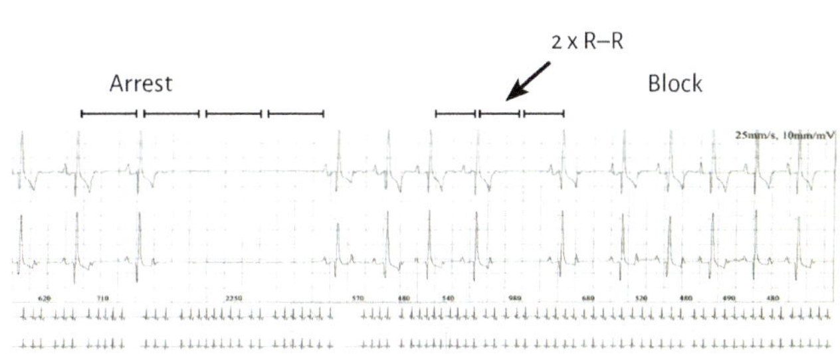

Figure 5. ECG obtained from Holter monitoring showing an episode of sinus arrest and sinus block. In both cases the absence of the P wave and the QRST complex can be seen. In the case of sinus block the RR interval is equal to double or multiple of the preceding RR interval.

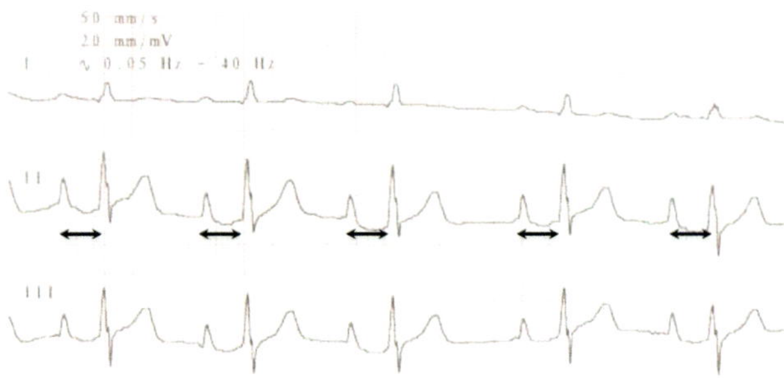

Figure 6. ECG in a cat including bipolar leads (I, II and III) showing sinus rhythm with first-degree AV block (50 mm/s and 20 mm/mV). A prolonged PR interval can be seen (0.15 seconds).

Second-degree AV Block

Due to the **intermittent failure of conduction of the impulse** through the AV node.

The ECG is **characterised by P waves that are not conducted** and, therefore, not followed by a QRS complex (Figure 7).

Second-degree blocks in turn are classified.

- **Mobitz I**: there is a gradual prolongation of the PQ interval that eventually gives rise to a non-conducted P wave (Wenckebach phenomenon). This is seen in some normal dogs due to elevated vagal tone and can occur in animals with sinus arrhythmia.
- **Mobitz II**: the PQ interval is constant (unlike the previous type) and there are non-conducted P waves. It usually follows a pattern (block 2:1, 3:1, 4:1). These blocks can progress to complete block. They are usually due to AV node disease but can also be caused by drugs that affect AV node conduction, such as digoxin, or potassium electrolyte disturbances.

Third-degree or Complete AV Block

There is a persistent inability to conduct through the AV node. It is usually associated with an escape rhythm generated below the AV node (junctional escape rhythm characterised by normal, narrow QRS complexes with a rate of 60–70 bpm or ventricular escape rhythm characterised by wide and bizarre QRS complexes with a rate of 30–40 bpm).

The ECG is characterised by the presence of **P waves that are not related to the QRS complexes** (atrioventricular dissociation), and an escape rhythm of variable frequency (depending on the origin of the escape rhythm) (Figure 8).

The treatment of choice for patients with high-grade second-degree AV blocks that are unresponsive to atropine and third-degree blocks is **implantation of a permanent pacemaker**.

Atrial Standstill

This is characterised by an absence of atrial activity, due to a lack of depolarization of the atrial muscles.

The ECG shows the absence of P waves accompanied by a slow escape rhythm. The escape rhythm usually consists of QRS complexes with narrow morphology (junctional escape rhythm), and only occasionally does the escape rhythm have wide and bizarre QRS complexes (ventricular) (Figure 9).

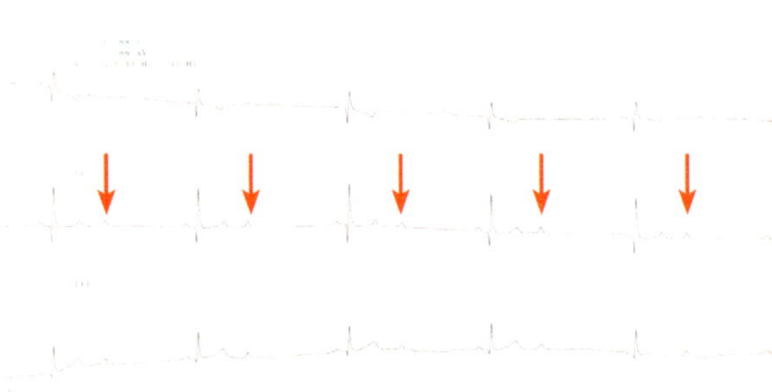

Figure 7. ECG including leads I, II and III showing second-degree AV block (50 mm/s and 10 mm/mV). The P waves are blocked intermittently (P waves which are not followed by QRS complexes) (red arrows) showing a 2:1 conduction ratio.

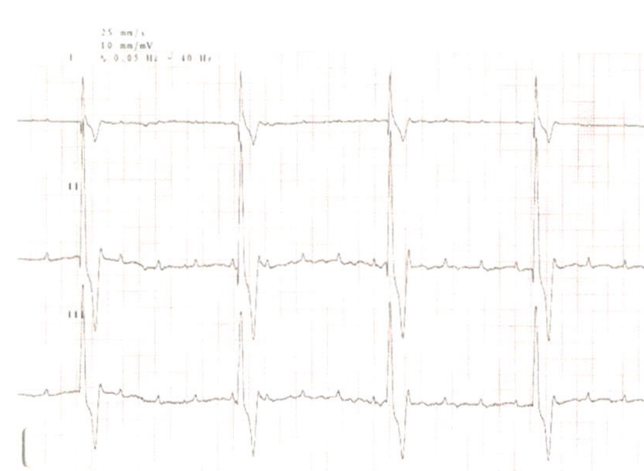

Figure 8. ECG including leads I, II and III showing third-degree AV block (25 mm/s and 10 mm/mV). A complete block of P waves with a slow ventricular escape rhythm with a heart rate of 30 beats/minute is present.

Causes

Persistent Atrial Standstill

Persistent atrial standstill is mainly due to **atrial myocardial dystrophy**, but the ventricle can also be affected, and it is irreversible. It affects both the musculature and the conduction system of the heart; therefore, an escape rhythm is generated in the junctional area or in the ventricles. In these patient's disease usually progresses until they develop heart failure. **Springer Spaniels** show a breed predisposition.

Transient Atrial Standstill

In this case the **condition is reversible** as it is caused by **hyperkalaemia** (Addison's disease, diabetic ketoacidosis, oliguric/anuric renal failure, iatrogenic), and by digitalis intoxication. When hyperkalaemia is present, impulses are generated and transmitted from the sinus node through the internodal conduction system to the atrioventricular node, therefore, the impulse continues to originate in the sinus node and is transmitted to the ventricles through normal conduction pathways, but there is no depolarization of the atrial musculature due to hyperkalaemia and, as a result, there is an absence of the P waves on the ECG.

Treatment

The treatment of transient atrial standstill caused by hyperkalaemia is to **correct the primary cause**.

In the case of **persistent atrial standstill, the treatment of choice is permanent pacemaker implantation.** This only covers clinical signs related to bradyarrhythmia, but not cardiac remodelling changes and heart failure. Therefore, if the patient has heart failure, this also requires treatment.

The prognosis of these patients, despite pacemaker implantation, is poor if they have already developed heart failure and guarded to poor if they have not yet progressed to heart failure.

Tachyarrhythmia

Sinus Tachycardia

Sinus tachycardia is a sinus rhythm generated at a faster rate than normal.

The ECG is characterised by an elevated heart rate with a regular rhythm and normal P–QRST complexes (Figure 10).

The most frequent causes are stress, anxiety, pain, hypovolaemia, anaemia, fever, congestive heart failure, hyperthyroidism, and the use of drugs such as atropine or adrenaline. Treating the primary cause is required to resolve the tachyarrhythmia.

Arrhythmias Caused by Premature Complexes

Premature complexes originate in an area outside the sinus node and appear ahead of time. When two appear in a row they are called **pairs**, three are called **triplets**, and if four or more are present they are considered **tachycardia (ventricular or supraventricular)**. This can be sustained (if it lasts more than

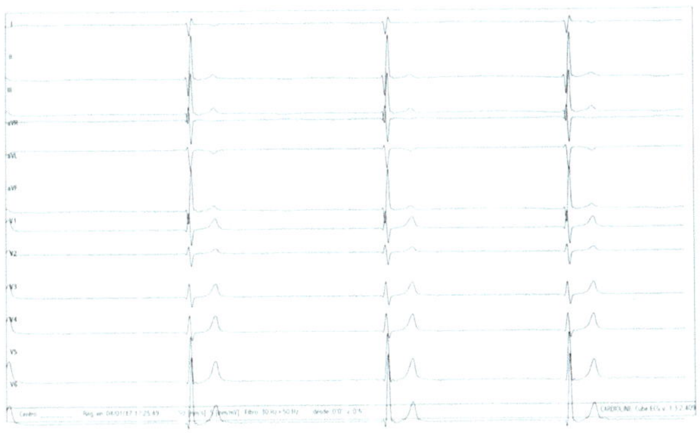

Figure 9. Twelve lead ECG showing atrial standstill (50 mm/s and 5 mm/mV). P waves are absent with an escape rhythm of 60 beats/minute.

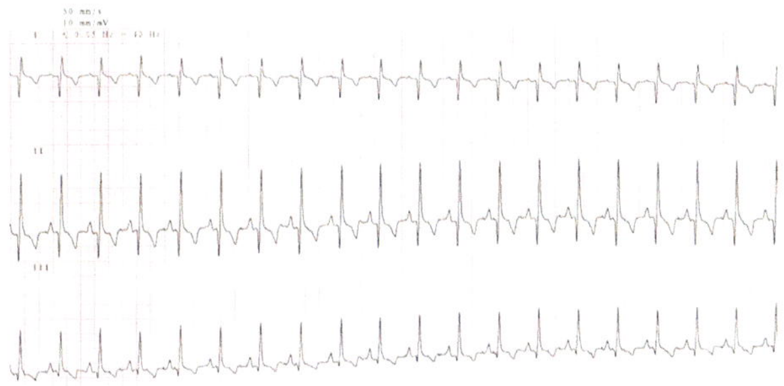

Figure 10. ECG of dog including bipolar leads (I, II and III) which shows sinus tachycardia (50 mm/s and 10 mm/mV). Sinus rhythm with a fast heart rate is present (220 beats/minute).

30 seconds), incessant (if it lasts more than 12 hours), non-sustained (duration less than 30 seconds) or paroxysmal (intermittent with abrupt onset and interruption).

Supraventricular Arrhythmias

This originates from an ectopic focus above the ventricles (atria, AV node, or bundle of His). Thus, the ventricles show normal depolarization, and the appearance of the QRS complexes on the ECG are normal (narrow QRS).

On the ECG, premature ectopic supraventricular complexes are **characterised by their premature appearance**. Ectopic P waves (P') may or may not be visible on the ECG and when present usually have an abnormal morphology (Figure 11).

Supraventricular premature complexes are often associated **with atrial dilation, atrial myocarditis**, or may be secondary to systemic diseases (e.g. hyperthyroidism).

A supraventricular arrhythmia (with narrow QRS) can be due to atrial fibrillation, atrial flutter, or supraventricular tachycardia.

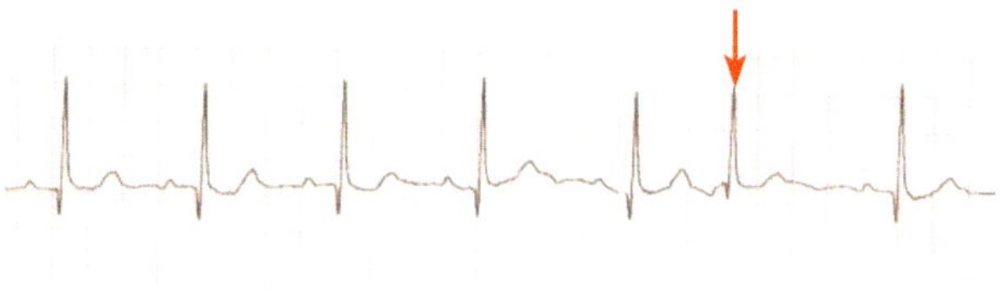

Figure 11. ECG including lead II which shows sinus rhythm interrupted by a premature supraventricular complex (red arrow) (50 mm/s and 10 mm/mV).

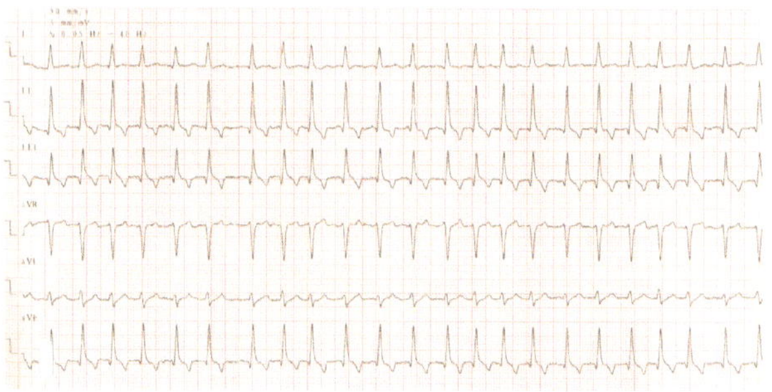

Figures 12. 6 lead ECG (I, II, III, aVR, aVL and aVF) in a dog showing atrial fibrillation (50 mm/s and 5 mm/mV). A chaotic rhythm can be seen (irregularly irregular) where the QRS complexes are normal with the absence of P waves and ventricular response rate of 260 beats/minute.

Atrial Fibrillation

Atrial fibrillation is **one of the most common arrhythmias in dogs,** although it is uncommon in cats.

The ECG is characterised as **an irregularly irregular rhythm (chaotic rhythm) with a normal QRS complex morphology in the absence of P waves** (f waves or atrial fibrillatory waves are sometimes seen on the baseline). The heart rate is usually high, although occasionally it is normal (Figure 12).

The most frequent cause is atrial enlargement. It can also be seen in some giant breeds of dog without obvious structural heart disease (lone atrial fibrillation), and these cases often have an almost normal heart rate. Some large breed dogs with lone atrial fibrillation progress to develop dilated cardiomyopathy.

There are two ways to treat atrial fibrillation.

1. Try to re-establish a normal heart rhythm through **cardioversion**. This option is normally reserved for patients with solitary atrial fibrillation or without obvious structural cardiac abnormalities.
2. **Reduce the ventricular response rate** to a mean heart rate of between 100–140 bpm.

The latter is the most common option since most patients with this arrhythmia present with enlargement of one or both atria. This means that, even if cardioversion is successful, they may develop atrial fibrillation again in the future. Antiarrhythmics used to control the ventricular response rate act by reducing the conduction through the AV node. The most commonly used antiarrhythmic agents are **digoxin, diltiazem (calcium channel blocker), or a combination of these**. β-blockers can also be effective in reducing heart rate during atrial fibrillation. However, they are not usually recommended in patients with systolic dysfunction and are contraindicated in patients with heart failure.

Atrial Flutter

The heart rate is fast or normal, usually irregular, although can also be regular; instead of P waves there are **F waves or flutter waves, which are usually observed on the baseline as saw-tooth oscillations** (Figure 13). The most common causes are like those of atrial fibrillation and are treated in the same way.

Supraventricular Tachycardia (SVT)

The heart rate is usually high (greater than 250 bpm) with a regular rhythm. There are different types depending on their origin (focal atrial tachycardia, accessory pathway, nodal or junctional tachycardia) and differentiating between them can be difficult. **SVT should be differentiated from sinus tachycardia**.

The ECG shows a regular rhythm (constant RR interval) with QRS complexes with normal morphology and a high heart rate (usually greater than 200–250 bpm) (Figure 14). P' waves are present, but not always visible on the ECG, although attempts should be made to locate them. To establish the origin of SVT, an ECG should be performed with at least six leads, ideally simultaneously. The morphology of the P' wave and the duration of the P'-R and R-P' intervals can help diagnose the origin of SVT and, therefore, be helpful in the management of the patient and target therapy.

The **most appropriate antiarrhythmic treatment depends on the mechanism and type of SVT** (focal atrial tachycardia, accessory pathway, nodal or junctional tachycardia). The most common antiarrhythmic agents used to manage SVT are calcium channel blockers or class IV (such as diltiazem PO or verapamil IV), class III (sotalol or amiodarone) and β-blockers or class II (such as atenolol PO or esmolol IV). **It is important to remember that β-blockers are not usually recommended in patients with systolic dysfunction and contraindicated in patients with congestive heart failure**. Mexiletine (class I antiarrhythmic) is not usually effective in treating SVT except for SVT caused by an accessory pathway (or bypass), since some patients with this type of SVT may respond to this antiarrhythmic agent.

Ventricular Arrhythmias

Ventricular premature complexes originate in an ectopic focus of the ventricular myocardium; thus, they do not use specialised conduction pathways and are conducted from cell to cell, giving rise to **wide and bizarre QRS complexes** (called wide QRS).

They are seen as **premature wide QRS complexes on the ECG**. The T wave goes in an opposite direction to the QRS complex,

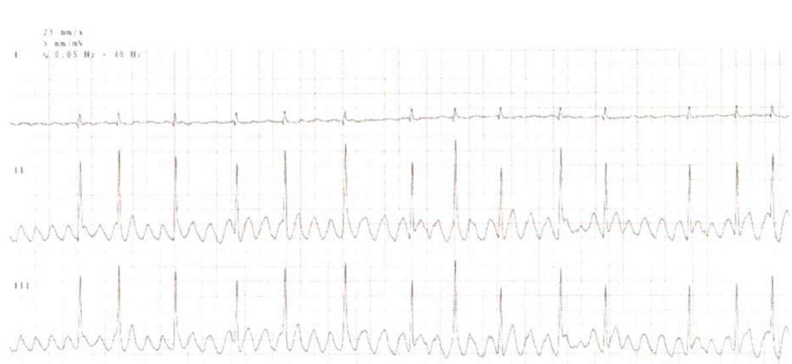

Figure 13. ECG including bipolar leads (I, II and III) in a dog (25 mm/s and 5 mm/mV). An irregular rhythm is present with F or flutter waves on the baseline with a ventricular response rate of 70 beats/minute.

which are not associated with a P wave. They may have a single morphology which are called **monomorphic** (all the same) or they can have a varied morphology which are called **polymorphic** (different from each other). When the QRS complexes have a positive appearance, this suggests a left bundle branch block morphology and they originate in the right ventricle; while those with a negative appearance are said to have a right bundle branch block morphology, which suggests they originate in the left ventricle (Figures 15 and 16). Premature ventricular complexes may present in **isolation**, in **pairs**, in **triplets**, or as **ventricular tachycardia** (four or more consecutive premature ventricular complexes) (Figures 16–18).

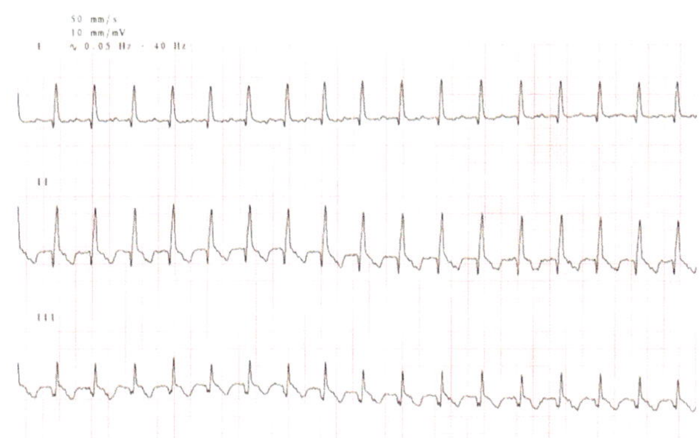

Figure 14. ECG including bipolar leads (I, II and III) in a dog showing supraventricular tachycardia with an average heart rate of 260 beats/minute (50 mm/s and 10 mm/mV).

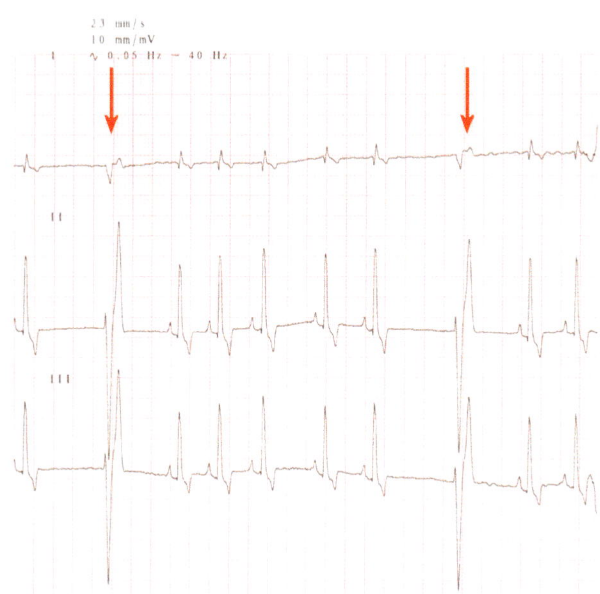

Figure 15. ECG including bipolar leads (I, II and III) which shows sinus rhythm interrupted by isolated ventricular complexes (red arrows) with right bundle branch block morphology, which suggests a right ventricular origin (25 mm/s and 10 mm/mV).

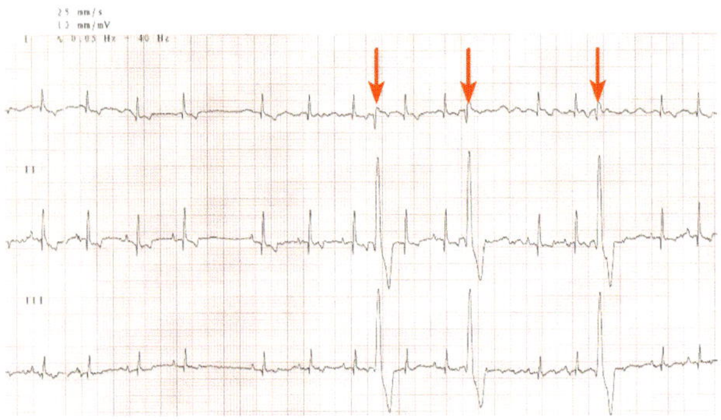

Figure 16. ECG including bipolar leads (I, II and III) which shows sinus rhythm interrupted by isolated premature ventricular complexes (red arrows) with left bundle branch block morphology, which suggests that they originate in the right ventricle (25 mm/s and 10 mm/mV).

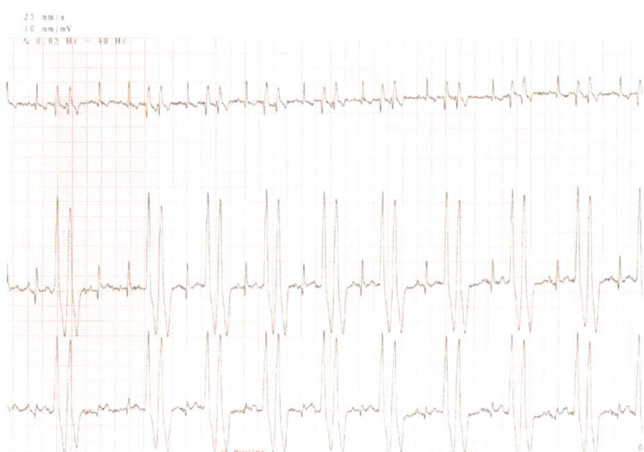

Figure 17. ECG including bipolar leads (I, II and III) which shows sinus rhythm interrupted by ventricular couplets with left bundle branch block morphology and R over T phenomenon (25 mm/s and 10 mm/mV).

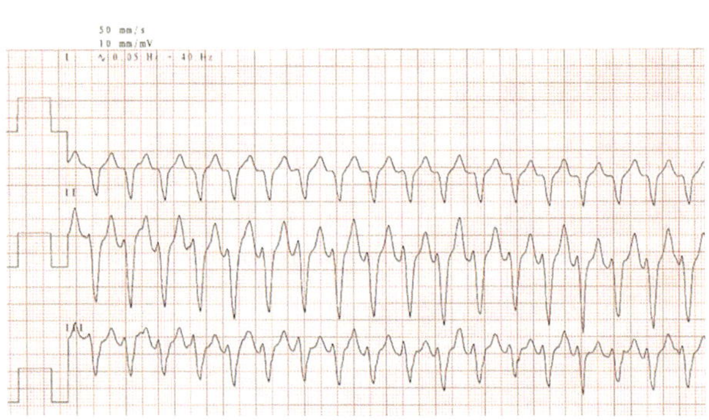

Figure 18. ECG including bipolar leads (I, II and III) showing an episode of ventricular tachycardia with a heart rate of 280 beats/minute (50 mm/s and 10 mm/mV). The morphology of the premature ventricular complexes suggests that they originate from the left ventricle.

When ventricular premature complexes are so premature, they overlap the T wave of the previous complex, **this phenomenon is called R over T** (Figure 17). The ventricles depolarize before completing repolarization, increasing the risk of ventricular fibrillation and **sudden death**. Ventricular premature complexes may be due to **extracardiac** (hypoxia, sepsis, prostatitis, pyometra, splenic neoplasia, gastric dilatation, pancreatitis, electrolyte imbalances, etc.) or **cardiac causes** (congestive heart failure, myocardial hypoxia, cardiomyopathy, advanced valvular endocardiosis, subaortic stenosis, cardiac trauma, myocarditis, cardiac neoplasia, etc.). They can also be associated with **digoxin poisoning**, the use of some anaesthetic agents, and other drugs.

Wide complex tachycardia may be due to ventricular tachycardia and ventricular flutter/fibrillation.

Ventricular Tachycardia

Ventricular tachycardia presents with **a high heart rate (>180 bpm) and a regular rhythm** (Figure 18). This is usually **associated with heart diseases such** as cardiomyopathies, congestive heart failure, myocarditis, pericarditis, neoplasia, myocardial trauma, intoxication (for example, with the antineoplastic agent doxorubicin or digoxin), myocardial infarct, etc. However, they are also associated with extracardiac diseases such as electrolyte disturbances, metabolic diseases, hypoxia, sepsis, abdominal diseases (splenic masses, prostatitis, gastric dilation, trauma), high sympathetic tone and drugs. The heart rate is usually high (>180 bpm) and if sustained, it is an emergency. As an additional note, occasionally, **supraventricular tachycardia can coexist with bundle branch block which mimics ventricular tachycardia**.

Accelerated idioventricular rhythm is a rhythm similar to ventricular tachycardia, but with a slower heart rate (typically less than 160–180 bpm in dogs) (Figure 19).

It is not always necessary to treat ventricular arrhythmias. However, **treatment is recommended of ventricular arrhythmias that are haemodynamically significant**, such as sustained ventricular tachycardia or those with clinical signs and/or hypotension. Also, those ventricular arrhythmias with significant complexity such as the presence of polymorphism, the R over T phenomenon, or a high number of premature ventricular complexes in 24 hours.

The drug of choice for managing haemodynamically significant sustained ventricular tachycardia causing signs of weakness and/or hypoperfusion is **lidocaine** (class I antiarrhythmic) injected intravenously (IV). This is administered in boluses of 2–4 mg/kg up to a maximum total dose of 8 mg/kg. As the duration of effect of lidocaine is short, the administration of a **CRI of lidocaine is usually necessary** after the administration of the initial

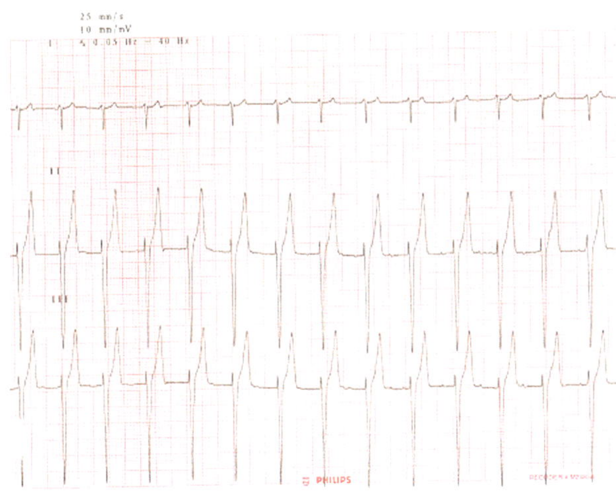

Figure 19. ECG including bipolar leads (I, II and III) showing an episode of accelerated idioventricular rhythm with a heart rate of 110 beats/minute (25 mm/s and 10 mm/mV). The morphology of the premature ventricular complexes suggests that they originate from the left ventricle.

bolus or boluses. If IV lidocaine fails to control sustained ventricular tachycardia with the risk of sudden death for the patient, intravenous administration of a class III antiarrhythmic such as **sotalol or amiodarone** (without preservatives, since otherwise there is a risk of an anaphylactic reaction when administered IV) should be considered, or, if not available, esmolol (β-blocker, class II antiarrhythmic). If pharmacologic cardioversion is not effective and there is concern for the patient's life, **electrical cardioversion with a defibrillator should be considered**.

However, in most cases when the animals present with ventricular tachycardia, they are stable enough (without signs of significant hypoperfusion or weakness) and do not to require emergency intravenous antiarrhythmic treatment. In these cases, **oral antiarrhythmic medication is recommended to initiate treatment**. The most commonly used drugs are **mexiletine** (class I antiarrhythmic), **β-blockers** (class II anti-arrhythmics), **sotalol or amiodarone** (class III antiarrhythmics).

When a single antiarrhythmic agent is insufficient to achieve adequate control of ventricular arrhythmias, **agents can be combined** (although never two agents from the same group of antiarrhythmics). **Sotalol and mexiletine** have a synergistic antiarrhythmic effect when combined, so this combination may be considered in those patients in whom a single antiarrhythmic agent is insufficient to control ventricular arrhythmias. It is important to remember β-blockers are not usually recommended in patients with systolic dysfunction and are contraindicated in patients with congestive heart failure. Also, lidocaine use should be avoided in cats, since they are very sensitive and the development of toxicity, accumulation and negative haemodynamic effects are common. The lidocaine dosages provided are for dogs.

Ventricular Flutter/Fibrillation

This arrhythmia is almost always associated with cardiac arrest. Ventricular depolarization waves are chaotic, so there is insufficient coordinated contraction to generate a stroke volume. In these cases, cardiopulmomary resuscitation should be initiated (the treatment of choice is electrical cardioversion with a defibrillator), but even so the success rate in animals is usually low. During ventricular fibrillation, the ECG is characterised by the presence of **fast, irregular, wide and bizarre or fine baseline waves without normal waves or complexes**.

Conduction System Disturbances

Conduction system disturbances include bradyarrhythmias such as sinus arrest and block, AV nodal block, and atrial arrest; those abnormalities explained in previous sections (bradyarrhythmias) are not repeated here. This section also includes **sick sinus syndrome and intraventricular conduction defects**.

Sick Sinus Syndrome

Sick sinus syndrome has breed predisposition including the **West Highland White Terrier, Miniature Schnauzers, and Terriers in general**, although any breed can present this pathology. There is a **widespread pathology of the conduction tissue of the heart** which can lead to its dysfunction. It usually produces bradyarrhythmia such as bradycardia and severe sinus arrest with failure to generate an escape rhythm. Some patients, in addition to bradyarrhythmia, also have supraventricular arrhythmias such as supraventricular tachycardia. In these cases, it is called **tachy-bradyarrhythmia syndrome**.

ECG characteristics are variable and include **persistent sinus bradycardia, prolonged episodes of sinus arrest, and/or second-degree AV blocks**, not followed by a rescue escape rhythm (Figure 20). In tachy-bradyarrhythmia syndrome, periods of bradyarrhythmia alternate with supraventricular tachycardia (Figure 20). In these patients, the bradyarrhythmia does not respond or has a partial response to atropine administration.

Patients with this pathology usually present symptoms associated with bradyarrhythmia and, less commonly, with tachyarrhythmia. The most common **clinical signs are weakness** including episodes of syncope or presyncope, and exercise intolerance.

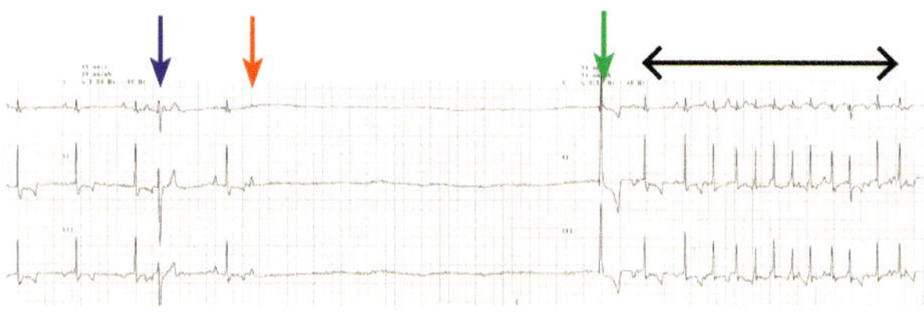

Figure 20. ECG including bipolar leads (I, II and III) from a dog with sick sinus syndrome (50 mm/s and 20 mm/mV). A blocked P wave is present (second-degree AV block) (red arrow) followed by a period of sinus arrest interrupted by a ventricular escape complex (green arrow). A short period of supraventricular tachycardia is also present (black arrow) as well as a premature ventricular complex (blue arrow).

The treatment of choice for symptomatic animals is **permanent pacemaker implantation** since medical treatment does not usually achieve sufficient control of arrhythmias or clinical signs. Occasionally, in patients with tachy-bradyarrhythmia, in addition to pacemakers, the use of antiarrhythmic agents to control periods of supraventricular tachycardia are necessary. If necessary, this would only be undertaken after pacemaker implantation, as treating tachyarrhythmias with antiarrhythmic agents would worsen bradyarrhythmia and increase the risk of sudden death for the patient.

Intraventricular Conduction Defects

The electrical impulse of the heart is generated in the sinus node and travels through the internodal tracts to the atrioventricular (AV) node. The base of the ventricular septum is then depolarised through the **bundle of His**. The bundle of His divides into the right and left branches, which conduct the electrical impulse to the right and left ventricle respectively. In turn, the left branch is subdivided into the anterior and posterior fascicles. When one or more of these conduction tissues present a conduction block it is called a **bundle branch block**. Isolated simple bundle branch blocks do not pose significant haemodynamic problems and, therefore, do not need to be treated.

The **most common intraventricular conduction defects** in small animals are the following.

- **Right bundle branch block**: this is due to a conduction block through the right bundle branch. Depolarization of the left ventricle is normal, but the right ventricle depolarizes cell by cell, causing a delay in conduction at this level, giving rise to a **prolongued QRS complex**. Therefore, the ECG is characterised by the presence of prolonged QRS complexes (>0.07 seconds) with deep S waves (negative) on leads I, II, III and aVF, and a positive QRS complex on aVR and aVL (Figure 21). The mean electrical axis (MEA) is deviated to the right. It is important to differentiate between right bundle branch block and the pattern of right ventricular enlargement. The right branch is more susceptible to injury than the left. Right bundle branch block is found in healthy animals, but can also be associated with the presence of cardiac disease or cardiac trauma.
- **Left bundle branch block**: this is due to a conduction block through the left bundle branch. The depolarization of the right ventricle is normal, but the left ventricle depolarizes cell by cell producing a delay in conduction at this level resulting in an increased duration of the QRS complexes. The ECG is characterised by the presence of wide QRS complexes (>0.07 seconds) with positive complexes on leads I, II, III, and aVF, and negative QRS complexes on aVR and aVL (Figure 22). This must be distinguished from a left ventricular enlargement pattern. Left bundle branch block, unlike right bundle branch block, is **rare in healthy animals** and is usually associated with cardiac disease, myocardial ischaemia, cardiac neoplasia, or trauma.

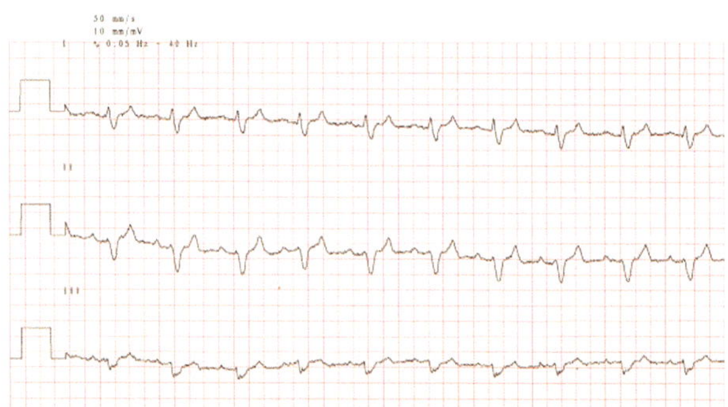

Figure 21. ECG including bipolar leads (I, II and III) showing a normal sinus rhythm with aberrant ventricular conduction due to the presence of a right bundle branch block (50 mm/s and 10 mm/mV). Normal P waves followed by wide QRS complexes, with deep S waves are present.

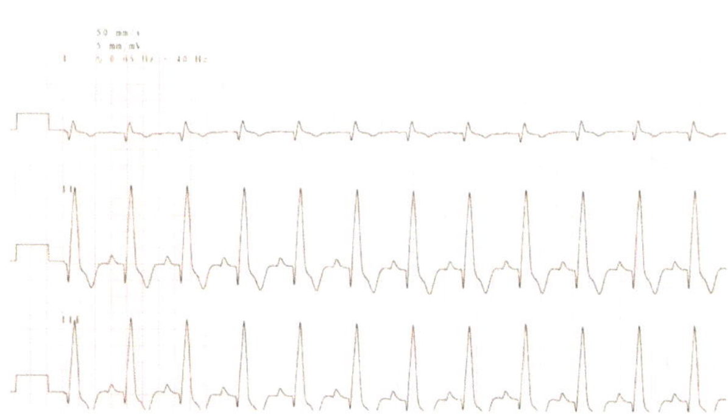

Figure 22. ECG including bipolar leads (I, II and III) showing a normal sinus rhythm with aberrant ventricular conduction due to the presence of a left bundle branch block (50 mm/s and 5 mm/mV). Normal P waves followed by positive, wide QRS complexes are present.

– **Left anterior fascicular block**: due to a conduction failure through the anterior fascicle of the left branch. It is found more frequently in cats than dogs, and its presence is suggestive of **cardiomyopathy**. The ECG is characterised by QRS complexes with a normal duration with positive R waves on leads I and aVL and deep S waves on leads II, III, and aVF. The MEA deviates to the left (Figure 23).

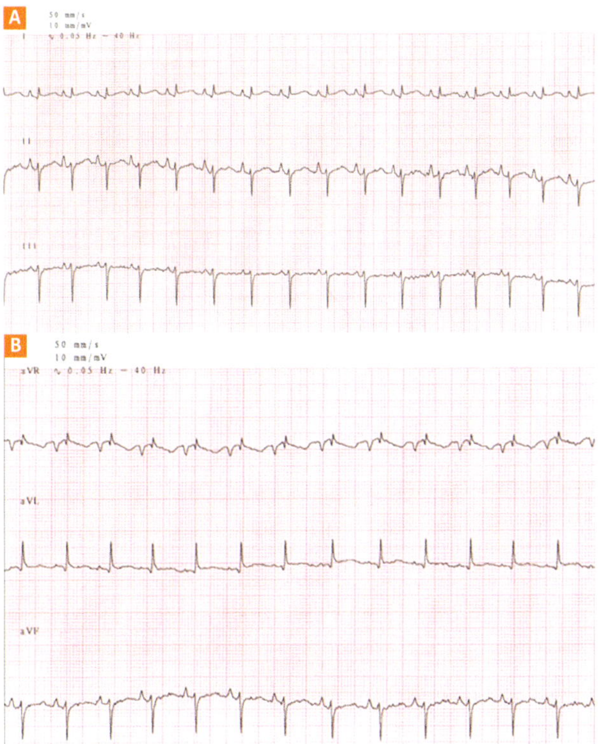

Figure 23. ECG including bipolar (**A**) and unipolar (**B**) leads in a cat showing sinus rhythm with left anterior fascicular block (50 mm/s and 10 mm/mV). Deep S waves are present on leads II, III and aVF and positive QRS complexes on leads I and aVL.

Antiarrhythmic Drugs

There are several classification systems for antiarrhythmic drugs. The most widely used in veterinary medicine divides these drugs into **four classes** according to the channels and/or receptors they affect.

Class I Antiarrhythmics

Inhibit fast sodium channels causing depression of phase 0 of the action potential. These drugs are classified into three subclasses according to their effect on the duration of the repolarization time.

Class IA (Quinidine, Procainamide)

This class depresses phase 0 of the action potential while prolonging its duration with a mild class III effect. They can have a **proarrhythmic effect** by prolonging the QT interval and/or depressing conduction and cause re-entry arrhythmias. In veterinary medicine, quinidine is used to treat atrial fibrillation in horses.

Class IB (Lidocaine, Mexiletine)

At the same time as inhibiting fast sodium channels, class IB drugs decrease the duration of the action potential in healthy tissue (there is no prolongation of the QT interval). These drugs **act selectively in diseased or ischaemic tissues**, inducing conduction blockages and thus interrupting re-entry circuits.

In veterinary medicine, **lidocaine is the emergency drug of choice for the treatment of ventricular tachycardia**. In cardiology the injectable form is used without additional adrenaline (used for local vasoconstriction in its use as a local anaesthetic). Lidocaine has a fast-acting effect, but of intermediate duration, a characteristic that determines its use. In case of haemodynamically significant sustained ventricular tachycardia, **intravenous boluses of 2 mg/kg are recommended**, with a maximum of four boluses (8 mg/kg dose), followed by continuous intravenous infusion. Side effects include hypotension, bradycardia, vomiting, and neurological effects (epileptiform seizures that require treatment with intravenous diazepam).

Mexiletine is similar to lidocaine, but in an **oral form**, so it is often used in patients with ventricular tachycardia that responded to intravenous lidocaine. In **combination with sotalol** it has a synergistic antiarrhythmic effect. Unfortunately, there are problems with the distribution of this medication as in many countries it has been withdrawn from the human market. Some studies suggest that some supraventricular tachycardias, such as macro-re-entrant circuits (or accessory pathways), may respond to treatment with lidocaine and/or mexiletine.

Class IC (Flecainide)

Class IC drugs are powerful inhibitors of fast sodium channels, markedly depressing phase 0 of the action potential, with a **powerful depression of conduction**. This effect predisposes the development of electrical heterogeneity which, in turn, has a proarrhythmic effect. In medicine they are used in supraventricular and ventricular tachyarrhythmias which do not respond to other treatments. Information regarding the use of these drugs in veterinary medicine is limited.

Class II Antiarrhythmics

β-blocking or β-adrenergic antagonist agents. This group of antiarrhythmic agents acts on adrenergic receptors in the heart, mainly β1, found in the sinus and atrioventricular nodes and in the ventricles. Effects include the reduction of myocardial oxygen consumption (due to a decrease in heart rate) and improving coronary perfusion. They are **the treatment of choice in arrhythmias caused by excess sympathetic stimulation**, for both ventricular and supraventricular arrhythmias. They have a negative inotropic effect that can significantly depress the heart's systolic function and, therefore, are contraindicated in patients with heart failure and are usually avoided when there is systolic dysfunction.

Treatment with β-blockers should be started at the low end of the dose range, and increased gradually (for example, over one to two weeks) until the desired effect or dose is achieved. During this period, the patient should be monitored closely. Bradycardia, weakness, and/or depression are side effects due to the excessive effects of the β-blocker. If these effects are observed, the dose should be decreased (if these effects occur when starting treatment with low doses, more gradual increases in dose should be attempted). Similarly, **these agents should not be stopped abruptly**, but the dose gradually tapered.

They are sub-classified according to the type of receptors they affect.

- **First generation** or non-selective β-blockers (propranolol, esmolol): block β1 and 2 receptors.
- **Second generation** or selective β-blockers (atenolol): relatively selective blockers of β1 receptors.
- **Third generation** (carvedilol): block β and α1 receptors. Carvedilol, in addition to an antiarrhythmic effect, has vasodilator properties mediated by the release of nitric oxide and the blockade of α1 adrenergic receptors.

Class III Antiarrhythmics

Potassium channel inhibitors. These agents increase the duration of the action potential and the refractory period and therefore **prolong the QT interval**. In the presence of hypokalaemia, hypomagnesaemia, or bradycardia, QT prolongation predisposes to torsades de pointes. In addition to their class III effect, both amiodarone and sotalol also have properties of other classes of antiarrhythmic drugs.

Sotalol is a class III antiarrhythmic (potassium channel inhibitor) which also possesses class II activity (β-blocker, approximately one third of the effect of propranolol). It is a racemic mixture of dextro- and levo- sotalol: dextro-sotalol has class III activity and the levo- isomer has class II activity. It is used for **supraventricular** (atrial fibrillation, atrial flutter, supraventricular tachycardia) and **ventricular arrhythmias**. In addition to QT prolongation, side effects include bradycardia, hypotension, depression, etc. It should be used with caution in patients with renal failure, as it is a water-soluble drug with renal excretion. It should also be used with caution in patients with myocardial dysfunction, as it can induce congestive heart failure due to its negative inotropic effect.

Amiodarone belongs to class III and blocks potassium channels. However, it also exhibits class I (sodium channel inhibitor) effects, with additional class II and IV (β-blocker and calcium channel blocker) effects. This medication is highly fat-soluble and has a prolonged half-life, so it can **take months to achieve a stable concentration** in the blood. It accumulates in liver and lungs, metabolised in the liver and excreted through the skin, tears, and bile. Like the rest of the class III antiarrhythmics, it can cause QT prolongation and lead to torsades de pointes type malignant ventricular arrhythmias. In addition, it has several important side effects (hepatotoxic properties, thyroid function alteration, and anaphylactic reactions with the IV formulation with preservatives).

It is used to treat **supraventricular** (atrial fibrillation, atrial flutter, supraventricular tachycardia) and **ventricular arrhythmias**, but due to side effects with long-term use, it is usually reserved for patients with severe ventricular arrhythmias or those refractory to other antiarrhythmics. It has also been successfully used to reverse patients with spontaneous atrial fibrillation to sinus rhythm. Due to its potential hepatotoxic effect and alteration of thyroid function, **blood tests should be undertaken before using amiodarone** to assess thyroid and liver function.

Class IV Antiarrhythmics

Calcium channel blockers. **Diltiazem and verapamil** belong to this group of antiarrhythmic agents. In addition to their antiarrhythmic effect, they have a negative inotropic effect (weaker than that of β-blocking agents), which should be monitored when used in animals with decreased systolic function. Calcium channel blockers belonging to the dihydropyridines group have a greater affinity for vascular tissue than for cardiac tissue and are used for the treatment of systemic hypertension (e.g. amlodipine).

Non-dihydropyridine blockers are those with affinity for cardiac tissue and exert their effect on the calcium channels of the sinus and atrioventricular nodes. It is the negative dromotropic effect (they slow down the conduction of the electrical impulse) that is used for the **treatment of tachyarrhythmias**, mainly of supraventricular origin (atrial fibrillation, supraventricular tachycardia, atrial flutter).

Other Antiarrhythmic Agents

Digoxin, a glycoside agent, exerts its action by inhibiting the Na^+/K^+ ATPase pump which secondarily increases intracardiac calcium concentration and the force of contraction (positive inotropic effect). As an antiarrhythmic it acts on the vagal centres and increases the sensitivity to parasympathetic stimulation at a cardiac level, thus reducing heart rate and speed of conduction through the atrioventricular node.

Although previously used as a positive inotrope in veterinary medicine, there are currently more effective products with fewer side effects (such as **pimobendan**). Its main use is the treatment of atrial fibrillation, to control ventricular rate. Sometimes it is combined with other antiarrhythmic agents for optimal control of ventricular rate during atrial fibrillation. A study carried out by Gelzer and colleagues suggests the combination of digoxin with diltiazem for the treatment of atrial fibrillation achieves better heart rate control than the use of either of these drugs alone.

Digoxin has a half-life of over 24 hours, so it takes about **a week to reach a stable concentration** in the blood. Its bioavailability is variable, depending on the format (tablets 60%, syrup 75%). Although partially metabolised by the liver, its main route of excretion is renal, so **it should be used with caution in patients with kidney disease** or failure. It has a **narrow therapeutic index**, with proarrhythmogenic side effects associated with toxicity (ventricular arrhythmias induced by increased intracellular calcium, AV blocks, bradycardia, etc.), plus gastrointestinal (anorexia, vomiting, diarrhoea) and neurological (depression) effects. In the event of suspected toxicity, the medication should be discontinued and blood digoxin levels evaluated. In addition, **renal function and electrolytes should be tested** prior to starting digoxin administration, since hypokalaemia exacerbates the toxic effects of digoxin. In geriatric, cachectic or animals with effusions (ascites, pleural effusion), digoxin should be used with caution since they present a greater risk of reaching a toxic dose.

As this agent has a narrow therapeutic index, its use must be accompanied by monitoring of serum levels. To do this, approximately a week after starting digoxin therapy, a blood sample should be obtained 6–8 hours after its administration to measure the serum concentration.

Electrical Therapy: Pacemaker Implantation

Pacemaker implantation is the **technique of choice in the treatment of arrhythmias**, which due to a severe reduction in heart rate **do not maintain adequate cardiac output and endanger the patient's life**. The implantation of the permanent pacemaker in the dog is a lifesaving technique, with a survival rate of 70–86% one year after implantation, 57–65% after 2 years and 39% after 3 years.

Pathologic bradyarrhythmias that require electrical treatment are generally due to abnormalities in impulse formation in the sinus node or to disorders involving sinoatrial, intra-atrial, or atrioventricular conduction.

The most common veterinary pathologies that require pacemaker implantation are **sinus dysfunction** (sick sinus syndrome), **atrial standstill, and advanced second-degree and third-degree atrioventricular blocks**.

The most common symptoms in patients with these arrhythmias are **weakness, exercise intolerance, and syncope**. Symptoms, in most cases, are associated with either a low ventricular rate (atrioventricular blocks) or long episodes of sinus and ventricular pauses (sick sinus syndrome). The persistence of abnormally low heart rates over time can lead to so-called arrhythmia-induced cardiomyopathy. A sustained low ventricular rate activates a series of pathophysiological mechanisms (neurohormonal activation, metabolic changes, etc.) in the myocardium causing myocardial dysfunction and lead to different degrees of heart failure. In some cases, signs are evident of left-sided congestive heart failure (such as pulmonary oedema) or right-sided congestive heart failure (such as ascites or pleural effusion). The phenomenon may be reversible depending on the duration of the arrhythmia and the myocardial damage caused. In these cases, the pacemaker makes it possible to artificially restore the average heart rate needed by each patient.

A pacemaker may be useful for other rhythm disorders such as neurally mediated syncope, which is a transient loss of consciousness due to an inadequate vasovagal reflex. Different stimuli (vomiting, coughing, excitement, etc.) generate this reflex arc which is characterised by an increase in parasympathetic tone and a decrease in sympathetic tone, inducing a progressive decrease in heart rate, sinus pauses, and vasodilation. The combination of both phenomena leads to a temporary decrease in cerebral perfusion with the consequent loss of consciousness. In this case, the pacemaker makes it possible to maintain a minimum heart rate during the episodes of syncope and avoid or reduce the duration of loss of consciousness.

Another use for pacemakers is the case of **cardiac resynchronization**. This technique is used in supraventricular arrhythmias which do not respond to medical treatment and cannot be treated by radiofrequency ablation. In this case, the atrioventricular node is ablated to achieve atrioventricular dissociation to prevent the supraventricular rhythm from activating the ventricle. To maintain an adequate ventricular rate, the pacemaker is implanted and programmed based on the patient's needs.

Equipment

The pacemaker is a closed circuit composed of an impulse generator and a lead with an electrode in direct contact with the cardiac chamber to be stimulated.

Electric Pulse Generator

The generator consists of a long-life lithium battery which emits pulses to **provide the electrical activity necessary to stimulate the myocardium** (Figure 24). This energy travels through the lead to the myocardium, stimulates it, and finally returns to the generator, completing the electrical circuit (Figure 25). In addition, the lead allows detection of the intrinsic electrical activity of the myocardium. This **dual role of pacemakers** is known as pacing followed by capture (depolarization of the myocardium) and detection (identification of the intrinsic activity of the heart).

Conduction Leads

Leads are classified according to **fixation type** (epicardial/endocardial, active/passive), **length, shape, and polarity** (unipolar/bipolar).

The lead fixation type is determined by the type of implant and positioning of the lead. Implantation of the pacemaker may be **endocavitary** through vascular access such as the jugular (Figure 26) or epicardial vein by **thoracotomy or transdiaphragmatic** access (Figure 27).

The latter technique was used in the first pacemakers described in veterinary medicine. Subsequently it has been replaced by the **endocavitary implant**, as it is less invasive. Currently, the epicardial implant is reserved for special situations such as the replacement of a contaminated endovascular implant or implants in the feline species or exotic animals such as the ferret. Each implant technique requires a specific type of lead.

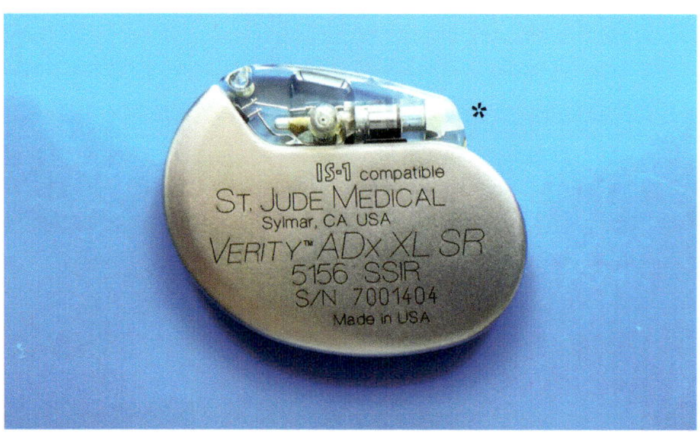

Figure 24. Mono-chamber pacemaker generator. The asterisk indicates the point of lead attachment.

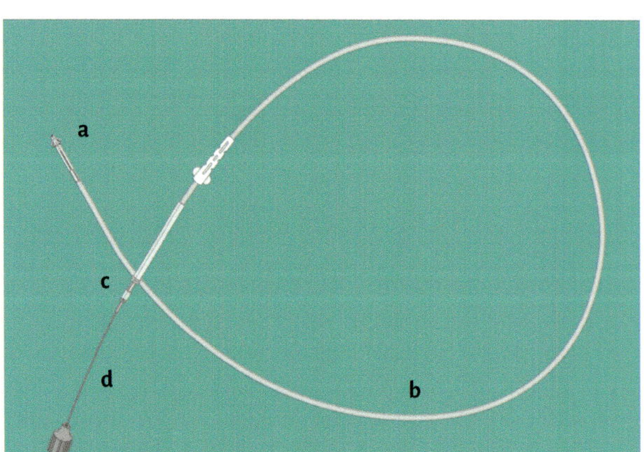

Figure 25. Ventricular lead with passive type fixation: (a) tip, (b) body, (c) connection portion and (d) stylet.

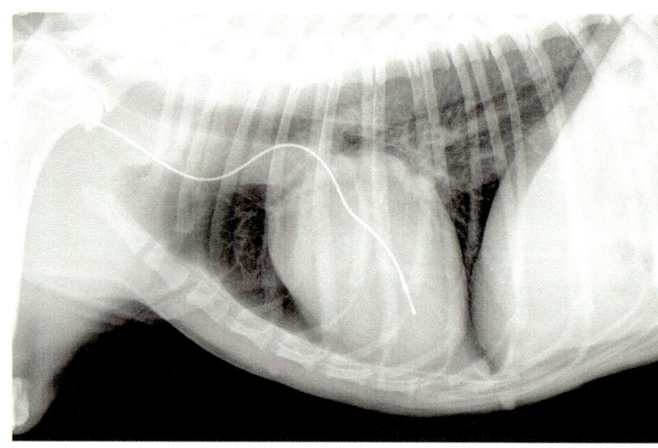

Figure 26. Thoracic radiograph (right lateral projection) in a patient with an endocavitary single-chamber pacemaker.

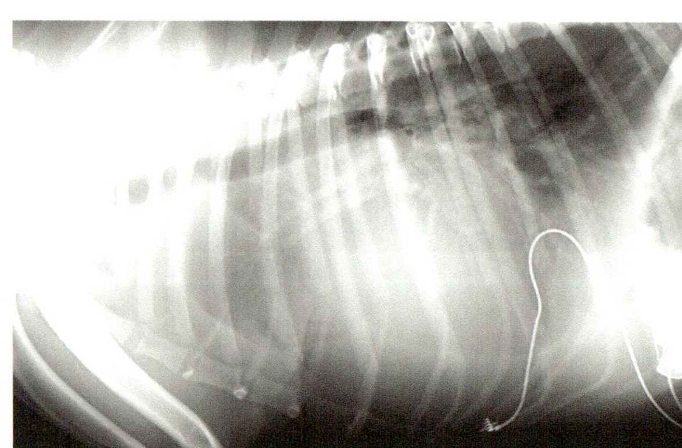

Figure 27. Thoracic radiograph (right lateral projection) in a patient with an epicardial pacemaker. In this case the surgical approach was transdiaphragmatic and the battery is placed in the abdominal wall. (Courtesy of Dr Roberto Santilli).

Fixation to the myocardium is determined by the type of tip on the lead and can be **passive or active** depending on which anchorage to the myocardium is more or less traumatic (Figure 28).

- **Active fixation leads feature a helix tip** that is fixed and penetrates directly into the myocardium.
- **Passive fixation leads have a tip with pins or wings** that attaches to the myocardial trabeculae.

The length is determined by the brand and the selection of one size, or another is determined by the size of the patient. Depending on the anatomical position of the lead and to facilitate fixation, there are different types of leads, such as the J-shaped lead for the atrium.

Lastly, the **leads can be monopolar or bipolar** depending on the type of electrode positioned at the tip of the lead.

- Monopolar electrodes are characterised by the cathode positioned at the tip of the lead and the anode at the generator.
- Bipolar electrodes, on the other hand, have both the anode and the cathode at the tip of the lead.

The drawback of monopolar electrodes is that, since the poles are further apart, the electrical circuit is subject to the greater effects of extracardiac electrical potentials and suffers more interference. On the other hand, the circuit is completed on the surface of the body so stimulation can result in involuntary movements of the neck muscles.

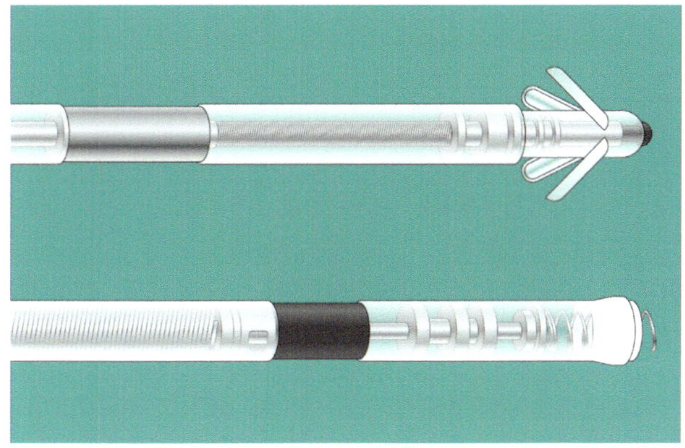

Figure 28. Tips of ventricular leads: passive fixation (above) and active fixation (below).

Pacemaker Control System

To program and assess pacemaker function, a **telemetry system** is connected to programming software (Figure 29) which allows external control of the pacemaker in a non-invasive, comfortable way. During implantation of the pacemaker, an alternative telemetry system called the **PSA module (pacing system analyzer)** is used, which offers the option for analysis of the endocardial electrocardiogram and direct stimulation through the lead before fixing it to the generator (Figure 30).

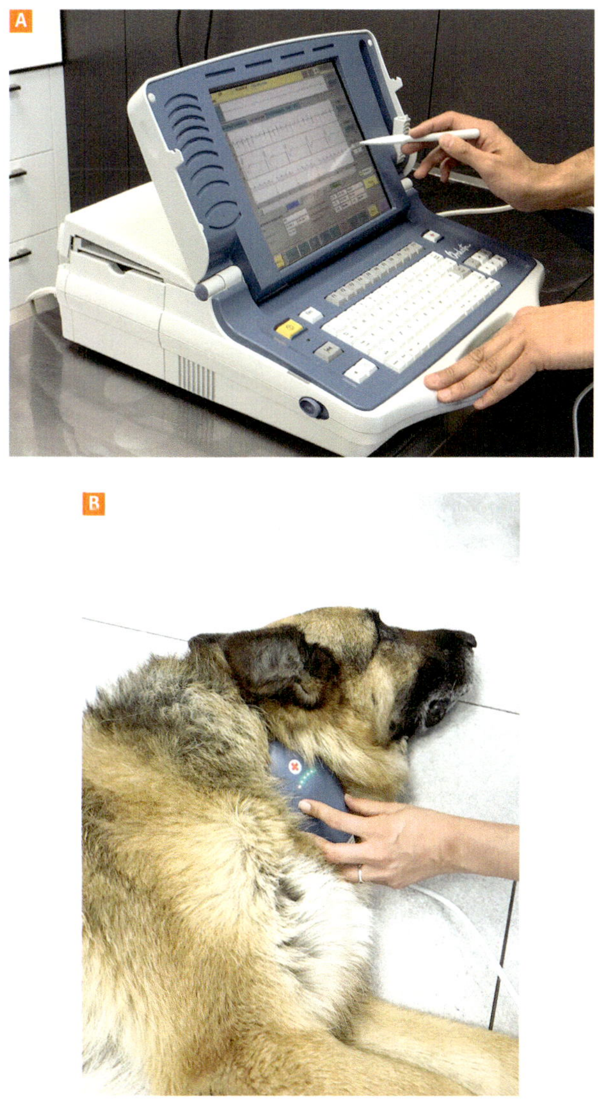

Figure 29. Telemetric programming of a pacemaker: programming (**A**) and magnet positioned on the patient's neck (**B**).

Temporary Pacemakers

Patients undergoing pacemaker implantation are generally unstable and present a **high anaesthetic risk**. In these cases, use of a temporary pacemaker during the preoperative and operative period is important (Figure 31). Depending on the location of the electrodes, temporary cardiac stimulation can be transvenous, epicardial, transcutaneous, transoesophageal, or transgastric.

Transvenous stimulation was widely used in veterinary medicine in the past. With the aid of a fluoroscope, the lead is positioned in the right ventricle through a venous access through the femoral vein and then connected to a generator. The epicardial technique requires a thoracotomy to position the electrode on the epicardium. Recently, both have been replaced by less invasive techniques such as **transoesophageal, transgastric, or transcutaneous stimulation.** Transoesophageal stimulation allows correct atrial stimulation, but transgastric ventricular stimulation does not, which seems to be less effective in the dog. Transcutaneous stimulation is a simple technique in which energy is released through special patches placed on the skin of the thorax.

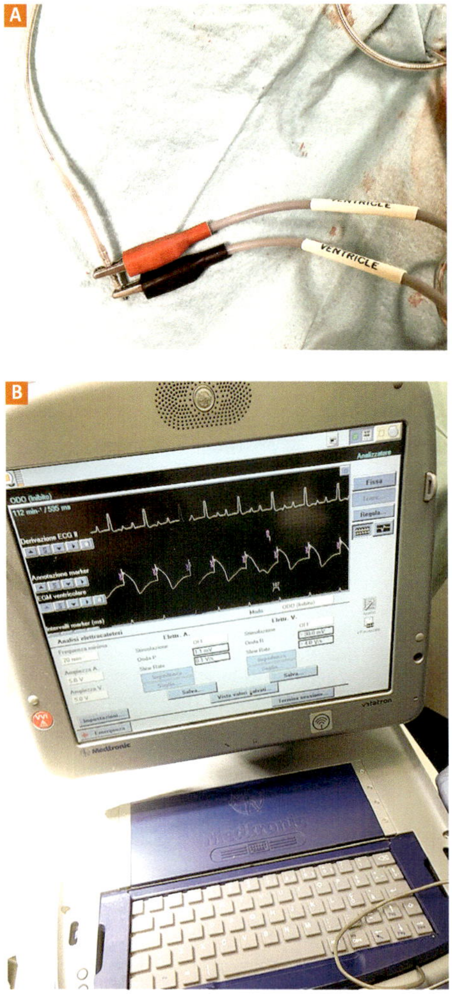

Figure 30. Analysis of an endocavitary electrocardiogram using a PSA module: connection of the pacemaker lead to the PSA module (**A**) and the PSA module (**B**).

Electrophysiological Principles of Pacemaker Stimulation

The energy required to depolarize the myocardium and create an electrical impulse depends on the stimulus released by the pacemaker. The energy of the stimulus is related to the **intensity of the current or voltage (volts), the duration of the stimulus (milliseconds)** and the **resistance to the flow of energy** generated by the pacemaker material itself and the tissues (called impedance-ohms). The combination of all these parameters is the basis for correct myocardial stimulation and optimization of other parameters, such as the duration of the generator battery.

The basic principle of successful pacemaker stimulation is to **use the minimum energy** required to achieve effective depolarization of the myocardium to maintain correct cardiac output and **extend battery life as long as possible**. The greater the current intensity or duration of the stimulus, the greater the battery consumption. Similarly, higher impedance (for example, by the presence of abundant scar tissue around the tip of the lead or breakage of the lead) requires higher energy consumption by the battery.

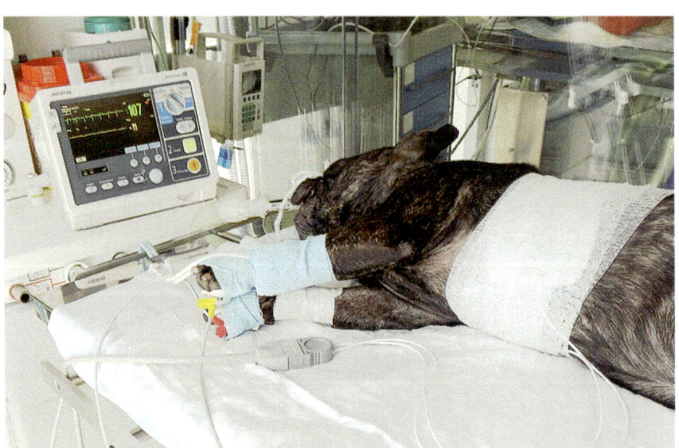

Figure 31. Temporary transcutaneous pacemaker with positioning of thoracic patches.

Type of Pacemaker

Different types of pacemakers are available, and the appropriate choice is determined by the arrhythmic disorder present, the patient and economic limitations (in veterinary medicine). **The objective is to achieve a normal atrioventricular activation sequence** (synchronous pacing) and to minimize the haemodynamic abnormalities of chronic artificial pacing (pacemaker syndrome).

Pacemakers are divided according to the cardiac chambers that stimulate the leads that compose them and the mode of generator stimulation and detection.

- **Single chamber**: the lead is positioned in a single cardiac chamber (atrium or right ventricle).
- **Dual chamber**: two leads are positioned in different cardiac chambers (atrium and right ventricle).
- **Triple chamber**: three paced cardiac chambers (right atrium, right ventricle, and left ventricle).

In turn, pacemakers are classified according to the **pacing and detection modality**, following the letter code developed by the North American Society of Pacing and Electrophysiology (NASPE) and the British Pacing and Electrophysiology Group (BPEG) (Table 1).

The sequence of letters is defined as follows:

1. the cardiac chamber being paced
2. the cardiac chamber sensed
3. the pacemaker's response to a detected stimulus
4. the pacemaker's ability to increase the heart rate in response to physical activity
5. whether or not the anti-tachycardia option is activated.

Table 1. Pacemaker classification by pacing and detection modality, according to the NASPE and BPEG code.

I	II	III	IV	V
Chamber(s) paced	**Chamber(s) sensed**	**Response to sensing**	**Rate adaptive**	**Anti-tachycardia**
O None	**O** None	**O** None	**O** No	**O** No
A Atrium	**A** Atrium	**T** Triggered	**R** Rate modulation	**P** Pacing
V Ventricle	**V** Ventricle	**I** Inhibited		**S** Shock
D Dual	**D** Dual	**D** Dual		**D** Dual

Stimulation Modalities

The most common stimulation modalities in veterinary medicine are **single-chamber or dual chamber stimulation**:

Single-chamber Pacing

A single lead stimulates and receives stimuli from the same cardiac chamber. There are two types.

- **AAI**
  - Characteristics: a single wire positioned in the right atrium senses the intrinsic activity of the atrium and stimulates only when this is absent.
  - Indications: in patients with abnormal sinus node function and normal atrioventricular conduction (for example, in cases of sick sinus syndrome).
- **VVI**
  - Characteristics: a single lead positioned at the apex of the right ventricle records the intrinsic activity of the right ventricle and paces when this is absent or below the limit at which the pacemaker has been programmed (Figure 32).
  - Indications: in patients with atrioventricular conduction abnormalities (such as atrioventricular block), atrial myocardial pathologies or as an alternative modality to AAI in cases of sinus dysfunction.

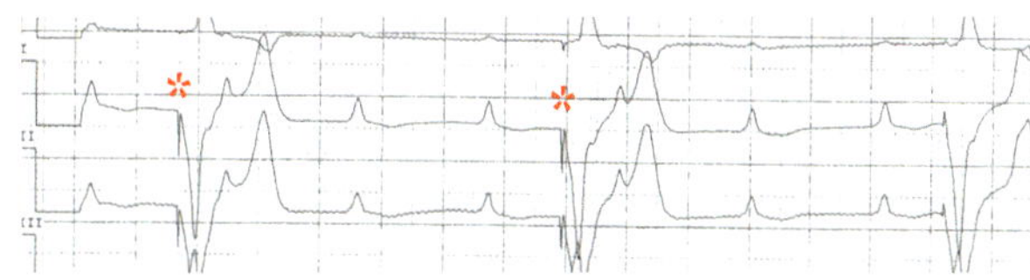

Figure 32. Surface electrocardiogram from a dog with third-degree atrioventricular block and a pacemaker in VVIR mode (lead II). The asterisks show the spicules generated by the pacemaker followed by ventricular stimulation (QRS complex). P waves appear dissociated from ventricular complexes. (Courtesy of Dr Roberto Santilli).

Heart rate may vary during pacing and may not be a fixed rate. Using the adaptive response option (R), thanks to the motion sensors which all generators have, the pacemaker discharge heart rate increases depending on the patient's physical activity. The pacing modality is called **AAIR or VVIR**.

Another feature that can be programmed into single chamber pacemakers is **hysteresis.** Rate hysteresis consists of **delaying the onset of pacemaker activation to promote the patient's intrinsic activity**. For this, a minimum rate is programmed below the base pacemaker rate. Periodically, the pacemaker reduces the pacing rate to the hysteresis rate. If there is a proper rhythm, the pacemaker is inhibited, and the dominant rhythm is the patient's natural rhythm. To the contrary, if the hysteresis frequency is reached and there is no physiological rhythm, the pacemaker is activated. This modality encourages the patient's natural rhythm to be present for as long as possible without endangering their life (Figure 33).

Dual-chamber pacing

One or two leads record activity and stimulate either one or two cardiac chambers.

- **VDD**
  - Characteristics: a single lead is positioned at the apex of the right ventricle. This lead has a sensor in the portion that remains floating in the right atrium, which detects activity in this chamber and consequently stimulates the ventricle with a predetermined atrioventricular conduction time (Figure 34).

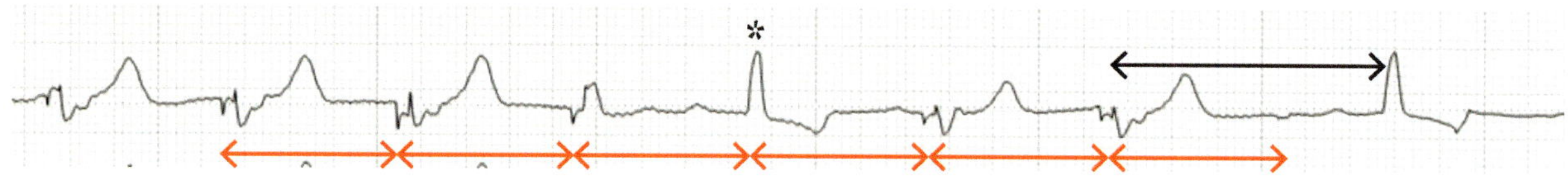

Figure 33. Surface electrocardiogram from a dog with a pacemaker in VVIR mode and chamber hysteresis (lead II). The arrow heads indicate the beats stimulated by the pacemaker (small spicules followed by aberrant ventricular complexes) with a constant rate of 60 bpm or cycle length of 1000 ms (red arrows). Pacing is inhibited when the pacemaker senses a sinus beat (asterisk), and pacing continues again until a new sinus beat interrupts it. In this case the interval between paced beats and sinus beats is greater because hysteresis has been programmed at 40 bpm (1500 ms) to favour the intrinsic rhythm. (Courtesy of Dr Roberto Santilli).

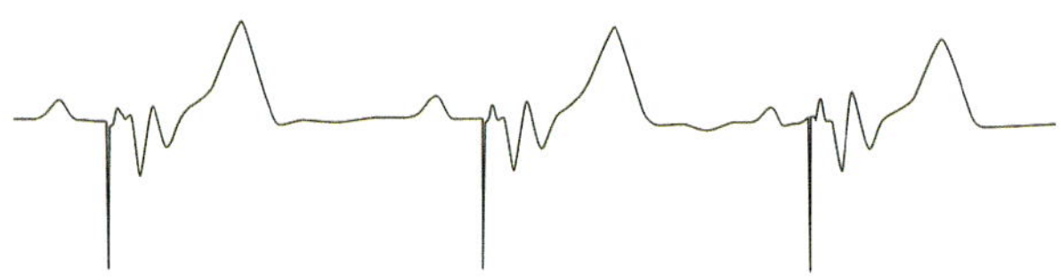

Figure 34. Surface electrocardiogram from a dog with a pacemaker in VDD mode. An intrinsic atrial rhythm (P wave) followed by spicules and the corresponding pacing of the ventricle represented by the QRS complex. (Courtesy of Dr Roberto Santilli).

In the absence of atrial activity, the ventricular electrode maintains the pacing rate. Similarly, the ventricular electrode inhibits pacing when it detects intrinsic ventricular activity.

- Indications: patients with atrioventricular conduction pathologies and normal sinus function (for example, atrioventricular block).

– **DDD**

- Characteristics: one lead is positioned in the right atrium and the other in the apex of the right ventricle (Figure 35). Function is similar to the VDD modality, but here the atrial lead records atrial activity and if absent stimulates it and guides the stimulus to the ventricular lead.
- Indications: patients with atrioventricular conduction pathologies and abnormal sinus function.

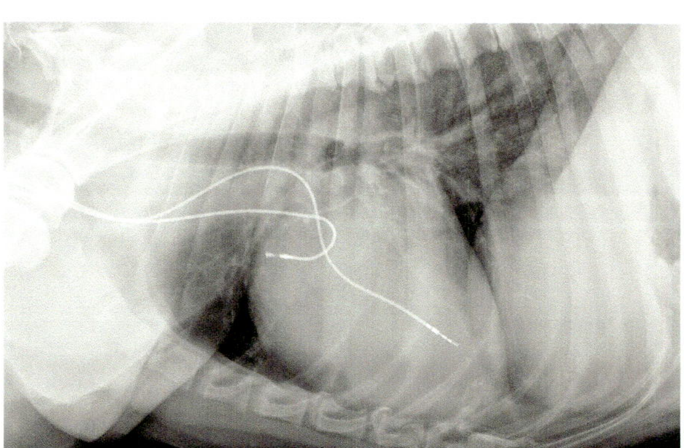

Figure 35. Thoracic radiograph (right lateral projection) in a patient with a dual chamber endocardial pacemaker.

Surgical Technique

The patient should be positioned in right or left **lateral recumbency**, depending on whether the implantation is via the left or right external jugular vein. The right jugular vein is recommended in case a vascular anomaly called persistent left cranial vena cava is present. This defect makes implantation difficult, since the abnormal vessel drains directly into the right atrium through the coronary sinus, making access to the right ventricle complicated.

The jugular vein is isolated through a surgical incision in the middle third of the neck (Figure 36). Cannulation of the vein is performed via venotomy or by using a special 8 Fr Peel-Away introducer using the Seldinger technique (Figure 37). The introducer technique is useful to position the leads of dual chamber pacemakers because it allows greater control in the movement of each lead and avoids friction between them. The lead should then be inserted; leads have a catch which gives a certain rigidity, shape, and facilitates their movement. The stylet should be removed, as the lead passes into the cardiac chambers to prevent the stiffened lead from perforating the myocardium. **Lead positioning should be carried out under fluoroscopic visualization** using different projections (lateral and dorsoventral).

Once the lead is in position, it is important to confirm that it is in the correct location by analysis of the endocavitary electrocardiogram and performing tests for the detection and pacing threshold with the PSA module. The endocavitary electrocardiogram detected at the level of the right ventricle shows a wide QRS complex with an R wave amplitude greater than 20 mV, a recording speed (dV/dt, change in amplitude with respect to time) of 4 V/s and a marked elevation of the ST-segment secondary to myocardial ischaemia (current of injury) (Figure 38).

Ischaemic damage is transitory, lasting approximately 10 minutes, and indicates a correct contact between the tip of the lead with the myocardium. Next, a stimulation test should be performed, which must present a threshold between 0.25 and 0.5 V. In the case of the P wave, the amplitude must be greater than 1.5 mV, the recording rate greater than 3 V/s, and the capture threshold between 0.25 and 0.5 V.

To check the correct fixation of the lead, (for leads with passive fixation), they should be pulled gently. With active fixation leads applying pressure to the endocardium with the tip is necessary and then, using a fixation tool, the proximal portion of the lead should be rotated clockwise until the helical tip is inserted into the endocardium. Finally, when the lead is correctly positioned, the stylet should be removed, and the lead attached to the jugular vein.

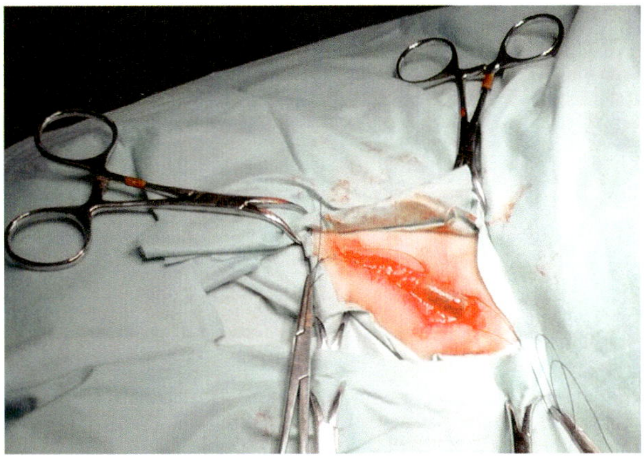

Figure 36. Surgical isolation of the left external jugular vein in a dog for pacemaker implantation.

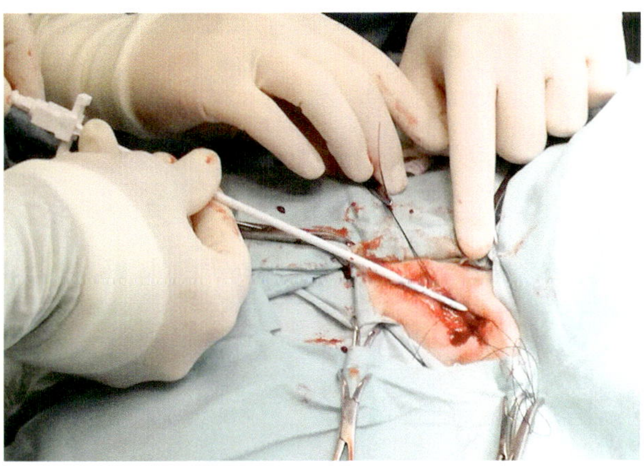

Figure 37. Cannulation of the left jugular vein in a dog using an 8 Fr Peel-Away type introducer with the Seldinger technique.

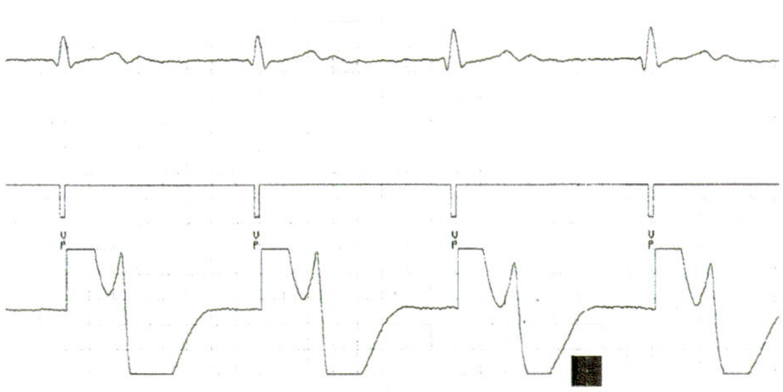

Figure 38. Surface and endocavitary electrocardiogram in a patient with grade II atrioventricular block during pacemaker implantation. (Courtesy of Dr Roberto Santilli).

The lead should then be attached to the generator and the generator positioned in a subcutaneous pocket near the incision point in the jugular vein. Finally, the muscle layers, subcutaneous tissue and skin should be closed.

After the surgery, a padded neck and chest bandage should be applied to try to immobilize the neck and avoid sudden movements which may dislocate the lead from the fixation point. The **bandage should be kept in place for a few weeks**, during which time broad-spectrum antibiotics should be prescribed.

Generally, it is advisable to carry out **telemetric control one month** after pacemaker implantation and, subsequently, **once a year**. Normally, pacemakers are initially programmed in VVI mode with a base rate of 60–70 bpm to promote correct lead fixation, and eventually changed to VVIR, DDD or VDD mode.

Complications

The main complications associated with the implantation of a pacemaker are those related to surgery (perioperative or postoperative) or the functioning of the pacemaker itself.

Complications During Surgery

The biggest complications during surgery are:

- heavy bleeding through the jugular vein;
- ventricular arrests which are unresponsive to external pacemaker stimulation;
- malignant ventricular arrhythmias that trigger ventricular fibrillation;
- myocardial perforation with the lead.

Complications During the Postoperative Period

In the postoperative period, the following complications may be seen.

- **Lead dislocation**: consists of lead displacement, which manifests with poor pacemaker function or directly with the loss of cardiac stimulus. Depending on the degree of dislocation, repeating the implantation may be necessary or pacemaker function can be restored by reprogramming the pacemaker.

- **Seromas or infections** of the surgical incisions or pocket where the generator is located. Treatment of serious infections at the insertion point of the generator or in the lead often requires removal of the infected material, specific antibiotic treatment, and replacement of the infected material with a new implant.
- **Cranial vena cava syndrome**: is defined as obstruction of the cranial vena cava secondary to pacemaker implantation. Possible factors that may contribute to this complication are not entirely clear, but it is suspected that pacemaker leads may induce endothelial injury in the vessel leading to fibrotic constriction and thrombotic obstruction of the vena cava. Other factors that favour the process are: a state of hypercoagulability, inflammation, or blood flow stasis. Clinical signs are due to increased hydrostatic pressure within the vena cava caused by the obstruction. Subcutaneous oedema occurs in the neck, forelimbs and, in more advanced cases, pleural effusion occurs. Medical treatment consists of the use of anticoagulants, platelet anti-aggregants, and thrombolytic agents. Generally, medical treatment is associated with surgical techniques such as thrombectomy, venoplasty, or stent placement.
- **Pacemaker syndrome**: this syndrome occurs in single-chamber pacemakers (e.g. VVI) due to asynchronous cardiac pacing (lack of synchronised atrial and ventricular activation). Over time this type of stimulation activates a series of neurohormonal mechanisms which lead to an increase in cardiac dimensions and loss of systolic function. Clinically, it is manifested by the appearance of signs of heart failure such as pulmonary oedema, which may or may not be associated with ascites, or signs of low cardiac output, such as weakness.

Problems Arising from Pacemaker Malfunction

Alterations in pacemaker function are most commonly due to errors in pacing or pacemaker detection.

Pacing Errors

Cases in which an **incorrect myocardial stimulation** occurs, despite the generator still emitting impulses.

Error detection: this can be verified on the surface electrocardiogram, from the presence of pacing spicules from the pacemaker but lacking ventricular complexes which should arise from it.

Causes:
- generator defect (e.g. the battery runs out)
- faulty leads (dislocation or damage to the electrode)
- abnormalities in lead contact with the myocardium (e.g. an increase in the stimulation threshold due to fibrosis).

Solution: in the case of dislocation or lead breakage, a new one must be implanted, either by endocavitary or epicardial techniques. A stimulation deficit due to an increase in the stimulation threshold should be corrected increasing the intensity or duration of the generator output pulse.

Sensing Errors

Due to the inability of the device to measure intrinsic activity in the chamber evaluated and differentiate it from noise or interference.

Undersensing

The device is unable to sense intrinsic activity in the patient and continues pacing at the programmed rate.

Error detection: on the surface electrocardiogram, paced beats are observed after intrinsic beats from the patient.

Causes:
- incorrect threshold programming (detection threshold too high)
- lead dislocation or breakage
- low myocardial potential quality due to metabolic or myocardial problems
- asynchronous mode programming (VOO). The generator paces without sensing the cardiac chamber.

Troubleshooting: this bug is corrected by lowering the sensitivity threshold of the device.

Oversensing

The device senses the presence of electrical signals as intrinsic activity which are not typical of the chamber evaluated (Figure 39).

Causes:
- external energy sources
- sensing of atrial activity: this phenomenon is called cross-talk
- oversensing of T waves or other waves.

Troubleshooting: the bug is fixed by increasing the sensitivity threshold of the device.

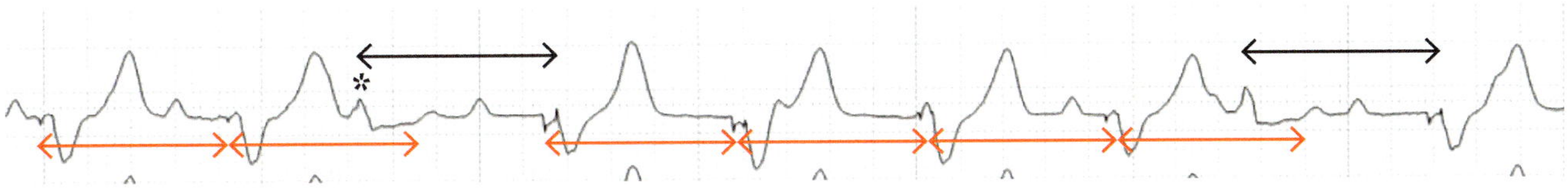

Figure 39. Surface electrocardiogram in a dog with a pacemaker in VVIR mode with poor function and oversensing. The interval between ventricular complexes paced by the pacemaker (red arrows) is constant until the third beat (black arrow). In this case the interval increases due to oversensing of the P wave which follows the paced ventricular complex (asterisk). (Courtesy of Dr Roberto Santilli).

Bibliography

■ Ellenbogen, K.A., Gilligan, D.M., Wood, M.A. et al. (1997) The pacemaker syndrome: a matter of definition. *Am J Cardiol*, 79, pp. 1226–1228.

■ Estrada, A.H. (2015) Cardiac pacing. In: Weisse, C., Berent, A. *Veterinary Image-Guided Interventions*, 1ª ed. John Wiley & Sons, Oxford, pp. 518–530.

■ Fine, D.M., Tobias, A.H. (2007) Cardiovascular device infections in dogs: report of 8 cases and review of the literature. *J Vet Intern Med*, 21 (6), pp. 1265–1271.

■ Fox, P.R., Sisson, D., Moïse, N.S. (1999) *Textbook of Canine and Feline Cardiology.* WB Saunders Company.

■ Fuentes, V.L., Johnson, L.R, Dennis S. (2010) *BSAVA Manual of Canine and Feline Cardiorespiratory Medicine.* BSAVA.

■ Johnson, M.S., Martin, M.W., Henley, W. (2007) Results of pacemaker implantation in 104 dogs. *J Small AnimPract*, 48 (1), pp. 4–11.

■ Lichtenberger, J., Scollan, K.F., Bulmer, B.J. et al. (2015) Long-term outcome of physiologic VDD pacing versus non-physiologic VVI pacing in dogs with high-grade atrioventricular block. *J Vet Cardiol*, 17 (1), pp. 42–53.

■ Martin, M. (2015) *Small Animal ECGs An Introductory Guide.* Wiley Blackwell.

■ Moise, N.S. (1999) Pacemaker therapy. In: Fox, P.R., Sisson, D., Moise, N.S. *Textbook of Canine and Feline Cardiology*, 2ª ed. Saunders, Philadelphia, pp. 400–425.

■ Mulz, J.M., Kraus, M.S., Thompson, M. et al. (2010) Cranial vena caval syndrome secondary to central venous obstruction associated with a pacemaker lead in a dog. *J Vet Cardiol*, 12 (3), pp. 217–223.

■ Noomanová, N., Perego, M., Perini, A. et al. (2010) Use of transcutaneous external pacing during transvenous pacemaker implantation in dogs. *Vet Rec*, 167 (7), pp. 241–244.

■ Oyama, M.A., Kraus, M.S., Gelzer, A.R. (2014) Rapid Review of ECG Interpretation in Small Animal Practice. *Taylor & Francis Group.*

■ Petrie, J.P. (2005) Permanent transvenous cardiac pacing. *Clin Tech Small Animal Pract*, 20 (3), pp. 164–72.

■ Ranjan, R., Dosdall, D., Norlund, L. et al. (2014) Diagnostic imaging and pacemaker implantation in a domestic goat with persistent left cranial vena cava. *J Vet Cardiol*, pp. 45–50.

■ Sanchis-Mora, S., Viscasillas, J., Mathis, A. et al. (2014) Anaesthetic management and complications of pacemaker implantation in dogs. *Vet Rec*, 175(12), p. 303.

■ Santilli, R., Perego, M. (2009) Elettrocardiogramma nei pazienti portatori di cardiostimolatori impiantabili (pacemaker). In: Santilli, R.A., Perego, M. *Elettrocardiografia del cane e del gatto*, 1ª ed. Elsevier: Milán, 213, p. 220.

■ Santilli, R., Perego, M. (2012) Terapia farmacologica ed elettrica delle aritmie. In: Santilli, R.A., Bussadori, C., Borgarelli, M. *Manuale di cardiologia del cane e del gatto*, 1ª ed. Elsevier: Milán, pp. 325–355.

■ Santilli, R.A., Perego, M. (2009) *Electtrocardiografía del Cane e del Gatto.* Elsevier.

Test

Answers on Page 336

1. Indicate which of the following is true regarding sinus arrhythmia:
   a. It is considered a normal finding in dogs and is secondary to increased vagal tone.
   b. It is considered a normal finding in dogs and cats, due to a high vagal tone.
   c. It suggests cardiac disease.
   d. It is common in patients with heart murmurs.

2. Indicate which of the following is true regarding third-degree AV blocks:
   a. Normal finding in cats.
   b. Normal finding in dogs.
   c. Treatment of choice is permanent pacemaker implantation.
   d. Patients with third-degree AV blocks usually show an adequate response to the atropine stimulation test.

3. Indicate which is true regarding cardiac arrhythmias:
   a. Supraventricular premature complexes do not differ from ventricular complexes on ECG.
   b. Sinus tachycardia causes different sized P waves on the ECG.
   c. Ventricular fibrillation is a pathognomonic arrhythmia of sick sinus syndrome.
   d. Atrial silence or arrest is characterised by an absence of atrial activity.

4. Indicate which is true regarding atrial fibrillation:
   a. It cannot be identified on the ECG.
   b. It is more common in cats than dogs.
   c. It can occur in dogs without structural heart disease.
   d. It does not cause haemodynamic problems.

5. When suffering from dilated cardiomyopathy, which dog breeds are predisposed to ventricular arrhythmias?
   a. Dobermann.
   b. Great Dane.
   c. Boxer.
   d. Dobermann, Boxer, and Great Dane.

6. In a patient with dyspnoea and a grade IV/VI systolic heart murmur with a PMI over the left apex, in whom the presence of sinus arrhythmia is detected on physical examination, the most likely cause of the respiratory symptoms is:
   a. Right-sided heart failure.
   b. Left-sided heart failure.
   c. Bilateral heart failure.
   d. Respiratory disease.

7. 8-year-old West Highland White Terrier with bouts of weakness and syncope during exercise, without the presence of other clinical signs. What additional diagnostic test should be chosed to try to reach a diagnosis?
   a. Holter monitoring.
   b. Thoracic radiography.
   c. Cardiac troponins.
   d. Biochemistry.

8. Which of the following antiarrhythmic agents could be used to treat a dog with supraventricular tachycardia?
   a. Lidocaine.
   b. Atropine.
   c. Diltiazem.
   d. Mexiletine.

9. Which of the following antiarrhythmic agents could be used to treat a cat with ventricular tachycardia?
   a. Sotalol.
   b. Lidocaine.
   c. Digoxin.
   d. Atropine.

10. For which of the following arrhythmias would the implantation of a pacemaker be recommended?
   a. Persistent ventricular tachycardia.
   b. Frequent ventricular premature complexes.
   c. High level/severe second-degree AV block.
   d. Supraventricular tachycardia.

11. A pacemaker in VDD mode is characterised by:

a. Detecting atrial activity with ventricular pacing.
b. Detecting atrial and ventricular activity with ventricular pacing.
c. Detecting atrial and ventricular activity with stimulation of the atrium and ventricle.
d. Does not record the activity of any cardiac chamber and only stimulates the ventricle.

12. What type of pacemaker does not allow atrioventricular synchrony?

a. DDD.
b. AAI.
c. VDD.
d. VVI.

13. What complication is uncommon during the postoperative period after pacemaker implantation?

a. Lead dislocation.
b. Infection or seroma of the pocket where the pacemaker battery is located.
c. Myocardial perforation with the electrode.
d. Pacemaker malfunction.

14. The presence of pacing spicules without QRS complexes on the surface electrocardiogram is indicative of a pacing error due to:

a. Partial lead dislocation.
b. Complete lead breakage.
c. T wave oversensing.
d. Battery depletion.

Clinical Case

Signalment. 5-year-old female spayed Labrador.

Reason for consultation. Lethargy, exercise intolerance, episodes of weakness and collapse over the last week.

Physical examination. Alert mental state. Good body condition (BCS 5/9, weight 27 kg). Slightly pale mucous membranes with a capillary refill time of 2 seconds. Heart rate 42 beats/minute, regular rhythm, good quality pulses without pulse deficits. Grade II/VI systolic heart murmur with maximum intensity over the left apex. Respiratory rate 26 breaths/minute, with a normal breathing pattern and sounds on thoracic auscultation. Rectal temperature 38.5 °C.

Electrocardiogram. See below.

1. **Provide a brief description of the ECG findings (including heart rate, heart rhythm, and electrocardiographic diagnosis).**

2. **Indicate which is the most probable cause of the symptoms in this patient.**

3. **Should further tests be recommended in this patient? Which ones?**

4. **Indicate which would be the treatment of choice for this patient.**

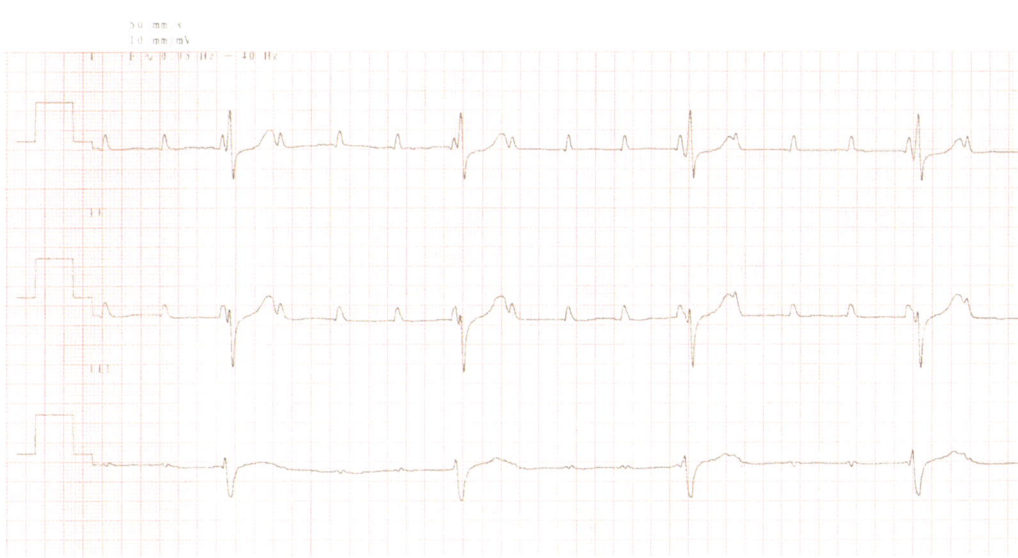

Correct Answers:

Test

1. a
2. c
3. d
4. c
5. d
6. d
7. a
8. c
9. a
10. c
11. b
12. d
13. c
14. a

Clinical Case

1. **Provide a brief description of the ECG findings (including heart rate, heart rhythm, and electrocardiographic diagnosis).**
   The ECG shows:
   - heart rate: 50 beats/minute
   - cardiac rhythm: ventricular escape complexes, regular rhythm
   - electrocardiogram diagnosis: third-degree block.

2. **Indicate which is the most probable cause of the symptoms in this patient.**
   Third-degree block (bradyarrhythmia).

3. **Should further tests be recommended in this patient? Which ones?**
   Further tests are recommended in this patient to try to find the cause of the bradyarrhythmia and heart murmur, as well as knowing the health status and prognosis should the owners decide to proceed with pacemaker implantation. Diagnostic tests initially recommended include the following.
   - Thoracic radiographs.
   - Echocardiogram.
   - Complete blood count and biochemistry.
   - Cardiac troponin I.
   - Arterial blood pressure.
   - If myocarditis is suspected, endomyocardial biopsies could also be considered, although these are currently only performed in a very limited number of centres.

4. **Indicate which would be the treatment of choice for this patient.**
   Permanent pacemaker implantation.

Notes

Cardiac Surgery

Oriol Domenech and Stefano Nicoli

Cardiac surgery is a discipline that includes **all procedures performed on the heart (ventricles, atria), aorta, pulmonary artery, vena cava, and pericardium**. From a technical perspective it is similar to other types of surgery, except the consequences of any errors can be immediately fatal and unlike abdominal or orthopaedic surgery, **performed on a moving organ** so its execution is more complicated.

Cardiac surgery is increasingly common in veterinary medicine and is becoming the **treatment of choice in patients with congenital or acquired cardiac pathologies.** Some surgical techniques have become routine and are performed in many veterinary practices, but others are only available in a few referral centres due to their complexity and requirement for specialist materials.

Most cardiac surgeries are performed using a **closed thoracotomy technique**, without opening or exposing the cardiac structures or great vessels. On other occasions the use of open thoracotomy techniques are necessary to expose one or more parts of the cardiovascular system. Cardiac surgery can be performed on a **beating or stopped heart**, interrupting the flow of blood for a varying length of time.

Interruption of circulating blood is achieved by:
- caval venous flow occlusion
- extracorporeal circulation (ECC) using a heart-lung bypass machine.

Closed Thoracotomy Cardiac Surgery

Cardiac surgery via closed thoracotomy does not entail opening of the heart or the great vessels and, therefore, does not interrupt circulation or cardiac movements. Common examples of procedures include:
- pericardiectomy
- closure of patent *ductus arteriosus* (PDA)
- extraction of extracardiac masses (heart base tumours).

Pericardiectomy is indicated for patients with pericardial effusion of an inflammatory, infectious, or neoplastic nature. Pericardial effusion around the heart causes an increase in intrapericardial pressure, with consequent cardiac compression and cardiac tamponade, which puts the patient's life at risk.

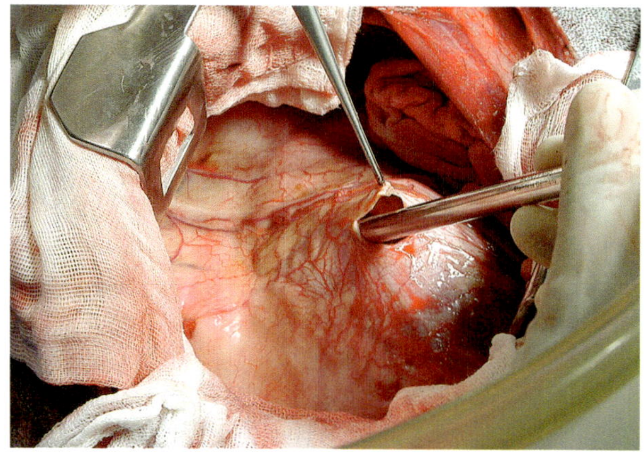

Figure 1. Magnified image of subphrenic access during pericardiectomy surgery. Immediately after access to the pericardial cavity, an aspiration cannula is introduced to aspirate pericardial effusion.

Pericardiectomy (Figure 1) and **surgical closure of the PDA**, are now considered routine procedures with good results and a low mortality or serious complication rate when carried out by experienced surgeons.

Open Thoracotomy Cardiac Surgery

Caval Venous Flow Occlusion Technique

Blocking the blood flow to the heart is achieved by **clamping the superior and inferior vena cava** so at to interrupt the blood flow and cause a brief period of circulatory arrest. This technique is only suitable for **brief surgeries to the right-side of the heart** (for example, excision of an intracardiac mass in the right atrium). It requires an expert surgeon and a well-prepared and preplanned surgical technique. Unlike cardiopulmonary bypass, if the intervention encounters a problem, it cannot be prolonged since the patient's life is at risk. In addition, the **heart continues to beat**, making surgery difficult from a technical perspective. This procedure carries a high risk of bleeding if the cardiac structures are not closed quickly or the vena cava not adequately occluded.

However, the methodology is simple since it does not require complex instrumentation and postoperative convalescence is reduced from a cardiocirculatory, metabolic, and haematological point of view; with a reduction in hospitalization times and total cost of surgery. **In normothermic patients the circulation can be stopped for two minutes**, minimizing the risk of ventricular fibrillation and brain damage. This time can be extended up to **eight minutes if the body temperature is 32–34 °C**. However, increasing the clamping time of the venous flow to the heart increases the risk of cardiac arrest. Likewise, it is important to avoid the temperature dropping below 32 °C because this increases the risk of ventricular fibrillation.

Whilst venous flow is clamped, **mechanical ventilation should be suspended** so as to avoid seepage of blood from the pulmonary vessels into the operative field during the inspiratory phase of the patient (Valsalva manoeuvre).

Use of Extracorporeal Circulation (ECC)

In veterinary medicine the use of cardiopulmonary bypass is fairly recent, used on and off since the 60's to surgically treat the most common heart diseases in dogs and to a lesser extent in cats. Recently, this technique is used with good results for mitral valve repair in patients with mitral endocardiosis.

In veterinary medicine, there are important considerations which should be taken into account compared to human medicine:

- anatomical differences
    - breed differences can considerably change the surgical approach, techniques, and instrumentation required
- limited blood volume
- differences in haemostasis and coagulation
- cost.

Extracorporeal circulation has two main objectives:

- replace the function of the heart (pump) and lung (oxygenation);
- allow the surgeon to operate in a stable, blood-free field with the absence of cardiopulmonary movements.

Cardiac arrest and myocardial protection are achieved through the administration of **cardioplegic solution, which allows cardiac arrest in diastole**. Cardioplegic solutions are high in potassium and may or may not mix with the blood.

There are two types of cardioplegic solutions, **crystalloid or haematic**:

- crystalloid solution:
    - inexpensive
    - readily available
    - a larger volume is required
    - does not transport oxygen.
- haematic cardioplegic solution:
    - transports oxygen
    - free radical scavenger
    - electrolyte composition and osmolarity are similar to that of the patient's blood
    - optimal buffering power.

The cardioplegic solution is administered via anterograde infusion through a cannula positioned in the aortic root or, in certain conditions (severe aortic insufficiency) administered by retrograde infusion through the coronary venous sinus. The objective of the cardioplegic solution is to eliminate electromechanical work and reduce the energy requirements of the heart.

Less frequently in veterinary medicine, ECC is performed on a beating heart to provide cardio-circulatory support during surgery, without the problems associated with cardiac arrest and its complications. In fact, cardiac arrest predicts an increased risk of ischaemic reperfusion damage, cannulation of the aorta (risk of rupture and haemorrhage), and postoperative defibrillation. However, the surgeon must operate on a moving heart, which makes the procedure more difficult. As a result, the preferred option is ECC with cardiac arrest for the surgical treatment of complex or acquired congenital heart disease.

ECC consists of a system of tubes and cannulas to facilitate extraction of the blood volume from the patient's venous circulation of the patient, pass the blood through pumps (heart, aspirators), the oxygenator (lung), and reintroduce the oxygenated blood volume via an arterial catheter into the patient's arterial circulation (Figures 2, 3, and 4).

A fundamental consideration is heparinization of the patient, especially as contact between blood and the ECC machine circuit leads to the activation of the coagulation cascade and thrombi formation.

Heparin is the main antagonist to antithrombin III (ATIII), binding to this molecule. The combination has a high affinity for thrombin, factor X, and other proteases responsible for coagulation; thus, reducing the procoagulant action. Heparin does not modify the circulating mass and its action is blocked by the antagonist, protamine sulphate, which is used at the end of the ECC procedure to reverse the effects of heparin and thus reduce the risk of bleeding.

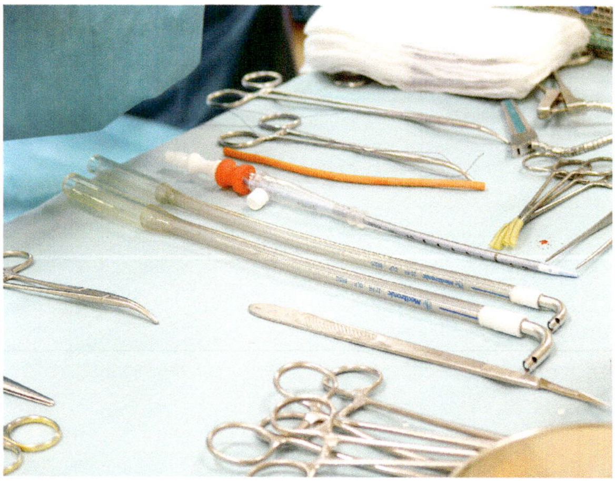

Figure 2. Image of the instrument table prepared for surgery with extracorporeal circulation. In the foreground the venous catheters with right angled metallic tips are seen and the straight arterial catheter. Behind, the material necessary for preparation of the tobacco-pouch in the large vessels, plus the forceps for clamping the aorta.

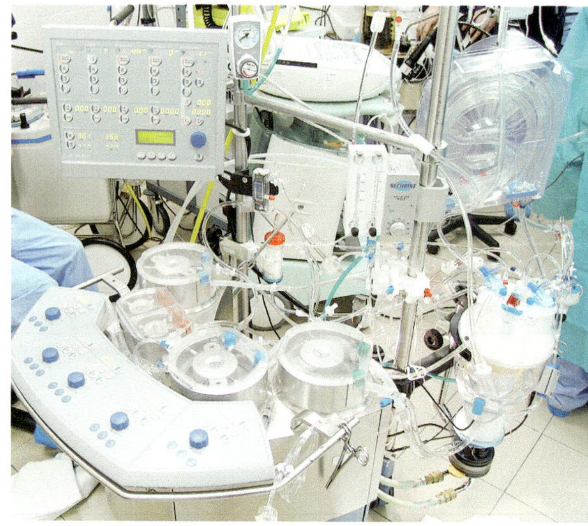

Figure 4. View of the extracorporeal circulation machine prepared for use, just before placement of venous catheters.

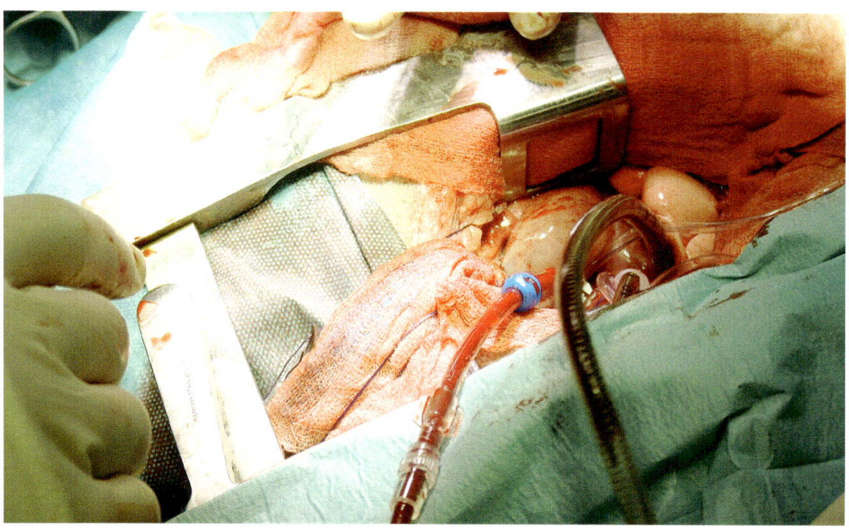

Figure 3. Image of the operating field during surgery with ECC where a venous and aortic catheter are present for cardioplegia.

Complications of Extracorporeal Circulation

ECC procedures present many complications, which is why control and monitoring of vital parameters, during and after surgery, are essential for patient survival. Considering all the potential complications and complexity of the procedures, it is important to mention that in surgical procedures with ECC, **collaboration between the different team members is important**: surgeon, perfusionist, cardiologist, anaesthetist, and intensivist.

In general, the duration of ECC and aortic clamping are directly proportional to intraoperative and postoperative complications. Before, during, and after ECC, the following parameters should be monitored:

- body temperature
- blood pressure
- acid-base and electrolyte balance
- renal, respiratory, neurological, and metabolic function.

During surgery, a cardiologist should monitor cardiac function using transoesophageal echocardiography and, after surgery, by transthoracic echocardiography, electrocardiogram, central venous pressure, and systemic blood pressure.

During ECC, blood pressure is reduced relative to normal reference ranges; likewise, protamine intake can cause **hypotension**. Surgery can result in a reduction in contractility and require the use of positive inotropes. The inflammation that occurs after ECC can lead to **vasoplegia**, with a drastic reduction in blood pressure which must be counteracted with vasoactive amines. It is also important to monitor **electrolyte alterations and acid-base balance**, assessed by arterial blood gas both during and after the procedure. Alterations in blood pH and concentrations of potassium, sodium, chloride, or magnesium are common and must be monitored to maintain a correct acid-base and electrolyte balance.

Other factors to consider in patients undergoing ECC interventions are haemodilution, blood trauma leading to red blood cell haemolysis, coagulation issues and thrombus formation, and embolic phenomena. **Emboli** can be composed of foreign materials (coming from the ECC circuit), air, and biological material (thrombi). Preventative measures to reduce emboli formation (during and after surgery) include:

- the use of filters
- good management of coagulation
- good ECC and surgical technique
- use of echocardiographic monitoring to remove all air from the left ventricle before the heart beats normally again in the final phase of the ECC procedure.

Another complication with a high mortality rate in both human and veterinary medicine is the **systemic inflammatory response syndrome (SIRS)**, which is described as a complication in ECC interventions. It is important to remember that **ECC and aortic clamping time are directly proportional to the postsurgical inflammatory response**.

Application Of Heart Surgery In Veterinary Medicine

Acquired Cardiac Pathologies

Mitral Valve Degeneration

Mitral valvular degeneration represents the most common cardiac pathology in the dog, representing about 80% of the cases seen in a cardiology department. The median survival time of a patient with severe disease is 6–12 months. Most of these cases are treated medically with diuretics, ACE-inhibitors, inodilators, and aldosterone antagonists.

The medical management of this pathology is a palliative treatment since patients with severe forms tend to present several episodes of left-sided congestive heart failure, reaching a point when some patients are refractory to medical treatment. Furthermore, unlike surgical treatment, medical treatment does not correct the degree of mitral regurgitation or the pathophysiological mechanism underlying this disease.

In man, this pathology is treated surgically, which gives better results compared to medical treatment. In recent years, there is an increase in the use of cardiac surgery for veterinary patients with mitral valve disease. These surgical techniques involve either **mitral valve repair or complete valve replacement with highly biocompatible synthetic material or with biological valves**. Mitral valve replacement has been carried out in the dog both with the use of mechanical valves and bioprosthetic material, but both techniques present the problem of requiring long term antithrombotic treatment due to the high risks of thrombus formation, a treatment that it is not necessary when performing valve repair.

In the study by Mizuno et al. (2013) three cases in which the mitral valve repair technique was performed by annuloplasty and replacement of the *chordae tendineae* with polytetrafluoroethylene fibres (PTFE, commercially known as Teflon) are described. Survival was two, five, and six years, which is much higher than the survival time for critically ill patients receiving medical treatment. This shows replacement of the *chordae tendineae* with PTFE material, together with the reduction of the mitral valve *annulus* by annuloplasty, is possible and an effective technique.

In another study carried out by Uechi et al. (2012) 48 cases of small dogs that underwent mitral valve repair surgery with good results for both intra-surgical mortality (<10%) and patient evolution, with a survival rate ≥12 months in 73.3% and ≥3 years in 26.6% of patients undergoing cardiac surgery are described.

Mitral valve repair consists of several steps:

- reconstruction of the *chordae tendineae*
- valvular annuloplasty
- valvuloplasty.

In valve degeneration, the *chordae tendineae* are often involved in the degenerative process and tend to rupture, further increasing the degree of valve prolapse and determining the lack of coaptation between several leaflets, causing secondary deterioration such as mitral regurgitation. The reconstruction of the *chordae tendineae* prevents severe valve prolapse, notably reducing or preventing mitral regurgitation.

Alternatively, **annuloplasty** reduces the circumference of the mitral valve *annulus*, restoring the normal anatomy of the valve *annulus*, to increase the coaptation of the leaflets, reduce the tension of the suture lines and prevent future dilation of the mitral *annulus*. Annuloplasty is performed using a circular suture with PTFE sutures or with a prosthetic ring. Use of the prosthetic ring represents a gold standard in human medicine because valve coaptation is better and prevents future dilatations of the ring more effectively.

Valvuloplasty allows the areas of rupture or laceration sites in the mitral valve leaflets to be sutured with polypropylene fibres, thus completing the valve reconstruction.

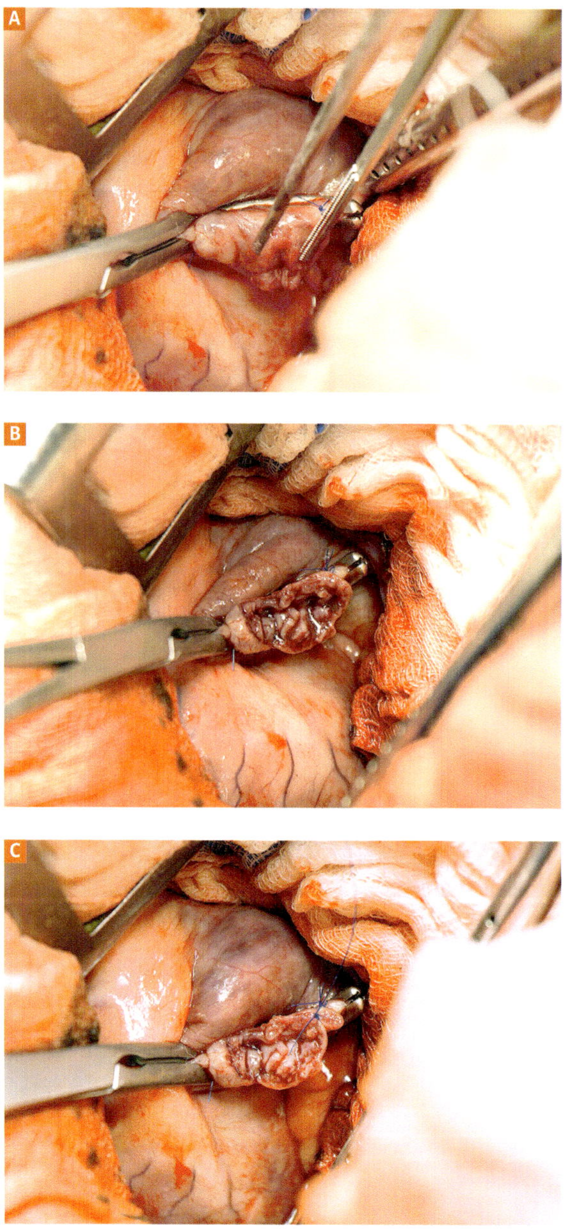

Figure 5. Right atrial tumour: the mass is isolated from the rest of the atrial tissue using placement of a Satinsky vascular clamp (**A**). The mass is extracted via an incision with a cold scalpel blade. The Satinsky clamp allows blood loss and haemorrhage of the rest of the atrial cavity to be avoided (**B**). Closure is by two layers of simple continuous sutures with non-absorbable monofilament suture material (**C**).

Cardiac Masses

In veterinary medicine **cardiac masses are rare** in the canine population and even more so in felines.

The most frequent neoplasms in dogs are haemangiosarcoma, chemodectoma, lymphoma, and ectopic thyroid carcinoma, and in cats, lymphoma. The palliative surgical treatment is pericardiectomy, which allows the pericardial effusion resulting from the presence of the masses to drain, not into the pericardium but into the pleural space. In fact, the continuous drainage of the pericardium through repeated pericardiocentesis can lead to its fibrosis, in addition to endangering the life of the animal, due to possible cardiac tamponade, leaving the patient in a possible emergency situation.

The treatment of choice for cardiac masses, when possible, is surgical resection of the mass together with pericardiectomy and, when indicated, chemotherapy (especially in cases of haemangiosarcoma and lymphoma). For example, for haemangiosarcoma, the mean survival time of patients who underwent mass removal, pericardiectomy, and chemotherapy is significantly longer compared to patients who only undergo surgery (189 days compared to 86 days).

The surgical plan is not without risks and requires careful **assessment with a transthoracic and transoesophageal echocardiographic study,** plus a thorough cardio CT, to evaluate the relationship of the neoformation with the cardiac structures and large vessels and the presence of possible metastases.

Cardiac masses that do not invade the heart chambers and are well encapsulated can be removed without the use of ECC, as can tumours at the base of the heart. For masses that invade the right-sided chambers, atrium or ventricle, surgical techniques with the heart beating that prevent the blockage of caval venous flow without the need for ECC are described in the literature (Figure 5).

Congenital Heart Diseases

Mitral Valve Dysplasia

Mitral valve dysplasia is a congenital heart disease characterised by a malformed valve apparatus which causes stenosis, insufficiency, or both. The most common features of mitral dysplasia include:

- reduced mobility of the septal and posterior leaflets
- elongated valves
- short *chordae tendineae*
- direct link between the papillary muscle and the valve
- fused and/or hypertrophied papillary muscles
- secondary dilation of the valvular *annulus*.

In severe forms with clinical signs and left-sided congestive heart failure that does not respond to medical cardiological treatment, surgical intervention is necessary. The latter includes valve repair or mitral valve replacement.

Depending on the case mitral valve repair envisages the reconstruction of the *chordae tendineae* and annuloplasty, reducing the component causing secondary insufficiency. In some cases, with highly hypomobile leaflets, fenestration of fused *chordae tendineae* and longitudinal excision between the papillary muscles and fixation of the *chordae tendineae* have been described.

Tricuspid Dysplasia

Tricuspid valve dysplasia is a rare congenital anomaly in dogs and cats and is characterised by a malformation of the valve apparatus, which may be stenotic and/or insufficient. Common features of tricuspid dysplasia include:

- long leaflets or those which are attached to the interventricular septum
- leaflet adhesions directly to the papillary muscle
- short or absent *chordae tendineae*
- fusion of papillary muscles.

Given the complexity of this congenital anomaly, it presents difficulties for surgical intervention, which are often reserved for patients with severe tricuspid dysplasia. In the literature, substitution of the tricuspid valve with a bovine and porcine bioprosthetic valve has been described with a high percentage of morbidity and mortality and a high rate of postoperative complications.

Patent *Ductus Arteriosus*

This **congenital heart disease is common in dogs**, with a prevalence of 20.9%, but rarer in cats. It is characterised by persistent flow through the *ductus arteriosus* after birth (this vessel connects the descending aorta with the pulmonary artery during foetal circulation). With the use of interventional cardiology procedures, patent *ductus arteriosus* (PDA) can be closed with an Amplatzer™ device, ACDO (Amplatz Canine Duct Occluder).

In very small sized dogs or those with PDAs with certain morphological characteristics (for example, of the tubular type), the PDA suture ligation technique by thoracotomy is used (Figure 6). Duct ligation is performed with the heart beating, with excellent results and a low mortality rate and low complication rates (1–2%), when performed by an experienced surgeon.

Pulmonary Stenosis

Pulmonary stenosis is a pathology characterised by **congenital malformation of the pulmonary valve** and can be valvular (the most common), subvalvular, or supravalvular. Valvular-type pulmonary stenosis represents one of the most frequent congenital heart diseases in dogs, making up for up to 32% of all these canine diseases.

Balloon catheter valvuloplasty is the technique of choice for severe forms, due to the low mortality and complication rate, plus the high success rate in cases of pulmonary stenosis, especially type A, which are the most frequent.

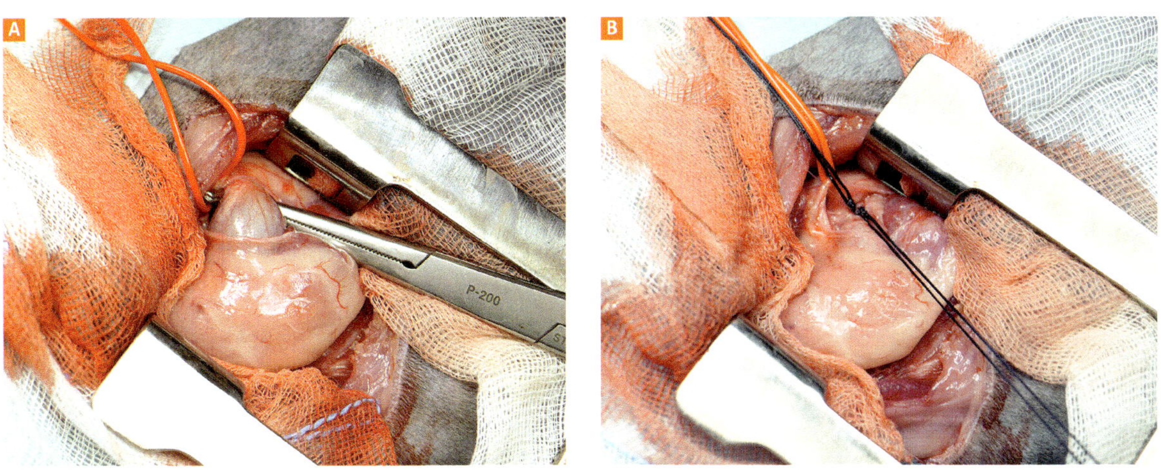

Figure 6. Patent *ductus arteriosus* (PDA) in a cat. The image shows how the large sized PDA has been isolated. Thanks to the clamp access to the medial side of the PDA is possible, which allows two silk sutures to be positioned and placed for posterior ligation and closure of the PDA (**A**). Once the sutures are in place around the PDA they are ligated: first the suture which is on the side of the descending aorta and then the one on the side of the pulmonary artery. It is important that the silk suture is of a large diameter to reduce the risk of a "cutting" effect by the suture thread against the wall of the PDA (**B**).

If the patient presents with a combination of PDA and pulmonary stenosis, pulmonary valvuloplasty followed by closure of the PDA with ACDO using an interventional cardiology procedure is indicated. Both can be undertaken during the same procedure (one-step procedure) or in two consecutive interventions 3–4 weeks apart (two-step procedure).

However, in some cases of pulmonary stenosis with highly dysplastic valves, severe infundibular hypertrophy, hypoplasia of the valvular *annulus*, or insufficient reduction of the transvalvular gradient with pulmonary valvuloplasty, open surgery may be considered. The surgical technique generally involves an arteriotomy of the valve with resection of the valvular *ostium* and the leaflets, a ventriculostomy, and application of a patch graft. The patch graft is a membrane that allows dilation of the right ventricular outflow tract and the valve *annulus*, which can be made of either a portion of the patient's pericardium or biosynthetic material (PTFE Gore-Tex®). To perform the arteriotomy and patch graft application, surgeries have been described that require the use of either the occlusion of caval venous flow or ECC.

The use of ECC (in contrast to occluding the caval venous flow), allows better visualization of the pulmonary valve and better suturing of the patch graft in the outflow tract of the right ventricle. Furthermore, it is the technique of choice in human medicine. Obviously, the intra-surgical mortality rate described is higher, around 20–40%, compared to for pulmonary balloon valvuloplasty, which is around 2–4%, with a higher risk of postoperative complications (33%). Despite this, this cardiac surgery technique is proven to be effective and achieves an average decrease in the transvalvular gradient of 83%.

Subaortic Stenosis

Aortic stenosis is the second most common congenital heart disease in dogs, representing 21.3% of congenital heart disease. The stenosis can be valvular, supravalvular, or subvalvular. Subvalvular stenosis is the most frequent in the dog and can be caused by the presence of subvalvular nodules (type 1), subvalvular fibrous ring (type 2), or a tunnel type fibromuscular structure (type 3).

Cutting-type balloon catheter valvuloplasty followed by high-pressure balloon catheter valvuloplasty is a viable interventional cardiology treatment option, especially for types 1 and 2 subaortic stenosis.

Surgery is appropriate when the patient has severe subaortic stenosis, especially with type 3 subaortic stenosis, when the gradient is >130 mmHg, or in cases of severe type 1 or 2 subaortic stenosis that do not respond favourably to balloon catheter valvuloplasty. The surgical technique involves aortotomy with resection of the subvalvular lesion and, occasionally, a partial myectomy of the interventricular septum. This requires ECC and although it appears to have advantages in terms of reducing the pressure gradient, it does not increase the survival times of these patients.

Interventricular Septal Defect

Ventricular septal defect (VSD) is characterised by a communication between the right and left ventricles, which can occur at various points in the interventricular septum. VSD is the **most common congenital anomaly in the cat** and fourth in the dog.

In most cases the interventricular septal defect is **haemodynamically insignificant** and the patient asymptomatic throughout their life. However, in a small percentage of patients, the ventricular defect is wide and non-restrictive, which leads to left-sided cardiomegaly and symptoms of left-sided congestive heart failure. Treatment in these cases is surgical using cardiac surgery techniques (with or without ECC) or interventional cardiology procedures. The two cardiac surgery techniques described in the dog are pulmonary artery banding and closure of the interventricular defect with open heart surgery (using ECC).

Bypassing the pulmonary artery allows an increase in right ventricular pressures with the consequent reduction of blood flow through the defect. This procedure is palliative, while open heart surgery via ECC resolves the problem since it closes the communication through the use of a Gore-Tex® or pericardial patch graft. There are also interventional cardiology techniques based on closure of the defect using coil or Amplatzer™ VSD occluder devices.

Interatrial Septal Defect

Interatrial communication (ASD) is characterised **by an abnormal communication between the two atria** which can occur at different anatomical points in the interatrial septum. It is a rare congenital heart disease in dogs and cats. As in VSD, most animals are asymptomatic and rarely present clinical symptoms. In some cases, where the ASD is large, and causes a haemodynamic impact on the patient and closure of the defect is advisable either by cardiac surgery techniques or by interventional cardiology procedures.

The cardiac surgery technique used generally involves the use of ECC to close the defect through a right atriotomy with the use of a Gore-Tex® or pericardial patch graft. This cardiac surgery technique is also used in the cat to repair a large defect with the use of beating heart ECC, thus reducing the haemodilution resulting from the use of cardioplegic solutions.

An alternative is to use the ASO device (Amplatzer™ Atrial Septal Occluder) introduced through an interventional cardiology procedure, with a high success and low mortality rate.

Double-chambered right ventricle

Double-chambered right ventricle is characterised by a mid-ventricular obstruction which leads to concentric hypertrophy of the right anterior ventricle to the point of obstruction and can lead to right-sided congestive heart failure. This is a **rare congenital heart disease**.

This obstruction is caused by a fibromuscular membrane which is not easily dilatable with a balloon catheter. For this reason, the chosen technique is cardiac surgery by means of ECC or by occlusion of caval venous outflow, which allows the complete resection of the fibromuscular band.

Sometimes, the marked hypertrophy affecting the right ventricle requires a myectomy. Elliptical removal of the free wall of the right ventricle over the fibromuscular band and the use of a patch graft using the caval venous flow occlusion technique have been described in cats.

Cor Triatriatum Dexter

Cor triatriatum dexter (CTD) is a congenital anomaly where there is persistence of the membrane corresponding to the embryonic venous sinus valve which divides the right atrium into two parts or chambers:

- a high-pressure posterior chamber communicated with the caudal vena cava and, sometimes, with the coronary venous sinus; and
- a low-pressure anterior chamber communicating with the cranial vena cava and tricuspid valve.

The residual membrane may or may not be perforated, allowing or restricting the limited passage of blood between the two chambers. This anomaly is treated with minimally invasive interventional cardiology techniques using balloon catheters of increasing diameters, which serve to dilate and break the membrane, especially when it is a perforated and easily dilatable membrane.

In addition, this membrane can be removed through cardiac surgery techniques by caval clamping, which is an efficient technique in veterinary medicine, especially when the membrane is thick and rigid, and difficult to expand with a balloon catheter.

CTD associated with other congenital heart diseases, requires hybrid interventional cardiology techniques and surgery, to optimize the results of each in terms of invasiveness, risk, and success rate. In cases where CTD is associated with ASD, consideration should be given to performing the interventional cardiology technique or the cardiac surgery technique using ECC, since it is inadvisable to clamp caval flow due to the risk of air embolism.

Cor Triatriatum Sinister

Cor triatriatum sinister (CTS) is a rare congenital heart disease characterised by the presence of a **membrane which divides the left atrium into two parts or chambers**:

- a high-pressure proximal chamber that receives blood from the pulmonary veins; and
- a low-pressure distal chamber communicating with the mitral valve.

This pathology is treated surgically with or without the help of ECC. In cats, a hybrid technique is described combining cardiac surgery and interventional cardiology using a balloon catheter. A thoracotomy is required to place an introducer in the left atrium. A series of balloon catheters with increasing diameters are passed through the introducer which serve to dilate and rupture the membrane. In some cases, in which the membrane hole is too small, or the anatomical position of the membrane makes it difficult or impossible to pass the catheters, the technique of choice is atriotomy with surgical resection of the membrane using ECC.

Tetralogy of Fallot

Tetralogy of Fallot is a complex congenital heart disease consisting of the combination of several congenital defects:

- pulmonary stenosis
- interventricular septal defect
- aortic dextroposition (aorta to the right)
- right ventricular hypertrophy secondary to pulmonary stenosis.

The pathophysiology of this malformation depends on the degree of right ventricular obstruction and, consequently, on the right-left shunt that causes the cyanosis and polycythaemia which are typical of this pathology.

Palliative and definitive surgical techniques are described to correct tetralogy of Fallot. Palliative surgery consists of creating an extracardiac shunt between the systemic and pulmonary circulation: a vessel is created forming a communication between the left subclavian artery and the pulmonary artery (Figure 7). The vessel used to create the shunt consists of a section of the patient's carotid artery or is synthetic (PTFE or Gore-Tex®) (Figures 7 and 8). The definitive surgical technique foresees the use of ECC and consists of the treatment of pulmonary or infundibular stenosis and the closure of the interventricular septal defect with a patch graft: a technique successfully performed in two patients.

Some cases, especially in puppies of small size, which implies a group of patients with a high intraoperative risk, may initially benefit from a mini-invasive palliative pulmonary valvuloplasty procedure using interventional cardiology techniques. This clinical improvement allows the patient to grow and reach an optimal weight to undergo more invasive cardiac surgery techniques.

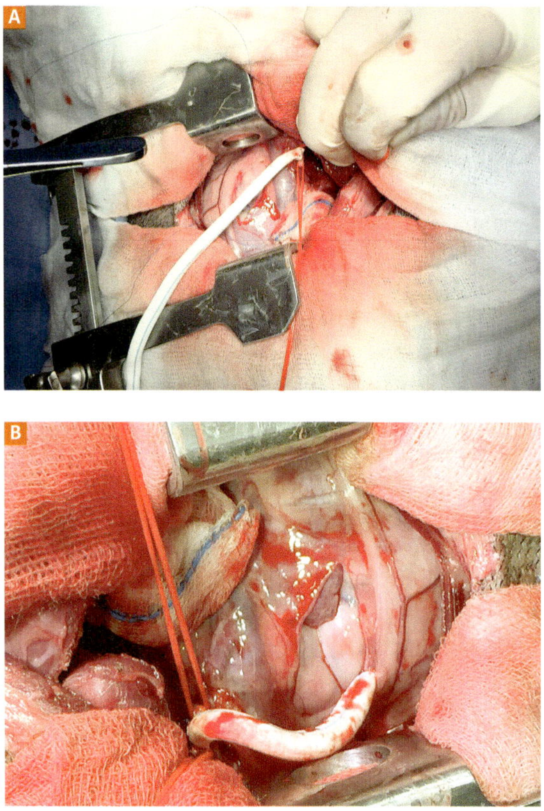

Figure 7. Tetralogy of Fallot: the use of a Gore-Tex® patch graft during anastomosis at the level of the subclavian artery can be appreciated (**A**). Final positioning of the bypass or shunt between the subclavian artery and the main pulmonary artery with the use of a Gore-Tex® patch graft (**B**).

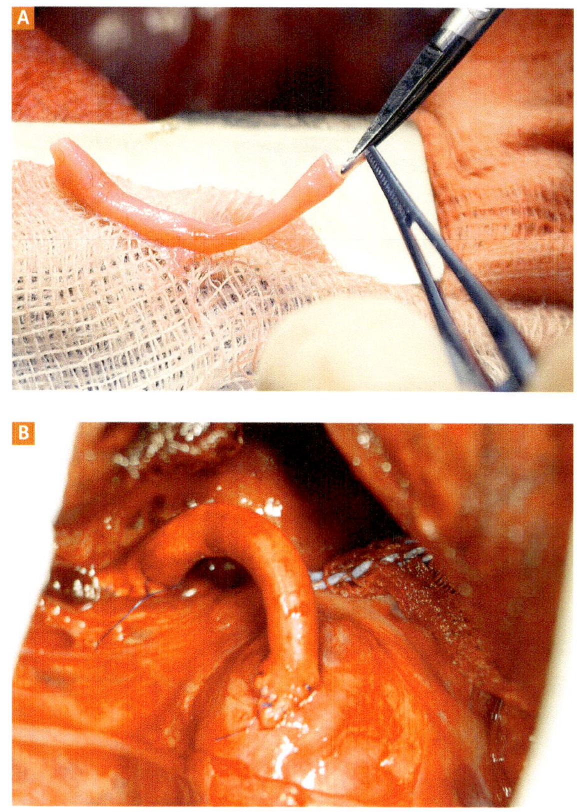

Figure 8. Tetralogy of Fallot: magnified image of the preparation of a patch graft on the carotid artery for subsequent bypass or shunt between the subclavian and main pulmonary artery (**A**). The patch graft on the carotid artery has been sutured into position (**B**). The distal portion of the anastomosis by the patch graft at the level of the main pulmonary artery can be appreciated in the foreground and further back the proximal portion of the anastomosis at the level of the subclavian artery can be seen with a Cobra head conformation.

Bibliography

- Arai, S., et al. (2011) Bioprosthesis valve replacement in dogs with congenital tricuspid valve dysplasia: technique and outcome. *Journal of Veterinary Cardiology*, 13, pp. 91–99.
- Behr, L., Chetboul, V., Sampedrano, C.C. et al. (2007) Beating heart mitral valve replacement with a bovine pericardial bioprosthesis for treatment of mitral valve dysplasia in a Bull Terrier. Vet Surg, 36(3), pp. 190–8.
- Borenstein, N., Gouni, V., Behr, L. et al. (2015) Surgical treatment of *cor triatriatum sinister* in a cat under cardiopulmonary bypass. *J Vet Surg*, 44, pp. 964–9.
- Bristow, P., Sargent, J., Luis Fuentes, V. et al. (2017) Outcome of bioprosthetic valve replacement in dogs with tricuspid valve dysplasia. *J Small Anim Pract*, 58, pp. 205–210.
- Bristow, P., Sargent, J., Luis Fuentes, V. et al. (2018) Surgical treatment of pulmonic stenosis in dogs under cardiopulmonary bypass outcome in nine dogs. *J Small Anim Pract*, 59, pp. 38–44.
- Brockman, D.J., Borer, K.E., Baines, S.J. (2009) Partial right ventriculectomy using the incised patch technique to treat double chambered right ventricle and chylothorax in a cat. *Vet Surg*, 38, pp. 631–5.
- Brockman, D.J., Holt, D.E., Gaynor, J.W. et al. (2007) Long-term palliation of tetralogy of Fallot in dogs by use of a modified Blalock-Taussig shunt. *J Am Vet Med Assoc*, 231, pp. 721–6.
- Bussadori, C., Carminati, M., Domenech, O. (2007) Transcatheter closure of a perimembranous ventricular septal defect in a dog. *J Vet Intern Med*, 21, pp. 1396–400.
- Domenech, O. (2018) Circulación extracorporea (CEC) en veterinaria. *Consulta Difusion Veterinaria.*
- Enriquez-Sarano, M., Akins, C.W., Vahanian, A. (2009) Mitral regurgitation. *Lancet*, 373, pp. 1382–94.
- Eyster, G.E., Whipple, R.D., Anderson, L.K. et al. (1977) Pulmonary artery banding for ventricular septal defect in dogs and cats. *J Am Vet Med Assoc*, 15, 170, pp. 434–8.
- Gordon, S.G., Miller, M.W., Roland, R.M. et al. (2009) Transcatheter atrial septal defect closure with the Amplatzer™ atrial septal occluder in 13 dogs: short- and mid- term outcome. *J Vet Intern Med*, 23, p. 995.
- Gordon, S.G., Saunders, A.B., Achen, S.E. et al. (2010) Transarterial ductal occlusion using the Amplatz Canine Duct Occluder in 40 dogs. J Vet Cardiol, 12, pp. 85–92.
- Gravlee, Glenn P., Davis, R.F., Stammers, A.H. (2008) Cardiopulmonary bypass. Principles and practice. Third Edition. *Wolters Kluwer.*
- Griffiths, L.G., Orton, E.C., Boon, J.A. (2004) Evaluation of techniques and outcomes of mitral valve repair in dogs. *J Am Vet Med Assoc*, 15;224, pp. 1941–5.
- Hunt, G.B., Malik, R., Bellenger, C.R., et al. (1992) Total venous inflow occlusion in the normothermic dog: a study of haemodynamic, metabolic, and neurological consequences. *Res Vet Sci*, 52, pp. 371–7.
- Hunt, G.B., Pearson, M.R., Bellenger, C.R., et al. (1995) Ventricular septal defect repair in a small dog using cross-circulation. *Aust Vet J*, 72, pp. 379–82.
- Johnson, M. S., Martin, M. (2004) Results of balloon valvuloplasty in 40 dogs with pulmonic stenosis. *Journal of Small Animal Practice* 45, pp. 148–153.
- Kerstetter, K.K., Krahwinkel, D.J. Jr, Millis, D.L. et al. (1997) Pericardiectomy in dogs: 22 cases (1978–1994). *J Am Vet Med Assoc*, 211, pp. 736–40.
- Martin, J.M., Orton, E.C., Boon, J.A. (2002) Surgical correction of double-chambered right ventricle in dogs. *J Am Vet Med Assoc*, 15;220, pp. 770–4, 768.
- Meurs, K.M., Lehmkuhl, L.B., Bonagura, J.D. (2005) Survival times in dogs with severe subvalvular aortic stenosis treated with balloon valvuloplasty or atenolol. *J Am Vet Med Assoc*, 1;227(3):420–4.
- Mitten, R.W., Edwards, G.A., Rishniw, M. (2001) Diagnosis and management of *cor triatriatum* dexter in a Pyrenean mountain dog and an Akita Inu. *Aust Vet J*, 79, pp. 177–80.
- Mizuno, T., Kamiyama, H., Mizuno, M. et al. (2015) Plasma cytokine levels in dogs undergoing cardiopulmonary bypass. *Res Vet Sci*,101, pp. 99–105.
- Mizuno, T., Mizukoshi, T., Uechi, M. (2013) Long-term outcome in dogs undergoing mitral valve repair with suture annuloplasty and chordae tendinae replacement. *J Small Anim Pract*, 54, pp. 104–7.
- Oliveira, P., Domenech, O., Silva, J. et al. (2011) Retrospective review of congenital heart disease in 976 dogs. *J Vet Intern Med*, 25, pp. 477–83.
- Orton, E.C., Bruecker, K.A., McCracken, T.O. (1990) An open patch-graft technique for correction of pulmonic stenosis in the dog. *Vet Surg*, 19, pp. 148–54.
- Orton, E.C., Herndon, G.D., Boon, J.A. et al. (2000) Influence of open surgical correction on intermediate-term outcome in dogs with subvalvular aortic stenosis: 44 cases (1991–1998). *J Am Vet Med Assoc*, 1;216, pp. 364–7.
- Orton, E.C., Mama, K., Hellyer, P. et al. (2001) Open surgical repair of tetralogy of Fallot in dogs. *J Am Vet Med Assoc*, 219, p. 1089.
- Pelosi, A., Anderson, L.K., Paugh, J. et al. (2013) Challenges of cardiopulmonary bypass-a review of the veterinary literature. *Vet Surg*, 42, pp. 119–36.
- Shimamura, S., Kutsuna. H., Shimizu, M. (2006) Comparison of right atrium incision and right ventricular outflow incision for surgical repair of membraneous ventricular septal defect using cardiopulmonary bypass in dogs. *Vet Surg*, 35(4), pp. 382–7.
- Soda, A., Tanaka, R., Saida, Y. (2009) Successful surgical correction of supravalvular pulmonary stenosis under beating heart using a cardiopulmonary bypass system in a dog. *J Vet Med Sci*, 71, pp. 203–6.
- Stern, J.A., Tou, S.T., Berker, P.C.A. et al. (2013) Hybrid cutting balloon dilatation for treatment of *cor triatriatum sinister* in a cat. *J Vet Cardiol*, 15, pp. 205–210.
- Treggiari, E., Pedro, B., Dukes-McEwan, J. et al. (2017) A descriptive review of cardiac tumors in dogs and cats. *Vet Comp Oncol*, 15, pp. 273–288.

■ Uechi, M., Harada, K., Mizukoshi, T. et al. (2011) Surgical closure of an atrial septal defect using cardiopulmonary bypass in a cat. *Vet Surg*, 40, pp. 413–7.

■ Uechi, M., Mizukosch, T., Mizuno, T. et al. (2012) Mitral valve repair under cardiopulmonary bypass in small-breed dogs: 48 cases. *J Am Vet Med Assoc*, 15, 240, pp. 1194–201.

■ Uechi, M. (2012) Mitral valve repair in dogs. *J. Vet. Cardio*, 14, pp. 185–92.

■ Verbeke, F., Binst, D., Stegen, L. et al. (2012) Total venous inflow occlusion and pericardial auto-graft reconstruction for right atrial hemangiosarcoma resection in a dog. *Can Vet J*, 53(10), pp. 1114–8.

■ Weder, C., Ames, M., Kellihan, H. et al. (2016) Palliative balloon dilation of pulmonic stenosis in a dog with tetralogy of Fallot. *J Vet Cardiol*, 18, pp. 265–270.

■ Worley, D.R., Orton, E.C., Kroner, K.T. (2016) Inflow Venous Occlusion for Intracardiac Resection of an Occluding Right Ventricular Tumor. *J Am Anim Hosp Assoc*, 52(4), pp. 259–64.

■ Yokoyama, S., Kanemoto, I., Mihara, K. et al. (2017) Treatment of severe mitral regurgitation caused by lesions in both leaflets using multiple mitral valve plasty techniques in a small dog. *Open Vet J*, pp. 328–331.

Test

Answers on Page 352

1. Cardiac surgery using the caval venous flow occlusion technique under normothermic conditions allows the blood circulation to be stopped for the following duration:

a. 2 minutes.
b. 5 minutes.
c. 8 minutes.
d. 10 minutes.

2. The caval venous flow occlusion technique, allows which of the following surgical procedures to be performed:

a. Excision of an intracardiac mass from the left atrium.
b. Excision of an intracardiac mass from the right atrium.
c. Closure of an interatrial septal defect.
d. Closure of an interventricular septal defect.

3. In which of the following procedures is a cardiopulmonary bypass not necessary?

a. Mitral valve repair.
b. Excision of a mass from the left ventricle.
c. Closure of patent *ductus arteriosus*.
d. Closure of an interventricular septal defect.

4. Which of the following refers to mitral valve *annulus* reduction?

a. Annulectomy.
b. Valvulotomy.
c. Valvuloplasty.
d. Annuloplasty.

5. The replacement of the broken *chordae tendineae* is carried out with the material known by the acronym:

a. PAME.
b. PTFE.
c. FTPA.
d. TAPSE.

6. Which technique is not recommended to treat a patient with *cor triatriatum sinister*?

a. Atriotomy with resection of the membrane by caval venous outflow occlusion.
b. Atriotomy with resection of the membrane using ECC.
c. Thoracotomy and balloon catheter dilation using a hybrid technique.
d. None of the techniques mentioned are recommended.

7. Palliative surgery for tetralogy of Fallot consists of creating a shunt between:

a. The subclavian artery and the right atrium.
b. The subclavian artery and the right ventricle.
c. The subclavian artery and the pulmonary artery.
d. The subclavian artery and the cranial vena cava.

8. Cardioplegia refers to:

a. Cardiac massage under normothermic conditions.
b. The solution that allows the heart to be stopped in diastole.
c. The solution that allows the heart to be stopped in systole.
d. Cardiac massage under hypothermic conditions.

Clinical Case

Signalment. 7-year-old, crossbreed dog, 20 kg.

Reason for the visit. The dog is getting more tired than usual and over the past week started coughing.

Physical examination. 5/6 continuous murmur under the left armpit, irradiating to the right heart base. Presents with irregularly irregular tachycardia with an alternating femoral pulse. Lung auscultation is normal, with a respiratory rate of 30 breaths per minute. Pink mucous membranes with CRT = 2 seconds.

Thoracic radiography:

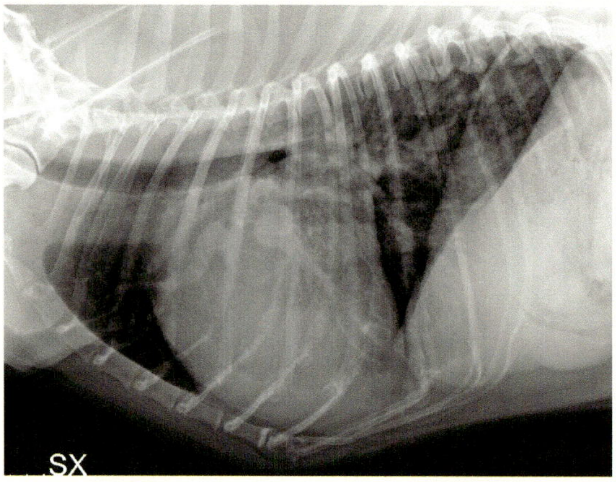

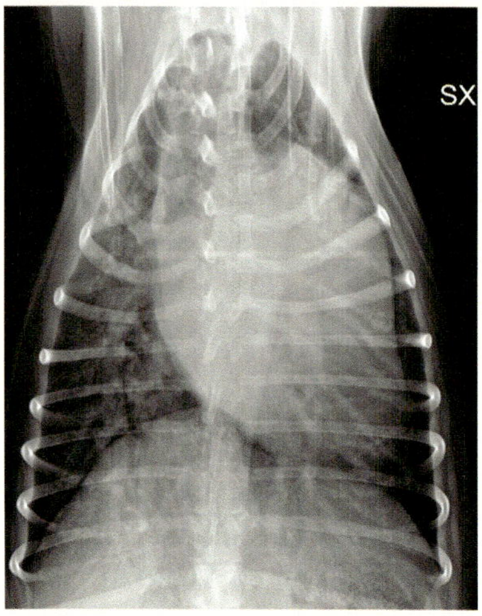

Electrocardiography. Paper speed 50 mm/second, sensitivity 5 mm/mV.

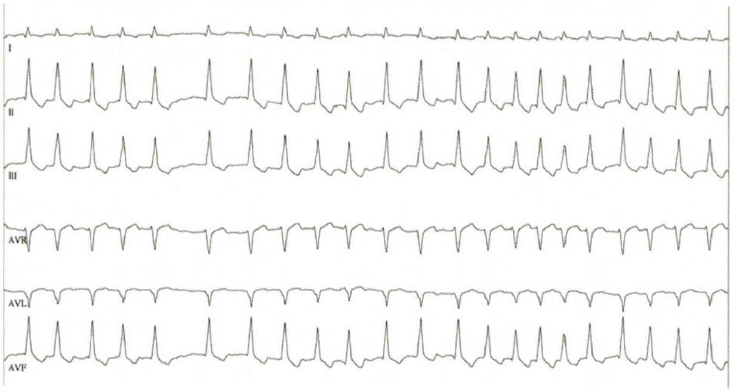

Echocardiography:

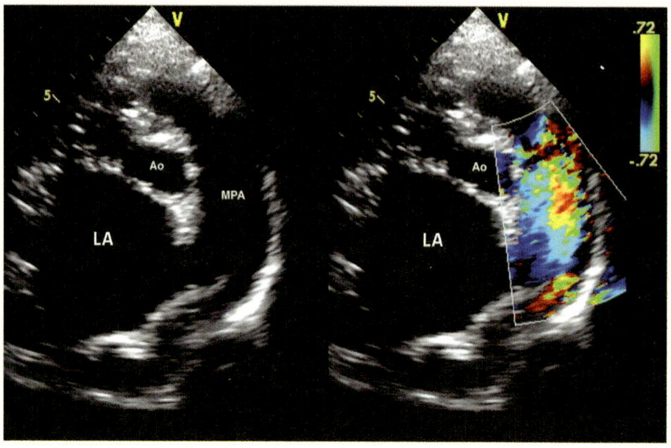

Electrocardiography just after treatment. Paper speed 50 mm/second, sensitivity 5 mm/mV.

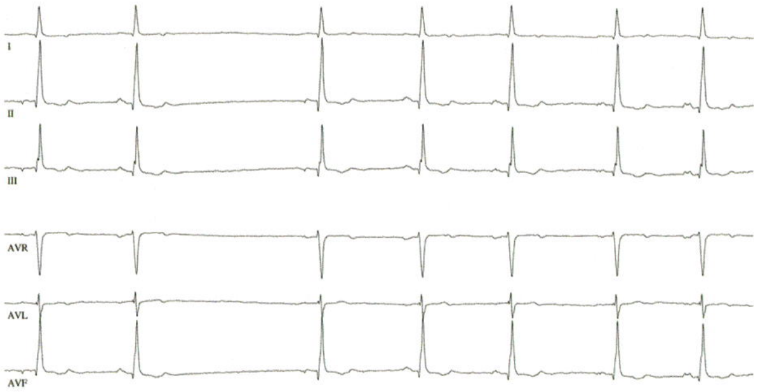

Questions:

1. What is the most likely cause of the murmur in this dog?

a. Patent *ductus arteriosus*.
b. Mitral dysplasia.
c. Interatrial septal defect.
d. Pulmonary stenosis.

2. Regarding cardiac auscultation, what is the most likely cause of this patient's alternating pulse?

a. Pericardial effusion with cardiac tamponade due to possible atrial rupture.
b. Atrial fibrillation due to possible enlargement of the right atrium.
c. Pericardial effusion with cardiac tamponade due to possible systemic venous congestion.
d. Atrial fibrillation due to possible enlargement of the left atrium.

3. Which of these options corresponds to the radiographic abnormalities in this patient?

a. The radiograph shows an image of left-sided cardiomegaly with pulmonary hypoperfusion.
b. The radiograph shows an image of left-sided cardiomegaly with a vascular pulmonary pattern.
c. The radiograph shows an image of right-sided cardiomegaly with protrusion of the projection area of the main pulmonary artery.
d. The radiograph shows an image of right-sided cardiomegaly with interstitial-alveolar pulmonary infiltrate.

4. Which of these options corresponds to the electrocardiographic abnormalities seen in this patient on the first ECG before treatment?

a. Atrial fibrillation with right deviation of the mean electrical axis of the QRS complex.
b. Atrial fibrillation with left deviation of the mean electrical axis of the QRS complex.
c. Atrial fibrillation with a mean HR >200.
d. Atrial fibrillation with a mean HR <200.

5. Considering the clinical history, physical examination, radiography, and electrocardiography, which of these pathologies is the patient most likely suffering from?

a. Pulmonary stenosis associated with atrial fibrillation with high ventricular penetrance.
b. Aortic stenosis associated with atrial fibrillation with low ventricular penetrance.
c. Mitral dysplasia associated with atrial fibrillation with low ventricular penetrance.
d. Patent *ductus arteriosus* associated with atrial fibrillation with high ventricular penetrance.

6. The 2D echocardiogram and colour Doppler (right parasternal projection, short axis at the cardiac base) is compatible with:

a. Type 2 subaortic stenosis.
b. Perimembranous interventricular septal defect.
c. Patent *ductus arteriosus* (PDA).
d. Pulmonary hypertension.

7. What is the most appropriate treatment for this patient?

a. Surgery or intervention + amiodarone + electrical cardioversion.
b. Surgery or intervention + atenolol + sildenafil.
c. Furosemide + ACEI + pimobendan + digoxin.
d. Furosemide + ACEI + pimobendan + digoxin + sildenafil.

8. What was most likely treatment used in this patient to obtain the ECG corresponding to the second electrocardiography?

a. Electrical cardioversion.
b. Atenolol-based treatment.
c. Diltiazem-based treatment.
d. Treatment based on digoxin + diltiazem.

Correct Answers:

Test

1. a
2. b
3. c
4. d
5. b
6. a
7. c
8. b

Clinical Case

1. a
2. d
3. b
4. c
5. d
6. c
7. a
8. a

Notes

Notes

Notes